Levison's Textbook for Dental Nurses

Eleventh Edition

Carole Hollins

General Dental Practitioner
Member of the British Dental Association
Former presiding examiner for the National Examining Board for Dental Nurses

WILEY Blackwell

This edition first published 2013. © 2013 John Wiley & Sons, Ltd
© 2004, 2008 Blackwell Munksgaard
© 1960, 1963, 1969, 1971, 1978, 1985, 1991, 1997 Blackwell Science Ltd

First edition published 1960; Second edition published 1963; Third edition published 1969; Fourth edition published 1971; Fifth edition published 1978; Sixth edition published 1985; Seventh edition published 1991; Eighth edition published 1997; Ninth edition published 2004; Tenth edition published 2008; Eleventh edition published 2013.

Registered Office
John Wiley & Sons, Ltd, The Atrium, Southern Gate, Chichester, West Sussex, PO19 8SQ, UK

Editorial Offices
9600 Garsington Road, Oxford, OX4 2DQ, UK
The Atrium, Southern Gate, Chichester, West Sussex, PO19 8SQ, UK
2121 State Avenue, Ames, Iowa 50014-8300, USA

For details of our global editorial offices, for customer services and for information about how to apply for permission to reuse the copyright material in this book please see our website at www.wiley.com/wiley-blackwell.

Library of Congress Cataloging-in-Publication Data

Hollins, Carole.
Levison's textbook for dental nurses / Carole Hollins. – 11th ed.
      p. ; cm.
   Textbook for dental nurses
   Includes bibliographical references and index.
   ISBN 978-1-118-50044-6 (pbk. : alk. paper) – ISBN 978-1-118-50043-9 (ePub) – ISBN 978-1-118-50042-2 (Mobi) – ISBN 978-1-118-50041-5 – ISBN 978-1-118-68990-5
I. Levison, H. (Henry). Textbook for dental nurses.   II. Title.   III. Title: Textbook for dental nurses.
[DNLM: 1. Dental Assistants.   2. Dental Care.   WU 90]
   RK60.5
   617.6'0233–dc23

                                              2013012752

A catalogue record for this book is available from the British Library.

Wiley also publishes its books in a variety of electronic formats. Some content that appears in print may not be available in electronic books.

Cover image: © Irfan Ahmad, BDS
Cover design by Meaden Creative

Set in 10/12pt Calibri by SPi Publisher Services, Pondicherry, India

1   2013

Contents

Introduction to the Eleventh Edition

Since the last edition was written, dental nurses have joined other members of the dental team to become registered professionals with the General Dental Council (GDC), and have at last been elevated to their well-deserved status as invaluable dental care professionals. With this professional recognition comes the necessity for set standards of attitude and behaviour outside the workplace, as well as suitable qualification, ethical work practices and the requirement for lifelong learning and continuous professional development during their careers.

This edition provides the underpinning knowledge required to cover the extensive curriculum contents of the National Examining Board for Dental Nurses' (NEBDN) new National Diploma qualification, which supersedes the old National Certificate. You can view the full curriculum for the NEBDN National Diploma in Dental Nursing at http://www.nebdn.org/diploma_in_dental_nursing.html. A similar textbook will be available to cover the City & Guilds' curriculum for its new Diploma in Dental Nursing qualification. Although the same register-able qualification is awarded to successful candidates following either route to registration, the training and assessment methods involved for each are quite different.

The revised and updated text of this latest edition embraces all the numerous legislative and regulatory changes that have occurred in the last 5 years, including issues around Health and Safety, infection control, information governance, quality assurance requirements and the expansion of the concept of continuous professional development into that of team members becoming 'reflective practitioners'. In particular, the text in relevant chapters puts particular emphasis on the standards to be attained in becoming dental professionals, and has been continuously cross-referenced to the GDC's own *Standards Guidance* booklets, as well as some of its other publications such as *Fitness to Practise*, in the hope that their content is easily absorbed into the understanding and knowledge base of the readers.

In addition and where appropriate, website addresses are included to allow readers to access further information on many topics covered throughout the text – especially links to the NEBDN's curriculum and charting booklet download facilities, and links to more information on subject topics with national variations, such as infection control.

It is hoped that the increased use of photographs and illustrations, as well as that of bullet points to highlight key facts throughout the text, makes this edition particularly user-friendly and easy to understand for all readers, without detracting from the high standards now expected of dental nurse students as they evolve into fully fledged dental professionals. Finally, and as always, I sincerely hope that this text stimulates at least some readers into becoming sufficiently inspired during their studies to continue their careers beyond their initial qualification, and consider extended duties, postregistration qualifications and further dental professional careers.

NEBDN National Diploma in Dental Nursing

You can view the full curriculum for the NEBDN National Diploma in Dental Nursing at http://www.nebdn.org/diploma_in_dental_nursing.html.

Carole Hollins

Introduction to the First Edition

This book is designed to cover the syllabus for the British Dental Nurses and Assistants Examination. Although written primarily for nurses preparing for this examination, it also provides an outline of dental surgery for those embarking on a career of dental nursing, thus helping them gain a greater understanding of the nature and aims of their duties. For examination purposes, the subject matter is deliberately presented in a dogmatic fashion and, to aid final revision, there is a summary after each chapter.

The text was prepared during a winter spent in the North Isles of Shetland with the School Health Service mobile dental unit; and for helpful advice and encouragement throughout, I am indebted to my former dental nurse, Miss M.E. Isbister. I wish to thank my wife for typing the manuscript; my sister, Miss B. Levison, for the drawings; the Amalgamated Dental Trade Distributors Ltd for providing some new blocks; and Mr P. Saugman of Blackwell Science for his guidance.

H. Levison

Acknowledgements

Sadly, since the last edition of this popular book was published, its original author Henry Levison has passed away. Therefore this edition is dedicated to his memory in grateful thanks, on behalf of the thousands of dental nurses whose careers are hopefully the better for his many years of dedication to their educational needs.

Once again, I must extend my grateful thanks to the patients and staff of Kidsgrove dental practice for their modelling skills, and give sincere thanks also to my sister (yet again!) for her technical and computer-related wizardry – thank goodness she knows what she's doing!

In updating this edition, I am very grateful to the General Dental Council and the Department of Health for their permissions to reproduce various documents and booklets throughout the text, and I hope I have done justice to their content. I must also express great appreciation for the continued support of previous illustrators too.

Finally, a huge 'thank you' to the various staff of Wiley Blackwell (past and present) for their superb help and support throughout the updating and publishing process, and especially the speedy professionalism with which they work.

Abbreviations

ADJ	amelodentinal junction
AED	automatic external defibrillator
AIDS	acquired immune deficiency syndrome
ALARA	as low as reasonably achievable
ALARP	as low as reasonably practicable/possible
ALS	Advanced Life Support
ANUG	acute necrotising ulcerative gingivitis
ARF	annual retention fee
BADN	British Association of Dental Nurses
BDA	British Dental Association
BDJ	*British Dental Journal*
BDS	Bachelor of Dental Surgery
BLS	Basic Life Support
BNF	*British National Formulary*
BPE	basic periodontal examination
BSA	Business Services Agency (previously Dental Practice Board)
CAL	computer-aided learning
C&G	City & Guilds
CG	clinical governance
CJD	Creutzfeldt–Jakob disease
COAD	chronic obstructive airways disease
COSHH	Control of Substances Hazardous to Health
CPD	continuing professional development
CPITN	Community Periodontal Index of Treatment Needs
CPR	cardiopulmonary resuscitation
CQC	Care Quality Commission
CRB	Criminal Records Bureau
CSF	cerebrospinal fluid
DCP	dental care professional
DDPH	Diploma in Dental Public Health
DDR	Diploma in Dental Radiology
DGDP	Diploma in General Dental Practice
DMF	decayed, missing, filled
do	distal occlusal
DOrth	Diploma in Orthodontics
DPF	*Dental Practitioners' Formulary*
DPT	dental panoramic tomograph
DRABC	dangers, response, airway, breathing, circulation
DRO	Dental Reference Officer
DVT	deep vein thrombosis
EAV	expired air ventilation
ECC	external cardiac compression
ECG	electrocardiogram
EMQ	extended matching question
F/	full upper denture
F/F	full upper and lower dentures
/F	full lower denture
FDI	World Dental Federation
FDS	Fellow in Dental Surgery
FGC	full gold crown
GA	general anaesthesia
GDC	General Dental Council
GDP	general dental practitioner
GI	gold inlay

GIC	glass ionomer cement	M Paed Dent	Membership in Paediatric Dentistry
GIT	gastrointestinal tract		
GP	gutta percha	MRSA	methicillin-resistant *Staphylococcus aureus*
GTN	glyceryl trinitrate (spray)		
HBV	hepatitis B virus	MSc	Master of Science
HCV	hepatitis C virus	NEBDN	National Examining Board for Dental Nurses
HIV	human immunodeficiency virus		
		NHS	National Health Service
HRT	hormone replacement therapy	NICE	National Institute for Health and Clinical Excellence
HSE	Health and Safety Executive	NME	non-milk extrinsic (sugar)
HTM 01-05	Health Technical Memorandum 01-05	NSAID	non-steroidal anti-inflammatory drug
IG	information governance	NVQ	National Vocational Qualification
IH	inhalation sedation (previously relative analgesia)		
		OHA	occupational health advisor
INR	international normalised ratio	OPG	dental panoramic tomograph (orthopantomograph)
IOTN	Index of Orthodontic Treatment Need		
		OSCE	objective structured clinical exam
IPA	isopropyl alcohol		
IR (ME) R	Ionising Radiation (Medical Exposures) Regulations	P/	partial upper denture
		P/P	partial upper and lower dentures
IRR	Ionising Radiation Regulations		
IT	information technology	/P	partial lower denture
IV	intravenous	PAT	portable appliance testing
LA	local anaesthesia (analgesia)	PBC	porcelain bonded crown
LDS	Licentiate in Dental Surgery	PCT	primary care trust
LPA	Laser Protection Advisor	PDP	personal development plan
LPS	Laser Protection Supervisor	PE	partially erupted
LSAB	Local Safeguarding Adults Board	PIDA	Public Interest Disclosure Act 1998
LSCB	Local Safeguarding Children Board		
		PJC	porcelain jacket crown
MAOI	monoamine oxidase inhibitor	PoM	prescription-only medicine
MCQ	multiple choice question	PPE	personal protective equipment
MFDS	Member of the Faculty of Dental Surgery	ppm	parts per million
		PV	porcelain veneer
MGDS	Membership in General Dental Surgery	QA	quality assurance
		RA	relative analgesia (now known as inhalation sedation)
MI	myocardial infarction		
MIMS	Monthly Index of Medical Specialities		
		RIDDOR	Reporting of Injuries, Diseases and Dangerous Occurrences Regulations
MJDF	Membership of the Joint Dental Faculties		
		RPA	Radiation Protection Advisor
MMR	measles, mumps and rubella (vaccination)	RPS	Radiation Protection Supervisor
		SCC	squamous cell carcinoma
mo	mesial occlusal	SWOT	strengths, weaknesses, opportunities and threats
mod	mesial occlusal distal		
MOS	minor oral surgery		

Abbreviations

TIA	transient ischaemic attack
TMJ	temporomandibular joint
TTP	tender to percussion
UE	unerupted

vCJD	new-variant Creutzfeldt–Jakob disease
WHO	World Health Organization
ZOE	zinc oxide and eugenol cement

How to use your Textbook and Companion Website

Welcome to the new and updated version of *Levison's Textbook for Dental Nurses*. These pages give you an overview of the key features in the book and companion website, and how to make the most of them to achieve exam success.

Features contained within your textbook

Every chapter begins with **Key Learning Points**. These outline the main learning outcomes you should have achieved by the end of the chapter.

Key learning points

A **factual knowledge** of
- the professional obligations of dental nurses
- Continuing Professional Development requirements and becoming a reflective practitioner

A **working knowledge** of
- the General Dental Council's professional standards guidance in relation to the dental team
- all aspects of patient records; including issues of confidentiality, information governance, and patient access to records
- patient consent to treatment
- raising concerns in the workplace

A **factual awareness** of
- the issues of protecting children and vulnerable adults
- patient complaints and their correct handling

Throughout the book you'll find useful illustrations, photographs and tables.

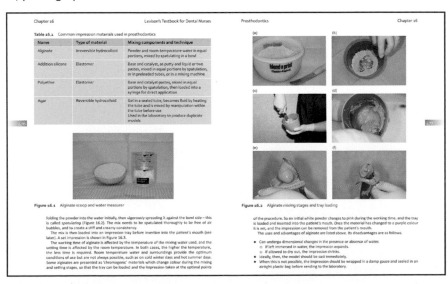

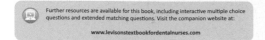

Further resources are available for this book, including interactive multiple choice questions and extended matching questions. Visit the companion website at:

www.levisonstextbookfordentalnurses.com

At the end of every chapter there is a helpful reminder to visit the companion website at

www.levisonstextbookfordentalnurses.com

On the website you can test yourself on the interactive multiple choice and extended matching questions.

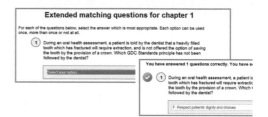

We hope you enjoy your new textbook. Good luck with your studies!

Copyright Information

1

Structure of the Dental Profession

Key learning points

A **factual knowledge** of
- the various members that make up the dental team

An **overview** of
- the key roles of each member as well as the dental nurse
- the National Health Service and its current involvement with the provision of dental care

The dental team is now made up of dentists and six categories of registered dental care professionals (DCPs), all of whom work together to provide oral healthcare for their patients. In hospital and clinic environments, some of the dentists may have gone on to become specialists in various fields of dentistry, while dental nurses are now able to train and become competent in various postregistration qualifications as well as 'extended duties'. With the introduction of a new National Health Service (NHS) dental contract and with a new commissioning system imminent, there has never been a more exciting time for dental nurses to push the boundaries of their profession and become recognised as vital members of every dental team, in every dental workplace.

An overview is given below of the roles of the various registrants, and that of the dental nurse is covered in detail in Chapter 2.

Levison's Textbook for Dental Nurses, Eleventh Edition. By Carole Hollins.
© 2013 John Wiley & Sons, Ltd. Published 2013 by John Wiley & Sons, Ltd. Companion website: www.levisonstextbookfordentalnurses.com

The dentist

Dentists undergo 5 years of undergraduate training at a university dental school. On passing their final examinations, students are awarded the degree of Bachelor of Dental Surgery (BDS), but they cannot use the title of dentist or practise the profession until their names have been entered onto the Dentists Register. In addition, dentists who have qualified in member states of the European Union may also join the Register, although they must have an adequate level of written and spoken English. Dentists from non-European Union countries must have their skills and knowledge assessed for equivalence with that required for UK dentists before they may work here.

The Register is kept by the General Dental Council and contains the name, address and qualification(s) of every person legally entitled to practise dentistry in the United Kingdom. Such persons may describe themselves as dentist, dental surgeon or dental practitioner – there is no difference between these titles. Dentists may also use the courtesy title of Doctor but must not imply that they are anything other than dentists. Following qualification, all dentists are legally required to continue their professional education until their retirement from practice, in order to maintain and update their skills.

Registered dentists have a wide choice of opportunities within the profession.

- General practice.
- Community dental service.
- Hospital service.
- University teaching and research.
- Industrial dental service.
- The armed forces.

They may also take additional higher qualifications and become specialists in a particular branch of dentistry. Some examples of such qualifications are as follows.

- Fellowship in Dental Surgery (FDS).
- Master of Science (MSc) in a specialty.
- Membership in the Joint Dental Faculties (MJDF).
- Membership in Paediatric Dentistry (M Paed Dent).
- Membership of the Faculty of Dental Surgery (MFDS).
- Diploma in Dental Public Health (DDPH).
- Diploma in Dental Radiology (DDR).
- Diploma in General Dental Practice (DGDP).
- Diploma in Orthodontics (DOrth).

These qualifications are provided by the joint dental faculties of the Royal Colleges of Surgery.

Having obtained the relevant higher qualifications, dentists may then join the Specialist List of the Register for their particular specialty, which includes the following areas.

- Oral and maxillofacial surgery.
- Surgical dentistry.
- Dental and maxillofacial radiology.
- Dental public health.
- Oral medicine.
- Oral microbiology.

- Oral pathology.
- Orthodontics.
- Periodontics.
- Prosthodontics.
- Restorative dentistry.

The General Dental Council

The General Dental Council (GDC) is the regulatory body of the dental profession and its duties are set out in legislation. It aims to promote high standards of professional education and professional conduct among dentists and DCPs, throughout their working career. It thereby ensures that the status of the profession in the general community is upheld and that a proper code of conduct is maintained, for the protection of the public. In essence, its remit is to:

- protect patients
- regulate the dental team.

In the performance of these duties, the GDC must be satisfied that courses of study at dental schools and the qualifying examinations are adequate, and the same applies to postgraduate education and to the register-able qualifications for all the DCP categories.

It is the policy of the GDC for all dentists, after qualification, to complete a year of foundation training (previously called vocational training) before starting independent practice. Such training schemes are already in force in NHS general practice, the community and hospital services, and also on a voluntary basis in non-NHS practice. As soon as adequate resources and facilities are available, it is likely to be mandatory for all newly qualified dentists to undergo foundation training soon after qualification.

The GDC is empowered to remove or suspend from the Register any dentist or DCP who has been convicted of a criminal offence or is guilty of serious professional misconduct. It may also suspend any registrant whose fitness to practise is seriously impaired because of a physical or mental condition. These issues are discussed further in Chapters 2 and 3.

Apart from registered dentists, the only other persons permitted to undertake dental treatment are registered dental hygienists and dental therapists, and registered clinical dental technicians may provide and maintain full dentures to edentulous patients. The GDC is responsible for these dental care professionals in much the same way as for dentists. The expected level of their competences by the time of their qualification is laid out in the GDC document *Preparing for Practice*, while those additional duties possible after a period of suitable training and assessment are laid out in its document *Scope of Practice*. This has particular relevance to dental nurses, and all GDC documents can be downloaded at www.gdc-uk.org.

The dental team

Dentists' training enables them to undertake, without assistance, all treatment necessary for patients, including construction of their dentures, crowns and bridges, provision of restorations and root fillings, extractions, etc. Except for the actual treatment performed within the mouth, much of the work which a dentist is qualified to do can be performed by other members of the dental team. For example, a chairside dental nurse provides an extra pair of hands for preparing and mixing filling and impression materials, and for helping with suction, retraction and illumination to keep the operative field clear and dry for the dentist and comfortable for the patient. A dental technician can make dentures, crowns and bridges ready for the dentist to fit, while dental hygienists and therapists are permitted to undertake limited forms of dental treatment.

By utilising all this assistance, a dentist becomes the leader of a team which can practise in the most efficient way. Dentists carry out all the treatment which they alone can perform, while the other members of the team – hygienist, therapist, dental nurse and technician – perform all the work which a dentist can delegate. Compared with a single-handed dentist, the dental team can provide far more treatment each day with less effort and fatigue for all concerned, and thereby give a better total service to the patient and the community. Dental team working is discussed in more detail in Chapter 3.

The full group of registered dental team members will eventually comprise:

- dental nurses
- dental hygienists
- dental therapists
- orthodontic therapists
- dental technicians
- clinical dental technicians
- maxillofacial prosthetists and technologists.

All except the last group are already required to be registered with the GDC, and must have specific training programmes, extended duties and professional responsibilities for continuing professional development and professional conduct similar to those of dentists. The issue of professionalism and its relevance to all dental team members is discussed in detail in Chapter 3.

Further information is also available at www.gdc-uk.org.

Dental care professionals

This is the new professional title for all members of the dental team besides the dentist. They were previously referred to as professionals complementary to dentistry (PCDs).

Dental nurse

This whole text is aimed at dental nurses and their training requirements, and their invaluable role and position in the dental team are discussed in detail in Chapter 2.

Dental hygienist

After 2 years' training at a dental hospital or in the armed forces, hygienists used to be awarded a Diploma in Dental Hygiene and could then become registered by the GDC. Dental hygiene training has now been combined with that of dental therapists as a dual qualification, so that all those who qualify have a much wider range of skills and competencies.

Hygienists are permitted to undertake a number of dental procedures for which they have been trained, under the prescription of a dentist. These duties include:

- scaling and polishing teeth
- use of infiltration local anaesthesia
- application of fluorides and fissure sealants
- treating patients under conscious sedation, provided that a dentist is present in the room

- emergency replacement of dislodged crowns, using a temporary cement
- removal of excess cement
- application of a temporary filling if one becomes dislodged while under their treatment
- taking impressions.

Apart from their treatment role, hygienists are also trained to be proficient dental health educators.

Dental therapist

Dental therapists undertake a 2-year course at a dental hospital and now become qualified in both hygiene and therapy. They are awarded a Diploma in Dental Therapy and Hygiene and can carry out a wider range of treatments once they have obtained GDC registration. They are permitted to carry out all of the same duties as a hygienist, and all of the following additional duties:

- simple fillings
- pulp treatment of deciduous teeth
- extraction of deciduous teeth
- fitting preformed crowns on deciduous teeth
- dental radiography (when taught as an integral part of the training course).

Prior experience as a dental nurse and possession of the relevant dental nursing qualification are requirements for admission to dental hospital training courses for dental hygiene and therapy training.

Dental technician

Dental technicians are highly skilled craftsmen and women who construct dentures, crowns, bridges, inlays, orthodontic appliances, splints and replacements for fractured or diseased parts of the face and jaws. They work to the dentist's prescription in a dental laboratory. Training consists of a full-time course in a dental hospital or technical college; or an apprenticeship with part-time attendance at a technical college.

Clinical dental technician

Clinical dental technicians are specially trained to provide and maintain full dentures for edentulous patients, and may do so without the involvement of a dentist.

Maxillofacial prosthetists and technologists

Maxillofacial prosthetists and technologists are technicians who have specialised in jaw and facial reconstruction and replacement, and work closely with maxillofacial surgeons in a hospital environment.

The National Health Service

Dental treatment in the United Kingdom is provided either privately or through the NHS. Private patients obtain treatment from a practitioner of their choice and pay a fee to the practitioner for professional services given, or they join one of the private registration and capitation schemes and pay a monthly or annual subscription to cover the majority of their treatment charges.

National Health Service dental treatment differs from private practice in the range of treatment provided and the method of payment for such treatment. Certain types of treatment available in private practice are currently restricted in the NHS (such as tooth-coloured fillings and crowns on posterior teeth), while payments to the dentist are set and controlled by the NHS, with patients' contributions ranging from nil to a set maximum.

Currently, NHS treatment available to the public is split into three bands, as follows.

- Band 1 – simple treatments such as examinations, radiographs, scaling.
- Band 2 – routine treatments such as fillings, extractions, root treatments.
- Band 3 – complex treatments involving laboratory work such as crowns, bridges, dentures.

A set fee is charged to the patient for each of the bands, regardless of the amount of treatment carried out, so for instance the same fee is paid for one filling or 10 fillings, if provided during the same course of treatment.

However, the system is due to change in the very near future, and while the final decision is not yet made on the replacement system to be introduced, it is highly likely that more emphasis will be placed on the role of DCPs within the dental team. The dentist will still be the only team member capable of providing all care and treatment for a patient, but much will be delegated to those DCPs with suitable training and qualifications to be carried out instead. So, dental workplaces may eventually consist of fewer dentists and more DCPs, but with the ability to carry out the same range of dental treatments between them.

The cost of the NHS is borne by the state, and the government department responsible for it is the Department of Health. This delegates operational management of the service to the NHS Executive. For administrative purposes, the country is divided into a number of large strategic health authorities for overall planning. These are currently subdivided at a local level into a large number of smaller authorities, called NHS trusts for hospital services and primary care trusts (PCTs) for community clinics and general practitioner services. PCTs have the responsibility of deciding the level of need for NHS dentistry in their area, as well as providing emergency out-of-hours dental care to the public.

In April 2013, PCTs are due to be replaced by another system of commissioning medical and dental care in their localities, and although the final details are unclear at this time, it is likely that local councils and general medical practitioners (GPs) will take responsibility for commissioning healthcare in their areas instead.

Community dental service

This was formerly called the school dental service, providing examination and treatment for children and expectant and nursing mothers. It still meets the same needs but has acquired additional responsibilities. These vary according to local demand but can include treatment for special needs patients of all ages, emergency treatment for patients without access to an NHS dentist, treatment of the elderly (especially those unable to attend a dental workplace), provision for general anaesthesia and conscious sedation, and dental health programmes for the community at large.

The community dental service is administered by the NHS trust or PCT and co-operates with hospital staff and general practitioners in planning and co-ordinating all dental services in the district. Salaried community dental officers provide treatment in clinics with equipment and materials supplied by the trust or PCT.

Hospital dental service

Hospitals are administered by an NHS trust. Dental services are provided by consultant oral and maxillofacial surgeons and orthodontists. They give specialist advice and treatment for patients referred by practitioners outside the hospital, and for patients referred from other departments of the hospital. They are also in overall charge of dental care for long-stay inpatients. In addition, most consultants provide postgraduate courses and part-time training posts for general practitioners.

General dental service

This is the general practitioner service which provides a significant share of all dental treatment in the UK. It is currently administered by the local PCT which holds dentists' NHS contracts and is responsible for NHS disciplinary procedures.

The Dental Practice Division of the Business Services Authority (previously the Dental Practice Board) authorises payment of NHS treatment fees to practitioners. It can also arrange for patients to be examined by its dental reference officers (DROs).

General practitioners set up and equip their practices at their own expense and are entitled to have private patients as well as NHS patients. However, if involved in NHS care of patients, they must also demonstrate compliance with various quality assurance measures, as follows:

- clinical governance
- clinical audit/peer review
- information governance.

There is no reason why a fully private practice cannot have the same quality assurance systems in place also, although they are only required to abide by any relevant legislation, rather than having to abide by NHS rules.

Clinical governance

This requires every NHS practice principal to have a quality assurance system for the practice, in order to ensure a consistent quality of care. It must cover the following areas to ensure the safety of its patients:

- infection control (Chapter 8)
- all legal obligations of health and safety law in the practice (Chapter 4)
- all legal obligations for radiation protection (Chapter 4)
- compliance with GDC requirements for continuing professional development (Chapter 3).

The practice must also:

- appoint a member of the staff to be responsible for operating the system
- display a written practice quality policy for patients
- provide the PCT with an annual report on the quality assurance system.

Clinical governance is discussed further in Chapter 3.

Clinical audit and peer review

Clinical audit is an essential feature of clinical governance that came into force for NHS dentists in 2001. Its purpose is to ensure that individual dentists assess different aspects of their practice, make changes where necessary, and thereby improve service and care for their patients. The running of quality assurance programmes within the dental workplace can often be delegated to suitably trained dental nurses, an example being retrospective clinical audits of dental radiographs.

Peer review is an optional alternative to clinical audit for dentists who prefer to undertake their practice assessments within a group of other dentists and thereby share the benefit of the group's combined experience.

As these are now clinical governance requirements, rather than optional activities, funding is no longer available to dentists for their completion.

Information governance

This is a quality assurance system that has been implemented for healthcare, corporate and information technology (IT) organisations that sets out to ensure the safety and appropriate use of personal and patient information. It is therefore linked to patient confidentiality, data protection and the freedom of information passing between various organisations and bodies.

The Department of Health has charge of the implementation of the system for healthcare organisations, including all dental workplaces, and has developed sets of information governance requirements in a toolkit (referred to as the IG Toolkit), which enables NHS healthcare providers to measure their own compliance.

Information governance is discussed further in Chapter 3.

British Dental Association

The British Dental Association (BDA) is the professional body representing the majority of dentists in the UK. It publishes the *British Dental Journal (BDJ)*, and many compendiums, toolkits and other literature to provide its members with up-to-date information and advice on the business of dentistry. It runs annual dental conferences which provide further update advice, as well as many continuing professional development (CPD) events aimed at the dental team rather than just dentists. The Association also negotiates for the profession with the government and other bodies, such as local dental committees, where dental interests are concerned. Membership of the BDA is voluntary, it is open to all dentists and allows its members access to a huge source of dental literature and research material.

Resources

www.gdc-uk.org.
General Dental Council, 37 Wimpole Street, London W1G 8DQ
Tel: 020 7887 3800
Fax: 020 7224 3294

 Further resources are available for this book, including interactive multiple choice questions and extended matching questions. Visit the companion website at:

www.levisonstextbookfordentalnurses.com

2

The Dental Nurse

Key learning points

A **factual knowledge** of
- the General Dental Council and its role in dental nurse training, registration, and regulation

A **working knowledge** of
- the overall role of the dental nurse in relation to administrative and chairside skills

A **factual awareness** of
- the National Examining Board for Dental Nurses' National Diploma examination structure

A **detailed explanation** of
- each element of the examination

An **overview** of
- available postregistration qualifications

History

Until 2008, any person wishing to work as a nurse or assistant in the dental surgery environment could do so without undertaking any form of training or passing any examination. Since 1943, the National Examining Board for Dental Nurses (NEBDN), previously called the National Examining Board for Dental Surgery Assistants, had been setting and running its voluntary examination for any persons working as nurses (assistants) in the dental workplace. Qualification in the National Certificate examination showed that successful candidates had achieved a set basic standard in dental nursing, were able to work unsupervised alongside the dentist and could call themselves a 'dental nurse' (previously a 'dental surgery assistant').

More recently, City & Guilds (C&G) introduced its Level 3 NVQ in Dental Nursing, as an alternative qualification for those students wishing to follow a vocational rather than a more academic career

Levison's Textbook for Dental Nurses, Eleventh Edition. By Carole Hollins.
© 2013 John Wiley & Sons, Ltd. Published 2013 by John Wiley & Sons, Ltd. Companion website: www.levisonstextbookfordentalnurses.com

pathway to becoming a dental nurse. Both qualifications ran successfully alongside each other, and were open to any students wishing to take them. In Scotland, students were able to access a Scottish equivalent of the NVQ, as well as the National Certificate.

In the last 5 years, dental nurses, along with all other dental care professionals, have gradually been brought under the regulatory umbrella of the General Dental Council (GDC). Following a period of 'grandparenting', during which unqualified but well-experienced dental nurses were allowed to register with the GDC without prior qualification, compulsory training and qualification for all were introduced.

Registration

Since 2008, any person wishing to work as a dental nurse has had to undergo a period of supervised training, and then pass a formal examination before being allowed to register with the General Dental Council. All unqualified dental nurses must be supervised and 'in training' to be able to work directly with patients, and all qualified dental nurses must be registered on an annual basis with the GDC, to be able to continue to work with patients unsupervised.

As with the other dental care professionals (DCPs) listed in Chapter 1, the necessity of registration for dental nurses has raised their role to that of a professional in the eyes of both the public and other members of the dental team. In addition, it has brought all members of the dental team into line with other healthcare professionals in the United Kingdom, so that all are now accountable to a regulatory body.

In line with other regulators, the purpose of the GDC in its regulatory role is to maintain the list – or Register – of those persons deemed suitable to work as healthcare professionals at their level of qualification. This is correctly termed their 'fitness to practise'.

As with all other GDC registrants, dental nurses are required to pay an annual retention fee to maintain their place on the Register, having behaved in a professional manner throughout the previous 12-month period. In other words, the GDC has to ensure not only that anyone joining the Register is fit to practise at the point of initial qualification but that they remain so throughout their career. Consequently, the GDC's own aims are summarised throughout its publications as: 'Protecting patients, regulating the dental team'.

Role of the General Dental Council in dental nurse training and qualification

To ensure that dental nurses are adequately trained and qualified to a suitable level in their chosen dental career, the GDC describes the learning outcomes that each student must be able to demonstrate by the end of their training, to be able to join the GDC Register. Originally, these outcomes were published in the GDC document *Developing the Dental Team* but they are now covered in the updated publication *Preparing for Practice – Dental Team Learning Outcomes for Registration*. This updated document has also superseded the equivalent publication for dental undergraduates, *The First Five Years*. All GDC publications can be viewed or downloaded by accessing its website at www.gdc-uk.org.

In summary, then, the GDC has a vital role to play in the regulation of the whole dental team, including dental nurses, from the time that they enter a formal course of training as a student, right through their professional career until they leave the GDC Register. The GDC's functions as a regulatory body and the way that this affects the dental nurse are as follows.

- Set standards to be followed – in relation to behaviour, education (pre- and postregistration) and ethics.
- Handle fitness to practise issues – in relation to poor health, poor professional performance or professional misconduct.
- Remove individuals from the Register and prevent them from practising as dental professionals, if they are considered to be 'unfit'.

In carrying out its role as a regulatory body for the dental profession, the GDC also promotes its own aims to.

- protect patients
- regulate the dental team
- promote public confidence in all dental professionals
- quality assure dental education for all dental professionals working in the UK
- ensure that all dental professionals maintain an up-to-date level of knowledge
- assist patients with serious complaints against dental professionals.

These fundamental aims of the GDC affect the working lives and careers of every dental professional on a day-to-day basis, and represent the standards that should be achieved by all. The GDC has conveniently published these principles and standards in booklet format, *General Dental Council Standards Guidance*, and made them available to all registrants. They are discussed in detail in Chapter 3. All student dental nurses are expected to be familiar with the detailed contents of these booklets by the time they sit their qualification examinations.

Learning outcomes and qualification

As mentioned previously, the GDC has set out the outcomes that dental nurses must be able to demonstrate by the end of their training period, in order to become a registrant and be deemed 'fit to practise'. Within a training course, demonstration of these outcomes is met through education, training and assessment, and they are therefore referred to as 'learning outcomes'. They are derived from the GDC's own *Standards for Dental Professionals* document, and include the requirements set by the GDC for lifelong learning to be achieved. In the UK, student dental nurses can meet the training requirements by following an approved course and passing either the NEBDN National Diploma examination or the City & Guilds Level 3 Diploma in Dental Nursing examination.

The GDC learning outcomes have been developed so that a student who achieves them can be said to be competent – they can practise safely, effectively and professionally as a dental nurse. The vast majority of the learning outcomes are actually set, word for word, for each dental professional category, from the dentist through to the dental technician. Once achieved, they demonstrate that the student has the knowledge, skills, attitudes and behaviours required to become a GDC registrant.

To understand what is required from student dental nurses during their training, education and assessment, the following interpretations of these key terms may be useful.

- **Knowledge** – the underpinning, theoretical information gained from learning or experience, which gives the student understanding of a subject.
- **Skills** – the special abilities acquired by learning and practice to be able to complete a task, often manually or verbally.

- **Attitudes and behaviours** – the moral and ethical beliefs held by the student which demonstrate their values and priorities, and guide their actions.

Students must exhibit all of these attributes to be considered as professional dental nurses after qualification, and be entered onto the GDC Register. They must then maintain and improve upon these qualities throughout their working life, to stay on the Register.

The GDC learning outcomes are grouped into four domains for all registrants, and their specific relevance to the dental nurse is as follows.

- **Clinical** – described as the range of skills required to deliver direct care, where registrants interact with patients.
- **Communication** – described as the skills involved in effectively interacting with patients, their representatives, the public and colleagues, and recording appropriate information to inform patient care.
- **Professionalism** – described as the knowledge, skills and attitudes/behaviours required to practise in an ethical and appropriate way, putting patients' needs first and promoting confidence in the dental team.
- **Management and leadership** – described as the skills and knowledge required to work effectively in a dental team, manage own time and resources, and contribute to professional practice.

The NEBDN National Diploma curriculum has been designed to follow these domains and learning outcomes very closely, with more detail given in many areas, as necessary. The glossary of terms has been reproduced in Appendix 1. Details of the qualification itself are given at the end of this chapter, together with information on the C&G Level 3 Diploma.

Student 'fitness to practise'

The GDC's role in regulating the dental profession begins when any student enrolls on a training course and is deemed to be 'in training'. This is irrespective of the category of the future registrant (whether a dentist, dental nurse and so on), or whether the training is being delivered in a dental hospital, further education college or in the dental workplace. All healthcare regulators are required to ensure the safety of patients while being treated by healthcare students, and to ensure that they are fit to practise at the point of registration. While the student dental nurse would not be in a position to 'treat' a patient as such, certain standards of professionalism are quite rightly expected of them, as with any other healthcare student.

Some of the areas of concern that may draw the attention of the GDC to a particular student in relation to issues surrounding their fitness to practise may come as a surprise to some, especially when events have occurred outside the training course or the workplace. While those allegations or areas of concern involving the police (whether resulting in a conviction or a caution) are bound to be considered by the GDC in fitness to practise hearings, other circumstances (such as cheating in an examination or having a poor work attitude) may be erroneously considered to have little to do with the regulator. However, actions and behaviours such as these latter examples may give an overall impression of an unprofessional attitude by the student to the public, and are therefore of great concern to the GDC. Further examples of the types of allegations or convictions that may cause concern and bring into question a student's fitness to practise are set out in Table 3.1 in Chapter 3.

The principles of professionalism that the student dental nurse must adhere to are clearly laid down in the GDC *Standards for Dental Professionals* document (see Chapter 3 for details), and fall into the following six categories.

1. Put patients' interests first and act to protect them.
2. Respect patients' dignity and choices.
3. Protect the confidentiality of patients' information.
4. Co-operate with other members of the dental team and other healthcare colleagues in the interests of patients.
5. Maintain professional knowledge and competence.
6. Be trustworthy.

The responsibility is on the education provider to inform students that unprofessional behaviour or serious health problems during their training may affect their ability to register with the GDC, if they are not considered to be 'fit to practise'. The provider must have transparent processes and procedures in place to communicate and investigate concerns when they arise, and determine whether the student could possibly put patients and the public at risk by their actions.

Full details of the guidance available from the GDC in these matters, for both education providers and students, are available from the GDC website at www.gdc-uk.org.

To ensure that student dental nurses fully appreciate the levels of professionalism expected of them as members of the dental team, examples of some of the potential areas of concern that may result in a fitness to practise investigation are shown in Table 3.1. The topic of professionalism is discussed in detail in Chapter 3.

Dental nurses and the law

The ethical and legal issues that affect dental nurses in their workplace and day-to-day duties are covered in detail in Chapter 3, and those related to safe working practices in Chapter 4.

Overall, the two Acts of Parliament that govern the whole dental profession, including dental nurses, are:

- The Dentists' Act 1984 (Amendment Order 2005)
- The Health and Social Care Act 2008.

The Amendment Order to the Dentists' Act stipulates that only those persons registered with the GDC, following success in a register-able dental nursing qualification, can legally call themselves a 'dental nurse'. This may seem a minor point but a breach of the Order is viewed as a serious legal matter involving an abuse of trust, as the person is seen to be misleading the public over their implied professional status. Qualified dental nurses who have failed to maintain their registration simply by not paying the GDC annual retention fee are therefore breaking the law, and can be prosecuted. Any other registrant (dentist or DCP) who employs such a person is also putting their own registration at risk.

The Health and Social Care Act was introduced in response to the apparent loss of trust in the healthcare professions (including the dental profession) by the public. This followed public inquiries into several notorious cases of serious harm being done to patients by their doctors, both in the hospital environment and out in the community. The most shocking of these was probably the case of Dr Harold Shipman, a GP in Manchester who was successfully convicted of murdering 15 of his patients. His actions were only uncovered after the solicitor daughter of one of his victims became suspicious of events surrounding the death of her mother, and contacted the police. The case highlighted just how uncontrolled and unaccountable a healthcare professional could be at the time, as Shipman is alleged to have killed over 200 of his patients over the years, without raising any suspicions until that point.

Finally, in addition to the above enactments, the same professional standards of behaviour listed previously for students also apply to those who are qualified, and must be adhered to throughout their working career. Now that all DCPs are individually registered with the GDC, the onus is on each team member to take full responsibility for their own actions and to act in a professional manner at all times. The issue of 'vicarious liability' no longer applies – the dentist is no longer personally responsible for the actions or omissions of other registered members of the dental team. However, they are still responsible for unregistered staff, including trainee dental nurses.

The practical application of the professional principles laid down in the GDC *Standards for Dental Professionals* document requires all members of the dental team to behave in the following manner, as professional individuals and on a day-to-day basis.

- Apply the principles in your work as a dental professional, whether or not you routinely treat patients.
- Understand that you are professionally responsible for your actions and must be able to account for them.
- Put patients' interests before your own or those of your colleagues.
- Apply these principles when handling queries and complaints from patients and in all other aspects of non-clinical professional service.
- Maintain your GDC registration and work only within the limits of your knowledge, professional competence and physical capability.
- Take effective action to protect patients if you believe they are being put at risk by your health, behaviour or professional performance, or those of a colleague, or by any aspect of the practice clinical environment.
- If in doubt, obtain advice from senior staff, appropriate professional body or the GDC.
- Treat patients with respect, courtesy and awareness of their dignity and rights.
- Understand and promote patients' responsibility for making decisions about their bodies, their priorities and their care, and obtain their consent before any treatment is undertaken.
- Provide all the information, including the risks, benefits, costs and alternative options, upon which they can make their decision.
- Ensure that there is no discrimination against patients regarding their race, ethnic origin, age, sex, disability, special needs, sexuality, lifestyle, beliefs or economic status.
- Treat all information about patients as confidential, and for use only for the purposes for which it was provided.
- Ensure that such material is kept securely to prevent any accidental or unauthorised access to it.

These points are discussed in detail in Chapter 3.

General Dental Council registration completes the first stage of the dental nurse's professional career. From that point on

- compliance with your legal obligations, knowledge, skills and professional competence must be maintained and updated by verifiable continuing professional development
- justify your professional status, and the trust of your patients and colleagues, by honesty and fairness in all your professional and personal activities
- apply all these ethical principles to clinical and professional relationships, and to any commercial or business dealings in which you may be involved

- maintain proper standards of personal behaviour in all aspects of your life, and thereby promote patients' confidence in you and public confidence in the dental profession.

Continuing professional development

Continuing professional development (CPD) and lifelong learning are now statutory requirements for the continuing registration of DCPs, and more recently the concept of becoming a 'reflective practitioner' has enabled dental professionals to understand how experiences in their daily working lives should guide their CPD achievements. Carrying out CPD activities should aim to guide an individual in updating their skills and education throughout their working lives, to ensure that they stay abreast of all the changes and updates involved in their chosen career. This should then ensure that they provide the best care and service possible to patients. A summary of information and knowledge is given here, but the subject is discussed in more detail in Chapter 3.

Continuing professional development is either verifiable or non-verifiable. Verifiable CPD is that offered formally, with specific learning outcomes given. Certificates of attendance and/or participation in verifiable CPD activities will be issued and must be kept as evidence of complying with the GDC's requirements; they may even have to be produced as evidence of verifiable CPD activity. Examples of verifiable CPD are as follows.

- Attendance on postgraduate courses.
- Attendance at local meetings organised by postgraduate tutors or deaneries.
- Distance learning programmes with learning outcomes.
- Computer-aided learning programmes (CAL).
- Attendance at conferences with stated learning outcomes.
- Studying and taking formal examinations in dentally related subjects.
- Completing tests set on articles published in dental journals.

Some topics of coverage are considered to be essential to the safe delivery of dental care, and are therefore called 'core subjects'. The GDC stipulates the amount of CPD that must be undertaken in these core subjects over a 5-year cycle, for each category of registrant. For dental nurses, the core subjects and the number of verifiable CPD hours for each are as follows.

- Medical emergencies – 10 h.
- Disinfection and decontamination – 5 h.
- Radiography and radiological protection – 5 h.
- Legal and ethical issues – if dealing with patients on a regular basis.
- Complaints handling – if dealing with patients on a regular basis.

Non-verifiable CPD is that done on an informal basis, often purely on a personal interest basis. Although new information may well be learned during these activities, it cannot be tested nor proved that specific learning outcomes have been achieved. Currently, the number of hours of non-verifiable CPD completed annually must also be stated in the registrant's CPD submission. Examples of non-verifiable CPD activities include the following.

- Reading dental journals, with no testing of the contents of any articles.
- Reading postgraduate handbooks.
- Accessing websites and downloading information.
- Attendance at staff meetings.

- Completion of 'in-house' training – although if aims and learning outcomes are stated, feedback is given and a certificate of attendance issued, these events can easily be turned into verifiable CPD activities.
- Completion of staff appraisals.

When carried out correctly, organised CPD events covering the mandatory areas of dental practice, as well as a wider range of subjects relevant to the role of the dental nurse, are of great benefit. It should enable recognition of areas that are of interest as well as areas where more knowledge is required, as dentistry, and therefore dental nursing, are ever-changing disciplines where new materials and techniques are introduced regularly. Completion of CPD should produce some of the following personal outcomes for all dental nurses.

- Increased job satisfaction.
- Identification of problem areas.
- Improved communication with colleagues.
- Improved efficiency.
- Improved career prospects.
- Greater commitment to the workplace.

The planning and undertaking of CPD should be given careful thought by dental nurses to ensure not only that the mandatory requirements of the GDC are met but also that any other CPD undertaken is of use to them. While the temptation exists to only attend courses of personal interest, a broader coverage of subjects is more desirable and useful to the development of the dental nurse.

A staff training and development system must be in place in all dental workplaces, whereby the skills held by all staff are reviewed on a one-to-one basis so that individual training needs can be identified. This is usually carried out as an annual staff appraisal process and is discussed further in Chapter 3.

In essence, records should be kept of the points discussed during the appraisal, as well as any needs that have been identified and any methods discussed for meeting these needs. These points can be developed into a personal development plan (PDP), where the necessary CPD requirements can be looked into and successfully accessed, and the individual PDP can be updated accordingly. This is then available to the GDC, or prospective new employers, as evidence that the staff member not only has ambitions and identified training needs, but that they have successfully carried them out.

The development and use of a PDP is now a requirement for completion of the Record of Experience for the NEBDN National Diploma qualification, while student dental nurses undergo their formal training.

Overall role of the dental nurse

The role of the dental nurse during specific chairside, or patient-orientated, activities is discussed in detail in each of the following clinically relevant chapters. However, as a key member of the dental team, there are many overall duties that must be carried out by the dental nurse on a daily basis to ensure the efficient running of the dental workplace, as well as administrative or reception duties. This is achieved by ensuring meticulous attention to detail during completion of the many background activities that allow the workplace to run smoothly, like a well-oiled machine. These background activities have traditionally developed as dental nurse roles, while the dentist (and now also the hygienist and therapist) have concentrated more on the patient-centred, hands-on activities of delivering treatment. The actions of all members of the dental team working together in this way culminate in a pleasant and successful experience for the patient at each attendance.

The activities specific to the dental nurse can be summarised under the following three areas.

- General duties.
- Administrative and reception duties.
- Surgery duties.

General duties

- Acceptable level of personal appearance and social cleanliness, in accordance with the dress code requirements of the workplace, to give an overall appearance of professionalism.
- Maintenance of a high standard of cleanliness and tidiness throughout the premises.
- Adequate levels of heating, lighting and ventilation, to ensure a comfortable environment for patients and staff.
- Full and accurate list of all contact details for suppliers, service and maintenance personnel, patient health and welfare organisations, and laboratories.
- Ordering and correct storage of dental stock and general supplies.
- Full knowledge of, and compliance with, all Health and Safety directives in relation to general issues (such as fire drill, location of fire extinguishers, waste disposal requirements, etc. – these are discussed further in Chapter 4)

Administration and reception

- Acceptable level of personal appearance and social cleanliness, in accordance with the dress code requirements of the workplace.
- Good level of communication skills.
- Reception of patients and dental company representatives.
- Full working knowledge of all appointment systems in use.
- Arrangement of current and recall appointments.
- Recording of all attendances and treatment.
- Completion and filing of patients' records, whether manual or computerised.
- Receipt and actioning of all correspondence.
- Knowledge of NHS and private regulations and organisation.
- Management of financial records.
- Running of computer entry back-ups, on a daily basis.
- Liaison with laboratories, to ensure work is collected and delivered as required.

A large part of the successful administration and reception duties of the dental nurse is related to good patient management skills, and involve all of the following areas.

- Reception of the patient into the practice.
- Appointments.
- Communication skills.
- Equality of dental care.
- Patients with special needs.
- Dental emergencies.

The dental nurse has a key role to play in ensuring that the dental experience of each patient is a pleasant one, whether working at the chairside or in a reception and administrative position.

Reception of patients into the practice

Most dental practices have one or more dental nurses who 'double up' as receptionists for at least part of their working week, although it is possible to have staff with purely administrative duties. However, since GDC registration of dental nurses has become mandatory, administrative staff without a dental nurse qualification can no longer 'double up' as dental nurses during periods of short staffing. The obvious problem with purely administrative staff manning reception occurs when patients are asking for dental advice or for further information about specific dental treatments, as they will have limited dental knowledge. For this reason, most practices prefer a dental nurse to carry out reception duties.

The word 'reception' illustrates the main role of these personnel – to 'receive' the patient into the practice as the first point of contact in the dental environment. It is vital that the dental nurse in this role has all of the following attributes.

- Pleasant disposition.
- Good communication skills (discussed further in Chapter 13).
- Friendly and welcoming attitude.
- Knowledgeable about dentistry but only to the limit of their training.
- Efficient and accurate at reception duties.
- Works well under pressure, without becoming flustered.
- Pleasant telephone manner.
- Caring and considerate attitude.
- Well presented, and neither too loud nor too softly spoken.

As very few dental practices, and no hospital clinics, are without computerisation of at least some part of their working system, IT skills are also an imperative requirement for the modern dental nurse to acquire. However, the increasingly extensive use of computers in dentistry and dental practice management does not replace the need for the dental nurse to have legible, neat and accurate handwriting skills, and this is especially important when giving written information such as appointment details to patients.

A friendly disposition is invaluable when greeting nervous and anxious patients onto the premises, and is often all that is required to allay the fears of most patients. While this tends to come naturally when dealing with younger patients, it should be remembered that many older patients are just as anxious, whether they try to hide their feelings or not. Being friendly and welcoming to all patients should come as second nature to all of the dental team, so that the patient's dental experience is of a consistently high standard for the whole visit.

Appointments

Booking appointments for patients takes up a large part of the working day, and during busy periods it can be an area that causes many problems. When several patients are hovering in a reception area, and one or more telephones are ringing with enquiries from other patients, it is quite easy for members of the dental team to be overwhelmed by the demands of their role and for mistakes to happen. In larger practices and hospital clinics, it is usual for more than one staff member to be responsible for appointment bookings, and without a written protocol in place for the task to be carried out in a consistent manner by all, mistakes can easily be made.

A successful apointments booking system can easily be established by any dental workplace if the following points are considered and adapted for use as necessary.

- Ensure that all staff working at the reception area have been fully trained in all of their necessary duties.
- Have written protocols to be followed by all staff.
- Ensure the booking system is sensible, easy to follow, and is explained clearly during training sessions.
- If manual appointment books are used, rather than a computerised system, ensure alterations and cancellations are deleted in a tidy manner, so that the daylist is still readable by all staff.
- If possible, delegate the simpler reception duties to other staff so that one senior person remains in control of appointment bookings, as this will lead to fewer mistakes.
- Ensure all staff are aware of how each dentist and DCP prefers their appointments to be booked, especially the length of time required for various procedures.
- Be considerate but firm with patients when booking appointments; sometimes it may not be possible for them to have the time slot they request.
- If a problem does occur, attempt to rectify it to everyone's satisfaction as soon as possible, but try to uncover the cause of the problem so that it will not be repeated in the future – this shows maturity and common sense.

Equality of dental care

As discussed in Chapters 3 and 13, the dental nurse has a legal responsibility to behave equally towards all patients without showing any form of discrimination. This can occur in all of the following areas.

- **Sex discrimination** – between male and female patients.
- **Age discrimination** – especially between elderly patients and others.
- **Ethnic discrimination** – between ethnic minorities and white British patients, especially where there is a language barrier too.
- **Socio-economic discrimination** – between the perceived social class and economic status of various patient groups.

In particular regard to sex discrimination, the development of inappropriate relationships between members of the dental team and patients is particularly frowned upon by the profession, and more importantly by the GDC. No favouritism should be shown towards any patient by a staff member because they are attracted to them – problems are likely to occur, which may result in dismissal or even a charge of serious professional misconduct. Staff only have to read the quarterly misconduct reports issued by the GDC to determine the seriousness of these charges.

The dental team needs to be aware of any likely cultural differences between ethnic groups, some of which are of dental relevance and are discussed further in Chapter 13. The team must accept these differences in an appropriate manner, while offering oral health advice as necessary. Religious beliefs may prevent a patient from undergoing oral examination at certain times, such as the Moslem period of Ramadan, and again the dental team must accommodate the belief to allow smooth running of the practice.

Patients with special needs

There are many patients who can be considered to have special needs in relation to dentistry and dental treatment, because of a physical, mental, social or medical problem. Some of these special needs patients who are likely to be treated in a general dental practice setting, rather than in a specialist dental clinic, are as follows.

- Elderly patients.
- Patients with learning disabilities.
- Patients with physical disabilities.
- Patients with certain medical problems.
- Patients from low socio-economic backgrounds.

This subject is also discussed further in Chapter 13.

Dental emergencies

Even with the very best dental care, emergencies do arise from time to time. Since April 2006 it has been the responsibility of the primary care trust (PCT) to provide out-of-hours emergency dental care to all patients, whether they are NHS, private, regular or irregular attenders. This is currently operated through a telephone triage system, by organisations such as NHS Direct, where calls are received from patients and categorised into a range of severity. Each PCT will determine the most severe incidents that require emergency treatment, but the following are likely to be included by all.

- **Severe dental pain** – which is not controlled by analgesics.
- **Severe swelling** – of the oral soft tissues, which is at risk of compromising the patient's airway.
- **Uncontrolled bleeding** – after an extraction or minor oral surgery procedure.

Less severe emergencies, such as swelling with no airway implications, are passed to the 'on-call' dentist for an opinion on whether the patient should be seen within 12 or 24 hours, by either their own dentist or by the emergency dentist. As the system is intended to operate during evenings, weekends and public holidays, it may be that treatment will be required before the patient's own dentist is available. In these cases, they will be directed to a local dental access centre for emergency treatment, such as lancing an abscess, placing a tooth on open drainage or placing a dressing. The patient can then seek full treatment from their own dentist at a later date, or find a dentist willing to undertake their treatment if they receive no regular dental care.

Private patients may be members of various private dental plans, such as Practice Plan or Denplan, and member dentists will often provide emergency care for less serious incidents, such as recementing a crown or bridge. Each practice will have its own emergency protocol to follow for all eventualities, and the dental nurse has a key communication role to play when dealing with patients in these situations.

When emergency calls are received during normal working hours, it is the responsibility of the practice to provide care as it deems necessary, although since the new NHS dental contract system began in April 2006, the situation has become less clear. This is because the new system indicates that NHS patients are no longer registered with a practice or a dentist, and can attend any practice they choose if the dentist is willing and able to provide treatment for them. It could be interpreted, then, that between courses of dental treatment, the practice has no responsibility towards any patient for the provision of emergency dental care. The vast majority of dentists tend to show good will to all regular attenders, however, and are happy to provide emergency care for them as necessary.

Various different management systems for dental emergencies during working hours may be operated, and some examples are as follows.

- **Double booking appointment slots** – this saves unbooked time slots but is disruptive to the running of the appointment system and often results in the dentist 'running late'.
- **Set aside emergency time slots** – this is less disruptive but can result in unbooked surgery time occurring.

- **In-house triage system** – the practice determines what constitutes an emergency, and the dentist decides which patients require treatment that day; the patient is then slotted into any unbooked appointment time or is seen after normal hours.
- ***Ad hoc* system** – all emergency treatment requests are received and slotted into any available appointment slots; again this saves unbooked time but can cause disruptions if a high number of calls are received.

Most dental workplaces will run a combination of the above management systems, but the most effective methods of reducing the number of emergencies is for the dental team to work as follows.

- Provide consistently good-quality dental care to all patients, to reduce the incidence of predictable emergencies; for instance, if a new crown does not fit well, it should be remade rather than fitted as a poor fitting cown is likely to fail.
- Have a written emergency dental call protocol for all to follow, and stick to it without exception.
- Have an accepted triage system in place, that is used by the whole dental team.
- Ensure that patients are made aware that they will only receive emergency treatment initially, and will have to reattend for further treatment in a routine appointment slot.
- Be aware of the regular patients and their dental histories; an emergency call from a regular attender is more likely to be a *genuine* emergency than one from a patient who routinely fails appointments and ignores oral health advice.

The dental nurse plays a vital role in running a successful emergency management system, as this team member is the first point of call for what is often a distressed and anxious patient, and one who is quite likely to be in pain. A sympathetic and caring attitude must always be adopted, but a firm hand may also be required for the successful management of those relatively few patients who will not accept advice alone, and insist upon an immediate appointment with the dentist. If all else fails, the handling of these patients may have to be transferred to a senior staff member or the dentist. No matter what, the dental nurse should not be intimidated into breaking the emergency call protocol of the practice by any patient.

Surgery duties

As stated above, the details of the surgery role for each type of treatment are covered in the relevant successive chapters, but there are many points that the dental nurse should follow which are common to all opening up, during treatment and closing down procedures for all chairside activities.

Thorough preparation of the surgery is essential before the day starts, between patients and at the end of a treatment session. In addition, a clinical level of personal appearance and cleanliness is required in the surgery areas, in accordance with the uniform and personal protective equipment (PPE) requirements of the dental workplace.

Beginning of the day, after switching on all power to the equipment

- Disinfect all working surfaces.
- Fit new disposable covers where necessary.
- Discharge water for 2 min through three-in-one syringe and all handpieces with water spray.
- Run, and record result of, autoclave test.
- Refill ultrasonic cleaner with fresh fluid.
- Check that all other equipment is working satisfactorily.

- Ensure that appointment book, day book, patients' notes, radiographs, laboratory work, emergency kit and all materials for the day are ready.
- Prepare records, instruments and materials for first patient.

During treatment

- Highlight any relevant aspects of the patient to the dentist before treatment begins, such as anxiety about treatment, special medical history, nausea during impressions, fainting tendency, etc.
- Always greet patients by name, in a friendly manner, and introduce them to the dentist by name.
- Seat the patient comfortably, and apply a protective bib and safety glasses if treatment is to be carried out.
- Maintain an atmosphere of relaxed efficiency and friendly communication with the patient.
- Maintain patient records and charts as required.
- Process and mount radiographs, if taken.
- Maintain a clear and dry operative field throughout treatment, using good retraction and aspiration techniques.
- Provide full chairside support throughout treatment in relation to instruments and materials used.
- Monitor the patient throughout for any signs of distress, and inform the dentist where necessary.
- Act as a chaperone and witness throughout the treatment session.
- Ensure the patient is cleaned and tidied before leaving the surgery, by removing material debris and offering a mouth rinse.
- Give postoperative and/or oral hygiene advice, as necessary.
- Correctly disinfect, package and label any laboratory work, ready for collection.
- Remove all used instruments to the decontamination area.
- Dispose of all waste in the correct manner.
- Prepare the surgery for the next patient.

End of the day

- All used instruments, waste and laboratory work are handled as detailed above.
- All disposable shields are removed from equipment and put into the hazardous waste container.
- Surgery hazardous waste containers are removed from the area to their place of storage.
- All surfaces are correctly disinfected and wiped down.
- All portable equipment is switched off, disconnected and put into storage cupboards.
- All sterilised instruments are returned to their correct place of storage.
- Spittoon and suction unit is run through with the correct disinfectant solution.
- The air compressor is switched off and the air tank is drained.
- All other electrical equipment is switched off and disconnected.
- Any locking drawers and cupboards are secured.
- Any paper records are written up and then filed appropriately or returned to reception.

Dental nurse qualifications

The basic, pre-registration qualifications available to anyone wishing to become a dental nurse are provided by the National Examining Board for Dental Nurses (NEBDN) or by City & Guilds (C&G). Although the same level of qualification is achieved by successful candidates with either awarding body, the route to qualification is different. The merits of each are discussed below.

National Examining Board for Dental Nurses

For almost 60 years, the NEBDN has been the awarding body solely responsible for the provision of a dental nursing examination – the National Certificate for Dental Nurses. The organisation is made up of GDC-registered examiners from all branches of dentistry, both dentists and dental care professionals, who are available on a voluntary basis to examine dental nurse candidates throughout the UK.

All examiners have been qualified themselves for a minimum of 2 years and have a history of dental nurse teaching and/or experience in dental clinical examinations. The position of examiner is held for a 3-year term, after which applicants are considered for reappointment in line with the organisation's reappointment criteria.

With the National Certificate qualification, examiners were responsible for marking candidates' written papers, as well as conducting structured practical and oral examinations. The new NEBDN National Diploma qualification only requires examiners to conduct objective structured clinical examinations (OSCEs) on the exam day, as the written paper is marked by an optical marking system beforehand.

All candidates wishing to sit the NEBDN National Diploma must have undergone a formal training course with an NEBDN-accredited training provider, while working as a trainee dental nurse in the dental workplace. In addition, every candidate must have successfully completed an NEBDN Record of Experience portfolio before entering for the examination, as this provides written evidence of the practical experience achieved within the dental workplace by the candidate.

Further information about the NEBDN National Diploma is given below, and full details of the qualification, the Record of Experience and postregistration qualifications available from NEBDN can be accessed from:

NEBDN, 108–110 London Street, Fleetwood, Lancashire FY7 6EU
Tel: 01253 778417
Fax: 01253 777268
E-mail: admin@nebdn.org
Website: www.nebdn.org

The National Examining Board for Dental Nurses National Diploma Examination

This new examination is composed of a written element and a practical element. The written element is currently held twice a year, in May and November, in various large regional centres throughout the UK. It is likely that this will be increased to four times a year in the future, to accommodate large candidate numbers and to improve career choices for students. The practical element is only available to those candidates who are successful in the written examination, and is also held twice a year, in June/July and January/February.

As stated previously, all entrants to the exam must have completed a formal training course first, as well as having their completed Record of Experience 'signed off' by both their course provider and a supervising workplace colleague. There is now, therefore, no longer a requirement for students to have worked at the chairside for a 24-month period, before they can receive their qualification. However, the formal examination must be passed in its entirety while the Record of Experience is still valid – this is currently for a term of 3 years from its date of purchase.

Training courses are currently run in dental hospitals, colleges of further education or privately in dental surgeries – a full list of accredited course providers is available from: admin@nebdn.org.

While there are currently no formal entry requirements imposed by NEBDN on student applicants, individual course providers may request them to have a minimum number of GCSE qualifications (or equivalent) or a minimum level of literacy and numeracy skills. In addition, as this is a UK qualification, all students must have a reasonable level of spoken and written English as well as a reasonable understanding of the English language.

An outline of the examination components is given below.

Written paper

The written paper has two sections which each contain one style of question – either one of five multiple choice questions (MCQs) or extended matching questions (EMQs). Unlike the old National Certificate examination, there are no diagrams to label, no short answer questions and no long answer questions. While there is no separate charting exercise to complete within the new examination, questions in either section may contain questions about charting.

Multiple choice questions

The new style of MCQ has the full title of one of five single best answer MCQ and is written as follows.

- The question itself is usually one or two sentences long.
- The first sentence introduces the topic of the question.
- The final sentence asks the question.
- They are designed to test the application of relevant knowledge.
- Key words or phrases are not highlighted.
- There are always five answer options.
- Only one of those five will be the 'best', and therefore the correct, answer.
- The answers are always homologous – of the same form (so, all micro-organisms, all periodontal instruments, all filling materials, and so on).
- They are always set out alphabetically or numerically in ascending order.

As the question style always follows the same pattern, it is not possible for candidates to 'work out by elimination' or 'guess' the correct answer; they must have the relevant knowledge and the understanding to be able to apply it to the scenario of the question. Only then can the single best answer be identified.

Similarly, as a logical alphabetical or numerical order is always followed in the answers, the correct answer cannot be determined by seeing how many times, say, option (d) has been an answer and therefore not choosing it again. The single best answer will be at whichever option letter it falls alphabetically or numerically only. So it is quite feasible for an examination to have option (d) as the correct answer for every question asked, if the correct answer happens to fall at the position of option (d) alphabetically or numerically. Consequently, the candidate is unable to guess the answer.

Candidates mark their single answer choice on an optical marking sheet for each question, by pencilling in a small box. Only one box must be filled in, otherwise the computer will reject that question. Similarly, the box must be filled in horizontally – drawing a circle around it or marking with a cross will also cause the computer to reject that question.

An example of the new-style MCQ is shown in Figure 2.1. The question clearly states that only the buccal gingivae of the upper premolar teeth will be involved in the procedure, so the nerve supplying this area simply needs identifying from the options listed. Only the middle superior dental nerve is relevant to the question.

A gingivectomy procedure is to be carried out on an epileptic patient. The technique will involve the removal of hyperplastic gingival tissue from the buccal side of the upper left premolar teeth. Which one of the following nerves must be anaesthetised to allow the procedure to be carried out painlessly?

(a)   Greater palatine nerve
(b)   Inferior dental nerve
(c)   Long buccal nerve
(d)   Middle superior dental nerve
(e)   Posterior superior dental nerve

The correct answer is (d).

Figure 2.1   An example of the new-style MCQ.

Extended matching questions

This style of question follows a similar layout to the MCQ in some respects, and was introduced to replace the short answer style question but with all candidates having the same definitive option list provided for each set of questions in the examination paper. There is no opportunity for candidates to create an answer, as they could with the old short answer style, as only the options listed can be used.

Each options list has several questions (a question set) attached to it.

The EMQ style questions are written as follows.

- The topic covered by the question set is stated, to help focus the candidate's thoughts.
- A lead-in statement is then given which explains what the candidate is required to do, and how many options they are required to choose from the list, for each question.
- The option list is then given, and will usually contain a minimum of eight options.
- The options are always homologous – of the same form (so all surgical instruments, all micro-organisms, and so on).
- They are always set out alphabetically or numerically in ascending order.
- The questions are set out as several sentences giving a detailed scenario.
- They are designed to test analytical and reasoning skills, as well as requiring a more detailed and concise application of knowledge.
- Key words or phrases are not highlighted.
- Each topical option list has several questions set to it.

The candidate is required to understand the question and apply detailed knowledge to be able to reason the answer(s) from the option list.

A simple example of an EMQ style question used in the new National Diploma examination is shown in Figure 2.2. The clinical scenario describes the signs and symptoms of the condition and then states the disease that is present. The candidate must then apply their knowledge of micro-organisms that cause this condition and locate it from the option list. With a more extensive option list, the lead-in statement could ask for two appropriate micro-organisms from the list, making it a harder question still.

Alternatively, the name of the disease diagnosed can be left out of the question, so that the candidate then has to determine it from the signs and symptoms themselves, before being able to choose the correct option from the list – again, this would become a harder question still. These

Topic: Dental Pathology
For each of the following dental pathology questions, select the single most appropriate micro-organism from the option list. Each option might be used once, more than once or not at all.

(a) *Bacillus fusiformis*
(b) *Candida albicans*
(c) Coxsackievirus
(d) Epstein–Barr virus
(e) Herpes simplex
(f) Paramyxovirus
(g) *Porphyromonas gingivalis*
(h) *Staphylococcus aureus*
(i) *Streptococcus mutans*

An 18-year-old patient attends the surgery as an emergency, complaining of severe gingival pain and halitosis. He admits to being a smoker, and brushing his teeth only once every few days. On examination, his oral hygiene is very poor and his gingivae are swollen and sloughing at the papillae. The dentist diagnoses acute necrotising ulcerative gingivitis. Which one of the options listed is a micro-organism associated with this condition?

The correct answer is (a).

Figure 2.2   An example of an EMQ.

styles of assessment questions are given at www.levisonstextbookfordentalnurses.com/ and a full revision aid is available as *Questions and Answers for Dental Nurses*, 3rd edition. Details are given on the back cover of this book.

Objective structured clinical examination

The practical component of the Diploma examination is an objective structured clinical exam, or OSCE. Candidates must pass the written paper first, before being allowed to take the OSCE element of the examination. Therefore the written paper and the OSCEs are held several weeks apart, so that the written papers can be marked first and a list of successful candidates produced for the OSCEs.

The OSCE has replaced the practical and oral sections of the old examination, where examiners had to ask candidates questions throughout both sections. However, candidates could be asked different questions, possibly at different knowledge levels, by whichever examiner they were allocated to within an examination centre. The old tests were therefore unstructured and were subjective rather than objective, so a candidate's performance was graded according to the opinion of the examiner at the time, rather than against set criteria.

The new style of practical examination, the OSCE, is completely different and provides a far more accurate and fairer assessment of every candidate. As its name suggests, it is both objective and structured in the way that it assesses the candidates – the examiner does not ask any questions but simply grades clinical performance against set criteria as the candidate carries out the task. The set criteria are the same for every candidate, throughout every examination centre, and cannot be altered in any way by the examiner.

Each examination sitting will typically have between 15 and 18 OSCE stations that every candidate must go through, and they are usually timed at 5 min each. Other than to welcome the candidate into each test area, and ask if they have read the candidate instructions for the test beforehand, the examiner merely observes their performance.

There are four general types of practical assessment that the OSCE will cover, and each is designed to test both the professional and practical skills of the candidate. Simplistic examples are given below.

- **Communication skills** – such as giving specific oral hygiene advice to a patient (who will be a professional actor).
- **Medical emergency** – such as an asthma attack scenario (again, possibly involving a professional actor).
- **Mixing** – any material from within the curriculum.
- **Clinical** – such as setting up instruments for a specific dental procedure or completing a charting exercise.

The candidate instructions will give the scenario relevant to the station, and the candidate is able to read these instructions before the 5-min timing starts. The instructions will be clear and concise, so that the task to be carried out is obvious.

Where a patient (actor) is involved in the scenario, the candidate will be scored by both the examiner and the patient.

To ensure that every candidate is assessed objectively, the following system is used.

- Every examination centre will carry out exactly the same OSCE assessments, using exactly the same resources.
- All candidate and patient instructions will be worded exactly the same, in every centre.
- All candidates will be marked against the same performance criteria, and in the same way, as the examiners have been trained and calibrated to each other.
- All candidates will rotate through the OSCE stations in a set order until they have completed the full cycle.
- A single timer is used for each cycle of stations (usually a bell), so candidates cannot have too little, or too much, time at any station.
- All candidates are allowed 1 min to read the scenario and candidate instructions for each station, before entering the station and beginning the assessment when the bell rings.
- No candidate is allowed to enter the station until the start of the 5-min session.
- The candidate may repeat the assessment within the 5-min time period if they wish.
- The examiner will not ask any questions of the candidate.
- The candidate may carry out the task while talking their way through it, if they wish – they will only be graded on the performance criteria listed on the examiner's mark sheet.
- There are no 'killer stations', where the candidate must pass that one station or be failed for the whole OSCE examination.

City & Guilds Level 3 Diploma in Dental Nursing

This is the alternative training pathway for students wishing to become qualified dental nurses, and is different in that it follows a more vocational, less academic route to qualification. The same curriculum topics are covered, but the C&G Diploma is entirely different in the way that knowledge is tested. Whereas the NEBDN National Diploma examination covers the vast majority of the learning outcomes, takes place in two parts (the written paper then the OSCEs), and only after the Record of Experience portfolio has been completed, most of the learning outcomes of the C&G Diploma are covered in the workplace, by the witnessed completion of a portfolio.

The C&G Diploma students attend a training course too, but only some of the learning outcomes for the qualification are covered by a formal examination, currently consisting of the old-style (one of four) MCQs and short answers. The written paper is currently held three times per year, in March, June and December, and students can be entered numerous times to sit the examination.

The learning outcomes covered in the workplace are witnessed by personnel holding a City & Guilds Assessor award, at prearranged workplace visits. As the student carries out their dental nursing duties, the assessor 'signs off' the performance criteria covered to a satisfactory standard as they are witnessed. Qualification is not given until the whole portfolio has been completed, and the candidate has passed the written paper too. There is currently no limit to the number of times that the examination can be taken, and the portfolio has no restriction on its period of validity.

Further details of the C&G Level 3 Diploma in Dental Nursing are available from:

City and Guilds
1 Giltspur Street
London EC1A 9DD
Tel: 020 7294 2468
Fax: 020 7294 2400
Website: www.cityandguilds.com

Postregistration qualifications

Once qualified (by whichever training route) and registered with the General Dental Council, the dental nurse can access various postregistration qualifications run by the NEBDN, in a variety of specialised areas of dental nursing. Currently, these higher level qualifications cover the following areas.

- **Dental sedation nursing** – for those students working in hospitals, clinics and practices where conscious sedation techniques are used (intravenous and inhalation).
- **Oral health education** – for those students wishing to take responsibility for advising and instructing patients on improving their oral health.
- **Special care dental nursing** – for those students working with patients who have special needs.
- **Dental radiography** – for those students involved in all aspects of dental radiographic techniques, including positioning and exposing patients.
- **Orthodontic dental nursing** – for those students working in hospitals, clinics and practices where orthodontic treatment is carried out.
- **Dental implant nursing** – for those students working in hospitals, clinics and practices where dental implants are placed; this qualification is currently work in progress.

Other specialised areas of dental nursing are being considered for future postregistration qualifications, including mentoring in the dental workplace and endodontic dental nursing.

Further details of any of these courses, including a list of accredited training providers for each qualification, are available from: admin@nebdn.org.

Extended duties

Since dental nurses have become GDC registrants, their roles and those of other dental team members have been assessed to determine if any additional duties could be safely carried out once additional training has been given in the workplace, but without having to sit an examination first. Various duties fall into this category and are collectively known as 'extended duties' – they do not include the specialised area of study and examination required for a dental nurse to position and expose a patient to ionising radiation. This skill can only be achieved by acquiring the dental radiography postregistration qualification.

In allowing dental nurses to acquire these extended duties, the GDC released its publication *Scope of Practice* to give guidance on how they can be achieved without the dental nurse working beyond their level of skill. Obviously, those skills that are specifically provided by other dental team members as part of their register-able qualification training are excluded as skills available to the dental nurse, without undertaking that additional, formal training and qualification.

In all areas of possible extended duties, the GDC publication states that: 'The scope of your practice is a way of describing what you are trained and competent to do'. The key words in this statement are 'trained' and 'competent'. To achieve both in an extended duty, a senior work colleague must provide supervised guidance and training in the chosen topic, produce a written record of the training given, and sign to say that in their opinion you are competent to carry out the duty.

Examples of extended duties available to the dental nurse include the following.

- Impression taking (alginate).
- Shade taking.
- Suture removal.
- Casting of study models from alginate impressions.
- Construction of tooth-whitening trays.
- Pressing the x-ray machine exposure button under the direct supervision of the operator.
- Intraoral photography.

Further information and advice is available from the GDC website: www.gdc-uk.org.

The impact of the publication *Scope of Practice* on the dental nursing profession and the relevance of extended duties for dental nurses are covered in more detail in Chapter 3.

Finally, as mentioned in Chapter 1, the dental nurse may also go on to study and become qualified as a dentist, therapist, clinical dental technician or orthodontic therapist. Qualification as a dental nurse beforehand is not always a requirement but it does give the student an excellent level of knowledge from which to expand their career.

 Further resources are available for this book, including interactive multiple choice questions and extended matching questions. Visit the companion website at:

www.levisonstextbookfordentalnurses.com

3

Legal and Ethical Issues

Key learning points

A **factual knowledge** of
- the professional obligations of dental nurses
- Continuing Professional Development requirements and becoming a reflective practitioner

A **working knowledge** of
- the General Dental Council's professional standards guidance in relation to the dental team
- all aspects of patient records; including issues of confidentiality, information governance, and patient access to records
- patient consent to treatment
- raising concerns in the workplace

A **factual awareness** of
- the issues of protecting children and vulnerable adults
- patient complaints and their correct handling

Until 2006, dentists were the only individuals who could carry on the business of dentistry, and although others (including dental nurses) were involved in the dental care of patients up to this point, the dentist was solely responsible for all acts and omissions on behalf of their staff. So, if anything was below standard or harmful to a patient, the dentist alone was held responsible.

The General Dental Council (GDC) is the regulatory body of the dental profession (see Chapter 1), and in 2006 it opened the Dental Care Professionals Register so that all other persons involved in the dental care of patients had to become registered with it. Dental nurses joined the register in 2008 and have become a profession in their own right, along with other registrants such as

Levison's Textbook for Dental Nurses, Eleventh Edition. By Carole Hollins.
© 2013 John Wiley & Sons, Ltd. Published 2013 by John Wiley & Sons, Ltd. Companion website: www.levisonstextbookfordentalnurses.com

therapists, hygienists and dental technicians. However, with registration comes professional responsibility and compliance with professional standards – registrants are now responsible for their own acts and omissions in relation to patient care, unless it is proven that their employer knowingly prevented the member of staff from acting professionally.

To become a registrant, the dental nurse must first qualify by passing a recognised examination in dental nursing; currently these are the National Examining Board for Dental Nurses' (NEBDN) Diploma or the City & Guilds Diploma in Dental Nursing. Until qualification, the staff member is a trainee dental nurse (but must be on an approved training course and studying towards qualification) and their employer is still responsible for them.

Once initially registered, the dental nurse must meet the following criteria to ensure their annual re-registration, and therefore be legally entitled to work as a dental nurse in the UK.

- Comply with all relevant legislation and regulations to ensure they act both ethically and legally at all times.
- Maintain a professional standard of behaviour at all times.
- Comply with continuing professional development (CPD) requirements in core topics and minimum hours over a 5-year cycle.
- Maintain indemnity insurance cover from one of the dental protection organisations.
- Pay the annual retention fee (ARF).

The relevant legislation and regulations are covered throughout this text, particularly in Chapter 4, and the text as a whole covers the full curriculum requirements for the NEBDN Diploma qualification. The City & Guilds Level 3 Diploma in Dental Nursing curriculum requirements are covered in the alternative textbook, due to be released in late 2013.

In addition, the GDC has published a set of *Standards Guidance* booklets for use by all registrants, and trainee dental nurses are expected to be familiar with their contents by the time they sit their final register-able qualification. Each booklet and its relevance to the trainee dental nurse will be discussed in detail here. Other useful GDC publications for consideration throughout the training course include:

- *Preparing for Practice* – formerly called *Developing the Dental Team* and giving details of the expected level of skills and knowledge of each registrant group upon qualification
- *Scope of Practice* – gives details of the additional skills, after qualification, that may be achieved by the various groups of registrants, following a period of suitable and recorded training, and forming the basis of the extended duties and postregistration qualifications available to registered dental nurses
- *Fitness to Practise* – gives details of the professional standards expected of all registrants, and the disciplinary procedures that should be followed when they are not upheld, some of which are also relevant to the trainee dental nurse.

Further details of all these publications can be found at www.gdc-uk.org.

In summary, the ethical and legal implications of the following topics will be discussed here, with those of particular relevance to the duties of the dental nurse being covered in greater detail.

- Duty of care and professional obligations – overview.
- Fitness to practise guidance.
- GDC *Standards Guidance* – overview and notes on its relevance in other sections.
- Impact of Care Quality Commission (CQC) registration on dental workplaces.
- Clinical governance.

- Record keeping:
  - confidentiality of patient records
  - information governance.
- Consent to treatment.
- Protection of children and vulnerable adults:
  - Criminal Records Bureau (CRB) checks.
- Complaints handling.
- Raising concerns.
- Continuing professional development, reflective practice and developing the dental team.

Duty of care and professional obligations

It is the responsibility of the employer to ensure that the dental workplace and its day-to-day running comply with all of the legislation and regulations pertinent to the practice of dentistry, but every registrant working in the premises also has a duty of care to their colleagues and the patients to work safely and responsibly at all times. This requirement comes under the Health and Safety at Work Act, and is covered in greater detail in Chapter 4.

In line with our medical colleagues whose professional responsibilities include the phrase 'First, do no harm', the dental professional's first duty of care can be said to be 'always act in the patient's best interests'. This theme runs throughout the various sections of this chapter, and it will be seen that at all times, the guidance from the GDC with regard to the expected standards of dental professionals is to always put the patient's interests first, and act to protect them. This is the duty of care that all registrants must uphold towards all patients.

The professional obligations of registrants are discussed in greater detail later, and can be summarised as the following.

- Maintain their professional registration.
- Ensure that all patients have equal rights.
- Work within their professional level of competence.
- Undertake lifelong learning in their areas of competence.
- Be able to demonstrate their fitness to practise.

Fitness to practise guidance

No one factor determines whether a registrant is 'fit to practise' or not – whether a dental nurse is suitable to work in the dental workplace is not solely based on their academic achievements. Their qualification indicates that they are competent to do so – they have demonstrated an adequate ability to carry out the duties of a dental nurse – but suppose they are consistently rude to staff and patients, or lazy and neglectful, or dishonest and untrustworthy? Are they still fit to practise simply because they have a qualification in the required subjects? Of course, the answer is 'no'.

The qualities required to be fit to practise are to have good personal skills and acceptable attitudes and behaviour, as well as successful academic qualifications – together they produce the professional dental nurse.

One definition of the word 'professional' as a descriptive term for a person is '... characterised by or conforming to the technical and ethical standards of a profession', so by becoming professional members of the healthcare team, all registrants are expected to behave in a suitable manner in public, whether working or not.

It may be surprising to some that registrants are expected to follow a high standard of behaviour not just in the workplace but while not at work too. So it is not acceptable to be seen as 'pillars of society' from 9am to 5pm, and then become drunk and disorderly or antisocial while out with friends in the evening, for example.

As a professional, the registrant's conduct, behaviour and personal qualities are open to scrutiny by the public at all times, and the public quite rightly expects anyone who is regarded as a professional to behave correctly and to set an example of good behaviour and conduct that others aspire to achieve. Any registrant who falls short of these expectations may have their fitness to practise called into question – by the public, their colleagues, their employer and ultimately by their professional regulator – the General Dental Council.

If the registrant is called before the GDC to attend a conduct committee and is found to be unfit to practise, they may be suspended, or even erased, from the Register. It is then illegal for that registrant to work as a dental nurse again in the UK, until such time as the GDC allows them to re-register – and that may require further training and requalification in some cases. Effectively, to be erased from the Register, the registrant would be considered to have brought the profession into disrepute.

Table 3.1 shows a list of potential areas of concern that would highlight a registrant and their behaviour to others, including the GDC, and prompt an investigation into their fitness to practise. Examples of the types of allegations that fall into each area are given, but they must not be assumed to be exhaustive.

The second column of examples of allegations lists some of the types of poor behaviour or poor attitude that would draw attention to the registrant, or student, in the first instance. All examples given range from disappointingly unexpected and unacceptable behaviour by a so-called professional (such as having an undeclared health issue that may affect their capability to deliver a good standard of care to patients) to actual criminal activity (such as abuse, fraud, drink driving).

The crux of the matter is that the public would not expect to see these types of attitude and behaviour in a professional person. Professionals are assumed to 'set a standard' of behaviour and attitude that others should aspire to, rather than be seen to be behaving in an irresponsible fashion.

While in training, and therefore before becoming a registrant under the regulation of the GDC, students may believe that their previous poor behaviour will go unnoticed. However, several sections of the registration documentation ask for declarations of good character and good health, to be signed by other professionals, and failing to declare any relevant details at the very start of the newly qualified dental nurse's professional career would not be advisable.

General Dental Council *Standards Guidance*

The GDC has published a set of booklets that are available to all registered dental professionals, which set out the professional standards expected of every member of the dental team. As new team members train and become qualified, and are then entered onto the Register by the GDC, their own copy of the standards will be issued to them. However, all dental nurses are expected to be familiar with their content by the time of sitting their final qualifications (indeed, some examination questions will be based on their content) so students are advised to access them directly from the GDC website at www.gdc-uk.org.

The main booklet in the *Standards* series, shown in Figure 3.1, explains the six key principles of professionalism that every dental registrant should follow, and how they should be applied to their day-to-day working life. Some of these principles are then further clarified and discussed in greater detail in the accompanying GDC booklets of the series.

Table 3.1   Fitness to practise issues

Potential areas of concern	Examples of allegations
Criminal conviction or caution	Child pornography Theft Financial fraud Possession of illegal substances Child abuse Any other abuse Physical violence
Drug or alcohol misuse	Drink driving or driving under the influence of drugs Alcohol consumption affecting clinical work or environment Dealing, possessing or misusing drugs (with or without legal proceedings)
Aggressive, violent or threatening behaviour	Assault Physical violence Bullying Abuse
Persistent inappropriate attitude or behaviour	Uncommitted to work Neglect of administrative tasks Poor time management Non-attendance
Cheating or plagiarism	Cheating in exams or logbooks Passing off another's work as own Forging a supervisor's name on assessments
Dishonesty or fraud, including outside the professional role	Falsifying research Financial fraud Fraudulent CVs or other documents
Unprofessional behaviour or attitudes	Breach of confidentiality Misleading patients about their care or treatment Culpable involvement in a failure to obtain proper consent from a patient Sexual harassment Inappropriate physical examinations, or failure to keep appropriate boundaries in behaviour Persistent rudeness Unlawful discrimination
Health concerns	Failure to seek medical attention or other support Refusal to follow medical advice or care plan including monitoring/reviews Failure to recognise limits and abilities

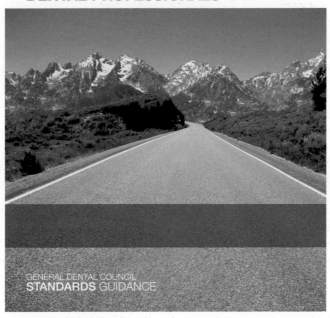

Figure 3.1   GDC Standards Guidance booklet cover. With permission from the GDC. Information correct at the time of going to press. Please visit the GDC website to check for any changes since publication: www.gdc-uk.org.

- *Principles of Patient Confidentiality*
- *Principles of Dental Team Working*
- *Principles of Patient Consent*
- *Principles of Raising Concerns*
- *Principles of Complaints Handling*

These topics are discussed in greater detail later in this chapter. The one area that is deliberately not covered by the documentation is clinical standards.

The six key principles of the over-arching booklet should be considered and followed at all stages of the registrant's education and practice, including their time leading up to registration as a dental professional. From that point on, they should be applied to every action they take as a dental professional, whether treating a patient or not. The GDC states that it is the responsibility of each dental professional to do the following.

- Be familiar with and understand:
    - current standards which affect your work
    - relevant guidelines issued by organisations other than the GDC
    - available sources of evidence that support current standards.
- Apply your up-to-date knowledge and skills ethically.

The importance of lifelong learning and participation in CPD activities becomes clear, as these are the methods used to ensure that updated information on relevant topics is made available to dental professionals. CPD is discussed later in this chapter.

The six key principles of practice in dentistry, which apply to all dental professionals, are listed below.

1. Put patients' interests first and act to protect them.
2. Respect patients' dignity and choices.
3. Protect the confidentiality of patients' information.
4. Co-operate with other team members and other healthcare colleagues in the interests of the patient.
5. Maintain your professional knowledge and competence.
6. Be trustworthy.

Depending on the level of qualification of the registrant, from dentist through all categories of dental care professionals (DCP) to trainee DCPs, the principles must be interpreted and followed accordingly – their application by a dentist will be different from that of a trainee dental nurse. Each registrant must use their own judgement to apply the principles to their daily work, and be prepared to justify their actions to the GDC if asked to do so. Failure to account for their behaviour satisfactorily is likely to result in their professional registration being at risk of suspension or even erasure.

The details and application of each key principle are further expanded in the *Standards* booklet, and the points raised are discussed below. Having a copy of the booklet to hand would be useful for this discussion. The following points are taken from Standards for Dental Professionals, © General Dental Council. Please visit the GDC website to check for any changes since publication: www.gdc-uk.org.

Put patients' interests first and act to protect them

1.1 Put patients' interests before yours, your colleagues or any organisation or business – the patients' interests can sometimes be forgotten, such as by providing unnecessary care to a patient for financial gain.

1.2 Follow the principles when handling complaints and in all other non-clinical activities – so information and accounts of events must not be altered to the benefit of the workplace or its staff, or to the detriment of the patient.

1.3 Work within your knowledge, professional competence and physical abilities – this refers to the levels of treatment that each category of registrant is enabled to carry out, in accordance with their qualification as set out in the *Preparing for Practice* document.

1.4 Make and keep accurate and complete patient records, at the time of treatment – these are then referred to as 'contemporaneous records' and should provide accurate evidence of the patient's treatment (clinical and non-clinical) in the workplace, and will form the basis of any defence required when complaints are made.

1.5 Respect the patient's right to complain – sometimes complaints are spurious, but often they are not. Responding in a helpful manner and in line with a formal complaints procedure is more likely to defuse and resolve the issue satisfactorily, rather than by being difficult and obstructive.

1.6 Make sure patients are able to claim any compensation they are entitled to – hence the need for all registrants (not just the dentist) to have professional indemnity insurance.

1.7 Take action if a patient may be put at risk – by your own health, behaviour or professional performance or that of a colleague, such as by alcoholism or drug use by a registrant. Reporting the concern to a professional body such as a defence organisation or the GDC may ultimately be necessary.

1.8 Find out about local procedures for child protection: this is discussed later in this chapter.

1.9   Never ask for, nor accept, any payment, gift or hospitality – this includes making or accepting referrals for financial gain.

1.10   Do not make any claims which could mislead patients – such as indicating that a registrant has skills beyond their qualification, or that they are the only registrant capable of providing certain treatments, for example.

Respect patients' dignity and choices

2.1   Treat patients politely and with respect – this should be self-explanatory to any professional.

2.2   Recognise and promote patients' responsibility for making decisions about their bodies – this is in reference to gaining a patient's consent for treatment, and is discussed in detail later in this chapter.

2.3   Do not discriminate against any patient on the grounds of sex, race, age, ethnicity, nationality, special needs or disability, sexuality, health, lifestyle or beliefs – to do so is illegal under equal opportunities law, and should be self-explanatory to any professional.

2.4   Ensure that your communication skills are effective so that patients can make informed decisions about their own treatment and oral health – again, this is covered later under patient consent.

2.5   Maintain appropriate boundaries in the relationships you have with patients – ideally, there should be no relationship between a staff member and a patient outside the workplace, other than a professional one.

Protect the confidentiality of patients' information

3.1   Treat all information about patients as confidential – patient confidentiality is discussed in detail later in this chapter.

3.2   Prevent unauthorised access to information, and from it being accidentally revealed – under information governance, there should be protocols and procedures in place to ensure the confidentiality of all patient information, and all team members must follow the workplace policies accordingly.

3.3   On the rare occasion that it is appropriate to release patient information without consent, do so only in accordance with the law – again, this is discussed later.

Co-operate with other team members and other healthcare colleagues in the interests of the patient

4.1   Co-operate with others and respect their role in caring for the patient – do nothing to contradict that care, unless the patient's safety is at risk.

4.2   Do not exhibit any type of discrimination against any colleague – to do so is against the law.

4.3   Communicate effectively at all times with all other team members, in the patient's best interests – this topic is discussed in detail later in this chapter.

Maintain your professional knowledge and competence

5.1   Recognise that your register-able qualification was the first stage in your professional education – it is the minimum level of competence required to become a dental care professional and must be expanded and developed throughout your career.

5.2   Continuously review your knowledge, skills and professional performance – this is the basis of reflective practice and the need for lifelong learning, and is discussed in detail later in this chapter.

5.3   Find out about current best practice in the fields in which you work – this can be achieved in many ways, especially by attending CPD events and reading relevant dental literature.

5.4   Find out about laws and regulations which affect your work, premises, equipment and business, and follow them – again, by attending relevant CPD events.

Be trustworthy

6.1   Justify the trust that your patients, the public and your colleagues have in you by always acting honestly and fairly – these characteristics should be evident not just in the workplace but in your private life too, and are self-evident to any professional.

6.2   Apply these principles to clinical and professional relationships, and any business or educational activities you are involved in – again, this should be self-evident.

6.3   Maintain appropriate standards of personal behaviour in all walks of life, so that patients and the public have confidence in you and the dental profession – so as stated previously, irresponsible and antisocial behaviour would not be expected from a dental professional, nor tolerated and accepted.

The Care Quality Commission

The Care Quality Commission (CQC) is the independent regulator of health and adult social care services in England, and since the empowerment of the Health and Social Care Act of 2008 it has been the organisation responsible for ensuring adequate standards in premises such as hospitals, nursing homes for the elderly, and care homes for such as those with a wide range of special needs.

From 1st April 2011, its powers of regulation were extended to include all providers of primary dental care services in England that carry on 'regulated activities' (in this case dentistry and oral healthcare), and all providers, whether NHS or private, have had to become registered with them from this point on.

Registration with the CQC has involved every primary dental care provider, as an individual or as an organisation, showing evidence of their compliance with new essential standards of quality and safety in all regulated activities. However, it should be noted that CQC registration is relevant in England only, and not in Scotland, Wales or Northern Ireland. Other laws and regulators are likely to perform a similar role in the future throughout the UK.

The stated aim of the CQC is to '… make sure that people get better care'. It achieves this by:

- driving improvement across health and adult social care
- putting people first and championing their rights
- acting swiftly to remedy bad practice
- gathering and using knowledge and expertise, and working with others.

In the dental workplace, the relevance of CQC registration is that all primary care providers are expected to comply fully with the essential standards of quality and safety – the vast majority found that they already did so, but that they had little or no evidence in place to prove it, while others found that they did not fully comply. In other words, a standard had been set that every dental workplace must achieve as a minimum to ensure registration. Although initially the registration process was partially a 'tick box' exercise for the workplaces, the CQC are currently inspecting those providers who are now registered to ensure that there is indeed evidence of their full compliance in all of the essential standards.

The regulations are set out in the Health and Social Care Act 2008 (Regulated Activities) Regulations 2010, and although the full content of the standards and outcomes is beyond the remit of the trainee dental nurse, further information is available for those who are interested at www.cqc.org.uk.

Areas of the essential standards of particular relevance to the trainee dental nurse are as follows.

- Those new procedures involved in infection control, such as the bagging and date stamping of all sterilised reuseable items (see Chapter 8).
- The necessity of resterilising unused bagged items within set time periods, to ensure their sterility at the time of use (see Chapter 8).
- The set-up and correct use of the decontamination area (see Chapter 8).
- The necessity of CRB checks for all staff – see later in this chapter.

Clinical governance

Clinical governance is the term used to refer to the NHS Framework for Quality Assurance that must be aspired to and followed by all those working in the delivery of NHS health and dental care. It defines the level of service quality that all NHS organisations (hospitals, clinics and practices) are expected to meet or be working towards, and those relevant specifically to dental services were set out in 2006. Although set out by the NHS and subject to compliance checks by primary care trusts (although these bodies will cease to exist from April 2013), it is good practice for private dental workplaces to follow the framework too.

The aim of the framework is not only to improve the quality of healthcare provided by standardising it, but also to make providers accountable for ensuring a consistency of care, thereby making the service they provide reliable for the patients.

As clinical governance has been around in dentistry for over 7 years now, it would be difficult to imagine that all workplaces do not already comply with its required standards, although many may not refer to it under this title. The 12 themes that are covered by the framework and examples of the key actions and policies necessary for compliance are listed in Table 3.2 and all trainee dental nurses should find equivalent examples of compliance in their own dental workplace.

The 12 themes in the first column indicate the clinical areas where the NHS expects every dental workplace to have evidence of how it ensures that the service provided is to a consistent standard for all patients. So with infection control as the example, there should be a written policy of how the workplace ensures that cross-infection does not occur – by stating the methods used for decontamination and sterilisation, that single-use disposables are used wherever possible, that staff and patients are provided with suitable personal protective equipment (PPE), and so on. All of these points should then tie in with the relevant sections of *Health Technical Memorandum 01-05* (HTM 01-05 or equivalent) (see Chapter 8) and be shown to do so, and then further evidence such as staff immunisation records are also held by the workplace as further evidence of compliance. An inoculation injury policy will demonstrate that all staff members are aware and trained to deal with this eventuality in an approved manner, by having a written policy readily accessible to all. Some workplaces may have other evidence of compliance besides those given as examples in the second column too.

Table 3.2   Clinical governance themes and compliance

Theme	Examples of key actions and policies
Infection control	Infection control policy Staff immunisation records Inoculation injury policy HTM 01-05 (or equivalent) policies
Child protection	Child protection policy Enhanced CRB checks Staff employment records Staff training records
Dental radiography	Ionising radiation policy Compliance with IRR and IR(ME)R Radiation protection file Local rules QA audits of radiographs

Safety assessment for staff, patient, public and environment	Health and Safety compliance requirements
	Risk assessments
	   Fire safety
	   COSHH
	RIDDOR compliance
	First aid and medical emergency training

Evidence-based practice and research	NICE guidelines on recall intervals Referral protocols to local hospitals
Prevention and public health	Oral cancer awareness Smoking cessation Fluoride application Dietary advice
Clinical records, patient privacy and confidentiality	Patient confidentiality Information governance Data protection Access to health records
Staff involvement and development	CPD and lifelong learning Personal development plans Staff appraisals and meetings Staff training and development Raising concerns
Clinical staff requirements and development	GDC requirements Patient consent Complaints policy Raising concerns

Table 3.2   (*Continued*)

Theme	Examples of key actions and policies
Patient information and handling, patient feedback	Handling complaints Patient information leaflets Patient surveys
Fair and accessible care	Disability access and compliance Access to emergency care
Clinical audit and peer review	Audits Record keeping

COSSH, Control of Substances Hazardous to Health; CPD, continuing professional development; CRB, Criminal Records Bureau; GDC, General Dental Council; IRR, Ionising Radiations Regulations; IR(ME)R, Ionising Radiations (Medical Exposure) Regulations; NICE, National Institute for Health and Clinical Excellence; QA, quality assurance; RIDDOR, Reporting of Injuries, Diseases and Dangerous Occurrences Regulations 1995.

Many of the examples of actions listed above are discussed in more detail later in this chapter and elsewhere in the text. None of the entries in the second column should be unfamiliar to the dental nurse.

Record keeping

The purpose of dental records is to provide an up-to-date case history of each patient's condition, and includes the examination findings and treatment given on each attendance at the surgery. By referring back to previous visits, the dentist can assess the results of earlier courses of treatment and thereby decide the best line of treatment on future occasions. Adequate records also facilitate the transfer of patients between dentists in the practice when absence or staff changes occur. When recorded correctly, another dentist should be able to determine all previous treatments for a patient and continue that care safely, without any risk of errors or omissions due to incomplete information.

In effect, the records are a communication tool which allows anyone reading them to determine what treatment was carried out, when and by whom, and how it was achieved. So the fullness and accuracy of the records are required for:

- patient safety
- evaluation of treatment
- basis for patient accounts
- monitoring of the provision of care
- probity enquiries.

Recording methods will be either manual or on computer, and the amount of detail recorded may vary considerably from practice to practice, but patients' records consist basically of personal and clinical information. They should include all of the following.

- Patient name, address, date of birth and telephone numbers.
- Doctor's details and contact information.
- Full medical history.

- Dental history.
- Contemporaneous clinical notes of each attendance (that is, written at the time or as soon as possible after, so that they are in date order).
- Tooth and periodontal chartings.
- Soft tissue assessments.
- Details of all appointments with other staff, such as the hygienist, therapist or oral health educator.
- All legally required NHS or private paperwork.
- Consent forms.
- Copies of all referral letters and response correspondence.
- Correctly identified and mounted radiographs.
- Photographs.
- Laboratory slips.
- Records of all payment transactions.
- Copies of all patient correspondence.
- Information on failed or cancelled appointments.

Where two or more patients exist with the same name or date of birth, the record should be clearly marked to alert all readers that a similar patient exists – otherwise there is a risk that one patient will receive treatment required by another.

For new patients, the personal details, reason for attendance, and medical and dental history are conveniently recorded by giving or sending a medical history form, such as the British Dental Association (BDA) Confidential Medical History Form, for home completion before their first visit. At that visit it would be assessed by the dentist, signed and dated, and placed in the patient's file. Clinical details of the visit, and subsequent ones, are entered on a dental chart and kept in the file.

A separate record of all attendances and treatment each day is kept in the daybook, or its computerised equivalent, and forms a valuable cross-reference system with the charts.

Apart from clinical records, those relating to practice administration are just as important. Such records concern the supply and purchase of equipment, materials and drugs used for treatment, batch numbers of drugs and medicaments over a set time period (so that those used on a certain date can be traced back where necessary), details of despatch and receipt of work done by dental laboratories, and staff personnel records.

Most practices use computers for dealing with the following.

- Stock records.
- Accounts.
- Patient recall systems.
- Standardised patient correspondence, such as account letters or appointment cancellation and rearrangement letters.

Importance of records

Accurate dental records are essential to ensure that patients receive necessary, appropriate and safe treatment. Poor record keeping often forms the basis of patient complaints that cannot be defended, and the dentist is ultimately responsible for their errors and omissions unless the notes were written to record treatment provided by a dental care professional. Errors or omissions in recording information may result in incorrect treatment being carried out, or failure to provide necessary treatment to maintain oral health. The dental nurse must accurately record information given by the patient or dictated by the dentist, ensuring that records are filed properly, made available at each appointment, and signed as necessary by the patient and the dentist.

Dental records are also extremely valuable as a means of establishing identity. In fatal accidents where facial features are destroyed, the teeth are often unaffected and can be compared with dentists' records to identify a victim.

Proper records allow correct treatment planning and provide a check on details of past treatment. They form the basis on which fees are calculated and accounts rendered to patients. Failed appointments and refusals of treatment are noted and the patient's attitude to oral health, as well as any risks factors to good oral health, can be assessed. Appropriate recall arrangements can then be made for each patient, in line with National Institute for Health and Clinical Excellence (NICE) guidelines.

Adequate records allow the practice to run with the greatest efficiency for all concerned, and should be retained for at least 11 years after completion of treatment, or to the age of 25 years in the case of children's records. Many difficulties concerning individual patients can be prevented altogether if complete records are available of all attendances at the practice, while no time is wasted in putting such information at the dentist's disposal. Recording and filing systems may vary considerably in different practices but whichever method is used, records must always be accurate, legible, comprehensive and easily accessible.

Clinical records

Clinical records consist of the past and present appointment and daybooks, as well as records of each patient attending the practice, and contain the information specific to the delivery of oral healthcare to that patient. They include the medical history, dental history, present oral health status (including chartings), treatment received on each date, and then the required estimate, consent and account paperwork. The relevance of each area of information to be recorded is discussed below.

Medical history

The importance of a full medical history in successful treatment planning is discussed in detail in Chapter 12, and summarised here.

Full details of any past and present illnesses, and other medical issues must be regularly updated, ideally at every recall appointment as a thorough run-through and update of the medical history form itself, which is then signed and dated as being updated at that time. A verbal confirmation of no changes at each treatment appointment is then satisfactory. The assessment of any updated entries or declarations is solely the responsibility of the dentist, although the information can be collected by the dental nurse. Medical history forms vary considerably, but the basic areas of questioning should include the following.

- Currently receiving any medical treatment – full details must then be given.
- Any history of steroid use within the last 2 years.
- Details of any current medications, including non-prescription ones – any unfamiliar drugs can be checked in the *British National Formulary*.
- Any allergies, with details.
- Any reactions to local or general anaesthetics.
- Currently pregnant or a nursing mother.
- Human immunodeficiency virus (HIV)-positive status.
- History of rheumatic fever, liver or kidney disorders.

- History of any heart or circulatory disorders.
- History of any respiratory disorders.
- History of diabetes, epilepsy or arthritis.
- Details of any medical warning cards issued, especially the use of anticoagulants.
- Smoking, tobacco and alcohol history.

In order to ensure complete confidentiality, a medical history must be taken and discussed in private where it cannot be overheard. Patients cannot be expected to provide full details unless they are satisfied about privacy. Confidentiality of patient records is discussed later in this chapter. Many conditions or drugs may influence the dental treatment plan.

- The method of pain control used may depend on the condition of the patient's heart, lungs and liver, and whether drugs are being taken for medical treatment (Chapter 14).
- If a patient has suffered from certain heart conditions it may be necessary to give antibiotic cover before extractions or subgingival scaling, as a precautionary measure against infective endocarditis and if requested in writing by the patient's cardiologist.
- Extractions may be inadvisable while a patient is being treated with certain drugs such as anti-coagulants and corticosteroids, or after irradiation treatment of the jaws.
- Special care is needed for patients with bleeding disorders such as haemophilia, and it is likely that these patients would receive dental treatment in hospital.
- Allergy to certain drugs and other products may cause a severe anaphylactic reaction (Chapter 6).
- Adverse reactions can occur because of an interaction between drugs being taken for medical treatment and drugs administered during dental treatment (Chapter 6).
- Patients may be allergic to certain dental materials, such as latex rubber, and a medical history of eczema and/or hay fever will alert the dentist to a potential risk of allergic reactions.
- Special care is necessary during pregnancy.
  - There must be no contact with staff or other patients who are rubella (German measles) contacts.
  - Local anaesthesia is safe but general anaesthesia and drugs of any other kind should be avoided, including sedatives and analgesics.
  - In the late stages of pregnancy, patients should not be treated in the supine position as they are likely to be extremely uncomfortable.
- Patients who have been in contact with infectious diseases such as mumps and rubella should not attend the surgery while these illnesses are still active.
- Careful observation of patients will detect signs which may affect treatment: breathlessness and pallor are suggestive of anaemia while cyanosis (blue complexion) and jaundice (yellowing of the skin and eyeballs) are indicative of heart and liver disease respectively.
- Special precautions are necessary for treatment of known hepatitis and HIV carriers, and for immune-compromised patients (Chapters 4 and 6).

The name of the patient's doctor should always be included in the records so that if any doubts arise, the doctor can be consulted before treatment is undertaken.

Dental history

Diagnosis of the present condition and determination of the treatment plan may depend on details of earlier dental disorders and their treatment. Knowledge of previous difficulties such as excessive bleeding, poor response to anaesthetics, difficult extractions, allergy to dental materials, latex gloves or rubber dam, or any other complications, will help the dentist to avoid their reoccurrence.

Present oral health status

The present condition of the teeth is recorded on the dental chart, and any other conditions, such as the state of existing restorations and dentures, level of oral hygiene, periodontal disease, malocclusion, tooth discolouration, etc., which may affect treatment are also noted. The dentist can then assess the patient's general attitude towards their oral health and accordingly advise the most appropriate treatment. Much of this information is conveniently set out in the Oral Health Assessment documents that are currently being piloted before NHS contracts change again in the near future, and can be used as prompts to gather the required information.

As described fully in Chapter 12, pertinent questions are asked and responses recorded about all issues that may affect the patient's oral health, especially diet, alcohol consumption and tobacco usage.

Treatment

Full details of dental treatment received and the date on which it was provided are recorded on the dental chart and in the notes. These will include the results of any special procedures carried out or events that happened, such as:

- radiographs, vitality tests, periodontal status, oral cancer check and orthodontic study models
- local anaesthesia, type of filling and lining, shades used for fillings, artificial teeth and crowns
- drugs and dosage and any prescriptions issued
- complications that occurred, for example excessive bleeding or retained roots after extractions
- treatment plans and options, cost estimates and the patient's choice of treatment
- missed appointments and refusals of treatment
- any accidents or complications, such as retained roots following extractions or breakage of an instrument, for example a root canal file, must be explained to the patient and its occurrence recorded, together with the measures and options offered, and emergency treatment arrangements.

National Health Service records

The NHS provides a large number of forms for detailing treatment plans, costs, emergency visits, orthodontic and periodontal treatment, exemption from payments and many other aspects of NHS procedure. Currently, the most commonly used forms include the following.

- A standard chart (Form FP 25) for recording patient visits, and treatment required and provided, together with a folder (Form FP 25a) to hold subsequent treatment forms and details.
- Form FP17 DC/GP17DC is given to the patient. It outlines treatment required and the NHS charges, as well as the details and costs of any agreed private treatment.
- The Dental Estimates Form FP17 is used by practitioners to record details of treatment required, and subsequently given, and provides a form of account for payment claimed.
- Form FP10D, for prescriptions.

With the expected introduction of the new NHS contract over the next few years, these details may well change.

Many practices are now partially or fully computerised with regard to patient records, but all the information held must be accessible to the dental team, the authorities and the patient, as necessary. Several software systems are available and the NHS records detailed above are compatible with many of them. Whichever system is used, and whether manual or computerised, the records must be written, handled and stored in full accordance with all relevant legislation. A good knowledge of the use of computers and information technology is required by, and expected of, the modern dental nurse.

Confidentiality of patient records

All members of the dental team have both an ethical and a legal duty to keep patient information gained in the course of their professional relationship confidential, and not to release it to others without the patient's permission, or in accordance with strict protocols if they do so without their permission.

As with the setting of minimum standards in clinical issues within the NHS under clinical governance requirements, a similar quality assurance process has been introduced in relation to record keeping and maintenance of record confidentiality. This is referred to as information governance and is discussed later.

The specific legislation that applies to issues of patient health information and confidentiality is as follows.

- Data Protection Act 1998
- Access to Health Records Act 1990
- Freedom of Information Act (passed in 1995 and came into effect in 2000)

The Data Protection Act aims to protect the confidentiality of sensitive personal data (including the personal health information held by the dental workplace) by placing obligations on the data controller (the dentist or organisation responsible for the data) only to make third party disclosures under the conditions of the Act, and to otherwise keep the data secure.

Data may be legally shared with certain organisations such as the Business Services Authority, the dental department of the local hospital or the salaried community dental services, but only on a 'need-to-know' basis. It must also only be shared in order to provide the patient with appropriate care and treatment, and for the provision of general health services.

The data must be kept for no longer than is necessary, and although NHS regulations require dental records to be retained for only 2 years (6 years in Northern Ireland), medico-legally they should be held for 11 years or to the age of 25 with child patients, whichever is the longer.

When in the dental workplace, all dental staff must adhere to the workplace confidentiality policy, but inadvertent breaches involving patients' health information can all too easily occur if common sense is lacking too. Examples of ways to avoid these non-deliberate breaches include the following.

- Patients must not be discussed in front of other patients – even when names are not used, some unusual or unique circumstance may make it possible to deduce a patient's identity, so such conversations must never take place in the hearing of others.
- Privacy must be maintained when discussing any personal matters with patients – this may involve taking them away from the reception area if other patients are around and using another room for private discussions.
- Attendance at the practice is private, and cannot be revealed to other patients, to employers, nor to schools, so phone calls asking for confirmation of a patient's attendance by an employer or a school must not be responded to by the staff. An appointment card may be issued to the patient to confirm the details instead.

- All written communications with patients should be sent in sealed envelopes – this includes examination reminders that traditionally were sent on postcards, as they reveal the confidential fact that the patient attends a certain practice.
- Dental records must be kept for the correct length of time by the practice and not be destroyed beforehand, either partially or wholly.

Disclosure without patient consent

Under normal circumstances, information about a patient can only be disclosed to a third party with the patient's written consent. However, there are some circumstances under which the dentist has a statutory obligation to disclose the necessary information, or has a legal right to do so.

- To assist in the identification of a driver or passenger(s) involved in a road traffic accident where facial trauma prevents identification otherwise – disclosure is allowed under the Road Traffic Act 1988.
- When requested to do so by the Dental Practice Division of the Business Services Authority (formerly known as the Dental Practice Board) – this is when an audit of patient records is to be carried out, rather than when a course of treatment is under way.
- To provide information about a child to their parent or legal guardian – although issues of age of consent to disclosure must also be considered (see later).
- When it is in the public's interest, such as with suspected or known criminals.
- When disclosure is requested by Court Order, under the Prevention of Terrorism Act 1989 or under the Police and Criminal Evidence Act 1984.
- When disclosure is necessary to a solicitor or debt collecting agency, to enable them to pursue a legal claim against the patient on behalf of the dentist.

Access to health records

Patients also have the right of access to their own manual or computerised health records, under the Access to Health Records Act 1990 and the Data Protection Act 1998. This covers all their medical and dental records written since November 1991, with the following provisos.

- Only the dentist, as the record holder, can approve access.
- The patient request must be made in writing, and there may be a fee to cover administration costs (usually around £10).
- The dentist must respond within 40 days of the fee payment.
- The patient identity must be checked before releasing their records, and records must be released to the patient only or their legal representative.
- Once viewed, the patient can request that any inaccuracies in their records are amended.
- Any dental terminology, abbreviations or jargon must be explained on request.

The dental nurse must therefore not release any records or parts of records themselves, nor alter them in any way before they are to be released. They must be true, accurate and contemporaneous (as written at the time), and contain no derogatory comments. If the dental nurse is responsible for writing the notes, they should be written exactly as dictated by the dentist and not altered in any way. However, it is the responsibility of the dentist to check that they have been recorded accurately.

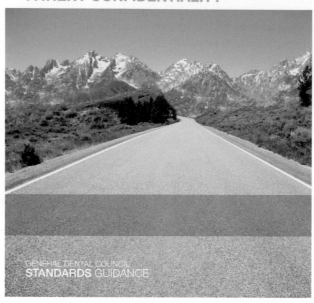

PRINCIPLES OF
PATIENT CONFIDENTIALITY

GENERAL DENTAL COUNCIL
STANDARDS GUIDANCE

Figure 3.2   GDC Standards – patient confidentiality. With permission from the GDC. Information correct at the time of going to press. Please visit the GDC website to check for any changes since publication: www.gdc-uk.org.

There are certain instances when the dentist can refuse to disclose the patient records to the patient.

- When disclosure would cause serious harm to the patient.
- When a second person is mentioned by name and has not given consent for disclosure (does not include the dental team).
- When access to their records after their death has specifically been refused by the patient beforehand.

The Freedom of Information Act excludes health records as a source of information that can be made available to a person on request, as other government-held information is subject to. The Access to Health Records Act allows the patient themselves or their legal representative to gain access to them, while preventing third parties from doing so.

General Dental Council Standards Guidance on confidentiality

One of the six key principles of the GDC *Standards Guidance* document states that dental professionals must 'protect patient confidentiality', and a separate booklet covering this topic is also available (Figure 3.2). In essence, its content reiterates all of the guidance and information given above, under the following four headings.

- Duty of confidentiality.
- Releasing information with the patient's consent.
- Preventing information being released accidentally.
- Releasing information in the 'public interest'.

The booklet gives additional information on protecting patient confidentiality from the perspective of the dental professional, and advises that further help and advice may be available from dental defence organisations when the action to take is not straightforward, and that it should be sought whenever necessary. In addition, it advises that the dental professional must always be prepared to explain and justify their decision in relation to releasing patient information, especially when doing so without the patient's consent.

Information governance

This is a quality assurance system that has been implemented to ensure the safety and appropriate use of personal and patient information. It brings together all the legal rules, guidance and information on best practice that apply to the handling of information. Compliance with information governance (IG) requirements by organisations should then show that they can be trusted to maintain the confidentiality and security of personal information.

For healthcare organisations, including dental workplaces providing NHS care for their patients, the Department of Health has developed a set of information governance requirements in the form of a toolkit, which enables NHS organisations to measure the level of their own compliance. These requirements cover the following areas.

- Data protection and confidentiality.
- Information security.
- Information quality.
- Health records management.
- Corporate information (where relevant).

The main points are that every NHS workplace must have a named IG lead person, who takes responsibility for:

- registering the workplace on the IG toolkit website
- accessing the toolkit requirements and completing them on behalf of the workplace's current sytems of data security and maintenance
- using the underpinning procedures and processes of the toolkit to develop the IG policy for the workplace
- ensuring that all other staff are aware of the organisation's approach to IG, and where further information can be found, including the IG policy itself – this should be a hard copy file kept securely on the premises, but accessible to all staff
- aiming for best practice by reviewing the policy and compliance with the requirements of the toolkit annually, and updating it as necessary. Where amendments have been made during this review process, they must be signed off by a senior person in the organisation
- confirming the named person at the primary care trust who acts as the Caldicott Guardian for the workplace – this is a person with specialist knowledge in the area of confidentiality and information governance issues, who can give help, support and advice to the workplace in matters of patient protection and confidentiality.

Templates are available from www.igte-learning.connectingforhealth.nhs.uk. to use as the basis of the organisation's IG document, or they can develop their own.

The IG policy must contain the following information.

- Why the policy is required – this may be stated as 'to ensure patient and data confidentiality, and the safe handling of sensitive information'.

- Give an overview of how information should be handled in the workplace, including:
  - storage of data
  - consent to view data
  - maintenance of patient confidentiality
  - situations where information disclosure may be required.
- Give a description of the accountability and responsibility for the policy:
  - name of the IG lead
  - job roles of support staff.
- State the process of policy monitoring.
- State the staff duties and their responsibilities in relation to IG.
- Describe how areas of the policy link together.
- Actions to take if the policy is breached:
  - sanctions against staff involved
  - remedial work for those responsible for IG procedures, to avoid future breaches.

Further information is available at www.igte-learning.connectingforhealth.nhs.uk.

Consent to treatment

The law concerning issues of consent to treatment is complicated and subject to change, so just a simplified overview of the topic and the issues it raises in relation to dental professionals and their working lives is given here. Further detailed information is available from the various dental defence organisations, and from the British Dental Association.

   The main points to be clarified here are as follows.

- What is consent?
- The key definitions of consent.
- Who can give consent?
- GDC *Standards Guidance* on patient consent.

Consent is effectively the patient, or their legal guardian, giving permission to the dental professional for treatment or physical investigation to be carried out. It is a legal and ethical principle that consent must be first given, and reflects the right of patients to decide what happens to their own bodies. It cannot be assumed that their attendance at the workplace is a signal for any type of 'hands-on' treatment to be carried out; indeed, without gaining consent to do so first before touching the patient is actually assault. The GDC would consider this occurrence as serious professional misconduct, and may suspend or erase the dental professional from the Register.

   To gain consent to proceed with a dental procedure, three key principles must be addressed.

- **Informed** – the patient must be given enough information to be able to make a decision, and in issues of treatment options this must include a host of information, as discussed below.
- **Voluntary decision** – the patient alone must make the decision to proceed, without coercion or threat.
- **Ability** – the patient must have the ability to make an informed decision.

These principles form the basis of the guidance issued by the GDC, and they are discussed in more detail later.

Key definitions

Legally, there are various definitions used depending on the type of consent required, and the three of relevance in this text are as follows.

- **Informed consent** – the patient must be given full information about the treatment offered to be able to make an informed decision as to whether they wish to proceed or not.
  - ○ The nature of the treatment (e.g. filling, crown, extraction).
  - ○ The purpose of the treatment (e.g. restore function, alleviate pain, remove infection source).
  - ○ The risks of the treatment (e.g. what can go wrong, what further treatment may be required).
  - ○ The consequences of not having the treatment (e.g. effect on oral health, effect on general health).
  - ○ The risks and benefits of any alternative treatment available.
  - ○ The longevity of success (will further treatment be required in weeks or months, or not for years if at all?).
  - ○ The cost of the treatment, whether NHS or private.
- The information must be given in a way that the patient understands, and this may involve the use of visual aids, an interpreter or sign language.
- The patient must have all their questions answered in a way that is understandable, without the use of dental terminology if it is not appropriate (communication skills are discussed in detail in Chapter 13).
- **Specific consent** – this is the consent gained expressly for each stage of the treatment, and not just consent assumed to be for a full course of treatment without the patient being aware of what is involved at each stage. For example, a symptomatic fractured tooth is to be restored initially with a filling, but it may require endodontic treatment too, and then restoration with a crown within 6 months, and the patient must give specific consent for each stage before it is carried out.
- **Valid consent** – for consent to be considered valid, it must be:
  - ○ informed
  - ○ specific
  - ○ given by the patient or their parent or guardian (if too young to give informed consent).

Consent does not have to be given in writing, especially for minimal and non-invasive procedures, but for more complicated treatment plans and for treatment provided under conscious sedation, a signed consent form is appropriate. Oral consent is adequate otherwise.

Although dental staff can be very helpful in assisting discussions to help the patient make a decision about whether they wish to proceed with treatment or not, it is the responsibility of the dentist alone to obtain that consent from the patient. It is not the duty of the dental nurse or any other DCP to do so. Where a patient is receiving treatment from a hygienist or other therapist that has been prescribed by the dentist, the dentist must first obtain the consent and then the DCP must check with the patient that they are still happy to proceed, before starting the treatment.

Who can give consent?

For consent to be valid, it must be both informed and specific. However, for consent to be informed, the patient must:

- be able to understand what is wrong
- be able to understand that it requires treatment to make it right

- be able to understand the consequences of both undergoing or declining the treatment
- be able to communicate their decision (not necessarily by speech).

Under these circumstances, it is perfectly feasible for some children under the age of 16 to be able to give informed consent for their own treatment. This is called 'Gillick competence' and is accepted by law as the right of the child to make the decision to proceed with treatment, which cannot be overruled by the parent or guardian. A child under 16 may also be perfectly capable of refusing to undergo treatment in contradiction to the wishes of their parent or guardian, but this can be overruled by the parent.

Similarly, a child under the age of 16 who is judged by the dentist to be mature and intelligent enough to understand the situation, and competent to make their own decisions, can also refuse the disclosure of their health records to their parent or guardian.

Children over the age of 16 and of sound mind can legally consent to undergo any treatment and cannot be overruled by their parent or guardian, but theoretically they can be overruled if they refuse treatment. However, in view of the complexity of the legal issues involved, the dentist would be advised to make an application to court for a decision in these cases. Alternatively, where a parent or guardian refuses treatment that is in the child's best interests, a court can be asked to make an order for the treatment to be carried out anyway, and lawfully.

In Scotland, the Age of Legal Capacity (Scotland) Act 1991 is quite specific and provides that a person under 16 who, in the dentist's opinion, is capable of understanding the nature and possible consequences of the procedure or treatment shall have legal capacity to consent on his or her own behalf to any dental procedure or treatment. In Northern Ireland the age of consent for medical and dental treatment is 16 years anyway.

Once a person reaches the age of 18 years and also has the capacity to reach decisions on their own behalf, they are judged to be a competent adult and can give or withhold consent. 'Capacity' in this context means the patient has the ability to:

- be able to understand, believe and retain the information provided about treatment
- consider the information appropriately in order to choose whether or not to proceed.

No-one else is able to consent to treatment on behalf of a competent adult, and all adults must be assumed to be competent and able to make their own decisions unless they demonstrate otherwise. Indeed, this does happen and there are some adult patients who may not have the capacity to give informed consent – these patients are referred to as 'incompetent adults'. Incompetent adults are those who, for reasons of mental incapacity or illness, cannot give informed consent to treatment because they do not have the capacity to reach an informed decision on their own behalf. However, not all mentally ill or incapacitated patients are incompetent, and the dentist has to assess the patient at that time and determine the validity of any consent that the patient has given. Sometimes the opinion of a second professional is required to determine the validity.

Whatever the decision, the dentist carrying out the treatment must always act in the best interests of the patient, and they must be able to justify their actions if necessary. Further information should be sought by viewing the provisions available under the Mental Capacity Act 2005.

In summary, then, those who can give consent are:

- parent or guardian of a child to the age of 16
- 'Gillick-competent' child to the age of 16 in England and Wales
- Scottish equivalent
- 16–18 year old of sound mind, in England and Wales
- 16 year old in Scotland and Northern Ireland

- competent adult
- dentist on behalf of an incompetent adult, when in the patient's best interest and with an agreeing second opinion from another professional.

GDC *Standards Guidance* on patient consent

One of the six key principles of the GDC *Standards Guidance* document states that dental professionals must 'respect patients' dignity and choices', and a separate booklet covering this topic is also available (Figure 3.3).

The guidance says that all dental professionals must treat patients politely and with respect, in recognition of their dignity and rights as individuals. So, the dental professional must not ignore the patient's wishes when offering or undertaking to provide dental treatment – they must not be overbearing or bombastic in their manner, with a 'doctor knows best' attitude towards the patient when they do not wish to take the advice on offer. It is particularly frustrating for the dental professional when the patient does not wish to follow their advice, especially when the known result otherwise will be damaging to their oral health, but it is the patient's right to refuse treatment and the team must accept that. They must also continue to support the patient to maintain their oral and general health in the meantime, and to the best of their abilities.

The guidance also says that the team must recognise and promote patients' responsibilities for making decisions about their bodies, their priorities and their care, and do nothing without their consent. In essence, its content reiterates all the guidance and information given above, and does so under the following three headings.

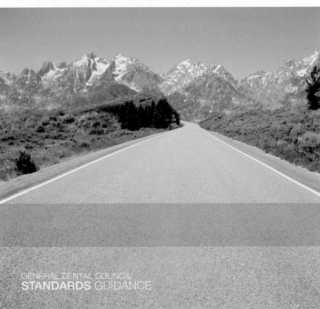

Figure 3.3   GDC Standards – patient consent. With permission from the GDC. Information correct at the time of going to press. Please visit the GDC website to check for any changes since publication: www.gdc-uk.org.

- Informed consent.
- Voluntary decision making.
- Ability to give consent.

The guidance specifically says that it does not attempt to give any legal advice, and that the dental professional must seek this advice from other sources, such as a dental defence organisation. Finally, the guidance reminds all dental professionals that it is their own personal responsibility to stay up to date with all the laws and regulations which affect their work, in this case with regard to the issue of consent.

Protection of children and vulnerable adults

Very few dental professionals will not come into contact with child patients on an almost daily basis, and this puts them in an almost unique position of being able to observe this group of patients and help prevent their abuse, or to suspect it and report their suspicions accordingly. On a lesser scale, many dental professionals will come into contact with vulnerable adults too, either in a hospital or special needs environment, and this group is at risk from the same types of abuse as children.

The CQC regulations require all dental workplaces in England to have systems in place for safeguarding children and vulnerable adults while on the premises, and to have knowledge of how to access local arrangements for child protection services. Further details of the requirements are available at www.cqc.org.uk.

No member of the dental team would be expected to make a diagnosis of abuse, but all would be expected to recognise potential causes for concern, document them, discuss their concerns with an appropriate senior colleague, and report them appropriately, when necessary. A very useful quick reference guide produced by NICE (Figure 3.4) is also available to download from www.nice.org.uk, and this gives further details on possible child maltreatment indicators and actions to take.

Types of abuse

There are four broad categories of abuse, and the possible indicators or areas of concern that should alert the dental team are discussed for each.

- Neglect
- Physical abuse
- Emotional abuse
- Sexual abuse

Neglect is the persistent failure to meet the child or vulnerable adult's basic physical and/or psychological needs – adequate food, clothing, shelter, supervision, medical and dental treatment, emotional support, and so on. Lack of any of these needs over a period of time is likely to result in the serious impairment of the victim's health, development or well-being.

Signs to look out for include the following.

- Failure to comply with dental professional advice that is in the best interest of the child or vulnerable adult.
- Malnourishment.

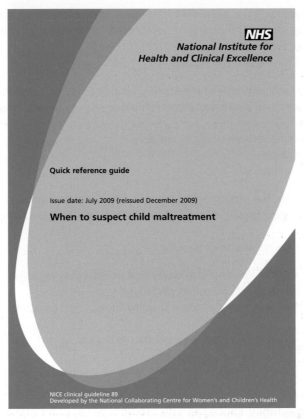

Figure 3.4   NICE reference guide. © National Institute for Clinical Excellence. Reproduced from http://www.nice.org.uk/nicemedia/pdf/CG89QuickRefGuide.pdf.

- Inappropriate clothing, especially in the winter.
- Persistently dirty, uncared for appearance (e.g. grubby skin, dirty hair, head lice, dirty or damaged clothing).
- Untreated illness, including severe dental caries involving several teeth.
- Difficult behaviour (e.g. attention seeking, distractive or withdrawn).

Physical abuse involves anything that causes physical harm to the victim – hitting, shaking, scalding, burning, biting; also the fabrication of symptoms or deliberately causing illness in the victim – forcing dangerous levels of salt intake on the victim to produce coma, for example.

Some children really are just accident prone but accidental injuries tend to occur on one side of the body and affect bony prominences such as the nose, chin, elbow, foot, etc. Some vulnerable adults may also be prone to frequent injury by having a physical disability, or by having no concept of danger due to a mental incapacity. Accidental injury must always be considered first.

Signs to look out for include the following.

- Orofacial trauma (e.g. the cheeks, intraoral soft tissues, the ears).
- Bilateral injuries (e.g. two black eyes, rather than one).
- Bite marks (these may be more obvious to dental professionals than others).
- Soft tissue injuries to the neck (e.g. scratches, bruises, cuts).
- Flinching away from sudden movements or noises (fearful).

Emotional abuse involves the persistent emotional maltreatment of the victim, causing severe and adverse effects on their emotional development – bullying, made to feel worthless, useless, unloved, unwanted, for example.

Signs to look out for include the following.

- Inability to cope with normal life events (e.g. unable to make decisions or being antisocial).
- Becoming agitated and distressed when left alone (e.g. especially by a parent or other known adult).
- Self-harm (e.g. cutting themselves, bulimia).
- Drug or alcohol abuse.
- Educational problems.

Sexual abuse involves the victim being forced or enticed to take part in sexual activities of a physical nature, or being forced or enticed to watch sexual acts or take part in producing pornographic material.

Signs to look out for include the following.

- Physical trauma to the lips and oral cavity that is not easily explained (e.g. soft or hard tissue trauma from having objects forced intraorally).
- Evidence of lesions that may indicate a sexually transmitted disease (e.g. ulceration and vesicle formation).
- Inappropriate sexual knowledge, beyond that expected for the age of the victim (e.g. use of sexual words or innuendos).
- Pregnancy in a child or vulnerable adult who is institutionalised and unlikely to be in a relationship.

Vulnerable adults are those who need community care services because they have a mental or other disability, or are old and/or infirm or suffering from an illness that prevents them from adequately taking care of themselves. They include those who are unable to protect themselves against significant harm or exploitation, including by financial methods, such as unwitting elderly victims being conned out of their life savings by fraudsters.

Practical steps

In all cases the dental professional must be prepared to make a judgement decision on whether to pass on their concerns and involve others or not. However, if a tragedy occurs that could have been prevented by a team member's intervention, difficult questions will be asked by their dental defence organisation, by the GDC and possibly by the police. The patient is always the most important person in any potential case of abuse, and as with all other situations, the dental professional has a duty of care to that patient and must put their interests first at all times.

The process to be followed may vary on a local level, but should follow a cascade of seriousness as indicated below.

- Document the concerns as soon as they are noticed, including any injuries present.
- Enable another team member to witness any injuries too, but without alarming the patient or their parent or guardian.
- Discuss the matter with a senior professional colleague in the practice (there should be a nominated child protection lead, for example).

- The senior colleague may decide to contact any of the following local colleagues for advice, especially if considering reporting the matter:
  - dental defence organisation
  - hospital consultant
  - dental advisor
  - consultant in dental public health
  - child protection lead at the primary care trust.
- Where abuse of a child is likely, the Local Safeguarding Children Board (LSCB) will be contacted, as well as the police.
- Where abuse of a vulnerable adult is likely, the Local Safeguarding Adult Board (LSAB)will be contacted instead, as well as the police.
- Where there is serious physical injury present, the victim should be referred to Accident and Emergency, and both social services and the police should be notified, especially if the parent or guardian refuses to consent to medical care.

Criminal records checks

It is now a requirement for all dental team members who have any contact with children or vulnerable adults to undergo an enhanced criminal records check, if they wish to work in the dental care professions. This is a requirement of both the CQC and NHS primary care trusts when recruits apply to work in a dental workplace, and has been carried out retrospectively on those who already work in the dental sector. Other independent 'umbrella' organisations may also be authorised by the CRB to carry out the same checks on those working, or applying to work, in private dental workplaces. Therefore, it is not possible for any dental professional to work without being sufficiently checked and scrutinised first.

The checks are carried out by the CRB in England and Wales, and enhanced checks will disclose convictions, police cautions and information on previous police investigations where a conviction or caution was not issued. The checks carried out by the CRB are particularly thorough in that they consider every adult patient to be vulnerable whilst undergoing dental treatment, and therefore no-one is exempt from their scrutiny – dental professionals who have no access to child or vulnerable adult patients are still subject to the same enhanced checks as their colleagues in other workplaces.

In Scotland, similar criminal records checks are carried out by Disclosures Scotland, and in Northern Ireland they are carried out by Access Northern Ireland.

The existence of a criminal conviction or caution does not itself prevent anyone from working in the dental professions, and each case must be judged on its merits. An example that would not be considered very relevant is having a conviction for having no car insurance – whilst not ideal for a professional to have this against them, it has no bearing on their suitability to work safely in the dental workplace.

Further information is available at:

- England and Wales: www.crb.homeoffice.gov.uk
- Scotland: www.disclosurescotland.co.uk
- Northern Ireland: www.accessni.gov.uk.

Complaints handling

All dental workplaces undertaking NHS dental treatment for their patients must handle complaints about NHS care according to a formal procedure that complies with the regulations. Also, dental professionals offering both NHS and/or private treatment must comply with the GDC's guidance on complaints handling. The GDC booklet *Principles of Complaints Handling* is discussed at the end of this section.

A complaint is any expression of dissatisfaction by a patient about a service or treatment, whether it is justified or not, so a complaint often results from the patient feeling that their expectations have not been met. Complaints can be about any part of the service the workplace provides, and many may not be about the technical skill of the dentist or the quality of care that the patient has received. When the patient feels that their expectations of a good level of service have not been met, more often than not it is merely due to a lack of communication. Good communication skills are discussed in detail in Chapter 13.

There have been changes to the legislation concerned with handling NHS complaints over the last few years, and unfortunately there are now slight differences between what is required in each of the four countries of the UK. A general overview of what is required from an 'in-house' complaints procedure is therefore given here, and is relevant to the level of knowledge required for dental nurses. Further information in greater detail can also be requested from the following sources, if required.

- **England** – Local Authority Social Services and National Health Service Complaints (England) Regulations 2009
- **Wales** – *Complaints in the NHS – A Guide to Handling Complaints in Wales 2003*
- **Scotland** – Directions to Health Boards, Special Health Boards and the Agency on Complaints Procedures 2005
- **Northern Ireland** – Health and Social Care Complaints Procedure Directions 2009

'In-house' complaints procedure

The GDC requires all dental practices (NHS and private) to have an 'in-house' patient complaint handling procedure, which should aim to fully resolve any complaint received to everyone's satisfaction and as quickly as possible. Ideally, the matter should be resolved without the need for other authorities, such as the primary care trust (or their replacement body after April 2013) or the GDC, becoming involved.

The procedure should include the points listed in Table 3.3.

The GDC require a procedure to be in place so that every complaint is handled in a similar fashion, rather than in an *ad hoc* manner. This is the same whether the complaint appears initially to be spurious in nature, or is unfounded and no action is required, or becomes a serious matter that is referred to the PCT or the GDC; until the complaint has been investigated, no-one knows what the end result will be. It is therefore very important that a system is in place to be followed in the same way each time, so that no information is lost and requirements such as acceptable timelines are adhered to. If the complaint is taken further by the patient after going through the in-house procedure, evidence of a suitable complaints procedure being rigorously followed by the workplace will show that the situation has been taken seriously, and has been fully and correctly investigated. This avoids the workplace being left open to criticism for its handling of the situation. The written records of the investigation procedure should be kept in a 'complaints file' rather than in the patient's records, although a reference to them in the patient records is acceptable.

Any patient complaint, if not spurious in nature, can be used by the dental team as an opportunity to review and change workplace procedures if necessary, with the aim of improving the standard of service being offered to patients.

Table 3.3 Complaints procedure

Procedure point	Action and necessity
Responsibility	A 'responsible person' must be delegated within the workplace who ensures that the complaints procedure is followed correctly – this should be a senior dentist. A complaints manager should also be delegated to receive any complaints on a day-to-day basis – this can be a dental care professional who liaises with the responsible person, or both roles can be carried out by the same person
Acknowledgement	Receipt of a complaint should be acknowledged within a few working days, and the complainant must then be kept informed of how the complaint will be dealt with, who will be involved, and the expected timescale
Investigation	Obviously a thorough investigation must be carried out, and the essential point to consider is 'what is the complaint about?'. Gathering this information may involve a meeting with the complainant to discuss the details, a meeting with those staff involved, and reading all relevant patient records A resolution meeting with the complainant and the relevant member of staff present together may be very useful, and with someone else present to take notes. Notes from the meeting should then be confirmed with all concerned afterwards
Timescale	The whole procedure should be completed promptly, and if delays occur due to the involvement of a defence organisation, the complainant should be kept informed of any likely extensions to the timescale

Report	A written report should be sent by recorded delivery to the complainant when the investigation is complete. It should contain the following information.
	• How the complaint was considered
	• Conclusions reached:
	  • no basis for the complaint
	  • no blame attributable, but explain what happened and why (for example, regulations prevented a different course of action)
	  • blame attributable, explain what happened and apologise, indicate measures taken to prevent a recurrence, offer reasonable redress (for example, re-do treatment for free). Make it clear that the offer of redress is not an admission of liability but a goodwill gesture only

Appeal	If the complainant is not satisfied, information should be given about the bodies to which a formal complaint can be made • Primary care trust, or future NHS commissioning body after April 2013 • Health Service Ombudsman for NHS patients • Dental Complaints Service for private patients
Records	Full written details of the procedure followed must be kept, from the point at which the complaint was made onwards. These records should be kept in a secure central complaints file, and not in the patient's records. Make a note in the patient's records that a complaint was received on a certain date. As always, the records must be contemporaneous, legible, accurate and remain unaltered in any way. Complaint reports must be submitted to the commissioning body on an annual basis in England, Wales and Scotland, and quarterly in Northern Ireland

Even if the workplace does not receive any complaints or negative comments, it is a good idea to encourage patients to comment on the care and service they have received, using a patient survey or feedback process. The professional relationship desired, with patients as customers, requires that complaints are answered satisfactorily so that the matter can be put right, and the information provided is used to improve the service and therefore the patient's future dental experience.

Good communication skills and an open, honest approach are important when dealing with a complaint, and a sympathetic and understanding manner will often diffuse what could be a tense situation. All complaints should be resolved at the earliest opportunity, and often all that is required by the patient is an apology. This can be given without fear of admitting liability or negligence.

General Dental Council *Standards Guidance* on complaints handling

One of the six key principles of the GDC *Standards Guidance* document states that dental professionals must 'put patients' interests first and act to protect them', and a separate booklet covering one aspect of this principle is also available (Figure 3.5). The guidance says that all dental professionals must give a timely and helpful response to a patient when they make a complaint, and that the right of the patient to complain must be respected. The team member must follow the complaints procedure of their workplace and co-operate fully with any formal inquiry into the treatment of the patient.

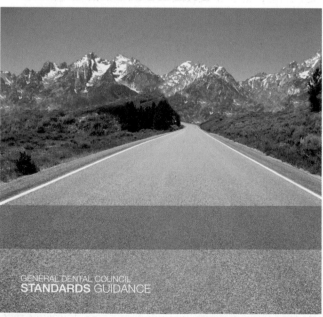

Figure 3.5   GDC Standards – complaints handling. With permission from the GDC. Information correct at the time of going to press. Please visit the GDC website to check for any changes since publication: www.gdc-uk.org.

The guidance provides a checklist to follow when a complaint has been received, and reiterates all of the guidance and information given above, under the following headings.

- Respect the patient's right to complain.
- Checklist to cover the following points:
  - that a complaints procedure is in place, and is suitable for purpose
  - that it follows certain regulatory requirements.
- The framework in place identifies who to contact when making a complaint, and that all team members are familiar with the complaints procedure.
- The process to be followed when handling a complaint.
- How to deal with the complaint correctly.
- Learning from the complaint.

It then summarises the main content of the booklet with seven 'punchy' statements, the three most pertinent of which are:

- do not make the complaints procedure unnecessarily complicated
- be polite and show consideration for the complainant at all times
- apologise that something has gone wrong.

Raising concerns

Throughout any team member's working life, a certain standard of behavior and competence is expected at all times from all dental professionals, by both the public and the regulators of the profession. Sometimes, it may become apparent to a team member that the actions of another are putting patients or other team members at risk – for example, if correct infection control measures are not being carried out or if the team member has an alcohol addiction. In these situations, all GDC registrants have a duty to 'raise concerns' over the matter, and the GDC has published the guidance booklet *Principles of Raising Concerns* which is discussed at the end of this section.

A dental professional's duty to raise a concern overrides any personal and professional loyalty to the colleague causing the concern, even if it is an employer. The concern the team member has should be acted upon as soon as possible, whether or not there is an immediate risk to patients. Raising a concern is not the same as making a complaint about the individual. A complaint may require the complainant to prove their case whereas raising a concern does not require proof of malpractice – the concern is being raised so that others can deal with it, as necessary.

Raising concerns does not always result from issues of underperformance, but may instead involve the health or behaviour of another team member or even yourself. Underperformance is usually defined as performance that puts patients at risk, fails to meet accepted and required standards, and/or is outside what is considered as normal practice. This therefore includes any issues where a dental professional works outside the limits of their qualification or competence.

Sources of help and advice

There may be instances when it is not clear whether or not to raise concerns, for fear of causing problems for a colleague unnecessarily or being considered a 'troublemaker' by others. This may be especially so for junior team members such as trainee dental nurses. At these times, various possible sources of help should be sought.

- Another colleague, especially a senior one.
- Employer.
- Professional association.
- Dental defence organisation.
- Health and Safety Executive.
- Healthcare Commission.
- Public Concern at Work.

Public Concern at Work is an independent authority that deals with whistle-blowing issues that are in the public interest, promoting compliance with the law and good practice in organisations across all sectors, not just healthcare. The authority focuses on the responsibility of workers to raise concerns about malpractice and on the accountability of those in charge to investigate and remedy such issues. It offers free advice to people concerned about danger or malpractice in the workplace but who are unsure of whether or how to raise the concern. Further details are available at www.pcaw.co.uk.

Otherwise, there are two stages for raising concerns, locally and then centrally. If a dental professional is concerned by the behaviour, health or professional performance of a colleague that does not pose an immediate risk to public safety, then they should try to deal with the issue locally by talking to their colleague directly and trying to persuade them to seek appropriate help. If this advice is ignored, they should then raise the matter with the appropriate local authority.

- Their mutual employer.
- The designated person within the local primary care organisation, if self-employed.
- The employing authority, if in a salaried position.

If the case appears to be serious or a local referral has been made and no action has been taken, the GDC should be contacted. Dentists have a responsibility to ensure that people they employ or manage are encouraged to raise concerns and are protected if they do so.

General Dental Council *Standards Guidance* on raising concerns

One of the six key principles of the GDC *Standards Guidance* document states that dental professionals must 'put patients' interests first and act to protect them', and a separate booklet covering one aspect of this principle is also available (Figure 3.6). The guidance gives advice and help on raising concerns when patients may be at risk, and gives useful information on the support that is available to dental professionals when doing so. It is set out in four sections covering the following topics.

- Your own health, behaviour or professional performance.
- The health, behaviour or professional performance of others.
- When to involve the GDC, and when to take action locally.
- Protection for people who raise concerns.

The fifth and final section summarises the content of the other four.

The first three sections expand on the information given previously, and the advice given on when to involve the GDC is particularly pertinent. The guidance says that the regulator should be referred to for advice under the following circumstances.

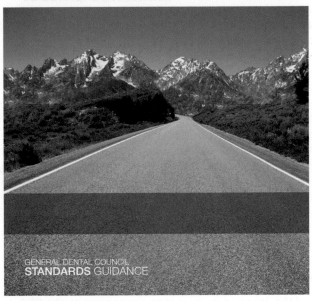

PRINCIPLES OF
RAISING CONCERNS

GENERAL DENTAL COUNCIL
STANDARDS GUIDANCE

Figure 3.6   GDC Standards – raising concerns With permission from the GDC. Information correct at the time of going to press. Please visit the GDC website to check for any changes since publication: www.gdc-uk.org.

- When taking local action would not be practical.
- When action at a local level has failed to resolve the issue.
- When the problem is of a serious nature:
  - issues of indecency
  - issues of violent behaviour
  - issues of dishonesty or fraud
  - when a serious crime may be, or has been, committed
  - when illegal practice has occurred.
- When there is a genuine fear of victimisation or a cover-up may occur.

The GDC booklet gives useful information on the issue of protection for people who raise concerns, as in the past 'whistle-blowers', the lay expression often used to refer to people who raise concerns, often were sacked from their employment after being identified as the source of leaks of disturbing information. To encourage people to continue to raise concerns without fear of retribution from their employers, the Public Interest Disclosure Act 1998 (PIDA) was passed which gives protection to employees who raise concerns about potentially dangerous or illegal practices in the workplace. The PIDA offers protection to all employed dental professionals (NHS or private) as well as to self-employed dental professionals working under NHS contracts. The Act applies more widely to employees in any workplace, not just to the health-care sector.

To ensure that disgruntled employees do not use protection under the Act as a means of causing problems for their employers by making spurious or groundless accusations, protection under the PIDA only applies under the following circumstances.

- When the whistle-blower is acting in good faith (not being malicious).
- When they honestly and reasonably believe that the information and any allegation in it are substantially true.
- When they are not raising concerns for the purpose of personal gain (such as gaining promotion by ensuring someone else is sacked).
- When they have initially been unsuccessful in raising concerns with the employer first, unless they have reason to believe that:
  - they would be victimised
  - the employer would ensure there was a cover-up
  - the matter is very serious.

So the concerns raised with any regulatory body, such as the GDC in the case of dental professionals, will be protected under the PIDA if they are about:

- crime (e.g. fraud, theft, assault)
- the breaking of a legal obligation (e.g. duty of care to patients)
- miscarriage of justice (e.g. an innocent colleague being prosecuted)
- danger to health and safety or the environment (e.g. any breaches of legislations covered in Chapters 4 and 8)
- a cover-up by the employer, involving any of the above issues.

When a member of the dental team does raise a concern with the GDC, they do not have to prove their concerns before action is taken but they must be made in good faith.

As citizens, we are all encouraged to report potential fraud and crime to various bodies, such as the police, the agency dealing with various benefits, the DVLA, and Trading Standards, and to avoid retribution from fraudsters and criminals we are encouraged to do so anonymously. However, when raising a concern under the PIDA, anonymity is discouraged as it makes the issue more difficult to investigate, as well as making it very difficult to offer protection to an anonymous whistle-blower. The whistle-blower can always ask for their name not to be revealed without their permission.

Continuing professional development and reflective practice

At the point of qualification for any dental professional, the memorised knowledge of their curriculum will be at a maximum, while their practical experience of the job will be at a minimum. Throughout their working career, each team member will then automatically retain information about topics they cover on a daily basis, while forgetting some of the more obscure facts that they were taught as trainees. Similarly, practical skills used daily will become routine and well performed, while those used infrequently will diminish.

None of the curriculum content for each professional group is taught unnecessarily (and cannot then just be forgotten), so the only way to retain the more obscure facts and skills and therefore have an acceptable level of competence is to undergo update training on a regular basis, with the aim of retaining knowledge and improving skills, as well as being made aware of new information since qualification. To avoid team members having to constantly retake examinations to achieve this, the GDC introduced a system of continuing professional development (CPD) for all registrants.

The GDC has determined topics that all categories of registrants must update on a 5-year cycle of CPD; these are called the core topics, and for dental nurses they are as follows.

- Medical emergencies.
- Disinfection and decontamination.
- Radiological protection.
- Legal and ethical issues.
- Complaints handling.

Lack of up-to-date knowledge by a registrant in any of these areas could result in patients or colleagues being harmed or worse, or the registrant being guilty of negligence or professional misconduct – that is why they are compulsory (core) topics of development. By undergoing CPD in accordance with GDC requirements, the registrant will then achieve lifelong learning; every time they attend a CPD event, they will learn new information or skills throughout their professional career.

In addition, dental professionals must also undertake general CPD in topics of their own choice, so those who work in mainly orthodontic workplaces are likely to attend orthodontic events, for example, while those who work with special needs patients are likely to attend events relevant to that specialty.

Continuing professional development is categorised as either verifiable or non-verifiable, and all of the core topics must be delivered as verifiable CPD.

Verifiable CPD is that offered formally, with written specific aims and learning outcomes given by the organiser/presenter. Certificates of attendance and participation in verifiable CPD activities will be issued and must be kept as evidence of complying with the GDC's hourly requirements for CPD events. The certificates may even have to be produced as evidence of verifiable CPD activity, when requested by the GDC at the end of each 5-year cycle (that for dental nurses ends in 2013). Random checks of CPD records allow the GDC to ensure that professional obligations are being met by its registrants, while taking a step back and allowing the profession to regulate itself.

Examples of verifiable CPD events including the following.

- Attendance on postgraduate courses.
- Attendance at local meetings organised by postgraduate tutors or deaneries.
- Distance learning programmes with learning outcomes.
- Computer-aided learning programmes (CAL).
- Attendance at conferences with stated learning outcomes.
- Studying and taking formal examinations in dentally related subjects.
- Taking postregistration qualifications.
- Attending training events in other than the CPD core subjects.

Non-verifiable CPD is that done on an informal basis, often purely for personal interest. Although new information may be learned during these activities, it cannot be tested nor proved that specific learning outcomes have been achieved. Examples include all of those listed below, although some can also count as verifiable CPD when assessments are set (in journals, for example) that are scored on completion and records kept. The greater variety will provide the better learning and development opportunities.

- Reading relevant articles in work-related journals – with or without assessments.
- Reading new textbook publications.
- Exploring relevant websites on the internet – with or without assessments.

- Diversifying your skill base by training in new areas of dental nursing.
- Attending seminars, conferences and other work-related events.
- Taking an active part in workplace events:
  - staff meetings
  - running of quality assurance systems
  - risk assessment analyses.

The types of knowledge gained from all these example sources will fall into one of the three broad knowledge categories recognised by the profession, and a suitable combination of the three is essential to good dental nursing skills.

- **Scientific knowledge** – models and theories that can be scientifically tested against data gathered and are therefore verifiable – scientific knowledge can be written down and learned by others.
- **Experiential knowledge** – that gained over time by intuition and repetitive practice, including reflection and self-evaluation (see later).
- **Ethical knowledge** – that considered to be morally correct, although it is based on beliefs and values rather than facts.

With reference to ethical knowledge, a good dental nurse will always follow the principles of 'best practice' in the interests of patient and colleague safety, irrespective of their own personal values and beliefs.

When carried out correctly, then, organised CPD events covering the mandatory areas of dental practice, as well as a wider range of subjects relevant to the role of the dental nurse, are of great benefit to the registrant. CPD should enable recognition of areas that are of interest as well as areas where more knowledge is required, as dentistry and dental nursing are ever-changing disciplines where new materials and techniques are developed regularly. Completion of CPD should produce some of the following for all dental nurses.

- Increased job satisfaction.
- Identification of problem areas.
- Improved communication with colleagues.
- Improved efficiency.
- Improved career prospects.
- Greater commitment to the workplace.

The planning and undertaking of CPD should be given careful thought by the dental nurse to ensure not only that the mandatory requirements of the GDC are met but also that any other CPD undertaken is of use to their lifelong learning. While the temptation exists to only attend courses of personal interest, a broader coverage of subjects is more desirable and useful to the development of the dental nurse. The following points should also be taken into consideration when planning CPD activity.

- It can be time consuming, and may involve personal expense.
- It requires self-discipline to carry out and complete.
- It must be structured and organised to be of any real value.
- There must be a real educational benefit to undertaking it.
- Appropriate courses may not be available locally.
- Courses may run during work time, so employers must be amenable to participation.
- Courses may also run outside work time, so personal leisure time will be affected.

Reflective practice

Learning can occur on a regular basis within the workplace by the dental nurse reflecting on their work performance – by constantly analysing, constructively criticising and evaluating themselves. The aim is to recognise their own shortcomings and act upon them to improve their overall work performance. In this way, the dental nurse becomes a *reflective practitioner*.

However, it is human nature to be subjective and tend towards being either overly critical or overly lenient when reflecting on your own performance, as your ideas are based on the perception you have of yourself. More constructive analysis is that carried out by others, especially more experienced colleagues who have gone through the learning and reflection process themselves previously. This is the basis for an appraisal system within the workplace, where a senior colleague acts as a mentor for a more junior colleague, and gives verbal and written feedback on their performance (see later).

This can be carried out on a daily basis initially, with new employees being 'shadowed' by senior colleagues so that problems and shortfalls can be identified and addressed early in the learning process. While completing the Record of Experience portfolio towards their course completion and examination entry, every trainee dental nurse aiming for the NEBDN Diploma qualification will also undergo this witnessed feedback and reflection process.

The two main types of reflection that occur are:

- **reflection in action** – occurs as a situation happens
- **reflection on action** – occurs after the event, also referred to as 'hindsight'.

Reflection enables the dental nurse to think about how learning occurs, especially from experience, so that their work performance becomes more effective. It should produce a thinking professional who can react effectively and appropriately to changing circumstances to produce a successful outcome for the patient and the dental team.

It is the duty of the employer to ensure that changes in legislation are followed and referred to in updated policies, but it is the duty of the dental nurse to ensure that the updates are known of, understood and adhered to.

An example of reflection on action in the dental nursing context is given here. Compare the competence of a dental nurse carrying out a certain procedure for the first time compared to their competence when performing the same procedure for the fourth or fifth time. Obviously they will feel more comfortable as experience is gained, because subconsciously their own techniques are bettered after each event. In other words, 'practice makes perfect'.

So for instance, when aspirating for an oral surgery procedure, the first time the following may occur.

- Unsure of all the instrument identifications, as some may be being handled for the first time.
- Aspiration is not fully effective, as there is uncertainty about when to intervene without blocking the dentist's vision.
- Hesitant when handling some instruments, because they are unfamiliar.
- Concentrating so much on the procedure that the patient is forgotten.

Whereas when performing the procedure for the fourth or fifth time the following may occur.

- Instruments are now known because they are more familiar.
- Aspiration is more effective, perhaps by learning from the first patient choking and the dentist being unable to see clearly.

- Confident when handling instruments because they are more familiar.
- Able to monitor and reassure the patient at the same time as performing the other duties.

Reflection on action occurs by being able to think back over the procedure at a later date. This allows realisation and identification of any problems encountered, with the natural continuation of thought being to recognise how to improve next time.

Most of us carry out this second type of reflection on a regular basis, for example when driving home from work and going over the day's events in our minds, or by discussing our day with a family member, friend or colleague. However, we often forget the full impact of our thoughts unless we write them down at the time and review them at a later date.

Therefore, it would be prudent for the dental nurse to keep a diary, or portfolio, on a daily or at least weekly basis. This helps to organise and clarify thoughts, so that the reason why problems occurred can be discovered and action plans can be developed to prevent their recurrence.

A suggested layout of a diary or portfolio could be as follows.

- **Describe** the event.
- **Record** your emotions and thoughts.
- **Evaluate** the event – giving both good and bad points.
- **Critically analyse** the event – why did it happen?
- Reach a **conclusion** – what could have been done differently?
- **Develop an action plan** – what will be done differently next time?

After going through this process, it is relatively easy to determine whether a gap in knowledge has been identified.

It can be seen that the points suggested above follow those used when carrying out a risk assessment after an event, such as an injury occurring in the workplace or a chemical spillage say (see Chapter 4). When a serious event happens, such as any covered by the Reporting of Injuries, Diseases and Dangerous Occurrences Regulations 1995 (RIDDOR), the evaluation process is often referred to as a significant event analysis. The key aim of any analysis is to identify what went wrong, and how to prevent it recurring under similar circumstances in the future.

Self-evaluation and reflection can also be recorded in more detail in the form of a personal development plan (PDP), and one is included in the Record of Experience document for completion during the course of training.

The PDP is used to effectively look at the following points on a personal basis.

- Professionally, where am I now?
- What qualifications, knowledge and special interests helped me to achieve this position?
- What learning needs do I have now, if any?
- Do I wish to acquire new knowledge or skills?
- What is preventing me? Carry out a SWOT analysis (see below).
- What can be done to overcome any obstacles identified?
- Collate all the information to develop a personal learning/development plan, with achievable time scales if possible.
- Evaluate the PDP at least annually, to determine whether the development needs that were identified have been met, and to what extent.
- Summarise the progress made, and use it to determine your desired future learning and development needs.
- Keep a written record of all CPD events for each year, both verifiable and non-verifiable (this is a GDC requirement anyway, once registered).

Strengths
These are personal to the individual, and may include previous achievements as well as points such as reliability or ambition

Weaknesses
These are personal, and may include a personal lack of ambition, or home circumstances that make studying difficult

Opportunities
These are beneficial external factors which will influence success, and may include a supportive employer who encourages and funds further training

Threats
These are harmful external factors, or obstacles to future success, and may include an unsupportive employer, or lack of training opportunities

Figure 3.7   SWOT analysis.

- Analyse the CPD events attended to ensure that the core subjects are covered, but also to determine the necessity and relevance of the others to your personal learning and development needs.

A strengths, weaknesses, opportunities and threats (SWOT) analysis is an excellent method of determining whether the obstacles to future learning and development are identified as being of a personal nature or involve external pressures. It is used as follows (Figure 3.7).

- **Strengths** – these are personal to the individual, and may include previous achievements as well as points such as reliability or ambition.
- **Weaknesses** – these are personal, and may include a personal lack of ambition, or home circumstances that make studying difficult.
- **Opportunities** – these are beneficial external factors which will influence success, and may include a supportive employer who encourages and funds further training.
- **Threats** – these are harmful external factors or obstacles to future success, and may include an unsupportive employer or a lack of training opportunities in the locality.

Once the relevant points have been identified and recorded, efforts can be made to determine how to overcome the obstacles to future development. In some instances, this may be as dramatic as determining that an unsupportive employer is holding you back, and that a change of workplace is required.

Staff appraisals

Private reflection carried out using diaries, portfolios or personal development plans can be distorted, however, because by definition they record our own perception of ourselves. Of far more value is the input of our professional colleagues, such as that provided by a system of staff appraisal where the employer or a senior colleague reviews the performance of the staff member in the workplace, to achieve the following aims.

- Identify the strengths and weaknesses of the staff member.
- Identify the strengths and weaknesses of the running of the workplace, to give valuable information for good workplace development.
- Disclose any barriers to the efficient working of the dental team.

- Improve communication amongst the dental team.
- Encourage problem solving.
- Reduce any negative tensions between staff members.
- Improve practice morale.

Annual reviews in the form of staff appraisals are a requirement of the CQC, and provide evidence of good practice in the workplace by the employer. Several areas of appraisal can be carried out at one time during an annual review, or just one area can be highlighted. Common areas to consider are the following.

- **Personal** – hygiene, attitude, punctuality, dress code.
- **Administrative** – policies and protocols, regulations, filing, knowledge of paperwork.
- **Clinical** – infection control, mixing techniques, nursing skills, patient management.
- **Team work** – ability to function as a team member, acceptance of authority, ability to take responsibility.
- **Communication** – interpersonal, telephone manner, patient management.
- **Development** – self-evaluation, self-study, attendance at courses, learning by experience.

Once the relevant areas to be appraised have been selected, discussed and agreed upon, an appraisal sheet can be drawn up which gives the dental nurse the opportunity to self-evaluate their performance in these areas, before being compared with the recorded comments of the workplace evaluation (Figure 3.8).

Differences of opinion on performance can be explored and resolved, and then an action plan can be developed to determine future goals and aims. All details should be recorded on the appraisal sheet and then copied so that both the dental nurse and the practice can refer back to it in future, to assess the level of success of that appraisal.

It should also serve as a record of the dental nurse's self-development and progression within the practice, and expose any areas which continue to cause problems in future appraisals.

The areas can be adjusted to suit individual workplaces as necessary. The frequency of appraisal will also differ between workplaces as well as for different staff members. Younger, less experienced staff members are likely to require more frequent appraisal while learning all the relevant practice policies and protocols, and how to put them into practice. More experienced staff will need to be supportive and non-judgemental during this period.

When run correctly, appraisals can be an invaluable tool for the development of the whole dental team, so that the end result is the best possible outcome for the patient. An appraisal should identify the strengths and weaknesses not only of the staff members but also of the workplace environment itself, indicating routes that can be taken for good workplace development. By relying on feedback and constructive criticism, it should remove any interstaff communication barriers and improve problem-solving techniques. Overall, appraisals should improve the workforce morale by providing an opportunity for discussion without recrimination by all.

General Dental Council *Standards Guidance* on dental team working

One of the six key principles of the GDC *Standards Guidance* document states that dental professionals must 'co-operate with other members of the dental team and other healthcare colleagues in the interests of patients', and a separate booklet covering this topic is also available (Figure 3.9).

Areas of appraisal	Self-appraisal	Practice appraisal	Notes
Personal hygiene Dress Punctuality			
NHS procedures Rules / regulations Medico-legal knowledge			
Materials techniques Infection control Patient management X-ray procedures Equipment handling			
Courses of study Self-study Experiential learning Problem-based learning Peer group learning			
Teamwork experience Innovation Originality			
Communication skills Interpersonal skills Administrative accuracy Telephone manner Complaints handling			
Appraisal summary			

Signed.......................... Signed...................... Date......................

Figure 3.8   Staff appraisal example sheet.

The guidance booklet reiterates that good dental care is not delivered by just one individual but by a dental team, and the quality of the teamwork is reflected in the quality of care that the team provides to the patient. The guidance lists the members of the dental team who must be registered to work legally in the UK.

- Dentists
- Dental nurses
- Hygienists
- Therapists
- Dental technicians

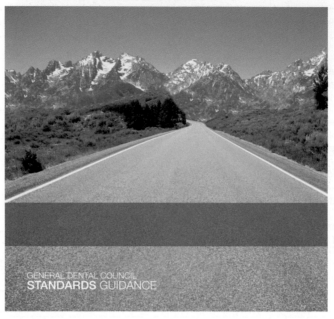

PRINCIPLES OF
DENTAL TEAM WORKING

GENERAL DENTAL COUNCIL
STANDARDS GUIDANCE

Figure 3.9   GDC Standards – dental team working. With permission from the GDC. Information correct at the time of going to press. Please visit the GDC website to check for any changes since publication: www.gdc-uk.org.

- Clinical dental technicians
- Orthodontic therapists

To be seen to co-operate with other team members, all dental professionals must do the following.

- Respect the role of others in caring for patients – no single team member is more important than another, or as the saying goes, 'there is no "I" in the word "team"'.
- Never discriminate against other team members or healthcare colleagues.
- Always communicate effectively with other team members so that patients are safe while undergoing treatment – the best interests of the patient must always be the first priority for everyone.

The booklet then goes on to discuss and give guidance on the principles of dental team working and how they should be followed, under the headings described below.

- The dental team – the professionals who make up the team, both on and off the workplace premises.
- How the team should work together.
  - The dentist must see all patients for a full oral assessment.
  - The only current exception to this is for a clinical dental technician to supply and maintain full dentures to an edentulous patient, without seeing a dentist first.
  - Otherwise, various treatments may then be delegated to other team members to be carried out under the prescription of the dentist, such as scaling, oral hygiene instruction, deciduous tooth extraction, for example (within their scope of practice).

- ○ The dentist carries out any treatment as necessary, assisted at the chairside by a dental nurse.
- ○ The patient may need referring to another dentist or a specialist for other treatments.
- ○ A recall interval is set for the patient to return to a team member within the workplace.
- Individual responsibilities within the team – a reminder that all registrants are responsible for their own actions, and must not work outside the sphere of their capabilities and competence, and also of their duty to raise concerns when appropriate.
- Working effectively as a team – the need for good communication skills with the patient and other team members, so that the patient can give valid consent and other team members are clear about their individual duties.
- Leading a team – the skills required to lead a team successfully, and the responsibilities of leadership, especially:
  - ○ encouraging members to raise concerns
  - ○ correct handling of complaints
  - ○ safe management of medical emergencies.

The final point raised, which is of interest to those team members who work in the specialty of maxillofacial surgery, is to note that general nurses registered with their own regulators (the Nursing and Midwifery Council) are legally allowed to assist in clinical procedures related to this specialty.

In summary, then, although many team leaders will be dentists, the team as a whole needs to work as a well-oiled machine to provide the best possible care for their patients at all times. Each team member is one important cog in that machine, without which it cannot properly function. A happy and well-functioning team is one that feels valued by its employers, respected by its patients, and treated as professionals while members carry out their day-to-day duties.

 Further resources are available for this book, including interactive multiple choice questions and extended matching questions. Visit the companion website at:

www.levisonstextbookfordentalnurses.com

4

Health and Safety in the Dental Workplace

Key learning points

A **factual knowledge** of
- health and safety requirements relevant to both employers and employees

A **working knowledge** of
- the legislative and regulatory requirements of the dental workplace and its staff
- risk assessment in the dental workplace
- occupational hazards and their avoidance in the dental workplace

A **factual awareness** of
- the actions to take in various first aid scenarios
- general safety and security issues in the dental workplace

Health and Safety at Work Act (1974)

All dental workplaces, their staff and patients are covered by the provisions of the Health and Safety at Work Act (1974), as is any other workplace. In addition, other legislation is relevant to the dental workplace due to the potentially harmful nature of the equipment and chemicals used, as well as the occupational hazards associated with delivering dental treatment or working in the dental environment.

The Health and Safety legislation seeks to protect staff and patients while on the premises by making the staff aware of any potential hazards at work, and encouraging them to find the

Levison's Textbook for Dental Nurses, Eleventh Edition. By Carole Hollins.
© 2013 John Wiley & Sons, Ltd. Published 2013 by John Wiley & Sons, Ltd. Companion website: www.levisonstextbookfordentalnurses.com

best ways of making their premises safer for all concerned. In legal terms, the employer has a statutory duty to ensure that, as far as is reasonably practicable, the health, safety and welfare at work of all employees and all visitors (including patients) are considered at all times. To do this, all the potential hazards first need to be identified, and then the likelihood of them actually causing harm to anyone must be determined. The chance that a particular workplace hazard could cause harm to someone is known as its risk, and the correct procedure to be followed by the employer (and their staff) to identify those hazards that could cause harm is called a risk assessment.

Compliance with the Health and Safety at Work Act is overseen and regulated by the Health and Safety Executive (HSE). This is a government body that provides guidance to employers on the correct enforcement of the Act, and investigates when any serious incidents occur in any workplace where someone suffers serious harm or is killed. Every dental workplace is required to be registered with the HSE.

Compliance with the additional legislation specific to the dental workplace is also required by the General Dental Council, under its *Standards for Dental Professionals* documentation.

To comply with the basic requirements of the Health and Safety at Work Act, every employer in the dental workplace must abide by the following requirements.

- Provide a working environment for employees that is safe, without risks to health, and adequate with regard to facilities and arrangements for their welfare at work.
- Maintain the place of work, including the means of access and exit, in a safe condition.
- Provide and maintain safe equipment, appliances and systems of work.
- Ensure all staff are trained in the safe handling and storage of any dangerous or potentially harmful items or substances.
- Provide such instruction, training and supervision as is necessary to ensure health and safety.
- Review the Health and Safety performance of all staff annually, be aware of and investigate any failures or concerns highlighted, when they occur.
- Display the official Health and Safety poster for all staff to refer to (Figure 4.1).

To comply with these statutory obligations, dentists must keep their staff informed of all the safety measures adopted. Practices with five or more employees must produce a comprehensive Health and Safety policy and provide all staff with a copy. The policy will classify the practice Health and Safety procedures and name the persons responsible. It should also list the telephone numbers of all dental, administration and equipment maintenance contractors, the local HSE contact, and emergency services.

Role of the dental nurse

All dental nurses have a legal obligation to co-operate with their employers in carrying out the practice requirements in respect of these safety measures. They are designed to protect not only the staff and patients, but anybody else using or visiting the premises. In a large dental workplace, a dental nurse may be appointed as safety representative under the Act for the purpose of improving liaison within the practice about Health and Safety matters.

However, many dental nurses begin their careers as young trainees in the dental environment, so the following two sets of regulations are specifically important in protecting their welfare.

- Health and Safety (Young Persons) Regulations 1997
- Management of Health and Safety at Work Regulations 1999

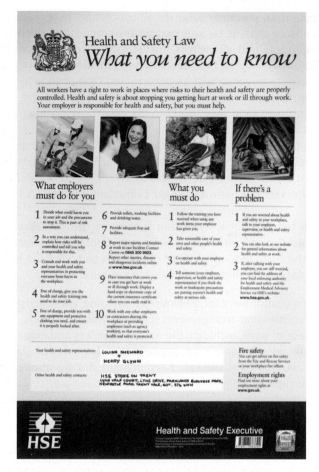

Figure 4.1 Health and Safety poster. © Crown Copyright 2009. Published by the Health and Safety Executive (HSE).

These sets of regulations dictate that a risk assessment of the dental environment has to be carried out, with particular regard to the protection of younger staff members, by taking into account the following points.

- The risks to young people before they start work.
- The psychological or physical immaturity and inexperience of young people.
- Their lack of awareness of existing or potential risks to their health and safety.
- The fitting and layout of the practice and surgery, with regard to the safety of young people.
- The nature, degree and duration of any exposure to biological, chemical or physical agents within the work environment.
- The form, range, use and handling of dental equipment.
- The way in which processes and activities are organized.
- Any Health and Safety training given, or intended to be given.

A summary of the risk assessment details, covering the various types of work activity that a student dental nurse is likely to undertake, to ensure their safety in the dental workplace is shown in Table 4.1. The risk assessment should take into account the likely activities that the student dental

Table 4.1   Risk assessment for student dental nurse

Work activity	Potential risk	Prevention with controls
Chairside assisting	Eye injury from projectiles during treatment Inhalation of aerosols during treatment	Explanation of risks, training in activities undertaken, initial supervision Provision and use of all personal protective equipment (PPE)
Instrument decontamination	Inoculation injury (clean or dirty) Contamination splash during cleaning	Explanation of risks, training in cleaning methods, initial supervision Additional PPE – plastic apron and thick rubber gloves
Use of autoclave	Burns from hot machine or instruments Scalds from steam	Explanation of risks, training in handling methods, initial supervision
Exposure to hazardous chemicals	Inhalation of vapours, skin contact, eye contact	Explanation of risks, training in handling methods, initial supervision Provision and use of full PPE Adequate ventilation
Use of x-rays	Accidental exposure to x-rays	Explanation of risks, inform of designated control area, avoid unauthorised entry to area

nurse will undertake while on the premises, and these are listed in the first column. To train effectively, they must always be involved in chairside assisting activities, so the potential areas of risk to the student during chairside working should then be considered – these are listed in the second column. The final column then needs to identify the methods required to ensure that the student is not exposed to these risks in the first place, and for each area it can be seen that suitable induction training is always required. This involves explaining why a certain activity is a risk to them, the provision of suitable training in the activity so that the risk is minimised as far as possible, and initial supervision when the activity is carried out for the first few times. Before dental nurses became registrants with the General Dental Council (GDC), and therefore before training and qualification were necessary, this supervision used to be referred to as 'shadowing' of a junior colleague by a senior colleague, until they were deemed able to carry out the activity unsupervised. The risk assessment procedure described here merely formalises the technique of shadowing.

Full compliance with Health and Safety legislation for all dental workplaces, whether a practice, a clinic or a hospital department, involves all of the following.

- Fire Precaution (Workplace) Regulations (1999)
- Health and Safety (First Aid) Regulations (1981)
- Control of Substances Hazardous to Health (COSSH) (1994)
- Reporting of Injuries, Diseases and Dangerous Occurrences (RIDDOR) (1995)
- Environmental Protection Act (1990)
- Special Waste and Hazardous Waste Regulations (2005)

- Ionising Radiation Regulations (IRR) 1999
- Ionising Radiation (Medical Exposure) Regulations (IR(ME)R) 2000
- Occupational hazards
- General safety measures
- General security measures

Since 2010, additional regulations have been introduced in the specific areas of decontamination and infection control in the dental workplace, although their implementation currently varies throughout the UK. Referred to collectively as HTM 01-05, their detail is discussed in Chapter 8. Finally, since 2011 a system of mandatory registration with the Care Quality Commission (CQC) has been introduced for all providers of health and social care, including all dental workplaces. The CQC is a regulatory body which ensures that all registrants comply with essential standards of quality and safety when dealing with patients. The impact of CQC registration on the dental workplace, and its relevance to dental nurses, is discussed more fully in Chapter 3.

Risk assessment

As stated above, the whole purpose of the Health and Safety legislation is to protect everyone within the dental workplace (staff, patients and visitors) from coming to any harm while on the premises. This is achieved by carrying out a risk assessment of every potential hazard that could occur. The aim is not necessarily to eliminate every risk completely (this is likely to be impossible in most workplaces, including dental surgeries) but instead to minimise those risks identified as far as possible, so that there is little chance of them causing harm to anyone.

For example, various chemicals must be used in the dental workplace to carry out dental treatment successfully – these include decontamination solutions, x-ray processing solutions, and mercury in amalgam fillings; all are potentially harmful but only if mishandled. So knowledge of their correct storage and usage by staff, and protection from misuse by all others, are key factors in avoiding a hazardous event.

The steps involved in carrying out a risk assessment on a hazard, whatever its nature, should always follow the same pattern.

1. **Identify the hazard** – a chemical, a piece of equipment, a procedure that occurs in the workplace, etc.
2. **Identify who may be harmed** – certain staff, certain patients, visitors, everyone, etc.
3. **Evaluate the risk** – is there a hazard only if misused, is there a hazard with every use, or is there a hazard if certain precautions are not followed?
4. **Control the risk** – train all staff in correct usage, improve precautions to prevent misuse, keep hazards away from untrained persons, install health monitoring where appropriate, remove the risk where possible, etc.
5. **Record the risk assessment findings** – to prove compliance, to provide a reference for all users, to ensure all staff are fully informed of the potential hazards in the dental workplace.
6. **Review the assessment process** – on a regular basis to ensure that hazardous events or injuries do not occur.

Although specialist knowledge of some hazards in the dental workplace is necessary to fully realise their potential for causing harm, many of the actions that should be followed to ensure the health and safety of everyone on the premises are common sense.

Table 4.2   Avoidance of hazards

Scenario of potential hazard	Common-sense actions to avoid harm
Injury sustained by falling down on the premises	Keep all access routes clear of debris and blockages Maintain floor covering adequately Avoid cleaning during work time Clear all spillages immediately Use hazard signs to highlight potential sources of injury (Caution – wet floor, etc.)
Child drinking harmful chemical	Keep harmful chemicals out of reach Keep chemicals in locked storage area Keep children out of storage area Keep children under control at all times
Person falling out of window on premises	Install window locks Install restricted opening device Keep staff-only areas locked
Injury sustained from slammed door	Keep doors locked when rooms not in use Install slow closure devices to prevent slamming Install safety glass

Consider the scenarios and relevant common-sense actions in Table 4.2. The table gives examples of various hazardous situations that may be encountered by patients and visitors to the dental workplace in the first column, in a similar way to those that may be encountered by the student dental nurse shown in Table 4.1. The second column then suggests common-sense actions to take that will minimise the potential risk in the first place. So, for example, there are several potentially harmful chemicals used in dentistry that cannot be avoided, such as bleach-based cleaning agents. When used for their specific purpose, there is no risk but if used contrary to that purpose (such as being swallowed by a child), their potential to cause harm is huge. The common-sense action is to prevent the child from having access to the chemical at all times, by locking it away in a cupboard or storing it in a locked room away from the public access areas of the workplace. The differing design and layout of each workplace will require that an individual risk assessment is carried out for each one.

These scenarios are not exclusive to the dental workplace – they could occur anywhere at any time and to anyone. However, if they do occur in the dental workplace then they are not merely an unavoidable accident but have become an avoidable risk that should have been prevented from happening. In other words, someone is to blame. If the simple common-sense actions have not been carried out initially, then the employer is to blame. If, however, a risk assessment has resulted in the necessary preventive measures being put into place and someone has flouted them, such as by leaving a door or cupboard unlocked to avoid the inconvenience of having to keep unlocking it, then that person is to blame instead.

All members of staff have a legal obligation under the Health and Safety at Work Act to co-operate with their employer by following the policies and procedures put in place to protect all persons while on the premises. They must also take reasonable care for their own and others' health and safety while on the premises. Failure to do so, as indicated above, will result in their possible investigation and prosecution by the HSE, and a fitness to practise hearing by the GDC, for those who are registrants.

The level of reasonable care expected to be taken for their own health and safety as an employee (and in line with 'fitness to practise' requirements by the GDC) requires all dental care professionals to abide by the following when in the dental workplace.

- Undergo suitable training in the use of dental materials and equipment.
- Always follow that training when using those materials and equipment.
- Always follow all policies in relation to health, safety and welfare issues.
- Never misuse any materials or equipment on the premises.
- In particular, never misuse or fail to use any materials or equipment that are specifically meant to reduce or eliminate hazardous risks.
- Always report any faults in procedures or equipment to a senior colleague immediately.
- Never enter certain designated 'hazardous' areas unless authorised to do so.
- Always report any suspected health problem that will affect their normal work to a senior colleague as soon as possible.

It is important, then, that a FULL risk assessment of the dental workplace is carried out and its findings reviewed on a regular basis, and that all staff follow the control measures that have been put into place, at all times. Advice and guidance are available on risk assessment generally, and in the dental workplace in particular, from both the HSE and from organisations such as the British Dental Association. Their website addresses for further information are:

- Health and Safety Executive: www.hse.gov.uk
- British Dental Association: www.bda.org.

Fire Precaution (Workplace) Regulations 1999

The above regulations were updated by the Regulatory Reform (Fire Safety) Order, which became law in 2006. This stipulates that the employer/owner of the premises (the dental workplace) must take reasonable steps to reduce the risk from fire, and to make sure that people on the premises can escape safely if there is a fire. They therefore require the employer/owner to risk assess the fire precautions that are needed for their own work premises, as these will vary from one work-place to another; a ground floor practice will be considered less dangerous to staff and patients in the event of a fire than one that is in a multistorey building, for instance.

A typical fire risk assessment should consider the following points, and in this order.

1. **Identify the fire hazards on the premises** – these will include flammable materials (liquids, vapours, textiles, paper products), heating appliances with naked flames, electrical equipment, static sparks from electrical equipment, flammable sedation gases, flammable rubbish.
2. **Identify who may be harmed** – anyone on the premises, paying special attention to children and vulnerable adults who may be attending, and where they may be on the premises.
3. **Evaluate the risk of a fire occurring** – the amount of various flammable materials on the premises, and where they are used or stored, the number of heating appliances and items of electrical equipment, any sedation gases, the amount of flammable rubbish at any time.
4. **Control the risk by taking precautions** – reduce the amount of flammable materials used where possible, and ensure they are stored away from heat sources, replace naked flame heat sources with safer alternatives (only likely exception will be portable burners used for denture

work), ensure electrical appliances are properly serviced and maintained, use and store sedation gas cylinders away from heat sources, avoid storing flammable waste near heat sources, consider if current fire detection methods, fire-fighting equipment and evacuation procedures are adequate or not.

5. **Record the risk assessment findings** – in particular, record all findings and details of the actions taken to improve precautions, ensure all staff are notified of the findings and any new actions to be followed.

6. **Review the risk assessment periodically** – annually is adequate, recording the date of the review and whether any revisions were made or not.

All dental workplaces then undergo a fire safety inspection, so that the premises can be formally recorded as having carried out the necessary risk assessment. Although several companies provide the means for this to be carried out by post, a visit by a suitably qualified inspector from the Fire Brigade will hold more weight if a fire does occur and the practice is held to account for its level of compliance.

The inspection will give advice with regard to the following.

- The number and positioning of smoke detectors.
- The number and positioning of fire extinguishers.
- Written records of staff training in the use of fire extinguishers.
- The types of fire extinguishers to be provided, with at least two types present in all workplaces.

Fire detection

The Regulatory Reform (Fire Safety) Order 2005 states that an electrical fire alarm system and/or an automatic detection system are only necessary on premises where these devices would be necessary to give warning in case of fire. The types of premises involved would be large workplaces, perhaps over several levels, where a fire breaking out in one area could go undetected by an ordinary smoke alarm or unnoticed by a person for some time. Hospital departments and health clinics are examples of places where these additional fire detection methods would be required.

In smaller workplaces (the majority of dental practices), a fire risk assessment should determine that adequate fire detection is provided by battery-operated smoke alarms around the premises (Figure 4.2). The local fire station, or the fire inspector, will give advice on the number required and

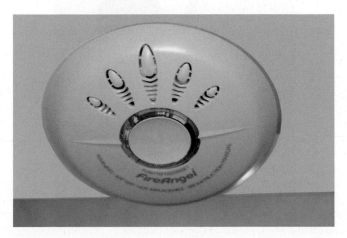

Figure 4.2   Smoke alarm.

their suitable locations at key points throughout the premises. They should be tested on a regular basis to ensure they are functioning correctly, and a record kept of these test dates and results. Obviously, the battery should be changed as soon as it begins to fail, or the alarm changed if any malfunctions occur.

Fire fighting

The main equipment available for use in fire fighting is the fire extinguisher (Figure 4.3), although some premises will have additional equipment such as fire blankets and hoses. To determine which fire-fighting equipment should be available, the classification of fires is considered as follows.

- **Class A fire** – caused by the ignition of carbon-containing items such as paper, wood and textiles.
- **Class B fire** – caused by flammable liquids such as oils, solvents and petrol.
- **Class C fire** – caused by flammable gases such as domestic gas, butane, liquefied petroleum gas (LPG).
- **Class D fire** – caused by reactive metals that oxidise in air such as sodium and magnesium.
- **Class E fire** – caused by electrical components and equipment.
- **Class F fire** – caused by liquid fats such as used in kitchens and restaurants.

In the dental workplace, the likeliest causes of fire shown above suggest that extinguishers to fight classes A, B, C and E should be available. The content of each fire extinguisher varies depending on its recommended use, and is identifiable by a coloured label or specific wording on the label of the

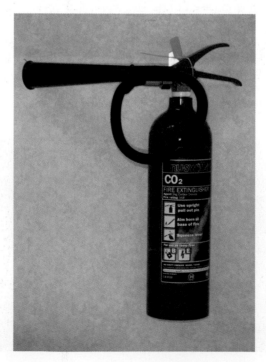

Figure 4.3   Fire extinguisher.

extinguisher. All extinguishers are coloured red so that they are easily visible, while the label and its wording describe the fire classification that it is suitable for, as follows.

- Red (water) extinguisher – for use on all except electrical fires.
- Black (carbon dioxide) extinguisher – for use on all fires.
- Blue (dry powder) extinguisher – for use on all fires.

The extinguishers must all be inspected and certificated by a competent person on an annual basis, and replaced as necessary. They should be located:

- within easy reach, ideally along escape routes
- in conspicuous positions (so not hidden by surrounding cupboards, for example)
- on wall mountings and signposted
- in a similar position on each level of the premises.

Evacuation and escape routes

During the risk assessment process, consideration should be given to whether, in the event of a fire, all persons on the premises could leave safely and reach a place of safety. There should be no possibility of anyone being cut off from escaping from the premises by either smoke or flames.

In particular, the following areas of fire safety must be complied with.

- Escape routes must be kept free from all obstructions to allow immediate evacuation from the premises if necessary. In particular, key-operated doors must be kept unlocked during normal working hours.
- Fire exits must lead directly to a place of safety, usually outside the building itself.
- They must be clearly marked by green 'Fire Exit' signs, with an accompanying pictogram of a running man (Figure 4.4).
- Emergency lighting should be provided if necessary – this applies to hospitals rather than individual practices, and will have been identified during the fire risk assessment.
- Emergency doors should open manually in the direction of escape, and should not be operated electrically.
- Sliding or revolving doors should not be used as fire exits.

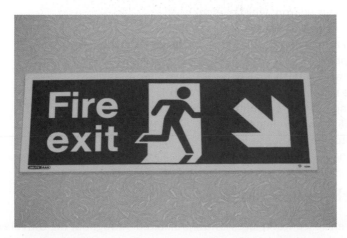

Figure 4.4   Fire exit pictogram.

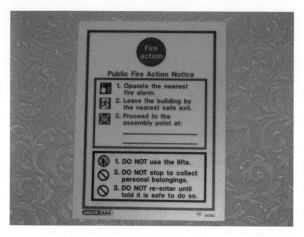

Figure 4.5   Fire escape poster.

- All staff must be aware of the fire safety and evacuation process, and the procedure for evacuation should be practised at least annually.
- In addition, some staff should be charged with certain actions during the evacuation procedure, such as checking certain areas are clear or closing certain doors to contain the fire.
- Special consideration also needs to be given to the needs of disabled persons, and in small workplaces they should only be treated in ground-floor surgeries so that they can be easily evacuated from the premises.

The culmination of the findings from the fire risk assessment will ultimately be the development of a written fire policy or an emergency plan. This is a legal requirement in workplaces with more than five employees, and must be available to all employees and to the fire inspector. It should detail what action everyone on the premises should take in the event of a fire, and may be covered by a simple 'Fire Action' poster displayed in the reception area (Figure 4.5). Larger premises will be expected to provide more detail still, and a suitable emergency plan should cover the following points.

- Action to take in the event of a fire.
- Alarm warnings (klaxon, whistle, etc.).
- How to call rescue services.
- Evacuation arrangements, including details for disabled persons.
- Assembly point.
- Method of accounting for all persons (daylist, for example).
- Key escape routes.
- Location and use of fire-fighting equipment.
- Responsibilities of nominated persons.
- Power shutdown methods.
- Staff training.

Smoking in the workplace

Smoking in all enclosed workplaces is now prohibited throughout the UK. All enclosed workplaces, which include all types of dental workplace, must display a 'No Smoking' sign at each entrance (Figure 4.6) and the sign must contain the following wording: 'No smoking. It is against the law to

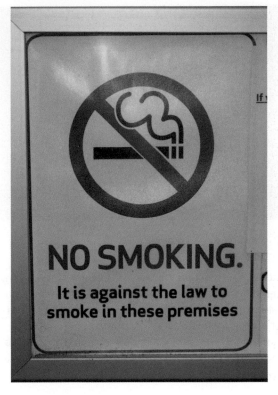

Figure 4.6   'No Smoking' sign.

smoke in these premises'. Before the ban, careless disposal of cigarettes was a significant cause of fires in the workplace, so future analysis of fires and their causes will hopefully show a reduction in their incidence.

Health and Safety (First Aid) Regulations 1981

In addition to the identification of the signs and symptoms of the medical emergencies that may occur in dental practice and their correct management (see Chapter 6), the whole dental team should be able to deal with basic first aid procedures too.

Under the First Aid Regulations, all workplaces must have adequate first aid provision available for all employees, although there is no legal requirement to provide first aid treatment and facilities for non-employees, including patients.

The risk assessment process carried out to comply with general Health and Safety requirements should identify the hazards and risks associated with the workplace itself, and the occupational hazards associated with the business of dentistry. The hazards and risks identified will determine the extent of the first aid provision that is required for the premises and the employees.

In line with clinical governance guidelines (see Chapter 3), every practice must comply with the following requirements.

- All staff must be trained and certificated in basic life support (see Chapter 6).
- All workplaces with more than five employees should have at least one person trained in emergency first aid.

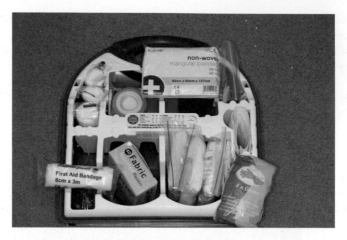

Figure 4.7   First aid box.

- All practices must have a first aid kit available, besides the full range of emergency drugs and emergency oxygen cylinders required under clinical governance guidelines.
- All practices must have an accident book, which is used to record all except major accidental events that occur on the premises to staff, patients or visitors.
- In the event of a medical emergency, the dental team must be able to reassure and help the casualty until the professionals arrive, and this may include basic life support (BLS) to maintain life if necessary.

The first aid kit that must be present in the dental workplace should be placed in an easy-access and signposted location. Regulations stipulate that it should be a green box with a white cross on (Figure 4.7), and should contain minimum requirements with regard to sterile dressings, eye pads, bandages, etc.

Specific training for emergency first aid is provided by various HSE-approved organisations, including the British Red Cross and St John Ambulance. The first aid emergencies that should be covered are as follows, and are summarised below.

- Severe bleeding
- Burns and scalds
- Poisoning
- Electrocution
- Bone fractures

Severe bleeding

- The first aid principle is to *restrict the blood flow to the wound and encourage clotting to reduce blood loss*.
- Arterial bleeding will spurt rhythmically and be cherry red in colour.
- Venous bleeding will gush quickly and be dark red or purple in colour.
- Capillary bleeding will ooze slowly and be dark red in colour.
- The required treatment is to raise the injured part above the level of the heart if possible, and apply direct pressure to the wound for up to 15 min using a clean dressing.
- Any foreign objects present should *not* be removed from the wound.

- As a last resort, severed arteries can be compressed against the underlying bone for up to 15 min, using a tourniquet.
- The casualty should be removed to hospital once the bleeding is under control, or the emergency services should be called if it cannot be controlled.

Possible causes of severe bleeding in the dental workplace include unexpected surgical trauma, traumatic falls, severe sharps injury, etc.

Burns and scalds

- A **burn** is an injury caused by dry heat, corrosive chemicals or irradiation.
- A **scald** is a wet burn caused by steam or hot liquids.
- The first aid principles are to *prevent infection* of the underlying tissues and to *prevent clinical shock developing* due to the loss of blood serum.
- The required treatment is to remove the casualty from the source of danger if possible, and to reassure them if they are still conscious.
- The injured part should be placed under cold water for a minimum of 10 min, to reduce blistering.
- Any restrictive jewellery should be removed before any swelling occurs, but clothing should be left in place as its removal may causing tearing of the tissues.
- Seek medical help for all but minor burns or scalds, and be prepared to carry out BLS if clinical shock develops in severe cases.

Possible causes of burns in the dental workplace include touching hot equipment or instruments, touching naked flames, various chemicals (etching gel, bleach products, other cleaning agents) and uncontrolled exposure to x-rays.

Poisoning

- The first aid principle is to *limit the exposure of the casualty to the poison*, and maintain life if necessary.
- Consult any available COSHH documentation for the required first aid advice.
- The required treatment is to remove the casualty from the source of the poison, without endangering other lives.
- Where vapours are the cause, provide good ventilation of the area immediately.
- Vomiting should not be induced, as caustic poisons will burn the digestive tract each time they pass through.
- Maintain the airway and carry out BLS if necessary.
- Seek urgent medical help.

Possible causes in the dental workplace include the ingestion or inhalation of various agents, such as corrosive chemicals (bleach products and acids), toxic chemicals (cleaning agents, processing chemicals, mercury), toxic vapours (processing chemicals, mercury, gases).

Electrocution

- This is caused by an electrical current passing through the body, causing burns and possibly affecting the electrical conduction of the heart itself.
- The first aid principle is to *remove the casualty from the electrical source and maintain life until help arrives*.

- The required treatment is to isolate the electrical supply if it is safe to do so, treat any surface burns and minimise the effects of clinical shock.
- The casualty should not be touched by the rescuer until the electrical source has been isolated, otherwise the rescuer could be electrocuted too.
- Carry out BLS if necessary.
- Seek urgent medical help.

Possible causes in the dental workplace are any faulty electrical equipment items, including portable appliances.

Fractures

- A fracture is a break of a bone, either contained within the surrounding soft tissues or puncturing through them to cause a compound fracture, where the bone ends are visible and soft tissue damage is severe.
- The first aid principle is to *prevent further tissue damage by restricting the movement of the casualty*.
- The required treatment is to not move any injured part of the body, to cover any open skin wounds with clean dressings, and control bleeding as necessary.
- Seek urgent medical help.

Possible causes in the dental workplace are external trauma or a fall, although violent assault of a person may also be a cause.

Basic life support techniques and medical emergencies are covered in detail in Chapter 6.

Control of Substances Hazardous to Health (COSHH) 1994

Many of the chemicals and other hazardous substances used in the dental workplace can be harmful to a person's health if they are misused or if adequate precautions are not taken to prevent access by unauthorised persons. However, without these substances the business of dentistry could not be carried out, so the continued use of the chemicals under safe conditions is the desired outcome. Again, the level of risk from any of the chemicals or substances involved, those who may be harmed and the necessary precautions to take are all determined by carrying out a risk assessment.

The risk assessment process to be followed in this case is determined by the COSHH regulations, which require all dental workplaces to carry out a risk assessment of all the chemicals and potentially hazardous substances used in the premises, to identify those that could harm or injure staff members. Harm may be caused if an accident occurs to expose personnel to an unusually large amount of a chemical, or if a chemical accidentally gains entry to the body (for example, by being inhaled), or merely just by the dangerous nature of even small amounts of a chemical (for example, mercury). The risk assessment process follows the usual steps but the written report produced must include every potential chemical hazard found, and the following specific information.

- The hazardous ingredient(s) it contains.
- The nature of the risk, ideally by indicating the risk category using recognised symbols (Figure 4.8).
- The possible health effects of the hazardous ingredient(s).
- The precautions required for the safe handling of the product.

Know your hazardous chemical products. Below are the four health categories:

 TOXIC
– can cause damage to health at low levels
for example, mercury is toxic by inhalation

 HARMFUL
– can cause damage to health
for example, some disinfectants / tray adhesives are harmful by inhalation

 CORROSIVE
– may destroy living tissue on contact
for example, phosphoric acid (etchant) causes burns in contact with skin

 IRRITANT
– may cause inflammation to skin and / or eyes, nose and throat
for example, some disinfectants and x-ray developer can irritate the eyes and skin

Note:
For packaged hazardous chemical products, the label (depending on the size) should contain a symbol (as above) and simple information about the hazard and the precautions required. The Safety Data Sheet will provide more detailed information and the supplier is obliged to provide this if the substance is hazardous to health and is used at work.

Figure 4.8   Symbols of COSHH risk categories.

- Any additional hazard control methods required for its safe use.
- All necessary first aid measures required in the event of an accident involving the product.

The reports are then kept in a COSHH file for quick reference and updated regularly. They should be available to the whole dental team for reference, and each staff member should sign to say they have read and understood the information. An example of a COSHH assessment sheet is shown in Figure 4.9.

The risk assessment follows the usual steps, with pertinent points to be determined as detailed below for each substance used in the dental practice, ranging from specific dental materials through to general cleaning agents.

- **Identify those substances which are hazardous** – by reading the manufacturers' leaflets and instruction sheets enclosed with the product, or shown on the label.
- **Identify who may be harmed** – this is likely to be anyone who uses the substance, although public access must be taken into consideration too.

Name of Substance						
Hazardous Ingredients						
Used for						
By whom						
Frequency						
Amount						
Nature of Risks	Chemical		Flammable		Poisonous	Biological
Exposure Limits	OES (MEL if applicable)			ppm		mg m^{-3}
	Long term (8 hr TWA)			–		
				–		
Other						
Health Effects						
Eye contact						
Skin contact						
Inhalation						
Ingestion						
Precautions for Safe Handling and Use						
Spillage						
Waste disposal						
Storage						
Control Measures						
Ventilation						
Eye protection						
Respiratory protection						
Gloves						
Health monitoring						
Staff training						
Other						
First Aid Measures						
Eye contact						
Skin contact						
Inhalation						
Ingestion						

Dentists and staff members to sign to confirm these Control Measures are carried out:

1 ....   4 ....   7 ....
2 ....   5 ....   8 ....
3 ....   6 ....   9 ....

Figure 4.9   Example of COSHH assessment sheet.

- **Identify how they may be harmed** – is the product hazardous on skin contact, or by inhaling fumes, or an eye irritant, etc.?
- **Evaluate the risk** – is the substance only harmful if misused, or is it harmful with every use?
- **Determine whether health monitoring is required** – for example, during exposure to mercury, or nitrous oxide gas used in inhalation sedation as a conscious sedation technique.
- **Control the risk** – by ensuring the substance is not misused, by providing suitable personal protective equipment (PPE), or reducing the risk as far as possible if it is harmful with every use – this may involve changing the product if the potential risk is considered too great.
- **Inform all staff of the risks** – by staff meetings, and introduction of the COSHH sheets to be read and signed by all team members.
- **Record the risk assessment** – keep documented evidence that the assessment has been carried out, with review and update dates recorded as necessary.

While the dental nurse is an integral part of the risk assessment procedure as a member of staff, more senior dental nurses may take over the role of maintaining the COSHH files and updating them as necessary, once suitable and documented training has been given. However, all student dental nurses must receive Health and Safety information covering these issues as part of their induction training with their employer.

Some general safety points with regard to hazardous substances likely to be found in the dental workplace are given below.

Storage

All chemicals should be stored in cupboards away from public access, with separate fire-resistant locked storage facilities available for inflammable substances and poisons. The manufacturer's instructions will indicate the ideal storage temperature required, and this is usually room temperature (20°C) or cooler, which is provided by refrigeration. Mercury must be stored in a cool cupboard in properly sealed containers.

Oxygen and nitrous oxide cylinders, used for treating patients under conscious sedation, should ideally be stored outdoors but if this is not possible a well-ventilated fire-resistant store should be used. Larger cylinders should be secured in an upright position so that they cannot fall over and puncture, or harm someone. An appropriate trolley should be available for moving heavy cylinders.

The exception to these storage requirements is emergency oxygen cylinders, which must always remain in easy-access locations throughout the dental workplace, at all times.

Ventilation and temperature control

Suitable ventilation in the dental workplace can be achieved simply by having windows open or by the use of extractor fans positioned so that they do not exhaust directly onto any passers-by. Air-conditioning units may also be installed, but the correct location of their vents and adequate system maintenance are crucial to prevent the risk of passers-by contracting legionnaire's disease. Units that use recycled air are not recommended for the dental workplace, as they will allow any airborne contamination to cross-infect other persons.

Where nitrous oxide gas is used during inhalation sedation, the waste gas must be removed by a suitable scavenging system to prevent the build-up of harmful levels of the gas in the surgery.

Conscious sedation is covered in Chapter 14.

In summary, then, adequate ventilation is essential to prevent the accumulation of hazardous vapours and gases, and therefore to minimise any risk of harm from them. This is particularly relevant to dangerous or irritant vapours from mercury, some disinfectants, nitrous oxide and some laboratory chemicals.

The temperature within the dental workplace is usually maintained by the central heating system in cooler months and by adequate ventilation throughout the summer. While the minimum working temperature should be no less than 16°C, there is no maximum temperature above which work should stop. However, higher temperatures usually allow for a greater volume of vapours, gases and fumes to develop, so in warmer periods the ideal is to maintain a temperature of around 20°C – this is called 'room temperature'.

Disinfectants

With the major emphasis on robust infection control in all healthcare environments nowadays, exposure to many types of disinfectant is the norm throughout the working day for all staff. Some disinfectants can irritate skin, airway and eyes when used carelessly, while others can cause irritation or initiate hypersensitivity or even allergic reactions in staff no matter how low their exposure to the disinfectant. PPE consisting of gloves, mask and glasses should be worn when handling them and working areas must be well ventilated to avoid irritation of the airway. Manufacturers' instructions must always be followed, in particular the first aid advice recorded in the COSHH file in the event of an accident.

Occupational hazards are covered later in the chapter.

Reporting of Injuries, Diseases and Dangerous Occurrences Regulations (RIDDOR) 1995

Accidents that occur in the workplace fall into one of two categories.

- **Minor accidents** – these result in no serious injury to persons or the premises, and are dealt with 'in house'. A written record of the minor accident must be made and kept in the accident book, under the Notification of Accidents and Dangerous Occurrences Regulations (Figure 4.10). Examples of minor accidents include a trip or fall resulting in no serious injury, a clean (non-infectious) needlestick injury or a minor mercury spillage that can be safely dealt with using the spillage kit.
- **Major accidents** – these result in a serious injury to a person or severe damage to the premises. They are classed as 'significant events' and are therefore *notifiable incidents* that must be reported to the HSE.

Notifiable incidents do not include those occurring to a patient while undergoing dental treatment but do cover all persons on the premises otherwise. Once notified, the HSE will carry out an investigation into how the incident occurred, to determine whether it was purely an accident or whether the practice or a staff member was at fault. Advice will then be given on how to avoid similar incidents in future, but in serious cases prosecution may follow.

Dental nurses should remember that once qualified and registered with the GDC, they are personally responsible for their own errors and acts of omission under Health and Safety law so it may be that they are the ones who are prosecuted. While in the dental workplace as a student, the trainee dental nurse is under the supervision of a more senior colleague and that senior person will be the one held accountable for any event under RIDDOR. The only exception to this would be if written records proved that the trainee had received the correct training in Health and Safety issues but had knowingly and blatantly disregarded them, resulting in the occurrence of the notifiable incident.

Once completed tear along perforation and store securely. '
Report Number

Accident Report Book

1 Person affected/injured

Name

Home Address

Postcode

Occupation   Works No.

2 Person reporting the incident - if other than injured person

Name

Home Address

Occupation   Postcode

Department   Date   /   /

3 Accident/incident

❦ Date   /   /   Time

❦ Place/Room

❦ Equipment/machinery involved

4 Description of incident - including cause and nature of injury

Action taken/recommendations

Signed   Date   /   /

Employer please initial box if accident reportable under RIDDOR
(Reporting of Injuries, Diseases and Dangerous Occurences Regulations 1995)

Figure 4.10   Accident book page.

The significant events covered by the regulations fall into one of three categories – injuries, diseases and dangerous occurrences. Further information is available at www.hse.gov.uk/riddor.

As with any other workplace, the occurrence of an accidental injury is a rare event in the dental world but nevertheless they can and do happen. Minor injuries, as discussed above, are handled 'in house' as they result in no serious harm to any persons. However, major injuries do result in serious harm or even death to the casualty.

The **injuries** that must be reported are as follows.

- Fracture of the skull, spine or pelvis.
- Fracture of the long bone of an arm or leg.
- Amputation of a hand or foot.
- Loss of sight in one eye.
- Hypoxia (oxygen deprivation to the brain) severe enough to produce unconsciousness.
- Any other injury requiring 24-h hospital admission for treatment.

The dental team may be exposed to common diseases in the workplace on a daily basis from patients (such as with simple colds or chest infections) or they may be exposed away from the workplace; in this case they are at risk of transmitting the infection to others in the workplace themselves. Dental personnel are also at risk of exposure to more serious pathogens by direct contact with infected blood and saliva from patients, and particularly by receiving an inoculation injury. The risk of infection by airborne diseases is increased significantly when the workplace is inadequately ventilated or poorly temperature controlled, and by cross-infection when the workplace is inadequately cleaned.

The **diseases** that must be reported under RIDDOR are any that cause acute ill health by infection with dangerous pathogens or infectious materials, such as:

- *Legionella* – causing legionnaire's disease
- hepatitis B or C infection – both linked to the development of liver cancer
- HIV – causing acquired immunodeficiency syndrome (AIDS).

In the hospital environment or when treating those with poor personal hygiene, dental personnel may also be exposed to, or even transmit, other dangerous pathogens such as methicillin-resistant *Staphylococcus aureus* (MRSA – referred to as one of the 'super-bugs' by the public) or *Clostridium difficile* (an intestinal micro-organism associated with diarrhoea and tetanus).

A dangerous occurrence is a significant event that could result in serious injury or death to anyone on the premises. It would result in the attendance of the emergency services (ambulance, fire and/or police) as well as specialists in service provision, depending on the cause (gas, electric, service engineer, environmental health officer, etc.).

The **dangerous occurrences** that must be reported are as follows.

- Explosion, collapse or burst of a pressure vessel (an autoclave or compressor).
- Electrical short circuit or overload that causes more than a 24-h stoppage of business.
- Explosion or fire due to gases or inflammable products that causes more than a 24-h stoppage of business.
- Uncontrolled release or escape of mercury vapour due to a major mercury spillage (see Chapter 15).
- Any accident involving the inhalation, ingestion or absorption of a hazardous substance which results in hypoxia that is severe enough to require medical treatment.

Most of the dangerous occurrences listed involve a catastrophic failing of an electrically operated equipment item, resulting in a fire or an explosion. Fire is a daily hazard that can occur in any workplace and as discussed previously, a risk assessment of the dental workplace will identify several specific fire hazards.

In addition to the fire potential from chemicals and gases, all dental equipment is electrically operated and may short circuit, malfunction or spark and cause a fire at any time, especially if not serviced and maintained correctly.

Larger electrical items of dental equipment, such as the dental chair and inspection light or autoclaves, have to be serviced and maintained by trained personnel on a regular basis. However, smaller portable items such as curing lights can be inspected for electrical safety by a general electrician or other approved person, in a process known as portable appliance testing (PAT). This should be carried out annually, with each appliance having the plug, fuse size and wiring inspected for wear and tear. If all is well, a sticky label is applied to indicate that the appliance is PAT compliant, and the due date of the next PAT inspection (Figure 4.11). A written record of the testing should be kept in the workplace if the 'other approved person' is a competent dental team member.

It is apparent, then, that RIDDOR should only be relevant when a serious, genuine and unforeseen accident occurs in the dental workplace, as all other incidents should be avoided by the correct instigation of policies and protocols covering the following.

- Waste disposal.
- Ionising radiation.

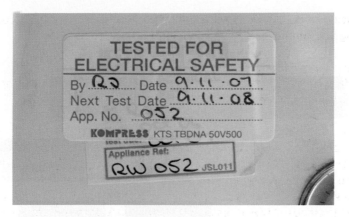

Figure 4.11   PAT inspection label.

- Recognition and management of occupational hazards.
- Infection control (see Chapter 8).
- Safe use of conscious sedation techniques (see Chapter 14).

Special Waste and Hazardous Waste Regulations 2005

Waste disposal

The safe storage, disposal and classification of waste have undergone several reviews and updates over the last 10 years. Yet more variation in terminology used occurs between the four countries of the UK as well as with that used in the Republic of Ireland, making this whole Health and Safety topic a difficult one to grasp for the trainee dental nurse.

During the time of compiling this text, a change in waste classification has occurred from the previous one shown in Figure 4.12, with which most students will be familiar. The previous dental workplace waste categorisation was split between three main areas – domestic waste, non-hazardous waste and hazardous waste. The final category was then split further into infectious waste and special waste, with various subcategories for each, as illustrated in Figure 4.12.

In addition, the guidance currently in place for the management of healthcare waste in hospitals and community dental workplaces may be different at a local level than that applying to dental practices. The information given in this section is correct at the time of writing but students are advised to check the relevant legislation affecting waste management in their area by accessing the following website: www.environment-agency.gov.uk for England and Wales or the equivalent agencies in Scotland, Northern Ireland or the Republic of Ireland. Further information may be available at www.opsi.gov.uk.

The current legislation and regulations apply to all healthcare waste producers, which includes all dental workplaces. Healthcare waste is of particular concern for environmental and personal safety because, by its nature, it is likely to be contaminated with body fluids or body parts and therefore poses a risk of cross-infecting anyone who handles it. This may be dental personnel or waste management contractors as well as the public, if it is not disposed of safely.

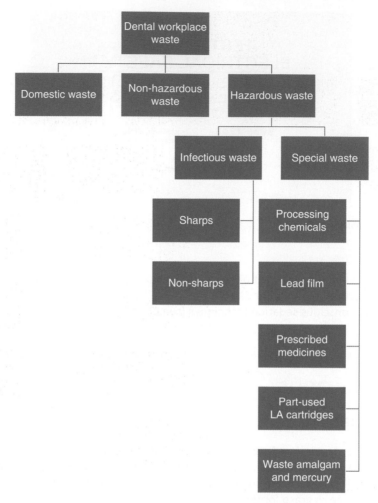

Figure 4.12 Old hazardous waste flowchart.

Some waste produced in the dental workplace will pose a greater risk of cross-infection, while other waste is hazardous by its chemical nature and possible toxicity. All must be correctly segregated, safely stored, and then handed over to a licensed waste contractor to be disposed of in a suitable manner.

Waste classification

Dental workplaces produce a wide range of both hazardous and non-hazardous wastes, and in order to segregate the waste correctly, it must first be identified and then classified in line with the current regulatory guidance. The legislation that sets out which wastes must be classed as hazardous is contained in the Special Waste and Hazardous Waste Regulations (2005).

The guidance in current use in England is based on the information contained in Appendix 1 (Waste Disposal) of the government's *Health Technical Memorandum 01-05* (HTM 01-05). Modified versions of this document are in use in Northern Ireland and Wales, while Scotland has its own system of compliance guidance. In addition, those providing dental treatment in a hospital or

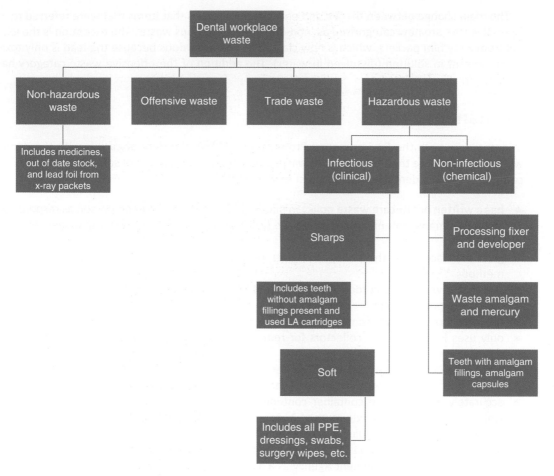

Figure 4.13   New hazardous waste flowchart.

community setting may be subject to local arrangements for the management of healthcare waste, which may have regional variations too.

The current classification of waste produced in the dental workplace (rather than that shown previously) is shown in Figure 4.13, with four broad types requiring segregation and storage on the premises. The new categorisation is divided between four main areas – non-hazardous waste, offensive waste, trade waste and hazardous waste. The final category is then split further into infectious (clinical) and non-infectious (chemical) waste, with subcategories for each, as illustrated in Figure 4.13.

Offensive waste is defined as 'wastes which are non-infectious, do not require specialist treatment or disposal but may cause offence to those coming into contact with it'. In the dental workplace this will include any PPE, cleaning towels, x-ray films and other similar items that have not been contaminated with body fluids, medicines, chemicals or amalgam, as well as toilet hygiene waste.

Trade waste includes items such as dental equipment (dental chairs, curing lights, portable suction units, etc.), as well as commercial electronic waste like computer screens, televisions, fluorescent lighting tubes and batteries.

The main change between the old and new classifications is that items that were referred to as 'special waste' are now categorised as 'non-infectious hazardous waste'. The exception is the lead foil from x-ray film packets, which is now classed as non-hazardous because the lead is only toxic when present in solution (dissolved in water). The addition of the offensive waste category has occurred in all workplaces.

Waste management

In accordance with the Environmental Protection Act 1990, the duty of care is with the dental workplace to ensure that its healthcare waste is managed and disposed of safely and correctly. To comply fully, every dental workplace must ensure that it:

- has a written healthcare waste policy in place which identifies a named person as responsible for waste management on the premises (referred to as the 'registered manager' in HTM 01-05)
- gives staff access to the policy, and gives recorded training in correct waste management methods
- segregates waste in accordance with Figure 4.13 and stores it safely while on the premises, away from public access
- uses the correct storage containers for each waste category – see later
- only uses licensed waste collectors for removal and disposal of the waste at an authorised disposal site
- accurately describes the container contents of all non-hazardous waste on transfer notes, which must be kept for a minimum of 2 years from the date of collection
- accurately describes the container contents of all hazardous waste on consignment notes, which must be kept for a minimum of 3 years from the date of collection
- receives and keeps the quarterly 'consignee returns' documentation which records the final destination of the hazardous waste consignment, and its disposal details
- registers with the Environment Agency as a hazardous waste producer if more than 500 kg of hazardous waste is produced annually.

Waste storage

For quick and easy identification of each category of waste produced in the dental workplace, various colour-coded containers are used to help segregate the various items. In addition, on all documentation the European Waste Catalogue (EWC) codes should be used; however, details of these codes are not relevant to the student dental nurse.

Details of the storage containers to be used are as follows.

- Offensive waste – yellow sack with black stripe, tied at the neck.
- Non-hazardous medicines and out of date stock – blue-lidded yellow rigid container (Figure 4.14).
- Soft infectious (clinical) hazardous waste – orange sack, no more than three-quarters full and tied at the neck (Figure 4.15).
- Sharps infectious (clinical) hazardous waste – all-yellow rigid container, no more than two-thirds full (Figure 4.16).
- Non-infectious (chemical) hazardous waste:
    ○ processing chemicals – separate securely lidded, rigid containers (Figure 4.17)

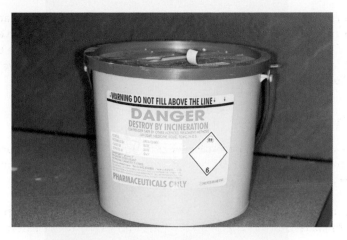

Figure 4.14   Blue top sharps box.

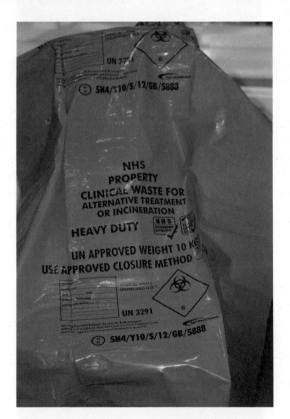

Figure 4.15   Orange hazardous waste sack.

- ○ waste amalgam/mercury – white, securely lidded container with a mercury vapour suppressant sponge insert (Figure 4.18)
- ○ amalgam-containing teeth and spent capsules – white, securely lidded containers with a mercury vapour suppressant sponge insert (Figure 4.19).

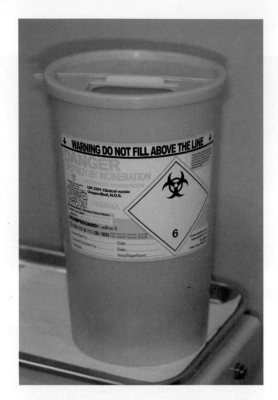

Figure 4.16   Sharps box.

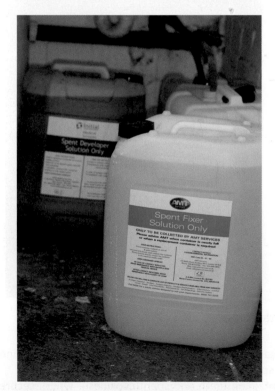

Figure 4.17   Processing chemical waste drums.

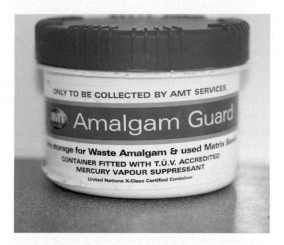

Figure 4.18   Waste amalgam tub.

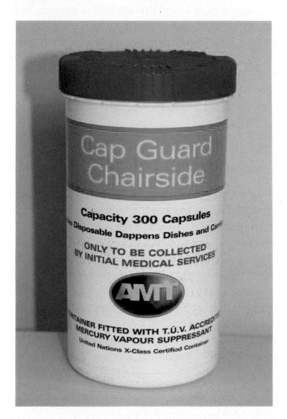

Figure 4.19   Waste amalgam capsule tub.

Waste handling training

All dental personnel who are likely to be involved in handling any healthcare waste must be correctly trained to do so. The training should cover all of the following points.

- Risks associated with each category of waste (such as sharps injury, exposure to toxic vapours, cross-infection, etc.).
- Correct classification, segregation and storage procedures, in line with the healthcare waste policy of the workplace.
- COSHH information on all non-infectious hazardous waste chemicals used on the premises.
- Safe handling, including the use of appropriate PPE and moving techniques.
- Correct procedures in the event of spillages or accidents.
- Correct completion of relevant documentation – transfer notes and consignment notes.

Ionising radiation legislation

The type of ionising radiation used in dentistry is that of x-rays, to produce images of teeth and their surrounding structures so that a diagnosis can be made and treatment carried out. However, despite its valuable uses, ionising radiation presents a hazard to the whole dental team, their patients and the general public.

X-rays cannot be seen, heard or felt, and therein lie the dangers as it can easily be forgotten that they are potentially hazardous to health. There is no 'safe' level of use – every exposure can cause some amount of tissue damage in the patient, or in anyone else in the imaging area that is exposed to the x-ray beam. An overdose can cause serious health effects, ranging from a mild burn to leukaemia and ultimately death.

For this reason, specific legislation is in place to ensure full compliance with the Health and Safety aspects of ionising radiation by all dental workplaces, under the following regulations.

- Ionising Radiation Regulations 1999 (IRR99)
- Ionising Radiation (Medical Exposure) Regulations 2000 (IR(ME)R2000)

While IRR99 is concerned with the protection of staff and IR(ME)R with the protection of patients, the aim of both sets of regulations is to keep the numbers of x-ray exposures, and their dose levels, to the absolute minimum required for clinical necessity, at all times. This principle is referred to as keeping radiation levels 'as low as reasonably achievable' (ALARA) or 'as low as reasonably practicable' (ALARP). This applies not only to the actual direct x-ray beam that is fired at the patient during the film exposure, but also to the 'scattered radiation' that inevitably occurs during this process. Scattered radiation, as its name suggests, is that which bounces off tissue cells during exposure in an uncontrolled manner, and can re-expose the patient several times over, thereby increasing their actual radiation dose.

In the dental workplace, three simple factors required for the ALARA/P principle to be achieved have helped to reduce by 40% the amount of scattered radiation that is created during a dental exposure.

- Use of 'fast' films – F-speed intraoral films require the shortest possible exposure time to create the radiographic image, once processed.
- Short exposure time – achievable with a combination of modern x-ray machines, fast films and fast intensifying screens in extraoral cassettes.
- Rectangular collimator tubes – these have replaced the old plastic aiming cones of intraoral machines, and provide a paralleled x-ray beam as it leaves the tube end, rather than a disorganised 'spray' effect with lots of scattered rays. The rectangular tube end has the same dimensions as a standard intraoral film too (Figure 4.20).

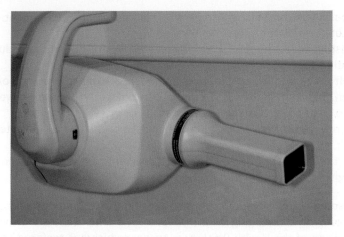

Figure 4.20   X-ray machine collimator.

Dental radiography and its use as an important diagnostic tool in oral health assessment is covered in detail in Chapter 12, while the Health and Safety aspects of its usage are covered here.

Compliance with IRR99

This set of regulations is concerned with the safety of staff in the dental workplace where ionising radiation is used, as well as the correct functioning of the radiation equipment, and the initial act of compliance is to inform the HSE of its use on the premises. This must be carried out whenever a dental workplace begins to use ionising radiation for the first time, and with each change of ownership thereafter.

Three formal appointments must then be made by the workplace owner.

- **Legal Person** – a designated person who ensures the workplace's full compliance with both sets of regulations (this is usually the employer).
- **Radiation protection advisor (RPA)** – a medical physicist who is appointed in writing by the dental workplace, and is available to give advice on staff and public safety in relation to both sets of regulations.
- **Radiation protection supervisor (RPS)** – a designated person within the workplace who can assess risks and ensure precautions are taken to minimise them, in accordance with IRR99 (this is usually a senior dentist or a DCP with a postregistration qualification in dental radiography).

The role of the RPA is to give advice on the actions the workplace must take to comply with both sets of regulations, and will cover the following points.

- The correct installation of all new x-ray machines.
- The regular maintenance and certificated checks that are required for each x-ray machine to ensure that the minimum exposure to radiation occurs.
- The contingency plans that need to be in place in case of a malfunction of an x-ray machine.
- The investigation of any malfunction of an x-ray machine.
- The designation of a 1.5 m controlled area around each x-ray machine and within the primary beam direction, where no-one but the patient may be present during an exposure.

- Advise on risk assessments with regard to restricting staff and patient exposure to ionising radiation, and review the assessments every 5 years.
- Advise on the necessary staff training required so that designated duties are carried out competently and safely.
- Assess staff protection with regard to the numbers of exposures carried out on the premises; if more than 150 intraoral films or 50 dental pantomographs are taken weekly, staff are legally required to wear a personal monitoring badge.
- Advise on the appropriate action to take if analysis of the badges indicates excessive exposure to any staff.
- Advise on the running of quality assurance programmes so that the principle of ALARA/P is maintained at all times.

The Legal Person is responsible for organising a 3-yearly assessment of radiation safety within the workplace. This involves arranging for an inspection by a competent authority such as the Radiation Protection Division of the Health Protection Agency (which has replaced the previous authority, the National Radiological Protection Board) or by using the workplace's own x-ray machine and processing test kit to carry out the necessary checks and then sending them to the competent authority for analysis.

In addition, the Legal Person must draw up a set of Local Rules which have to be displayed at each x-ray machine, so that they can be referred to by all staff. The Local Rules must give all of the following information.

- The name of the designated RPS and RPA.
- The identification of each controlled area to all staff and patients, to limit unauthorised entry during exposure; this is usually an area of 1.5 m from the machine head and the patient, and directly in the primary beam of the radiation during exposure. The designation of a 2 m safety zone from the machine head will then ensure that only the patient remains within the controlled area during x-ray exposure (Figure 4.21).
- Show the standard warning sign at each controlled area, indicating the use of ionising radiation – this is a black sign on a yellow background (Figure 4.22).
- A summary of the correct working instructions for each controlled area, including a 'no entry' rule for the designated 2 m safety zone around the x-ray machine head.
- A summary of the contingency plan to be followed in the event of a machine malfunction.
- Details of the dose investigation level.
- The use of a red light and an audible buzzer to indicate the actual exposure time.
- The arrangements in place for the safety of pregnant staff.

The role of the RPS is to carry out the following.

- Ensure all staff have suitable training according to the level of their legal responsibility.
- Carry out risk assessments with regard to restricting radiation exposure.
- Ensure the Local Rules remain current, or are updated as necessary.
- Maintain the contents of the necessary radiation protection file.
- Organise and run quality assurance programmes in relation to the safe use of ionising radiation.
- Organise and run quality control tests, or delegate the tests to suitably trained staff.
- Can also be made responsible for ensuring that all staff receive the necessary hours of continuing professional development (CPD) in relation to dental radiography, as it is one of the core subjects for all qualified staff working in the dental surgery environment.

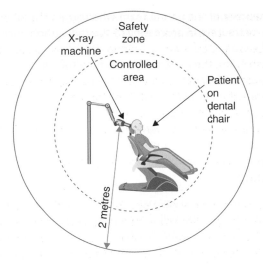

Figure 4.21   Safety zone and controlled area.

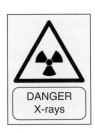

Figure 4.22   Radiation warning sign.

Compliance with IR(ME)R2000

This set of regulations is concerned with the safety of patients in the dental workplace, and with their protection during exposure to ionising radiation. They are of most concern to those dental personnel who have the qualifications and legal right to actually expose the patient to ionising radiation – that is, the dentist and any DCP holding a recognised dental radiography qualification. The regulations are therefore of less importance to the trainee dental nurse, and consequently only the basics are covered here.

Roles and responsibilities

The regulations set out the responsibilities of the various dental personnel who may be involved in taking and processing radiographs within the dental workplace, and restricts those responsibilities by referring to each category with specific appointment titles.

- **Referrer** – the dentist who refers the patient for radiation exposure, either to themselves or to another dentist or specialist dental radiographer who can carry out that exposure.
- **IR(ME)R practitioner** – the dentist or specialist dental radiographer who takes responsibility for *justifying* the taking of the radiograph, by determining that the diagnostic benefits gained will outweigh the risks of the exposure to the patient.

- **Operator** – any member of the dental team who carries out all or part of the practical duties involved with the exposure and processing of the radiograph, including:
  - ○ patient identification
  - ○ positioning of the film, the patient, the machine tube head
  - ○ setting the exposure controls
  - ○ pressing the exposure button
  - ○ processing the film
  - ○ evaluating the quality of the radiograph
  - ○ carrying out test exposures for quality assurance purposes
  - ○ running quality assurance programmes.

Except in the hospital setting, then, only a dentist can be a referrer and/or an IR(ME)R practitioner. Therapists and hygienists are likely to have undertaken study and qualification in dental radiography as part of their training course, and will therefore be able to carry out all of the above duties as operators. With suitable and authenticated training, or qualification, the dental nurse can also carry out a variety of duties under the title of 'operator', as shown in Table 4.3.

The table lays out the various duties involved in the exposure of patients to ionising radiation in the dental workplace, and the processing of the images into radiographs. The four other columns then identify which duty can be carried out by each level of experienced dental nurse, from those holding a postregistration qualification in dental radiography, through a qualified registrant to

Table 4.3   Details of duties allowed to operators

Duty	Radiography qualified DN	NEBDN qualified DN	NVQ qualified DN	Trainee DN
Patient identity	√	√	√	√
Positioning	√	No	No	No
Setting exposure	√	No	No	No
Pressing exposure button	√	√ in the presence of the 'set-up' operator	√ in the presence of the 'set-up' operator	√ in the presence of the 'set-up' operator
Processing	√	√	√	√
Quality audit	√	√	√	√
QA test exposures	√	√ in the presence of the 'set-up' operator	√ in the presence of the 'set-up' operator	√ in the presence of the 'set-up' operator
QA programmes	√	√	√	√

DN, dental nurse; NEBDN, National Examining Board for Dental Nurses; NVQ, National Vocational Qualifications; QA, quality assurance.

a trainee dental nurse. It can be seen that there is no difference between the final three categories – there is no suitable 'extended duties' training that will allow any additional duties to be carried out by a registered or 'in training' dental nurse. The risk of potential harm to a patient and others from unnecessary exposure to ionising radiation is so great that only further specialised qualification is recognised as enabling a qualified dental nurse to carry out the additional duties of positioning the patient and setting the exposure. While all categories can press the exposure button, only those dental nurses holding the dental radiography qualification can do so unsupervised.

A dental nurse holding the basic, register-able qualification will have received documented training in the majority of these duties throughout their training course, supplemented by documented 'in-house' training in any additional duties allowed (under the GDC *Scope of Practice* document) within the workplace. Similarly, the trainee dental nurse must receive the same documented training to be allowed to carry out any of the duties listed above.

The ability of suitably trained personnel to 'press the button' during radiation exposures is of great help in reducing cross-infection risks, as the 'set-up' operator would otherwise contaminate the exposure button unless they repeatedly removed and replaced their gloves between setting up and retrieving each film from the patient's mouth.

The medico-legal importance of all personnel receiving adequate, documented training in these operator duties cannot be stressed too highly.

Patient protection

The IR(ME)R is mainly concerned with the protection of patients while undergoing ionising radiation exposure in the dental workplace, so that they are not exposed unnecessarily and so that all exposure levels are as low as possible, to reduce the chance of any tissue damage occurring. The key points covered are summarised below.

- **Patient identification** – of particular importance when the referrer is not also the IR(ME)R practitioner, as occurs when patients are referred to hospital. To avoid the wrong patient being exposed, name, address and date of birth should be used as a minimum.
- **Referrer and IR(ME)R practitioner** – can only be dentists (unless the patient is referred to a specialist dental radiographer), as only they have the training to determine when an exposure is required for diagnosis and treatment, and when the exposure is justified.
- **Justification** – the benefit of exposing the patient should outweigh the risk of causing tissue damage, so every exposure should be expected to provide new information to help the patient's treatment or prognosis as a minimum requirement, otherwise it should not be undertaken.
- **Optimisation** – the dose of radiation should be kept as low as reasonably achievable/practicable (ALARA/P) at all times; this topic is discussed in detail in Chapter 12.
- **Pregnant patients** – routine dental exposure techniques do not irradiate the pelvic area and involve such low doses that pregnancy is not considered a contraindication to irradiation, and for similar reasons, lead aprons are also not required.
- **Staff training** – written evidence of all necessary training pertinent to ionising radiation techniques must be kept for all personnel in the radiation protection file, as documented proof of their competence in the duties that they undertake.
- **Quality assurance** – QA programmes and audits provide a valuable tool in determining whether the systems in place to protect patients (and staff) from any potential harm from ionising radiation are actually working, by looking at the procedures, the results achieved, and analysing any problems encountered so that policies and techniques can be suitably adjusted and updated where necessary.

- **Accidental exposure** – all x-ray machines must have an isolation switch outside the controlled area, an illuminated control panel or switch to indicate when the mains power is on, and an additional light and an audible buzzer that are activated during the exposure time itself. If a machine malfunctions during use, it will then be obvious by the lights and buzzers, and the mains power can be switched off without the operator having to enter the controlled area.

Radiation protection file

Effectively, this acts as a summary document that holds as much information as possible about the procedures in place to ensure radiation protection within the particular workplace, and should be reviewed and kept updated annually to ensure that it remains relevant and effective. It should contain all of the following information and have references included for any information that is kept elsewhere (such as qualification and relevant training details that are kept in personnel files).

- Formal appointments of staff on the premises – including referrers, IR(ME)R practitioners and all operators (with details of the range of their duties).
- Reference to the initial risk assessment carried out by the Legal Person, in consultation with the RPA.
- Local Rules for each x-ray set on the premises.
- Procedures for ensuring patient protection, as required under IR(ME)R.
- Information on how ALARA/P is achieved.
- Details of protocols followed in relation to justification and authorisation of exposures (usually referenced to the GDP booklet *Selection Criteria for Dental Radiography*).
- Details of protocols followed in relation to clinical evaluation of radiographs (so written notes are kept of each radiograph taken and what the findings were).
- Details of QA programmes to ensure consistently accurate radiographs, including their frequency and the named persons who run them.

Quality assurance of films

All the faults that may occur during the taking or processing of a radiograph, which may result in the patient having to undergo a retake, are avoidable. However, it may not be realised by the dental team that a recurring problem exists unless radiographs are regularly checked for quality, and this is especially so in large, multi-dentist workplaces. A processing fault may affect the radiographs of several dentists but unless someone is analysing the radiographs from all surgeries, it can easily be overlooked. This is the purpose of a quality assurance system, in which all radiographs are analysed and scored according to a universal system of quality so that commonly occurring problems will be identified.

With suitable training, a QA system of radiograph analysis can easily be run by the dental nurse, the aim being to reduce all faults to a minimum or to eliminate them completely. Indeed, in line with the relevant ionising radiation legislation and with clinical governance, the running of a QA system in dental workplaces is now a legal requirement.

The types of faults that may occur during the exposure, handling and processing of radiographs are detailed in Chapter 12. To protect both patients and the dental team from unnecessary ionising radiation exposure, it is everyone's duty to ensure that the occurrence of these faults is kept to a minimum or eliminated completely. To do this involves assessing the quality of the films processed to determine the following points.

- How readable is the film?
- Is a fault present?

- What is the fault?
- How has it occurred?
- How can it be prevented from recurring?
- Is re-exposure of the patient necessary?

When run correctly, the QA system should achieve the following results.

- Involve a simple-to-use scoring system that is understood and followed by all staff.
- Easily identify any areas of concern.
- Develop solutions to the problems identified.
- Limit the number of patient exposures to the minimum required for clinical necessity.
- Therefore, to achieve ALARA/ALARP.

A simple-to-use scoring system set out in clinical governance guidelines is as follows.

- **Score 1 – excellent** quality radiograph with no errors present.
- **Score 2 – diagnostically acceptable** quality, minimal errors present that do not prevent the radiograph from being used for diagnosis.
- **Score 3 – unacceptable quality**, where errors present prevent the radiograph from being used for diagnosis, and will therefore involve a retake.

Score 1 should be at a minimum of 70% of all exposures, while score 3 should be at a maximum of 10%. The results need to be easily recorded after every exposure so that they can be analysed on a regular basis and any problems identified.

A typical recording system is shown in Figure 4.23. The simple record sheet shows, at a glance, all the information required to enable a retrospective QA audit of the workplace

Date	Operator	Patient ID	Radiograph	QA score	Details
4.4.12	DTH	4173	L/R BWs	1 and 1	N/A
4.4.12	JM	854	PA UL6,7	2	Coned, unable to use holder
5.4.12	TNL	1559	DPT	1	N/A
5.4.12	DTH	6212	PA UR2	1	N/A
5.4.12	CSH	377	AO-maxilla	2	Elongated but canines visible
6.4.12	JM	5458	L/R BWs	1 and 2	R BW coned
6.4.12	TNL	905	PA UL4	3	Missed apex for endo - retake
6.4.12	TNL	905	PA UL4	1	N/A

Figure 4.23   Quality assurance radiograph record sheet.

radiographs to be carried out. As the operator is identified (by their initials), the audit can be used to track the performance of individuals, while the identification of the views used (detailed in the fourth column) also allows an audit of each type of radiograph to be carried out. The final column should give the information required to explain the QA score of 2 or 3 that has been awarded in each case, so that trends can be identified. For example, if an operator takes periapical radiographs without using a holder and regularly scores 2 or 3 due to coning or elongation, the audit will identify that this is a recurrent problem and that it can be resolved by the suitable use of film holders. Similarly, when all radiographs begin to score 2 or 3 due to poor processing from a certain date onwards, it may indicate a faulty machine or that the processing chemicals are spent.

A similar QA system can be set up to monitor other areas of dental radiography, such as equipment, working procedures or staff training.

Dangers of ionising radiation

X-rays cannot be seen, heard or felt, and therein lie the dangers of their use. As they cannot be perceived by any of the senses, it is easily forgotten that they are potentially dangerous to health and it is just as easy to ignore every safety precaution. An overdose can give rise to serious health effects, ranging from a mild skin burn to the onset of leukaemia. This is why the special legal requirements described previously are in force for dental workplaces.

In the course of dental radiography the patient never receives an overdose. It is the operator, not the patient, who is most at risk, as the former is continually taking x-rays and must therefore take strict precautions to avoid their own accidental exposure.

- Radiation safety must be checked at least every 3 years to ensure that x-ray sets are adequately shielded to prevent stray radiation and that processing equipment and procedures are satisfactory. All sets must have regular professional maintenance.
- Use of the fastest film (E and F speed) will allow the shortest possible exposure time. Indeed, there is no justification for using anything but the fastest available film. Cassettes should be fitted with the fastest (rare earth) intensifying screens.
- Plastic aiming cones on x-ray sets are no longer acceptable and must be replaced by rectangular collimator tubes to further reduce beam size to the safest level.

This combination of fastest film, shortest exposure and narrowest beam will alone reduce the amount of scattered radiation by 40%. In addition:

- the special film-holder/beam-aiming devices should be used for periapical and bite-wing radiographs, and the paralleling technique used in preference to the bisecting angle method
- the operator must stand well clear of the x-ray beam during exposure, at the full length of the cable on the time switch; this should be not less than **2 m**. On no account must a dental nurse hold the film in place for a patient; if a child cannot keep still during the exposure, the parent must hold the film packet in place and wear a protective lead apron
- exposure of the reproductive organs to x-rays has produced abnormalities in the offspring of laboratory animals. Similar exposure of humans may occur from scattered radiation during dental radiography. Although it is insufficient to produce such genetic changes in the case of pregnant dental patients, any possibility can be excluded by strict adherence to all the required safeguards
- every radiograph must not only be necessary but also of diagnostic value. There should be no need for retakes because of faulty technique or processing. Retakes mean unnecessary

additional exposure of patients and staff. To ensure perfect results the films must be in good condition, taken correctly, processed carefully and mounted properly
- x-ray sets should be disconnected from their electricity supply when not in use
- the amount of stray radiation received by staff can be checked by means of a film badge. This is an intraoral film which is worn at waist level for up to 3 months. It is then processed to indicate whether an excessive dosage is being received. If so, expert advice must be sought immediately to trace and eliminate the cause. Staff working in rooms adjacent to the surgery should also wear badges as x-rays can pass through walls.

Film badges are called personal monitoring dosemeters and details of suppliers are available from the Radiation Protection Division (RPD) of the Health Protection Agency or a local medical physics department. The RPD will process the badges, notify the dosage received and can arrange appropriate investigation if it is too high.

Occupational hazards

By definition, occupational hazards are those that a staff member may encounter during their normal working day, due to the nature of the work that they carry out while in the workplace. Those that are specific to the modern dental workplace may include all of the following.

- Exposure to ionising radiation (see above and Chapter 12).
- Cross-infection and inoculation injuries (Chapter 8).
- Exposure to hazardous chemicals, in particular:
  - mercury (see below and Chapter 15)
  - acid etchant (see below and Chapter 15)
  - sodium hypochlorite and other disinfectants (see below and Chapter 8)
  - nitrous oxide (Chapter 14).
- Exposure to hazardous waste (see above).
- Exposure to lasers, curing lamps and tooth whitening lamps.
- Use of display screen equipment such as computers.

Most of these occupational hazards are covered elsewhere in the text, but several are summarised here to help convey the importance of their safe use and the potentially serious consequences of their misuse.

Hazardous chemicals

Mercury

Mercury is a liquid metal that is mixed with various metal powders to form dental amalgam – this is a material used to fill teeth. It is classed as a hazardous substance because it is toxic, and it can enter the body in the following ways.

- **Inhalation** – toxic vapours are released from uncovered sources at room temperature and above, and are particularly hazardous because they are colourless and odourless and therefore difficult to detect.
- **Absorption** – particles can be absorbed through the skin, nail beds and eye membranes, and eventually become lodged in the kidneys.

- **Ingestion** – particles can contaminate foodstuffs and drinks, and be taken into the digestive system and eventually lodge in the kidneys.

Dental amalgam is still the material most commonly used to fill teeth, so mercury is present in significant amounts in the majority of dental workplaces. Exposure to the hazards mercury poses cannot easily be avoided, but the risks can be minimised by following simple rules designed to limit the chances of staff contact.

Inhalation

- Ensure that the workplace is adequately ventilated and kept at a reasonable working temperature, so that fumes do not build up.
- Avoid placing mercury and waste amalgam near heat sources (including sunny windowsills), as more fumes are given off at higher temperatures.
- Use capsulated amalgam so that bottles of mercury do not have to be stored on the premises.
- Store all waste amalgam in special sealed tubs containing a mercury absorption chemical (see Figure 4.18).
- Similarly, used amalgam capsules must be stored in special sealed tubs, as it is likely that tiny amounts of mercury will remain in them after use (see Figure 4.19).
- Ensure every trace of amalgam is removed from instruments before they are sterilised in the autoclave, otherwise fumes will be released as the autoclave heats up.
- If a mercury spillage occurs, wear appropriate PPE including a facemask, to avoid inhalation.

Absorption

- Always wear the correct PPE when handling amalgam capsules and waste amalgam, to avoid skin, nail and eye contact.
- Open-toed shoes must not be worn in the surgery area, to avoid absorption through the feet if any amalgam or mercury is spilled.
- Always wear safety goggles or a face visor when old amalgam fillings are being removed, so that stray specks do not enter the eyes.
- If a mercury spillage occurs, wear gloves and safety goggles to avoid skin or eye contact.

Ingestion

- Food and drink must never be consumed in the surgery environment.
- Stocks of mercury and amalgam capsules must not be stored within the staff rest room.
- Waste amalgam containers must not be stored within the staff rest room.

Handling of mercury spillages

The use of capsulated amalgam products will limit the likelihood of a large mercury spillage, but the capsules themselves can rupture during use, releasing liquid mercury into the environment although on a much smaller scale.

All spillages of mercury, no matter how small, must be reported to the senior dentist and recorded in the workplace accident book (see Figure 4.10). This will provide a written record of any accident or incident that has occurred on the premises, and that could have potentially harmed someone. It must include details of the following:

- the date and location of where the accident/incident occurred
- who was affected
- the names of any witnesses
- details of the accident/incident
- actions taken to assist those affected.

In the unfortunate event of any long-term health effects, this report will provide valuable evidence about whether correct procedures were followed, and whether the accident/incident was unavoidable or not.

If mercury is spilled, it tends to form into liquid globules or small balls. In this shape, the liquid can easily roll around and be difficult to pick up; indeed, larger globules often break into smaller ones when attempts are made to handle them. The correct actions to take after a mercury spillage are therefore very important, to prevent further contamination and spread into the workplace environment.

If a small spillage occurs:

- wear suitable PPE
- suck up small globules into a disposable plastic syringe or a dedicated bulb aspirator (Figures 4.24 and 4.25)
- put the particles into the waste amalgam special waste container.

Never use the dental suction unit or the cleaning hoover to suck up spilt mercury – their use will release toxic mercury vapours into the workplace. Alternatively, the lead foils present in intraoral x-ray film packets can be used to gather the globules together and scoop them up.

To avoid the release of small globules into the workplace, the amalgamator machine should have a lid on and be stood on a foil tray to collect any spillages without them contaminating the workplace (Figure 4.26). Any globules collected by these methods can be simply tipped into the waste amalgam store.

If a larger spillage occurs:

- wear suitable PPE
- open windows to ventilate the area

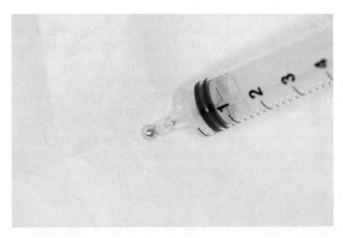

Figure 4.24   Droplets of mercury.

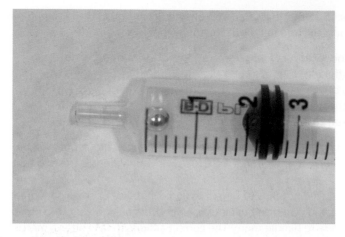

Figure 4.25   Droplet collection in syringe.

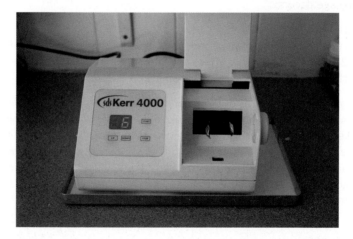

Figure 4.26   An amalgamator.

- inform senior staff
- use the contents of the mercury spillage kit to control the spread of the spillage (Figure 4.27)
- mix the powders of flours of sulphur and calcium hydroxide with water to make a paste, and paint this around the spillage to contain it
- the remaining paste can be painted over the spillage
- once dry, the contaminated paste and spillage are wiped up thoroughly with damp paper towels, and disposed of in the waste amalgam store.

If the size of the spillage is significant, such as a full bottle of mercury, or if globules have rolled into inaccessible areas, the work area must be sealed off and closed down. The HSE must be informed of the spillage and Environmental Health will attend to clear away the contamination professionally and safely.

Acid etchant

This material is used during the placement of composite (tooth-coloured) fillings. As the name suggests, it is acidic and can therefore chemically burn soft tissues, such as within the patient's

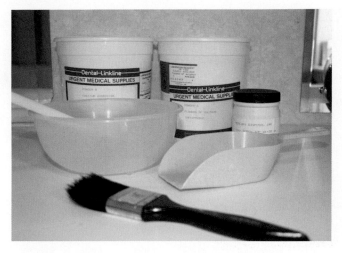

Figure 4.27   Mercury spillage kit.

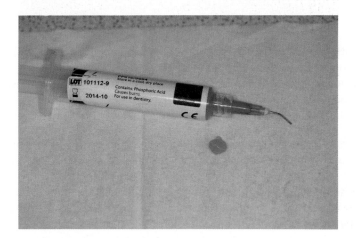

Figure 4.28   Acid etchant gel.

mouth or the skin of those handling the substance. The material itself is 33% phosphoric acid, in either a liquid or gel form (Figure 4.28).

All staff handling the etchant must be wearing the correct PPE, and when placed within the patient's mouth, it must be confined to the tooth undergoing restoration. Very careful aspiration must be used while the material is washed off the tooth, so that it does not fall elsewhere and burn the patient's oral mucosa. To aid this, the acid etchant is usually brightly coloured so that it is easily visible – some manufacturers produce a bright pink liquid, others a bright blue gel, for instance. The manufacturer's instructions for use will show the necessary symbol indicating a hazardous substance, and will provide details of the first aid actions to take if an accident occurs, in accordance with COSHH regulations.

Bleach (and other disinfectants)

All disinfectants have a major role to play in the decontamination of work areas and fixed equipment in the dental practice (see Chapter 8). Bleach, which is sodium hypochlorite, is used in many situations.

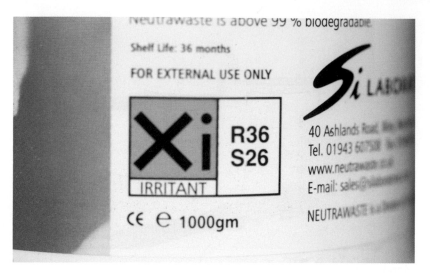

Figure 4.29   Hazardous substance label.

- Fresh solution of 10,000 parts per million (ppm) (approximately 1%) to disinfect all non-metallic, non-fabric surfaces within the surgery.
- Fresh solution (as above) to disinfect impressions and removable prostheses before transferring between the patient and the laboratory.
- Fresh solution (as above) to clean away blood spillages within the surgery.

Other disinfectants used for surface and laboratory item decontamination include a variety of antimicrobial and isopropyl alcohol solutions, often also sold as spray solutions or presoaked wipes.

Bleach has an unpleasant taste and smell, and is chemically irritant to soft tissues. It can cause tissue damage to the mouth and digestive tract, the eyes and lungs if strong vapours are inhaled. Appropriate PPE must be worn whenever it is handled, and fresh solutions made daily for the uses indicated above should be held in lidded containers, so that the noxious chlorine vapours do not become overpowering.

Disinfectant bottles of any solutions used will show the necessary hazardous substance symbol, and give the necessary first aid actions in the event of an accident, in line with COSHH regulations (Figure 4.29).

Lasers, curing lamps and tooth whitening lamps

These devices have various uses in the dental workplace but all can cause harm, especially to the eyes, if they are not used in a safe manner.

Lasers

These devices generate an intense narrow beam of light or other electromagnetic radiation that can be used as a cutting tool on hard and soft tissues, such as teeth and oral soft tissues. The danger they pose is that they can damage the eyes if viewed directly, and can burn other tissues if the beam used is too intense.

Figure 4.30   Laser warning sign.

They are categorised into four classes (1–4) depending on the increasing amount of damage that they can cause, and those used in dentistry are usually in the more powerful classes 3 and 4. There is no specific legislation relevant to the use of lasers but general safety legislation will apply (including Health and Safety at Work Regulations), and as always the employer will be expected to have carried out a risk assessment before the devices are used.

In a similar fashion to the use of ionising radiation in the dental workplace, the use of lasers in class 3 and 4 should include the following.

- Access to a Laser Protection Advisor (LPA) with a similar role to the RPA where x-rays are used.
- An appointed Laser Protection Supervisor (LPS) with a similar role to the RPS, as above.
- A set of Local Rules, including a controlled area with limited access during use, methods of safe working, register of authorised users, etc.
- Provision of an isolation switch in case of emergency.
- Use of a warning symbol outside each controlled area (Figure 4.30).

The use of lasers is still relatively limited in the dental workplace.

Curing lamps and tooth whitening lamps

These devices use blue halogen bulbs as their electromagnetic radiation light source. While they are less damaging to the eyes than a laser beam, they can still cause retinal damage if viewed without the required orange-tinted safety glasses or the orange-tinted safety shield. Both the patient and the dental team must use the appropriate eye protection while either of these devices is being used.

Display screen equipment

The use of computers in the dental workplace is now commonplace and the majority of staff will access patient details and workplace information via a computer on a daily basis. Problems may arise when the staff member has to sit viewing a screen for prolonged periods of time, so employers are required to make certain provisions under the Health and Safety (Display Screen Equipment) Regulations, to avoid muscle strain, fatigue, eyestrain and headaches.

A risk assessment should be carried out to determine who is likely to suffer from these problems, and how they can be prevented. Simple points to be considered are listed below.

- Adequate training for staff, including correct posture and the use of any devices to prevent problems occurring.
- Workstation issues – adequate space to work, including leg room, correct adjustable seating, mouse pads with wrist support where necessary, foot rests where necessary.
- Computer screen issues – adjustable contrast and brightness controls, use of anti-glare screens where necessary, clean screen, use of suitable font that is easy to read.
- Regular breaks from the workstation, so that muscles and eyes have relaxation periods.
- Eyesight tests for staff who experience headaches and eyestrain, and the provision of spectacles specifically for display screen work if necessary.

The cost of eyesight tests and any spectacles required exclusively for display screen work should be borne by the employer.

General safety measures

These relate to any work premises where staff are employed to provide a service to the public, and therefore apply to all dental workplaces, whether they are practices, clinics or hospital departments. The measures listed are all common-sense precautions aimed at preventing injury to anyone using or visiting the premises.

- A safe means of entry which is adequately lit and unobstructed, including for disabled people.
- Non-slip floor coverings which are secure, to prevent tripping.
- No dust traps in the décor of surgical areas, such as those present with embossed wallpaper coverings.
- No sharp edges on furniture and fittings.
- Guards around fires and heaters to avoid burns.
- No trailing electrical cables that could cause tripping.
- All portable electrical appliances must be inspected yearly for wear and tear problems – this is called PAT testing, and may be carried out by any approved person as long as written records are kept.
- All electric appliances should be disconnected overnight as a matter of routine, although this may not be possible with some items such as a fridge or the main computer server.
- A fully stocked first aid kit should be available for minor injuries.

Manual handling

The other important area of general safety for staff is that involving any moving or lifting work, which may cause personal injury if not carried out correctly. This is collectively referred to as manual handling.

In the majority of dental workplaces, the usual manual handling that occurs is the transport of boxes containing stock items or the movement of waste containers in and out of storage. Hospital departments and dental clinics may also require staff to be involved with the movement of disabled, sedated or unconscious patients too, and separate and specific training must be given in these areas by the employer.

Lifting heavy or awkward items incorrectly can result in all kinds of injuries to staff and employers must ensure that, as far as reasonably practicable, they adhere to the Manual Handling Operations

Regulations 1992. These were further revised in 2002, and state the following.

- All hazardous manual handling should be avoided, as far as is reasonably practicable.
- Any hazardous manual handling that cannot be avoided must be correctly risk assessed.
- All efforts must then be made to reduce the risk of injury as far as possible.

While carrying out the risk assessment of any manual handling and lifting that has to be carried out in the dental workplace, the following points must be considered when deciding whether the task is hazardous or not.

- The weight and dimensions of the object being moved or lifted.
- The likelihood of staff having to reach, bend, twist or stoop while moving or handling the object.
- The frequency of the task.
- The likelihood of excessive movements being required, such as pushing or pulling.
- The distance that the object has to be moved.
- The need for the object to be carried up or down stairs.
- The physical ability of the staff involved in moving and handling.
- The existence of any medical conditions that contraindicate staff from moving or handling objects (this includes pregnancy).
- The need for any training to be given in the correct techniques of moving and handling.

If each point is taken separately, it can be seen that much can be done to avoid injury to staff during moving and handling activities.

Weight and dimensions

The heavier the load and the greater its dimensions, the more difficult will be its handling and the more likely injury will occur, so consider the following points.

- Split the load to make it lighter.
- Ask other staff to help while lifting and moving it.
- Use a trolley or other handling aids, if available.

Awkward movements and frequency

Examples include twisting and bending while lifting or moving a load, and the more times the move is carried out, the more likely it is to cause injury, so consider the following points.

- Clear the path of travel before lifting, to avoid having to twist.
- Move the feet to change direction, rather than twisting the body.
- When precise positioning is required, put the load down and then adjust its position.
- When loads have to be moved frequently, use a trolley or other handling aid to avoid straining the back.

Excessive movements

Pushing and pulling lighter loads is not usually a problem, but when heavier loads are involved they must either be split into smaller units first or a trolley or other handling aid must be used.

In most instances, large boxes of stock can be opened and put into their place of storage individually, to avoid having to push or pull them into position.

Distance and stairs

It makes sense to move objects the minimum distance whenever possible, and to avoid having to carry them up and down stairs manually. The place of storage for stock should be carefully considered, to avoid repetitive strain injuries to staff, and a lift must always be used if available. Otherwise, a trolley or other handling aid needs to be provided.

Physical ability and medical conditions

Elderly or unfit staff are more likely to injure themselves while moving and handling, by overestimating their own capabilities, and the following must be considered.

- Elderly staff tend not to be as strong as younger staff, and may have less stamina to hold a load for any length of time.
- Overweight staff will find it difficult to hold loads as close to their centre of gravity as they need to for stability, and this will put unnecessary strain on their arms and back.
- Short staff will lift and carry loads less easily than taller staff.
- Male staff tend to be stronger than female staff, although this cannot be assumed.
- Various medical conditions will prevent some staff from being capable of moving and handling objects without risking injury to themselves, such as back problems, heart and respiratory conditions, hernias, etc.
- Pregnant staff should not be involved in moving and handling heavy objects.

Training

A correct handling technique should be taught to all staff involved in moving and lifting objects in the dental workplace, and this may involve:

- sending the staff (and the employer) on a well-run training course to learn the best posture to adopt while lifting and moving loads
- acquiring trolleys and other handling aids for the premises
- changing the location of storage rooms, to make them closer to the delivery point and ideally at ground level
- acquiring more storage cupboards or shelves at waist height for heavier items
- acquiring step ladders for the placement of light loads in storage spaces above shoulder level.

General security measures

Although it is unlikely that dental practices will have just one or two members on the premises during normal working hours, this situation can occur during holiday times or when several staff are attending courses so no patient appointments are set. In the interests of staff safety, it would be advisable for the premises to be locked during these times so that staff are not left vulnerable and open to attack.

All employers have a responsibility to maintain the security of the workplace premises and the safety and security of their staff. In addition, all staff have a responsibility to uphold the security procedures that have been put in place by their employer, to ensure that the safety of the workforce and the security of the premises are never compromised.

Maintaining security during the day

Security of the premises and safety of the staff during the day are achieved by ensuring that the premises are only accessed by those who have a right of entry. This is more difficult to achieve in large hospital departments and dental clinics than it is in general practice, where the majority of people attending are regular patients who are known by the staff. However, procedures must be in place to ensure that all visitors to the premises have to pass through a reception point, so that they can be seen and identified by staff. Several methods can be used to achieve this.

- Locked entry point with a speaker phone.
- Fire exits that can only be opened from inside the premises.
- Entry way that has to pass directly through reception, so that all visitors have to report there.
- CCTV system.
- Trained staff manning reception at all times, with an appointments system in place to identify any unexpected visitors to the premises.
- Security screening in place so that the reception area cannot be breached.
- Panic button in case any threatening behaviour occurs.

When expected visitors attend, such as booked patients, maintenance or repair workers, or stock sales representatives, they will be checked off against the appointment book and then usually held in the reception waiting area.

Patients will have appointment details to be confirmed, while other visitors will have usually phoned to book their attendance with a staff member. In any instance, the following should be the norm to eliminate the risk of any violence towards staff.

- Ensure all staff are trained to be caring and sympathetic towards patients.
- All visitors to the workplace should be treated with respect, and spoken to courteously.
- This is especially important when a patient attends unexpectedly, or without an appointment, and highlights the need for a robust dental emergency policy to be in place.
- Ensure all staff are aware of the practice protocols in relation to assault and violence towards themselves.
- Ensure all patients are aware of these too – this should be nothing less than a statement of 'zero tolerance' in cases of violence towards staff.

While working at reception, it is important that all cashboxes or tills are out of the reach of other persons and are locked unless in actual use. This reduces the risk of opportunistic thieves attempting to steal from the premises.

Similarly, all patient records, whether written or computerised, must be held securely and out of view of anyone attending the premises – the confidentiality of patient details is a legal requirement in the dental workplace. Filing cabinets or the record storage room should be locked at the end of each day, and computer records should be password protected. In larger dental workplaces, passwords are often only given to senior staff members.

Staff rooms should not be accessible to anyone except staff, and can be made so by the use of locks or security code entry systems. Ideally, lockers should be provided for all staff too, so that valuables and personal belongings are never at risk of being stolen.

Maintaining security out of hours

It is of great importance that the dental workplace is always securely locked when not in use. Not only are expensive portable items of equipment on the premises, but also drugs, syringes and needles, which may attract break-ins by drug users, for instance. In addition, the security of patient records and the data protection of their contents must be maintained at all times.

Several methods of maintaining the security of the premises are available.

- Adequate alarm system in place, which is ideally manned by a security company, so that unusual entry times or alarm activation can be acted upon immediately.
- Only senior staff should be given the alarm code, to reduce the number of persons who may open the premises.
- Similarly, key holder numbers must be kept to a minimum.
- The loss of a key by any member of staff must be reported to the employer immediately.
- All keys must be handed in when staff leave their employment.
- Ensure that alarms are set correctly at the end of each day, so that break-ins are detected immediately.
- Change the alarm code on a regular basis, and ensure that only senior staff are notified of the new code.
- Ensure that all monies are banked daily, to remove the incentive for opportunist burglary.
- Ensure that all doors are locked and bolted at the end of each day, especially the fire exits.
- All windows should have locks on them, and be closed and locked at the end of each day.
- Ground-floor windows are usually required to have metal screens placed over them by insurance companies.
- Most dental employers will have a policy to limit staff access to the premises to their normal working hours only, and this must be upheld by all.

 Further resources are available for this book, including interactive multiple choice questions and extended matching questions. Visit the companion website at:

www.levisonstextbookfordentalnurses.com

5

General Anatomy and Physiology

Key learning points

A **factual knowledge** of

- the normal structure and function of the human body
- the circulatory system and associated medical conditions relevant to the dental team
- the respiratory system and associated medical conditions relevant to the dental team
- the digestive system and associated medical conditions relevant to the dental team
- the nervous system and associated medical conditions relevant to the dental team

Dental nurses must have a good underpinning knowledge of the normal structure and function of the human body, and especially of the oral cavity and its surroundings, to be able to understand the subjects of human health, the processes involved in the onset of human disease, and the methods available to prevent disease or to treat it when already present.

The anatomy and physiology of the head and neck structures and the oral cavity are discussed in detail in Chapters 9 and 10 respectively. This chapter deals with the anatomy and relevant physiology (that is, the functioning) of the main organ systems, to provide the necessary underpinning knowledge and understanding of the human body as a whole in relation to dentistry and dental nursing.

Levison's Textbook for Dental Nurses, Eleventh Edition. By Carole Hollins.
© 2013 John Wiley & Sons, Ltd. Published 2013 by John Wiley & Sons, Ltd. Companion website: www.levisonstextbookfordentalnurses.com

Definitions

The scientific discipline that deals with the life processes of living organisms is called *biology*. The study of the structures of the human body and their relationships to one another is called *human anatomy*, and the study of how the body actually functions is called *human physiology*.

The subject of anatomy covers not just the gross structure of the human body – muscles, bones, organs, etc. – but the equally important microscopic structures of the cells and tissues themselves that make up these gross structures. The microscopic anatomy of the tissues is not relevant to this text, but is covered in detail for those interested in *Basic Guide to Anatomy and Physiology for Dental Care Professionals*.

Cell biology

The basic unit of living organisms is the cell, and all (except red blood cells) contain a nucleus that holds the individual genetic material (DNA) that makes each of us unique. The DNA is held as chromosomes which separate and duplicate during cell division and growth.

Most cells are specialised in their roles and actions, and perform certain functions within the body. When similar specialised cells are grouped together to carry out these particular functions, they are called tissues. Groups of tissues that perform different functions are called organs – such as the heart or the liver – while those that have related functions are called systems – such as the digestive system or the respiratory system.

There are four basic types of cell in the human body.

- **Muscle cells** – these generate forces and produce motion; they may be attached to bones to allow limb movement or enclose hollow cavities so that their forces cause expulsion of the cavity contents (such as the movement of food through the digestive tract).
- **Nerve cells** – these can initiate and carry electrical impulses to distant areas of the body along their length to produce many actions, such as to cause muscle cells to contract or glands to release chemicals or fluids in the body (such as the salivary glands).
- **Epithelial cells** – these cover the body surface as skin or surround organs or line hollow structures within the body; they act to separate areas of the body from each other and from the external environment, to prevent the uncontrolled movement of harmful micro-organisms.
- **Connective tissue cells** – these connect various parts of the body together by anchorage and support, as in the whole bony skeleton and tendons and ligaments, and also contain the specialised connective tissue cells making up the blood and lymph systems.

All these cells require a source of fuel to produce the energy they need to work and carry out their individual functions, and this fuel is provided by the food that we eat. The energy it contains is released for use by the cells by the action of food digestion in the digestive system, and is used for any of the following actions.

- Maintain body temperature above or below that of the surroundings – this is called *homeostasis*.
- Produce movement to allow food gathering, and therefore the production of more energy.
- Allow reproduction to occur, for the survival of the species.

In addition, the body cells require oxygen to be able to burn the food eaten to produce the energy they require to function. Oxygen is brought into the body through the respiratory system, and transported around the body to every cell that needs it by the circulatory system.

Table 5.1   The body systems

System	Composed of	Functions
Cardiovascular	Heart, blood vessels, blood	Transport of blood to lungs for oxygenation Transport of oxygenated blood to body Transport of deoxygenated blood back to lungs
Respiratory	Nose, throat, larynx, trachea, lungs	Exchange of oxygen and carbon dioxide between the body and the atmosphere
Digestive	Mouth, salivary glands, pharynx, oesophagus, stomach, intestines, pancreas, liver, gall bladder	Digest, process and absorb nutrients from food Excrete waste products
Nervous	Brain, spinal cord, nerves, sensory organs	Give consciousness Regulate and co-ordinate body activities
Musculoskeletal	Bone, cartilage, tendons, ligaments, joints, skeletal muscle	Support and protect internal organs Allow movement
Immune	White blood cells, lymph, spleen, bone marrow, thymus	Defend against infection Produce red and white blood cells
Endocrine	All glands that secrete hormones	Regulate and co-ordinate body functions
Urinary	Kidneys, ureter, bladder, urethra	Regulate blood plasma Excrete waste products
Reproductive	Male or female sex organs	Reproduction
Integumentary	Skin	Protects against injury and dehydration Maintains body temperature

The human body has 10 organ systems, each with various components and specific functions to allow the continuation of life, as shown in Table 5.1. The 10 body systems are identified in the first column, with those of particular relevance to the dental nurse listed as the first four. The second column identifies the structures that make up that system, while the third column states the function(s) of the system as a whole. These functions help to illustrate how the systems work together to enable the body to work effectively and maintain life. So for example, the circulatory system is responsible for the transport of oxygen around the body but the cells that actually carry it are made by structures within the immune system.

The four main body systems of relevance to the dental nurse are the circulatory system, the respiratory system, the digestive system and the nervous system.

Circulation

The main component of the circulatory system is the heart, a muscular pumping organ situated in the thorax (chest cavity). It is connected by blood vessels to every tissue in the body, and carries out the following actions.

- Pump oxygenated blood from the lungs to the body tissues so that they can work.
- Collect deoxygenated blood from the body and transport it to the lungs where the waste products it contains are excreted, by being breathed out.

The heart has four chambers within its structure; the upper two are called the atria and the lower two are the ventricles. The atria and ventricles are separated by one-way valves that allow blood flow in the direction of atria to ventricles only, and the left and right sides of the heart also have no communication between them. The right side of the heart transports only deoxygenated blood, from the body to the lungs, while the left side of the heart transports only oxygenated blood, from the lungs to the rest of the body again (Figure 5.1).

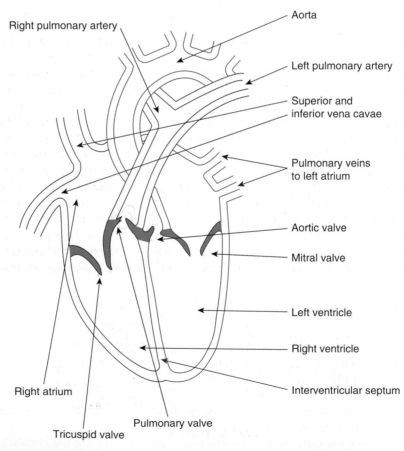

Figure 5.1   Gross anatomy of the heart.

Action of the heart

Deoxygenated blood is collected from the whole body through the veins and transported to the right atrium via the inferior and superior venae cavae. As the heart beats, it pumps this blood through the one-way valve between the two right heart chambers (tricuspid valve) and into the right ventricle. The next beat pumps it out of the right ventricle and into the pulmonary artery where it passes to the lungs for reoxygenation.

Once oxygenated, the blood returns to the left atrium through the pulmonary vein, then it is pumped through the one-way valve (mitral valve) into the left ventricle. The next heartbeat pushes this blood out of the heart into the aorta, and then back around the whole body to reoxygenate all the cells and tissues and allow them to continue their normal functions.

The heartbeat itself begins on the top surface of the right atrium in a group of specialised muscle cells called the sinoatrial node or *pace-maker*. These cells receive electrical stimulation from two sets of nerves from the brain; one set speeds up the rate of the heart beat and the other set slows it down. In this way the heart rate is regulated to allow both exercise and rest as necessary. After each heartbeat, the blood is prevented from flowing backwards again by the one-way valves within the heart itself, which snap shut as the blood pressure increases within the successive heart chambers.

Circulatory system

The circulatory system is an enclosed loop of blood vessels, with the heart at its centre. The blood vessels taking oxygenated blood around the body are the arteries, the largest of which is the aorta, and these gradually decrease in size away from the heart to become arterioles and then capillaries. The capillaries are just one cell thick, and this allows the oxygen that they carry to be released into the surrounding tissues so that it can be used to burn food nutrients and create energy.

As oxygen passes out of the capillaries, the waste product of the energy production – carbon dioxide – passes from the surrounding tissues into the capillaries. This gas exchange process is called internal respiration (Figure 5.2). The deoxygenated blood then travels from the capillaries into small veins called venules, then into larger veins until it reaches the heart in one of the largest veins, the venae cavae. Deoxygenated blood from the upper body is transported to the superior vena cava, and that from the lower body to the inferior vena cava. This is the systemic circulation.

At the same time, and with each heartbeat, the deoxygenated blood in the right side of the heart is pumped to the lungs through the pulmonary artery (the only artery to carry deoxygenated blood). Here, the carbon dioxide is released into the lungs to be breathed out while oxygen that has been breathed in travels from the lungs into the blood capillaries, so that the blood is

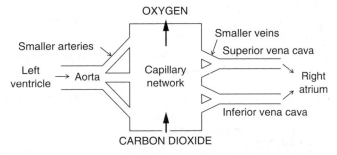

Figure 5.2   Internal respiration.

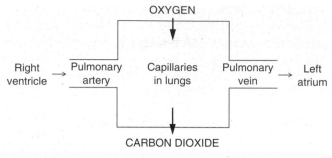

Figure 5.3   External respiration.

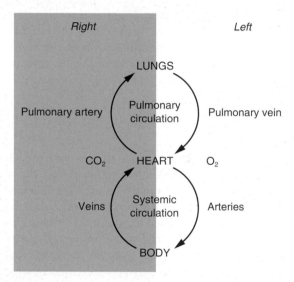

Figure 5.4   Circulation (deoxygenated blood shaded blue).

reoxygenated again. This gas exchange is called external respiration (Figure 5.3). The oxygenated blood is then transported to the left side of the heart in the pulmonary vein (the only vein to carry oxygenated blood) so that it can then be pumped back around the body. This is the pulmonary circulation (Figure 5.4).

Blood vessels

When the blood leaves the heart in the arteries, it is under greatest pressure as a result of the heartbeat, so the walls of the arteries are elastic to allow them to expand as the powerful surge of blood passes along them. Once the initial wave of the pumped blood has passed, the artery walls relax back to their normal size again until the next heartbeat. This difference in pressure within the arteries can be measured and recorded as a person's blood pressure. The maximum pressure of the blood in the arteries occurs during the peak of ventricular contraction, or *systole*, while the minimum pressure occurs at the end of ventricular contraction, or *diastole*.

So, blood pressure is recorded as systolic pressure over diastolic pressure, and in a healthy adult at rest it is usually around 120/80 millimetres of mercury, and is measured using a

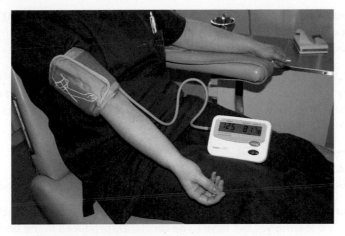

Figure 5.5   Measuring blood pressure.

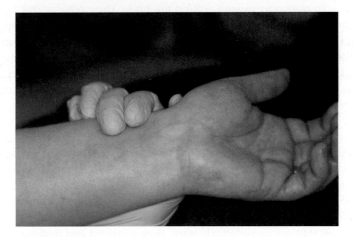

Figure 5.6   Taking the radial pulse.

sphygmomanometer and a stethoscope, or an automated device (Figure 5.5). Also, when the artery passes over bone, the blood surge can be felt as the pulse at various sites around the body.

- **Carotid pulse** – at either side of the neck where the carotid arteries lie across the neck vertebrae, and above the surrounding muscles.
- **Brachial pulse** – at the inner surface of the elbow where the brachial arteries lie over the elbow joints.
- **Radial pulse** – at the inner surface of the wrists as the radial arteries lie over the radius bone of the lower arms (Figure 5.6).
- **Femoral pulse** – at the top of the inner thighs as the femoral arteries lie over the femoral bone of the upper legs.

In comparison to the arteries, the veins contain little elastic tissue. It is not required because the pressure of the blood surge is greatly reduced by the time it reaches the venous side of the circulatory system, as it is so far away from the source of the heartbeat. Indeed, the larger veins contain one-way valves along their length to prevent the blood from flowing backwards between heartbeats, in a similar action to that of the valves within the heart itself.

Blood

The circulatory system is filled with about 5 litres of blood in an adult, and it is regulated and kept at a temperature of around 37°C by the process of homeostasis. It consists of several cell types floating in a straw-coloured fluid called plasma.

- **Erythrocytes** – red blood cells.
- **Leucocytes** – white blood cells.
- **Platelets** – thrombocytes, which are fragments of larger blood cells called megakaryocytes.

Erythrocytes are biconcave disc-shaped cells (like a doughnut) with no nucleus, so they cannot divide and replace themselves but have to be constantly produced in the body by the red marrow of certain bones, such as the pelvis and the spinal vertebrae.

Their lack of nucleus and their shape provide the maximum space available for them to carry out their main task – to transport oxygen around the body. They achieve this by attaching oxygen to the red pigment they contain – haemoglobin. As discussed previously, oxygen is vital to all cells to be able to produce energy and carry out their various functions. It is picked up by the erythrocytes in the capillaries of the lungs during external respiration, transported around the body by the circulatory system to wherever it is needed, and then released into the tissues during internal respiration. The presence of the red iron-based protein haemoglobin within the erythrocytes gives blood its characteristic red colour. When the haemoglobin is bound to oxygen molecules, as in arterial blood, it has a bright cherry-red colour, and when there is little oxygen present, as in venous blood, it has a dark reddish-purple colour.

Leucocyte is the collective name for a group of several cells that are mainly concerned with defending the body against attack by micro-organisms and disease. They are made in several areas of the immune system, such as the lymph nodes and bone marrow, and circulate throughout the body at all times. However, when the body comes under attack from micro-organisms, massive numbers of leucocytes pass around the circulatory system to the area of disease, and then squeeze through the capillary walls to the body tissues that are under attack. Here, they surround and destroy the micro-organisms so that the disease is stopped from spreading. In very severe infections, the leucocytes are helped to destroy the invaders by the presence of antibodies released from the body's immune system.

Platelets (or thrombocytes) also contain no nucleus, as they are just separate fragments of a larger blood cell found in the red bone marrow. Platelets are concerned with the coagulation of blood at the site of injury to prevent excessive blood loss. They achieve this by physically helping to plug damaged blood vessels by acting as a meshwork for the successful formation of a blood clot, as well as by releasing powerful chemicals that assist further in clot formation.

Plasma is the fluid part of the blood that carries the blood cells within it. It consists of about 90% water, with powerful chemicals called plasma proteins floating within, as well as the three types of blood cells. Plasma acts as the transport system of the body, by carrying numerous cells and chemicals from one area to another as they are needed. A summary of its functions is as follows.

- Transport of erythrocytes to allow oxygenation of the body tissues.
- Transport of waste carbon dioxide, dissolved in the plasma, from the body tissues to the lungs for exhalation and removal from the body via the respiratory system.
- Transport of digested food nutrients from the digestive system to the body tissues, for use as fuel to create energy.

- Transport of waste products from these cells to the kidneys, where they are filtered out as urine which is then excreted from the body through the urinary system.
- Transport of leucocytes to the site of any micro-organism attack, to allow the body to defend itself from disease.
- Formation of antibodies and antitoxins from special plasma proteins called globulins, which help the body resist against more severe infections.
- Transport of powerful chemicals called hormones, from the glands where they are made to the area of the body where they are required.
- Transport of the plasma protein fibrinogen to the site of any injury, to assist in blood clotting.

Relevant disorders of the circulatory system

Several disorders affecting the circulatory system are relevant to the dental nurse, as they may have an impact on the particular dental treatment offered. They may affect the suitability of local anaesthetics or conscious sedation techniques used, and patients suffering from some disorders may even present as a medical emergency during treatment. The recognition and management of medical emergencies are discussed in Chapter 6.

In particular with disorders of the circulatory system, the disclosure of any of the following points by the patient during medical history taking should be taken into full consideration by the dental team, with regard to the patient's dental treatment.

- **Heart conditions** – any medical condition that affects the efficiency of the heart may prevent it from coping adequately during stressful situations, such as when experiencing pain, anxiety and fearful events like undergoing dental treatment.
- **Blood disorders** – in particular, those blood disorders that prevent adequate clotting of the blood, as the patient may then experience an uncontrolled haemorrhage; also, any disorders affecting the oxygen-carrying capacity of the blood which contraindicates the provision of dental treatment under some types of sedation techniques.
- **Medications** – certain medications may react with some types of local anaesthetics used in dentistry, especially those containing *adrenaline* as a vasoconstrictor, and possible interactions may occur with:
  - thyroxine – for an underactive thyroid gland
  - some antidepressants.
- **Other medications**
  - Hormone replacement therapy (HRT) for menopausal women is often linked to a raised blood pressure, so adrenaline should be avoided.
  - Elderly patients may be on a complicated cocktail of various medications, and the more drugs taken, the more likely an adverse reaction is to occur.
  - Some antihypertensive drugs have an unwelcome side-effect of causing gingival tissue over-growth, or gingival hyperplasia, which can make good oral hygiene levels difficult to achieve.
  - Diuretics given to patients with hypertension act by encouraging fluid removal from the body; unfortunately this can result in reduced salivary flow and the patient will experience a dry mouth, or xerostomia.

Any medication (prescribed or 'over the counter') can be investigated for any potential side-effects or contraindications to dental treatment, by looking them up in the *British National Formulary* (BNF – Figure 5.7). This book is provided to all registered dentists by the Department of Health, and further information on how to receive copies is available at www.pharmpress.com.

The most relevant disorders of the circulatory system are outlined below.

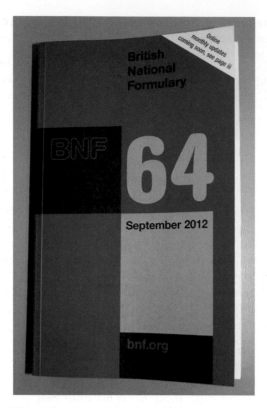

Figure 5.7   *British National Formulary.*

Heart failure

This occurs when the pumping efficiency of the heart itself is inadequate, resulting in its inability to pump enough blood with each beat to allow the body to function normally, and to carry out its normal metabolic activities. It may involve either one of the ventricles or both together.

Heart failure occurs either due to a problem with the heart itself or due to a medical condition that increases the workload of the heart as it pumps blood around the body (that is, something that makes the pumping action less efficient or something that restricts the flow of blood away from the heart, so that more effort is required to achieve blood flow).

Those due to a problem with the heart itself include those listed below.

- **Myocardial infarction** – a 'heart attack', where there is a sudden reduction in the oxygenated blood supply to the heart itself through a coronary artery, often due to blockage by a blood clot (thrombus), and causing a section of the heart muscle itself to die – this is acute heart failure and often (but not always) results in cardiac arrest (the cessation of the pumping action of the heart).
- **Myocarditis** – inflammation of the heart muscle itself, usually as a result of a viral infection.
- **Valvular disease** – affecting any of the heart valves so that the filling or emptying of the heart itself is inadequate, and it has to work harder to overcome the resistance to efficient blood movement that the diseased valve causes.

Those due to a medical condition elsewhere that causes an increased heart workload include the following.

- **Angina** – a condition of myocardial ischaemia (reduced blood flow) caused by the narrowing and partial blockage of the coronary arteries, due to the presence of fatty deposits or athero-matous plaques. This is often referred to as 'coronary artery disease'. When the heart workload increases, especially during exercise or at times of increased anxiety, the narrowed arteries are unable to supply sufficient oxygenated blood to the cardiac muscle, and symptoms similar to (but not as intense as) a heart attack are felt.
- **Renal failure** – kidney failure results in the sufferer being unable to remove sufficient waste fluids from the body (during urination). This fluid retention causes an increased blood/fluid volume which requires more work by the heart to pump it around the body. Eventually, a point is reached where the coronary arteries are unable to supply sufficient oxygenated blood to the cardiac muscle for it to work effectively, resulting in myocardial ischaemia.
- **Hypertension** – raised blood pressure at rest (rather than during exercise) means that the heart has to pump more strongly to move blood from the left ventricle into the aorta and so out to the body tissues, putting a constant strain on the cardiac muscle itself. In some cases the coronary arteries are unable to supply sufficient oxygenated blood, and myocardial ischaemia develops.

All these conditions except myocardial infarction (MI) are categorised as chronic heart failure, as the ineffectiveness of the pumping action of the heart deteriorates over time, rather than occurring suddenly as it does during an MI.

The plaques of fatty cholesterol that become deposited within the coronary arteries of an angina sufferer cause turbulence in the blood flow through these blood vessels. This not only restricts the volume of blood that can flow through them but it also allows any freely circulating platelets to become attached to the fatty deposits, causing the formation of a blood clot inside the blood vessel itself. This clot is correctly called a *thrombus*.

If the thrombus becomes detached from the blood vessel wall, it will naturally be carried by the circulating blood until it becomes trapped at a narrower point in the circulatory system, causing a sudden obstruction of blood to the tissues beyond. Once circulating, the clot is referred to as an *embolus*, and depending which blood vessel is obstructed, the results may be catastrophic.

- **Angina** – partial obstruction of one or more coronary arteries.
- **Myocardial infarction** – full obstruction of one or more coronary arteries.
- **Stroke (cerebrovascular accident)** – full obstruction of an artery supplying the brain.
- **Pulmonary embolism** – full obstruction of one of the pulmonary arteries supplying the lungs, often by an embolus originating as a deep vein thrombus (DVT) in the leg veins.

Cardiac arrest

The sudden failure of the heart to beat at all (asystole) or to beat ineffectively without pumping the blood (fibrillation) is called cardiac arrest, and is often the end result of a myocardial infarction. A cardiac arrest may also occur due to respiratory arrest, electrocution, severe blood loss, anaphy-laxis, drug overdose or for other reasons including severe anxiety – a state that can be seen in some patients who have a profound fear of dental treatment.

Rheumatic fever

This occurs when a patient has suffered a previous illness that has caused damage to the heart valves. Any future episodes of bacteraemia (bacteria in the blood) such as those that can occur following invasive dental treatment, including scaling, can cause inflammation of the inside of the heart (bacterial endocarditis) with possibly fatal consequences. Until recently, these patients were routinely prescribed prophylactic antibiotics at the time of dental treatment, to avoid developing a bacteraemia. However, this is no longer considered necessary unless specifically requested by the patient's cardiologist, as the possibility of the bacteria developing a resistance to antibiotics and being more difficult to control in future is considered more likely than the patient developing a dangerous bacteraemia.

Anaemias

This is a group of disorders that affect the oxygen-carrying capacity of erythrocytes, so that insufficient oxygen is available for use by the body tissues. This may occur due to heavy blood loss, lack of sufficient erythrocyte production by the red bone marrow (including due to iron deficiency), excessive destruction of erythrocytes by the body, or the production of abnormal haemoglobin as occurs in sickle cell anaemia. The ultimate result is that the patient has poor tissue oxygenation, which may result in a simple faint or may be life-threatening if they undergo dental treatment using sedation or general anaesthetic techniques, where the drugs used often reduce the respiratory rate of the patient anyway, so that in combination with an anaemic condition, tissue oxygenation becomes dangerously low.

Haemorrhage

Excessive bleeding may occur in patients with clotting disorders (such as haemophiliacs) or in patients prone to thrombus formation who have been prescribed anti-clotting drugs such as aspirin or warfarin. Patients who have suffered a stroke or a DVT are routinely prescribed these anticoagulants, and it is normal to find that most elderly patients take a low dose of prescribed aspirin too, to avoid a stroke in the first instance. Routine invasive dental treatment in these patients (especially extractions and other surgical procedures) could result in uncontrolled and life-threatening blood loss.

The completion of a comprehensive medical history form and its routine updating at the start of every course of treatment will identify any patients with relevant circulatory medical conditions that require careful consideration by the dental team, to ensure that appropriate treatment is provided safely.

Respiration

The main components of the respiratory system are the two lungs, which are immense air-filled sacks situated in the thorax. The heart lies partially over the upper surface of the left lung (Figure 5.8). The lungs are connected to the external environment by a system of air sacs and tubes deep within their structure called alveoli and bronchioles respectively, which join to larger tubes that ultimately become the two main bronchi, and these in turn connect to the trachea or windpipe (Figure 5.9). This travels up the neck and joins the respiratory system to the atmosphere through the larynx in the throat, which connects to the nasopharynx at the back of the mouth and nose (Figure 5.10).

The functions of the respiratory system are as follows.

- Inhalation of air to provide oxygen for absorption into the circulatory system.
- Expiration of the respiratory waste product, carbon dioxide, from the body.

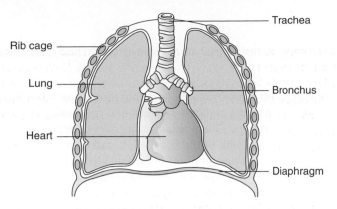

Figure 5.8   The chest.

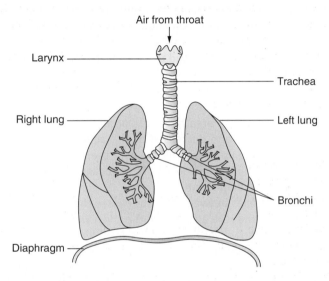

Figure 5.9   Respiratory system.

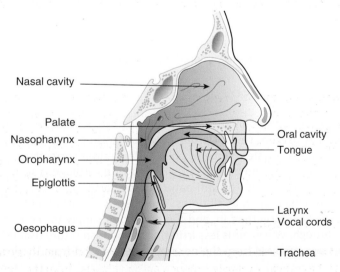

Figure 5.10   Upper respiratory tract.

- Filtering and warming of the inspired air, to remove foreign body particles and prevent irritation of the lung tissues.

The exchange of oxygen and carbon dioxide (external respiration – see Figure 5.3) occurs within the alveoli, which are microscopic air-filled sacs just one cell thick and surrounded by capillaries from the two pulmonary arteries. These vessels transport deoxygenated blood from the whole body to the alveoli, via the right side of the heart. Air breathed in (inspired) from the atmosphere contains around 21% oxygen and tiny amounts of carbon dioxide, while that breathed out (expired) contains around 16% oxygen. The average 5% difference in oxygen levels is used by the body tissues to help produce energy to function. Expired air contains 4% carbon dioxide too.

The deoxygenated blood contains carbon dioxide dissolved in the plasma as a waste product formed when the energy was produced by the body tissues. This gas has no function in the body; indeed, its presence can cause considerable damage to the cells and organs if not removed, so it passes out of the capillaries into the alveoli and is exhaled with each breath. At the same time, oxygen passes from the alveoli into the lung capillaries and binds itself to haemoglobin in the erythrocytes, and is then transported around the body as oxyhaemoglobin.

Breathing

The action of inspiring and expiring – breathing – can occur because the thorax is a sealed chamber whose volume can be increased and decreased by the action of the muscles involved with the chest cavity. The thorax is made up of the ribcage with the sternum (breast bone) between, and connected at the back to the spine. The bottom of the ribcage is sealed from the abdominal cavity by a sheet of muscle called the diaphragm.

The contraction of the muscles between the ribs causes them to expand outwards, pulling the lungs out with them because they are attached to the chest wall. At the same time, the diaphragm contracts and pulls the lungs downwards so that the overall result is an increase in the volume of the chest cavity, and therefore also the lungs that are attached to it. This creates a lower atmospheric pressure within the lungs than that of the surrounding environment and consequently air rushes into the expanded lungs and the process of external respiration occurs. Relaxation of the chest muscles and the diaphragm causes a reduction in the volume of the lungs, and expired air is pushed out of them as the person breathes out.

This process of ventilation occurs approximately 16 times a minute in an adult at rest, with an exchange of about a half litre of air at each breath. Both the rate and depth of breathing increase dramatically during exercise and also when the person is exposed to fearful or anxious situations.

Protective mechanisms

The respiratory system is the only means of supplying the body tissues with oxygen, and as life cannot exist without oxygen, several protective mechanisms have developed as humans have evolved to ensure that the system remains open and functions correctly.

The nose, larynx, trachea and bronchi are all lined with cartilage, a stiff gristly material that is derived from connective tissue. The stiff nature of the cartilage ensures that these areas of the respiratory system remain open at all times. The nostrils are also lined by hairs to trap foreign particles that have been breathed in, and the rich blood supply to the nose helps to warm the air as it passes through. Warm air is less irritating to the respiratory tissues than cold air. Larger foreign particles are removed from the nose by sneezing, and from the lower respiratory tract by coughing.

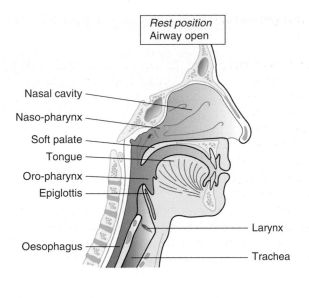

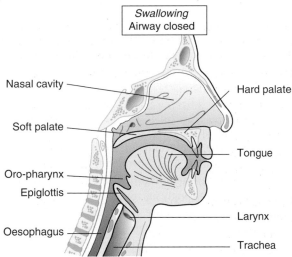

Figure 5.11   Swallowing.

Above the larynx in the throat, the respiratory and digestive systems split off into their own routes, with air passing down the trachea and food and drink travelling into the oesophagus and so to the stomach. A special flap of cartilage called the epiglottis falls across the top of the larynx during the action of swallowing, so closing the trachea momentarily and preventing food or drink from passing into the lungs (Figure 5.11).

In addition, the whole respiratory tract is lined by cells that produce a sticky coating called mucus, and these cells have microscopic hair-like projections called cilia that together trap any finer particles of dust and dirt, and then gently waft them back up the respiratory system away from the lungs and towards the mouth and nose. The foreign particles can then be expelled from the body by coughing or blowing the nose, or they can be swallowed and enter the digestive system to be expelled that way.

Relevant disorders of the respiratory system

Again, several disorders are of relevance to the dental nurse as they may affect the choices available for dental treatment as well as the manner in which the treatment can be provided. In particular with disorders of the respiratory system, the disclosure of any respiratory disease during medical history taking that may compromise the patient's ability to oxygenate their body tissues, or any specific allergies to dental products (such as latex) that may result in breathing difficulties, should be taken into full consideration by the dental team when considering the patient's dental treatment.

The most relevant disorders of the respiratory system are outlined below.

Bronchial asthma

This is a hypersensitivity response to inhaled particles that compromises the patient's breathing by constricting their airways. Asthma attacks can be brought on by anxiety (including the prospect of dental treatment) and can be life-threatening if the airways are not quickly reopened with the use of the appropriate drugs.

Anaphylaxis

Although not strictly a respiratory disorder, the severe allergic reaction of anaphylaxis has a catastrophic effect in shutting down the airways and preventing adequate breathing and tissue oxygenation. Death can occur quickly from either suffocation or cardiac arrest.

Bronchitis

This is inflammation of the bronchi, following a respiratory infection (acute bronchitis) or more usually as a slow-onset disease, especially in smokers and those living in areas of heavy industrialisation (chronic bronchitis). Acute bronchitis sufferers are unlikely to be seen in the dental workplace, as they are often bed-bound with the short-lived illness. In chronic bronchitis sufferers, the airways become increasingly narrowed and copious amounts of sputum are coughed up on practically a daily basis. Sufferers are prone to repeated chest infections, which further damage their respiratory system and compromise their breathing abilities. They are unsuitable patients for treatment under conscious sedation in practice, and should only undergo treatment under general anaesthetic as a last resort.

Emphysema

This condition is characterised by abnormal widening and enlargement of the alveoli, preventing the adequate occurrence of external respiration without the additional help of oxygen supplies. This occurs in response to damage by inhaled pollutants, such as tobacco smoke and industrial fumes and smoke. Bronchitis and emphysema occurring together is called *chronic obstructive airways disease* (COAD).

Inhaled foreign body

This event can occur at any time, but the dental patient is especially vulnerable during treatment, as fine instruments are used and the patient is often lying supine (laid back flat in the dental chair). If a foreign body is inhaled, it tends to fall into the right bronchus as this lies in a near vertical line with the trachea. The patient will exhibit sudden signs of choking as the foreign body passes into the laryngeal region of the throat, and if it passes further into the respiratory system its removal may involve chest surgery. Details of the emergency actions to take in the event of a patient choking are discussed in Chapter 6.

Digestion

The digestive system is composed of the following structures.

- The **mouth** and associated **salivary glands**.
- The **pharynx**, where swallowing occurs.
- The **oesophagus**, which transports food from the mouth to the stomach.
- The **stomach**, where the majority of ingested foods are stored while being broken down for absorption.
- The **small intestines**, where the final stages of digestion and absorption of various nutrients occur.
- The **large intestines**, where digestive waste products are stored before elimination, and water and salts are reabsorbed into the body.
- Accessory digestive organs – the **pancreas, liver** and **gall bladder**.

The oesophagus runs through the thorax and connects the head and neck structures of the digestive system to those lying in the abdominal cavity – from the stomach downwards. The digestive system is more correctly referred to as the *gastrointestinal tract* (GIT), and is illustrated in Figure 5.12.
    The various digestive organs act to:

- break down and absorb the nutrients within food
- transfer these nutrients to the circulatory system for transport to all areas of the body
- detoxify (make less harmful) any substances not required by the body
- remove any solid waste products from the body during defaecation.

All living organisms need food:

- for growth
- for replacement of worn and damaged cells
- as a source of energy to enable normal bodily functions to occur, for the organism to live and survive.

The food we eat cannot be used directly by the tissues to produce energy, but has to be physically broken down and chemically digested into nutrients by the action of powerful chemicals called enzymes. The enzymes involved are very specific for the classes of food eaten, and these classes can be grouped as follows.

- **Proteins** – these are found in meat, fish, eggs, milk, cheese, beans and some cereals; they are necessary for cell growth and repair.
- **Carbohydrates** – these are found in sugars from fruit, vegetables and processed foods, or in starch from bread, cereals and potatoes; they are necessary for cell energy production.
- **Fats** – these are found in meat, milk, cheese and butter from animals or seed and fruit oils from plants; they are necessary for energy production and when stored beneath the skin, they act as insulation against the cold environment and so help to maintain the body temperature.

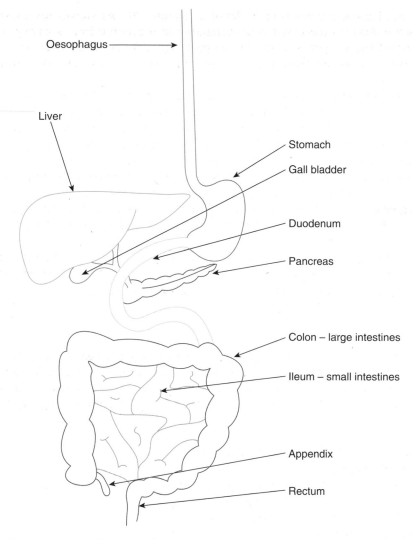

Figure 5.12   Gastrointestinal tract and accessory organs.

- **Vitamins** – several different vitamins are required for health but only in small quantities, specifically vitamins A, B group, C and D.
- **Minerals** – in very small quantities again; specifically calcium, phosphates, fluoride, sodium and iron.
- **Water** – more than 80% of the body is made up of water, and it is required by all cells and tissues for normal bodily functions.

Digestive system

All food and drink enters the body through the mouth, where it is masticated (chewed) by the teeth and mixed with saliva to begin carbohydrate digestion, before being swallowed. The correct term for swallowing is deglutition. The anatomy of the teeth and the biology and physiology of saliva are covered in detail in Chapter 10. As shown previously, swallowed particles are directed towards the oesophagus and prevented from entering the trachea by the action of the epiglottis in the larynx (see Figure 5.11). In a similar way, the particles are prevented from entering the nose by the sealing action of the soft palate across the nasopharynx.

The wave-like muscular action of the oesophagus (called peristalsis) pushes the swallowed foods down the throat, through the thorax (behind the heart and lungs) and into the abdominal cavity to the stomach. The acid and enzymes in the stomach begin digesting any proteins and fats, and removing any iron available for haemoglobin production, before the food passes out into the small intestines, where digestion is completed. The acidic stomach contents (with a pH value of 2) are neutralised by alkaline bile, which is made in the liver and stored before use in the gall bladder. The pancreas also assists digestion by manufacturing and passing various enzymes into the small intestines, where they act on proteins, carbohydrates and fats to aid food digestion. This organ is also responsible for the release of the hormones insulin and glucagon, which control the blood glucose levels in the body.

The indigestible mass that remains at the end of the small intestines is moved by peristalsis into the large intestines, where water and minerals are reabsorbed into the blood before the remaining semi-solid mass is excreted through the rectum during defaecation.

Liver

As the foods are broken down and digested, they are absorbed through the stomach and intestines into the underlying blood capillaries. The capillaries join to become the portal vein which carries the nutrient-rich blood to the liver for storage. The nutrients are then released by the liver as required by the body cells. The liver acts as the chemical factory of the body, and its functions are as follows.

- Storage and distribution of carbohydrates.
- Storage of vitamins.
- Manufacture of bile for fat digestion and neutralisation of stomach acid.
- Manufacture of plasma proteins for the blood.
- Detoxification of drugs and alcohol.
- Disposal of waste products.
- Storage and distribution of iron.

Relevant disorders of the digestive system

In particular with disorders of the digestive system, the disclosure of any of the following points by the patient during medical history taking should be taken into full consideration by the dental team, with regard to the patient's dental treatment.

- **Regurgitation conditions** – any condition likely to cause acid reflux of the stomach contents has the potential to cause enamel erosion of the teeth, in a similar way to consuming acidic foods and drinks regularly.
- **Vomiting** – any medical condition, or pregnancy, that results in regular vomiting over a period of time will have an erosive effect on the teeth.
- **Liver disease** – any medical condition or lifestyle choice (such as high alcohol consumption or drug taking) may affect the ability of the liver to carry out its detoxification role, so that

the effects of any drugs given during dental treatment are increased (potentiated) and/or take longer to wear off.

- **Malnourishment** – any medical condition affecting the ability of the digestive system to absorb nutrients from food, or having a poor diet, may result in the patient becoming malnourished over time so that they may be prone to infections, have poor wound healing abilities, and appear listless and lethargic – this is especially so with elderly patients.

- **Medications** – the use of long-term steroid medication for some digestive conditions may make the patient less able to cope with trauma and stressful situations, as their body's own ability to cope with these events becomes inactivated due to the drugs prescribed; this can result in the patient's collapse during times of anxiety, such as when attending for dental treatment.

The most relevant disorders of the digestive system are outlined below.

Dysphagia

Difficulty in swallowing (dysphagia) is usually due to an actual underlying medical condiditon, including any of the following.

- Dry mouth (xerostomia).
- Mucosal damage due to acid reflux conditions.
- Poor muscular control during swallowing.
- Oesophageal tightening, due to scarring from reflux or from oesophageal tumours.
- Poor nervous control during swallowing, due to a stroke or other central nervous conditions.

Dysphagia does not tend to refer to the intermittent inability to swallow due to psychological reasons, as can occur when the patient is anxious or fearful, especially when taking medicinal tablets, for instance.

Gastro-oesophageal reflux

This regurgitation effect occurs when the stomach contents pass back (reflux) into the oesophagus, and results from an increased abdominal pressure over the thoracic pressure, or when the junction with the oesophagus remains relaxed for extensive periods.

The pressure difference often occurs in the following instances.

- After a heavy meal.
- Eating just before lying down or bending.
- In the late stages of pregnancy, when the size of the foetus displaces the other abdominal contents and pushes against the stomach.

The burning sensation of the acidic stomach contents passing into the oesophagus causes the typical pain of indigestion or 'heartburn'. In severe instances, this can be mistaken for the pain associated with angina or even a heart attack.

Hiatus hernia

The oesophagus passes through the diaphragm to join the stomach in the abdominal cavity at a natural opening called the hiatus.

When a hiatus hernia occurs, the junction of the oesophagus and the stomach moves up through the opening in the diaphragm and becomes trapped there, so that a portion of the stomach is lying above the diaphragm itself, and in the thoracic cavity. This restricts the normal digestive movements and emptying of the stomach, and causes a reflux of stomach contents into the oesophagus. Again, the pain of indigestion will be felt by hernia sufferers, especially after a meal has been taken.

Hiatus hernias usually require surgical intervention to repair the diaphragm.

Gastric ulcers

During normal function, the stomach protects itself from acid damage by producing a protective layer of mucus and alkaline fluid from its specialised cells, and by preventing acid leakage into the deeper layers of the stomach walls.

Any drug or condition that increases acid production, or slows down mucus production, may allow acid leakage into these deeper layers, resulting in inflammation of the inner lining of the stomach – gastritis. When the acid damage is severe enough, the stomach wall is eroded and an ulcer develops.

A similar condition can also affect the first section of the small intestines – the duodenum – and develop as a duodenal ulcer.

Drugs and conditions associated with gastric and duodenal ulcers are:

- caffeine, especially from strong coffee
- nicotine
- non-steroidal anti-inflammatory drugs (NSAIDs) such as aspirin and ibuprofen
- stress
- infection with the micro-organism *Heliobacter pylori* within the stomach itself.

Bulimia

This is a psychological condition where the sufferer has a profound fear of becoming overweight, and prevents this by self-inducing vomiting after each meal. The constant acidic vomit in the mouth will eventually cause classic signs of erosion on the palatal surfaces of the upper anterior teeth, and this may often be the first signs of the condition that are detectable.

Crohn's disease

A chronic inflammatory disease that can affect any part of the gastrointestinal (GI) tract (including the mouth, as recurrent apthous ulcers) but which usually occurs in the small intestines, particularly at the end where they join the large intestines.

The cause is unknown, but it may be an allergic reaction to an infectious agent. With time, the walls of the intestines become thickened and their ability to absorb nutrients from food diminishes, so that the sufferer becomes generally unwell and loses weight.

In severe cases, the intestinal swelling is bad enough to restrict normal peristalsis and GI tract obstructions occur. Abscesses and fistulas (abnormal passageways) also occur in a significant number of sufferers.

Many sufferers are prescribed long-term steroid treatment for the condition. In severe cases, surgery may be required to remove sections of the GI tract that have become badly diseased or obstructed.

Ulcerative colitis

A chronic inflammatory disease that affects the lining of the colon and rectum only, rather than affecting any section of the GI tract as does Crohn's disease.

Its cause is unknown, and symptoms tend to be more severe than with Crohn's disease. Anaemia may occur due to extensive blood loss from the ulcerated colon, and in long-standing cases there is an increased risk of developing bowel cancer.

Again, many sufferers are prescribed long-term steroid treatment to help control the symptoms. In severe cases, and at the first indication of bowel cancer, the colon may have to be surgically removed – a procedure called a colectomy.

Diabetes

This is a disorder caused by reduced or non-existent production of insulin by the pancreas. There are two types of diabetes.

- **Type I insulin-dependent diabetes** – the more severe form, and developing in younger sufferers, it occurs rapidly following the destruction of the specialised area of the pancreas where insulin is produced, often following a viral infection.
- **Type II non-insulin-dependent diabetes** – develops gradually in older sufferers, and is the result of insufficient insulin production; there is often a genetic predisposition to the disease.

The reduced, or absent, levels of insulin in the undiagnosed sufferer allow a rise in blood glucose levels, which produce the following symptoms to a greater or lesser degree.

- **Excess urine production** – as the body attempts to eliminate the free glucose, because it cannot be stored or used by the body tissues.
- **Excessive thirst** – as a result of the increased loss of fluid from the body by urination.
- **Prone to infection** – as the excess glucose levels impair the ability of the body cells to fight infection.
- **Weight loss** – as the body cells release stored fat in an attempt to generate some energy.
- **Fatigue** – as the body cells are unable to take up and use the circulating glucose for energy production.
- **Peripheral neuropathy** – tingling and numbness in the extremities, as peripheral nerves and blood vessels degenerate more rapidly.

Many people with type II diabetes are unaware of their disorder, although obesity is the main factor that generates medical intervention and a diagnosis. Once diagnosed, a combination of diet control and/or medication and/or insulin injections will maintain acceptable blood glucose levels, so that the sufferer does not become either *hyperglycaemic* (high blood glucose) or *hypoglycaemic* (low blood glucose). Both of these conditions can result in the patient slipping into a coma if not diagnosed and treated rapidly.

People with diabetes also have a tendency to develop infections easily and to experience poor wound healing generally, including with conditions such as periodontal disease.

Sensible dietary measures combined with controlled weight reduction are often all that many people with type II diabetes require to keep their symptoms under control.

Liver disease

No matter what the cause, liver disease is likely to affect the ability of the patient to store and use food nutrients efficiently, and to be unable to detoxify many drugs, including local anaesthetics, sedatives and general anaesthetics. The following liver disorders may come to light during the taking of the patient's medical history.

- **Cirrhosis** – chronic damage of the liver cells, producing scarring and gradual loss of liver function; may be associated with high alcohol consumption, but also with diseased bile ducts and with cystic fibrosis.
- **Hepatitis** – inflammation of the liver, and can be due to alcohol and other drug abuse or to viral infections such as hepatitis A, B or C (as these can be transmitted sexually, they are often not declared by the patient).
- **Cancer of the liver** – both of the above conditions can develop into primary liver cancer.

Hepatitis B is of particular concern to the dental team as it is a bloodborne virus, and it is now mandatory for all clinical staff to be vaccinated against the 'B' virus throughout their working lives.

Nervous system

The nervous system is composed of the following parts.

- The brain and spinal cord, forming the **central nervous system**.
- The peripheral nerves, autonomic nerves and enteric nerves, forming the **peripheral nervous system**.
- The **sensory organs** of the eyes, ears, tongue (taste) and nose (smell).

The brain is the organ responsible for the continuation of life, by acting as the control centre of the body. All basic life functions, such as maintenance of the heart rate, respiration and the control of body temperature (*homeostasis*), are controlled by the brain. Damage to the brain, when severe enough and when affecting the areas responsible for these basic life functions, will result in the death of the patient.

Information required by the brain to maintain these functions is received from the body and its surroundings via certain types of peripheral nerves, and the necessary adjustments required to allow the body to respond to this information are then transmitted from the brain to the body by other types of peripheral nerves.

Types of peripheral nerves

The peripheral nervous system is composed of various types of nerves, each with their own specific functions. The cells of the brain receive information from the body and its surroundings via one type of nerve, and specialised central nerve cells found only in the brain analyse and interpret this information, ready to instruct the body on how to respond to it.

Once the message has been interpreted and a suitable response formulated, the brain sends messages to the relevant parts of the body to act on the information accordingly, via various other types of peripheral nerves.

The types of peripheral nerves involved are as follows.

Sensory nerves

These carry information from the body to the brain, to be interpreted and acted upon. The information they carry includes the following sensations.

- **Pain**
- **Temperature** – both hot and cold

- **Touch**
- **Specialised sensations** – sight, sound, taste, smell

The peripheral nerves of relevance to the dental nurse are sensory nerves which send information from the oral cavity to the brain, and they are discussed in detail in Chapters 9 and 10.

Motor nerves

These carry information from the brain to the body, to allow the body to respond to the information received accordingly. The motor nerves can be subdivided further, depending on their function.

- **Somatic nerves** – carrying impulses to the **musculoskeletal system**, to allow voluntary movement (controlled by conscious thought) of the body by the co-ordinated contraction and relaxation of relevant muscle groups.
- **Autonomic nerves** – carrying impulses to blood vessels and internal organs, to effect involuntary actions (cannot be controlled by conscious thought), such as blood vessel constriction or dilation.
- **Enteric nerves** – carrying impulses specifically to the gastrointestinal tract, to effect peristalsis and digestive secretions, and to regulate blood flow to the area during digestion; these are also involuntary actions.

The motor nerves of particular relevance to the dental nurse are those somatic nerves that supply the muscles associated with the oral cavity (muscles of mastication and facial expression), and the autonomic nerves that control the flow of saliva from the salivary glands.

Throughout the body, the sensory and motor peripheral nerves travel together and with blood vessels, in what are known as *neurovascular bundles*.

Nerve transmission

All information that passes from the body and the external environment to the brain, its analysis, interpretation and the actions that are generated as a consequence are transmitted as *simple electrical impulses* throughout the nervous system.

These electrical impulses are able to be transmitted due to the difference in chemicals on the inside and the outside of each nerve cell (neurone) – mainly potassium on the inside and sodium on the outside of the nerve cells. At rest, there is more potassium and sodium outside the neurone than inside, and this means that there is an electrical difference between the outside and the inside of the nerve cell too. When the neurone is stimulated, by a sensation such as the skin being gently touched or a cold drink stimulating the teeth, this electrical difference changes in a wave-like surge along the neurone from the point of stimulation all the way to the brain, as the potassium and sodium flow back into the neurones. This wave-like surge of electricity is called the *nerve impulse*.

The central nerve cells in the brain then analyse the nerve impulse that they have received, and send out a corresponding electrical surge through the motor nerve cells, all the way back to the area of initial stimulation, with instructions for the necessary action that needs to be taken by the body. In the examples given, the gentle touch sensation of the skin will be recognised as pleasant (with no avoidance action to be taken), while the cold sensation on the teeth will be recognised as painful, and avoidance action will be taken to move the cause of the cold away from the teeth. The whole process takes just a tiny fraction of a second to occur.

Once the nerve impulse has passed, the potassium and sodium chemicals will move back out of the neurone and restore the chemical levels to how they were before the nerve was stimulated.

The effect that local anaesthetics have on this nerve transmission process is discussed in Chapter 14.

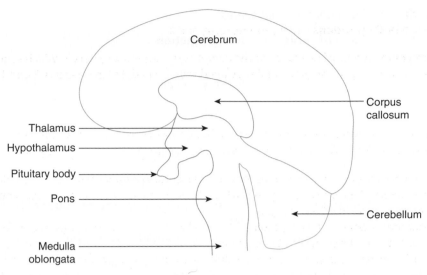

Figure 5.13   Areas of the brain.

The brain and spinal cord

The brain and spinal cord are encased respectively within the skull and the vertebral column of the spine. They are both covered by three membranous layers called the *meninges*, the inner two layers being separated by the *cerebrospinal fluid* (CSF). This clear fluid is secreted by specialised areas within the brain itself, and it acts in a shock-absorber capacity to protect the brain and spinal cord. During normal head movements, both structures float gently in the CSF and are therefore prevented from 'bouncing around' and becoming damaged within the confines of the skull and vertebral column.

The brain consists mainly of two *cerebral hemispheres* which take up the vast majority of the skull, and these are formed from four lobes in each hemisphere, named as follows and in line with the bony plates of the skull itself (see Chapter 9).

- **Frontal lobes** – forming the forehead region.
- **Parietal lobes** – forming the top sides of the head.
- **Temporal lobes** – forming the lower sides of the head in the ear region.
- **Occipital lobes** – forming the back of the head.

The areas of the brain are shown diagrammatically in Figure 5.13.

The cerebral hemispheres appear as vastly convoluted folds of nerve tissue, the layout of which provides a huge surface area of specialised nerve cells appearing as the characteristic 'grey matter' of the brain itself. It is here that thought, learning, memory and understanding of the world and the environment occur.

At the back of the brain, beneath the occipital lobes of the cerebrum, lies the 'hindbrain' or *cerebellum*, which is concerned with the control of balance and posture and the co-ordination of movement. Beneath the middle region of the brain the cerebral hemispheres lie over a structure called the 'brainstem' or *medulla oblongata*, which is the control centre for all the basic brain functions necessary for life – respiration, heart rate, control of body actions during times of stress, etc.

At the very base of the medulla oblongata, the nerve tissue forms into the top end of the spinal cord, and this then passes out of the skull through the large opening called the *foramen magnum* and runs down the length of the vertebral spine to the pelvis.

Table 5.2   Twelve pairs of cranial nerves

Roman numeral	Name of nerve	Nerve function
I	Olfactory	Sensory – smell
II	Optic	Sensory – sight
III	Oculomotor	Motor – external eye muscles Parasympathetic – pupil size
IV	Trochlear	Motor – external eye muscles
V	**Trigeminal**	**Sensory – pain, temperature, touch of teeth and oral soft tissues** **Motor – muscles of mastication**
VI	Abducens	Motor – external eye muscles
VII	**Facial**	**Sensory – taste from anterior two-thirds of tongue** **Motor – muscles of facial expression** **Autonomic – salivary glands**
VIII	Auditory	Sensory – hearing and balance
IX	**Glossopharyngeal**	**Sensory – taste from posterior tongue** **Motor – control of swallowing** **Autonomic – salivary glands**
X	Vagus	Sensory – from the abdominal region Parasympathetic – to the thorax and abdomen
XI	Accessory	Motor – neck muscles and the larynx
XII	**Hypoglossal**	**Motor – tongue muscles**

As the spinal cord runs down the bony spine, it gives rise to sequential pairs of nerves at each vertebral joint along its full length – sensory nerves entering the column and motor nerves leaving it. These form the *systemic nerves*, which receive sensations from the whole body except the head and neck region, and transmit motor impulses to the same body areas.

The nerves supplying the head and neck region leave the brain directly from its undersurface through various natural bony openings called *foramina*, emerging as the 12 pairs of *cranial nerves*.

The cranial nerves

The 12 pairs of cranial nerves are numbered with Roman numerals, but each has its own name too.

Some of the cranial nerves are of particular importance to the dental team because they supply the oral cavity and its surrounding structures. Those relevant to the dental nurse are shown in bold in Table 5.2, which lists the 12 pairs of cranial nerves in full.

The first and second column list the relevant Roman numeral and name of each nerve respectively, while the third column identifies the types of peripheral nerve that are present in each – whether sensory, somatic motor or autonomic. None of the cranial nerves is concerned with enteric impulse transmission to the gastrointestinal tract. The cranial nerves of particular importance to the dental team are highlighted in bold, and are the trigeminal (V), the facial (VII), the glossopharyngeal (IX) and the hypoglossal nerves (XII). All except the hypoglossal nerve are composed of both sensory and motor components, and their various functions are discussed in detail further in the text.

Relevant details of the four cranial nerves that are dentally important are given in Chapters 9 and 10. The specialised sensation of taste is covered in detail in Chapter 10. Full details of all the cranial nerves are available in the publication *Basic Guide to Anatomy and Physiology for Dental Care Professionals*.

Relevant disorders of the nervous system

Some disorders affecting the nervous system are relevant to the dental nurse; as they may have an effect on the dental treatment offered, they may cause difficulty in providing dental treatment or in allowing an adequate level of oral hygiene to be maintained, or sufferers may present as a medical emergency during treatment. The recognition and management of medical emergencies are discussed in Chapter 6.

In particular with disorders of the nervous system, the disclosure of any of the following points by the patient during medical history taking should be taken into full consideration by the dental team, with regard to the patient's dental treatment.

- **Previous stroke** – this may have resulted in poor speech and/or muscular control that may make communication and oral hygiene maintenance difficult for the patient.
- **Epilepsy** – a patient with poorly controlled epilepsy may have a seizure at any time, and this is a medical emergency that the dental team should be able to manage successfully.
- **Medications** – stroke sufferers will be taking some form of anticoagulation therapy to prevent a recurrence of their condition, and epileptics may be taking medication that has a detrimental effect on their oral soft tissues.

The most relevant disorders of the nervous system are outlined below.

Stroke (cerebrovascular accident)

The blood supply to the brain is well controlled by numerous normal body mechanisms. In fact, at times of severe blood loss or reduced blood oxygenation, the body will deliberately divert blood from other organs to the brain, in an attempt to maintain the cerebral circulation.

A stroke occurs when there is a sudden alteration in cerebral blood flow, due to one of three events.

- **Cerebral thrombosis** – the formation of a blood clot within a brain artery, reducing or cutting off the oxygenated blood supply to that region (in a similar fashion to the onset of a heart attack when a coronary artery is blocked).
- **Cerebral embolism** – the blockage of a brain artery by a loose blood clot formed elsewhere in the body, that detaches from the blood vessel wall and circulates to the brain.
- **Cerebral haemorrhage** – when a cerebral blood vessel ruptures and bleeding occurs within the skull, causing increasing pressure on the brain.

The effects of a severe stroke are of sudden onset, but the signs that occur will depend on the area of the brain affected. Also, the nerves supplying the left side of the body cross over to the right side of the brain and vice versa, so a left-sided stroke will show as a range of right-sided neuromuscular weaknesses and a right-sided stroke will have the opposite effects. The speech centre is located in the left side of the brain and can be affected to varying degrees following a left-sided stroke.

Stroke victims who survive the actual medical emergency are routinely prescribed the powerful anticoagulant warfarin, to prevent the formation of another thrombus and therefore another stroke. As the taking of this drug can allow uncontrolled haemorrhage to occur during surgical procedures (including dental treatment), these patients have routine blood tests to monitor the clotting ability of their blood. The results are recorded as an *international normalised ratio* (INR) score, and this is currently advised to be between 2 and 4 if surgical dental treatment is to be carried out safely.

Transient ischaemic attack

When a small, partial blockage of a cerebral artery occurs, the signs and symptoms are far less dramatic – often exhibiting just as a mild visual disturbance or a brief memory lapse lasting minutes. This is known as a transient ischaemic attack or TIA.

The sufferer will make a full recovery but the experience is actually a warning signal that a full-blown stroke could occur in future, in a similar way to angina attacks having the potential to develop into a full myocardial infarction. The TIA indicates that part of the brain has a reduced blood flow.

These patients are usually prescribed aspirin as a mild anticoagulant, to prevent further TIAs or an actual stroke, and again, the potential for uncontrolled haemorrhage to occur must be recognised and managed by the dental team during the provision of dental treatment.

Epilepsy

When the usually well-organised and regulated electrical activity of the nerve cells in the brain becomes temporarily abnormal and disorganised, the sufferer is said to have a *seizure*. During a seizure, the normal electrical discharges of the nerve cells become completely chaotic and random, and are often started by a stimulus such as flashing lights or certain sounds.

Sufferers experiencing a tendency to seizures are diagnosed as having epilepsy.

The two main types of generalised seizure, where consciousness is lost, are as follows.

- **Grand mal seizure** – the sufferer falls down unconscious, the body stiffens and becomes rigid, and then twitches and jerks uncontrollably – these signs are referred to as **tonic-clonic seizures**.
- **Petit mal seizure** – the sufferer has only a momentary loss of consciousness, with no associated abnormal movements; indeed, they often are thought to be just daydreaming for a period of just seconds – the alternative name for this mild form is therefore **absence seizures**.

While petit mal seizures last just seconds, grand mal seizures can last several minutes before the tonic-clonic phase ends and consciousness returns. In both cases, the sufferer has no memory of the seizure and, especially after a grand mal event, is often confused and disorientated for a time.

The occurrence of a grand mal seizure is a medical emergency that the dental team should be able to recognise and manage successfully. However, when a grand mal seizure lasts for more than 5 min or repeat seizures occur rapidly after the first, the sufferer is said to be in *status epilepticus* – an often fatal condition requiring urgent emergency medical treatment.

The commonly prescribed antiepileptic drug Epanutin (phenytoin sodium) has the unwelcome side-effect of causing the gingival tissues to overgrow – a condition called *gingival hyperplasia*, which makes gingival plaque removal and satisfactory oral hygiene levels difficult to achieve for the patient.

Bell's palsy

This is a (usually) temporary paralysis of the VII cranial nerve – the facial nerve. It often occurs following any condition causing inflammation in the region of the facial nerve, and results in a one-sided weakness of the facial muscles.

In particular, any inflammation associated with the parotid salivary glands can result in Bell's palsy, as the facial nerve runs across and through this gland to reach the oral cavity. It does not supply the gland itself though.

The condition of Bell's palsy is self-limiting and subsides as the inflammation resolves, although while present it can be difficult for the patient to communicate adequately with the dental team, and treatment may need to be postponed until the patient has made a full recovery.

The trigeminal nerve

Of all the cranial nerves, the trigeminal (cranial nerve V) is the one that is most dentally relevant, and while discussed in detail in Chapters 9 and 10, it is also summarised here. It is composed of divisions and branches, and the nomenclature used to name the various nerves follows that used in other areas of anatomy so *anterior* and *posterior* refer to front and back, respectively, and *superior* and *inferior* refer to upper and lower, respectively. The areas of supply in relation to the teeth and their surrounding soft tissues follow the dental terminology used in naming tooth surfaces, as discussed in Chapter 10.

The name of this nerve indicates that it splits into three divisions, each of which has several branches.

- **Ophthalmic division** – sensory supply of the soft tissues around the eye and the upper face.
- **Maxillary division** – sensory supply of the upper teeth, the maxilla and the middle area of the face.
- **Mandibular division** – sensory supply of the lower teeth, the mandible and the lower area of the face, and motor supply to the muscles of mastication.

The maxillary and mandibular branches of the trigeminal nerve are of most importance to the dental nurse, as together they relay sensory information from the whole of the oral cavity to the brain, and provide the motor supply to the muscles of mastication, to effect jaw closing and chewing movements.

Maxillary division

The maxillary division of the trigeminal nerve splits further, into five branches, all of which are sensory (Figure 5.14). By definition, then, they transmit sensations (such as heat, cold, pressure and pain) from this area to the brain, including from the upper teeth. It is these branches that have to be anaesthetised before painless dental treatment can be carried out on the upper teeth. The five branches are as follows, and their general anatomical paths are described below.

- **Anterior superior dental (alveolar) nerve** – supplies sensation from the upper incisor and canine teeth, and their labial gingivae. In addition, it supplies sensation from the soft tissues of the upper lip and around the nostrils of the nose.
- **Middle superior dental (alveolar) nerve** – supplies sensation from the upper premolar and the anterior half of the upper first molar teeth, and their buccal gingivae.
- **Posterior superior dental (alveolar) nerve** – supplies sensation from the posterior half of the upper first molar and the second and third molar teeth, and their buccal gingivae.

151

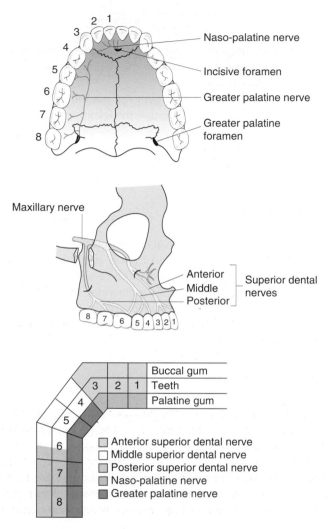

Figure 5.14　Maxillary division of trigeminal nerve.

- **Greater palatine nerve** – supplies sensation from the palatal gingivae of the upper molar, premolar and posterior half of the canine teeth.
- **Nasopalatine nerve** – previously called the **long sphenopalatine nerve**, this supplies sensation from the palatal gingivae of the upper incisor and anterior half of the canine teeth.

The maxillary nerve emerges from the base of the brain, leaves the skull through the foramen rotundum and passes forward through the floor of the eye socket (orbit). Before entering the orbit, it gives off its posterior superior dental and palatine branches. Within the orbit, it gives off the middle and anterior superior dental nerves. It emerges from the orbit through the *infraorbital foramen* on the front of the maxilla to supply the skin and mucous membrane of the lower eyelid, cheek and upper lip.

　The posterior superior dental nerve enters the back of the maxilla to reach its destination, while the greater palatine nerve also passes through the back of the maxilla and reaches the surface of the hard palate through the *greater palatine foramen*, opposite the third molar tooth.

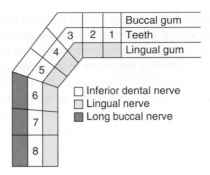

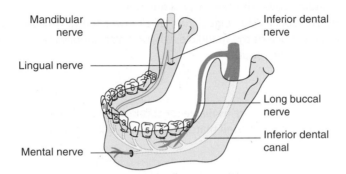

Figure 5.15   Mandibular division of trigeminal nerve.

The nasopalatine nerve passes through the floor of the nasal cavity to reach the surface of the palate through the *incisive foramen* behind the central incisors, and the anterior and middle superior dental nerves branch off from the maxillary nerve in the floor of the orbit. They pass down inside the maxilla, in the walls of the maxillary sinus, to reach the teeth. The sensory nerve impulses from the upper teeth and their surrounding soft tissue structures pass from the nerve endings back along these nerve pathways to the maxillary nerve trunk, and then enter the skull and join the other two divisions to form the trigeminal nerve trunk, which then enters the brain itself.

Mandibular division

The mandibular division of the trigeminal nerve emerges from the skull through the foramen ovale and splits into four branches which carry both sensory and motor components (Figure 5.15). The sensory branches of this nerve require anaesthetising before painless dental treatment can be carried out on the lower teeth. The four branches are as follows, and their general anatomical paths are described below.

- **Inferior dental (alveolar) nerve** – supplies sensation from all the lower teeth, and from the buccal or labial gingivae of all *except* the molar teeth. In addition, it supplies sensation from the soft tissues of the lower lip and the chin.
- **Lingual nerve** – supplies sensation from the lingual gingivae of all the lower teeth, the floor of the mouth, and touch sensation from the anterior two-thirds of the tongue.
- **Long buccal nerve** – supplies sensation from the buccal gingivae of the lower molar teeth.
- **Motor branch** – supplies stimulation to the muscles of mastication, to effect jaw closing and chewing movements.

The mandibular nerve passes down from the base of the skull on the inner side of the ramus of the mandible, between the medial and lateral pterygoid muscles, and divides into the above branches.

The *inferior dental nerve* supplies all the lower teeth and enters the mandible through the *mandibular foramen*. This is situated at the centre of the inner surface of the ramus and is guarded on its front edge by a small bony projection called the *lingula*. After entering the mandibular foramen, the nerve passes through a canal running inside the mandible, below the apices of the teeth. The end branch of the inferior dental nerve emerges on the outer surface of the mandible through the *mental foramen* which is situated below the apices of the premolars. From this point, it is called the *mental nerve* and supplies the buccal gum of the incisors, canines and premolars, plus the lower lip and chin.

The *long buccal nerve* supplies the buccal gum of the molars. It passes into the gum on the outer surface of the mandible, over the external oblique ridge.

The *lingual nerve* supplies the lingual gum of all lower teeth. It passes along the floor of the mouth on the inner surface of the mandible, where it also supplies the anterior two-thirds of the tongue and the floor of the mouth.

 Further resources are available for this book, including interactive multiple choice questions and extended matching questions. Visit the companion website at:

www.levisonstextbookfordentalnurses.com

6

Medical Emergencies

Key learning points

A **working knowledge** of
* the incidence of medical emergencies in the dental workplace

A **factual awareness** of
* basic life support procedures and resuscitation techniques

A **factual knowledge** of
* the use of emergency resuscitation equipment in the dental workplace

A **working understanding** of
* the actions to take in the event of various medical emergency scenarios

Medical emergencies can occur anywhere, at any time, but some may be more likely to occur in the dental surgery setting due to the nature of dental treatment and the anxiety it evokes in some patients. The anxiety that some patients experience may have the following effects.

* Lowers the pain threshold so that 'discomfort' is experienced as 'pain', producing an agitated or even unco-operative patient.
* Perception of being about to feel pain, so that stress levels and anxiety are raised – this can then put a huge strain on the patient's body, especially the heart and circulatory system.
* Fear and anxiety at the prospect of dental treatment may worry the patient enough to prevent them eating beforehand, for fear of vomiting – the patient will then have a low blood sugar and be more prone to fainting, and in those with diabetes the low blood sugar is likely to precipitate a hypoglycaemic attack.

In addition, the following points also have to be considered.

* Many dental treatments involve the injection of a local anaesthetic, and these drugs may interact with some common patient medications.

Levison's Textbook for Dental Nurses, Eleventh Edition. By Carole Hollins.
© 2013 John Wiley & Sons, Ltd. Published 2013 by John Wiley & Sons, Ltd. Companion website: www.levisonstextbookfordentalnurses.com

- Any of the dental materials, antibiotics or local anaesthetics used in dentistry have the potential to cause an allergic reaction in the patient, the worse-case scenario being a full anaphylactic reaction.
- Many dental treatments are carried out with the patient lying *supine* (flat) in the dental chair, and this leaves their airway potentially vulnerable to foreign object inhalation, choking and a full respiratory obstruction emergency.

The dental team can do much to reduce the anxiety levels of their patients merely by creating a friendly, welcoming and pleasant atmosphere within the workplace. Showing sympathy to an anxious patient helps to reduce their stress levels and alleviates their concerns over appearing 'foolish' to the staff and to other patients. For those patients whose anxiety is so great that it borders on *phobia* (an exaggerated and illogical fear), all methods of pain and anxiety control techniques should be considered by the dental team, and offered where appropriate. This ensures that these patients will still attend and undergo dental treatment routinely.

However, those patients who pose the greatest concern with regard to medical emergencies are those with diagnosed risk factors.

- **Heart conditions** – any abnormality or disorder of the heart may potentially allow unexpected problems to arise during stressful episodes, such as when undergoing dental treatment.
- **Hypertension** (high blood pressure) – anxiety often causes a raised systolic blood pressure, which can then put a considerable strain on an already malfunctioning heart.
- **Liver or kidney disorders** – both these organs are responsible for eliminating waste products and toxins from the body, and any amount of malfunction due to disease could result in drugs not being detoxified and removed adequately.
- **Diabetes** – uncontrolled diabetes or failure to take medications accurately may result in a hypoglycaemic attack. In addition, those with diabetes tend to heal poorly and be more prone to infections, including those involving the oral cavity.
- **Allergies** – these patients are often sensitive to, or even allergic to, more than one allergen, so great care must be taken to avoid the use of known potential allergens in the dental workplace, such as latex and penicillin-based antibiotics.
- Certain **medications** known to react with some local anaesthetics – these are drugs that can be potentiated by adrenaline-containing local anaesthetics, and include some types of antidepressants, thyroxine and any medication that may cause hypertension, such as some contraceptives and hormone replacement therapy.
- Previous history of **complications** during dental treatment – depending on the complication and its cause, it is possible for some to be a regular occurrence with the same patient.
- **Long-term steroid treatment** – this treatment tends to override the body's own production of the hormones required to react to and survive stressful events, resulting in shock and a potentially fatal crash in the patient's blood pressure when stressful events do occur.

These patients will be identified by the accurate completion and recording of a medical history before dental treatment begins. This medical history can then be stored with the patient records (computerised or paper, or both) and updated at the beginning of every course of treatment.

Nevertheless, medical emergencies can and do occur in the dental surgery environment and the dental team must be able to recognise them and support life where necessary until specialist help arrives (that is, paramedics). All members of the dental team are expected to hold a *Basic Life Support* (BLS) certificate if working with patients, and to undergo the necessary continuing professional development (CPD) requirements to update their medical emergencies knowledge as laid down in the General Dental Council (GDC)'s *Standards Guidance* documentation.

Casualty assessment

The correct recognition of the cause of any emergency is vital if the casualty is to be correctly treated and their life supported until the emergency services can attend. This is done by being able to recognise the 'signs' and 'symptoms' of an emergency.

The *signs* are what the rescuer can see.

- Skin colour – is it pink, grey, red, pale?
- Breathlessness – are they gasping, breathing quickly, struggling to inhale or exhale?
- Suddenness of any collapse – did the casualty fall straight to the ground or did they slowly slump down?
- Actions before collapse, such as clutching the chest.
- Condition of the pulse – is it fast, slow, weak, absent?

At the same time, the casualty will feel *symptoms*, which may be asked about if they are not unconscious.

- Any pain – is it sharp, dull, throbbing, made worse by anything?
- Location of pain – where is it felt exactly?
- Nausea – does the casualty feel sick or have they vomited?
- Drowsiness – do they feel sleepy, are they struggling to respond to verbal commands?
- Difficulty breathing – are they struggling to breathe in, out or both?
- Dizziness – does the person feel like they will fall over, is the room spinning?

By assessing the casualty and noting the signs and symptoms exhibited, the rescuer can determine their next course of action, and often this will be to reassure the conscious casualty and to summon more experienced help.

However, there are two signs that should prompt any rescuer to begin BLS immediately.

- **Unconsciousness**
- **Abnormal breathing**

These two signs indicate that the casualty's life is at risk, as sudden unconsciousness may indicate that the heart has stopped beating (*asystole*) or is beating ineffectively (*fibrillating*), and abnormal breathing indicates a compromised airway and possible lack of oxygen to the brain (*hypoxia*). The presence of any of these signs may result in the death of the casualty if not dealt with quickly by the rescuer.

The aim of BLS is to maintain a flow of oxygenated blood to the casualty until one of the following happens.

- They recover and begin to circulate oxygenated blood by breathing unassisted.
- Their life support is handed over to specialists, usually paramedics.
- The rescuer is too physically exhausted to continue.
- Their death is confirmed by an authorised practitioner, such as a doctor, at the scene.

Oxygen is the atmospheric gas that is vital for life. It is breathed into the respiratory system through the nose and mouth, and then passes down the trachea to the two bronchi which enter the right or left lung. In the lungs, the oxygen passes out into the circulatory system during external respiration, and is transported around the body in the arterial bloodstream by the continual pumping action of the heart. Where required, the oxygen passes out of the blood vessel and into the body tissues during internal respiration, where it is used to provide energy for the cells to work.

The actions of the respiratory system in taking up oxygen from the atmosphere and absorbing it into the blood, and the circulatory system in transporting that oxygen around the body to the cells, are carefully controlled by the brain. If any one of these three vital organs fails, the other two will also fail shortly after.

Without oxygen, the cells, and therefore the body, cannot function and death will occur. After only 3–4 min without oxygen, the brain cells can suffer irreversible damage which, if not fatal, will lead to some degree of permanent brain damage. The quicker that the need for BLS is established and begun, the better the chances of survival for the casualty – and ideally this should be within seconds of their own life support system failing.

So, the fundamental aims of BLS are to maintain the life of the casualty by achieving the following.

- Provide oxygen to the lungs – by some form of **rescue breathing**.
- Circulate the oxygen to the body tissues – by **external chest compressions** to mimic the pumping action of the heart.

Death occurs when there is a permanent cessation of the function of the heart and lungs, and these are the criteria by which a medical doctor will diagnose and certify death. Other specialists, such as paramedics, are able to diagnose and determine that death has occurred by the absence of:

- spontaneous breathing
- heartbeat
- pupillary response to light (pupils of the eyes remain dilated when exposed to light).

The lack of pupil response to light indicates brain death.

However, only a medical doctor can certify that death has occurred and issue a death certificate, so all rescue attempts must continue until this has been established, or until any rescuers are too physically exhausted to continue in their efforts to resuscitate the individual.

If there is more than one rescuer able to provide BLS, it is important that the compression and ventilation roles are regularly swapped between them, as chest compressions are physically tiring to perform and the rescuer will soon become exhausted.

Current Basic Life Support guidelines

In the United Kingdom, the general guidelines to be used for BLS are issued by the Resuscitation Council (UK) and should be followed nationally. Local protocol amendments may exist in some areas or in some workplaces (especially hospitals), and readers should ensure that they are aware of these. However, the current Resuscitation Council advice is that rescuers need to apply 30 chest compressions for each two rescue breaths given, no matter how many rescuers are present. This gives the current compression:ventilation algorithm of 30:2.

The two important signs that should be looked for when determining the need to provide BLS to a casualty are:

- **unconsciousness**
- **abnormal or absent breathing**.

Unconsciousness indicates that the casualty is unresponsive to all stimuli, and that their heart may have stopped beating – they have gone into cardiac arrest. There is no instance where the heart can have stopped beating and a person remain conscious, as the body cells (especially the brain) will become starved of oxygen very quickly and will be unable to function.

Abnormal breathing, such as infrequent noisy gasps, indicates that there is a possible obstruction in the casualty's respiratory system which is making normal breathing difficult. This will gradually reduce the oygen supply to the body cells, and once breathing ceases completely, the oxygen supply is cut off immediately. The casualty's skin colour will change from pink, through pale to blue or grey as their body tissues become starved of oxygen. This is more difficult to determine in those with darker skin tones, so the lips, nailbeds and mucous membranes of the mouth may also be checked for signs indicating lack of oxygenation or hypoxia.

The actions that may be required to help the casualty cannot be determined until the rescuer has fully assessed the situation, and although swift action is necessary to avoid brain damage or death, the following questions must be quickly considered by the rescuer in an effort to realise the correct medical emergency.

- **Why has the individual become unconscious?** Are there any external causes such as trauma, electrocution, poisonous fumes, drowning?
- **How is unconsciousness established?** Are they alert or moving, are they responsive to noise or voices, are they responsive to pain, are they completely unresponsive?
- **Is their breathing abnormal?** Are they gasping, coughing or even clutching at their throat?
- **Are there any breath sounds?** How is this established?
- **What does the rescuer do next**? At what point should help be summoned, and what actions are required immediately?

The accepted order to follow when assessing an emergency situation and determining whether BLS is required can be summarised and easily remembered by the following code.

- **D** for **Danger**
- **R** for **Response**
- **S** for **Shout for help**
- **A** for **Airway**
- **B** for **Breathing**
- **C** for **Circulation**

This is best remembered as **DRSABC** (referred to as 'doctors – a – b – c').

Valuable time can be wasted during this assessment by attempting to open or remove clothing from the casualty while trying to establish their condition, which should not be attempted by the rescuer. The casualty may actually sustain further injury while clothing is being removed. In addition, many individuals would become very distressed at finding themselves partially clad and surrounded by strangers. The dignity and rights to decency and privacy of the casualty must be maintained at all times, by all rescuers.

DRSABC in detail

Danger

Check the immediate area for possible dangers, such as electric wires running through pooled water, punctured gas canisters, spilt chemicals giving off strong fumes, etc. If hazardous chemicals are suspected of being involved in the emergency situation, the workplace COSHH file must be consulted at some point for information on first aid actions that may be necessary. This action is best delegated to a spare rescuer, while BLS is being carried out by others.

If possible, any dangers should be made safe by the rescuer before approaching the casualty, but not at the risk of endangering themselves in the process. Ideally, this should not involve moving the individual except in extreme circumstances, such as rising water levels that may cause drowning. This is to prevent any further injury being caused.

Response

The level of responsiveness will determine whether the casualty is unconscious or not. Call loudly to them, asking if they can hear you or if they are all right, while gently shaking them. Their responsiveness can quickly be assessed and determined by a system referred to as the AVPU code.

- **Alert** – the casualty is fully conscious and able to communicate fully and spontaneously.
- **Verbal** – the casualty is not fully conscious but is able to respond to verbal commands and prompts.
- **Painful** – the casualty is semi-conscious at best, but able to respond to painful stimuli such as a gentle pinch.
- **Unresponsive** – the casualty shows no response to verbal prompts nor painful stimuli, they are unconscious and unable to be roused.

If the casualty shows no response whatsoever, then they are in need of help urgently. Wherever possible, the level of responsiveness should be determined without moving the individual from the position in which they were found, to avoid any further injury.

Shout

If the casualty is unresponsive and therefore unconscious, the rescuer will need help with any attempt at BLS if it is required, as well as to summon specialist help if necessary. If only one rescuer remains to aid the individual while help is being sought, they may need to continue BLS for a prolonged period of time, and ultimately this may result in their physical exhaustion. If attempts at BLS have to then be abandoned before specialist help arrives, the casualty is likely to die.

Shout very loudly to alert anyone else in the vicinity that an emergency situation has arisen. In the workplace, there may be internal communication systems in place for just such an event, such as intercoms, alarm bells or coded calls, and these must be known and used appropriately by the rescuer.

Airway

The airway needs to be checked for any obstruction, such as vomit or debris or the tongue itself, which may have fallen back and blocked it. Any loose obstruction should be removed by rolling the casualty's head to the side to encourage it to drop out of the mouth. In the dental surgery there

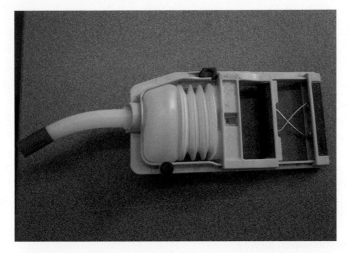

Figure 6.1   Portable suction unit.

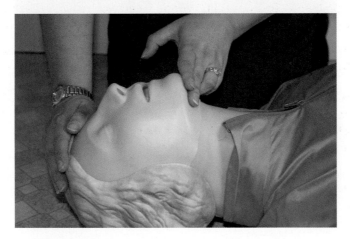

Figure 6.2   Head tilt to open airway.

will also be electrically operated suction equipment available at the chairside or a manually operated suction device within the emergency kit that all dental workplaces have to have on the premises (Figure 6.1). However, these must only be used by those rescuers who have been trained to do so, as they can push debris further down the airway or cause soft tissue injury if not used correctly.

The casualty's airway can then be opened to allow breathing to occur. This can be achieved by tilting the head back by placing the palm of one hand on the casualty's forehead and lifting the chin with the fingers of the other hand at the same time (Figure 6.2). However, this technique must never be used when an individual has a suspected neck or spinal injury, as to do so would almost certainly cause further damage to the spinal cord. This could result in permanent paralysis. In these cases, the airway can be opened by thrusting the lower jaw forward with both hands, without any head tilting occurring (Figure 6.3). This should avoid any further neck or spinal injury.

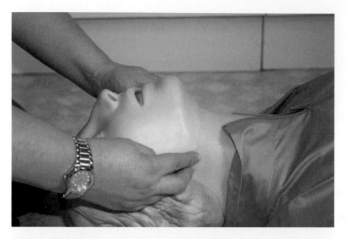

Figure 6.3   Jaw thrust to open airway.

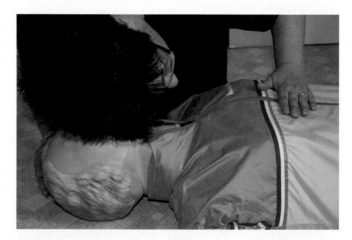

Figure 6.4   Look, listen, feel for signs of breathing.

Breathing

With the airway open, breathing is assessed quickly over a 10-sec period. The rescuer needs to determine if any spontaneous breathing attempts are being made, and their quality, by checking for the following (Figure 6.4).

- **Look** to see if the chest is rising and falling.
- **Listen** to any breathing sounds.
  - ○ Are they regular or infrequent?
  - ○ Are they quiet or noisy?
  - ○ Are they normal or gasping in nature?
- **Feel** for air flow by placing the cheek close to the casualty's mouth.

If breathing is absent or abnormal, the emergency services must be called as specialist help is required. Ideally, a second person can be sent to do this but if necessary, the lone rescuer must leave the casualty and go to call for emergency help.

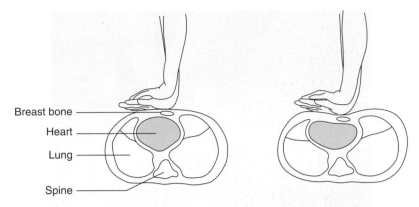

Breast bone
Heart
Lung
Spine

Figure 6.5 External cardiac compression.

If it is now decided that BLS is required to maintain the casualty's life until specialist help arrives, they may require moving to a position where this can be carried out effectively. This is usually achieved by very carefully rolling the individual onto their back with a firm surface beneath them, in a safe area and with enough room to manoeuvre as necessary, as BLS may need to be carried out correctly for a prolonged period until specialist help arrives.

Circulation

Any residual oxygenated blood within the casualty now needs to be quickly pumped around their body to the brain, and this is achieved by the rescuer carrying out chest compressions. These will only be effective if the heart is adequately compressed between the breastbone (sternum) and the spine, on a firm surface, and at a sufficient rate to actually cause the blood to flow through the circulatory system as required, rather than just swishing back and forth (Figure 6.5).

If any spinal or neck injuries are suspected, it would be ideal not to move the casualty from the position in which they were found, to avoid further injury. However, this may not always be possible, especially if their position prevents successful BLS from being carried out. Ideally, several helpers should be used to very carefully roll the casualty onto their back on a hard surface, keeping their head in line with their spine at all times – this is referred to as a 'log roll' technique.

In the dental surgery, dental chairs are designed to be firm enough to carry out chest compressions without having to move the casualty onto the floor.

The correct point at which to apply the compressions is quickly located by:

- kneeling at the side of the casualty, or standing if they are still on the dental chair
- run a finger along the lower border of the individual's ribcage, towards the midline
- once in the midline, the breastbone will be felt with the finger
- place the heel of the other hand adjacent to the finger, towards the head of the individual
- interlock the fingers of both hands over this compression point (Figure 6.6)
- lean over the individual, keeping the arms straight and the elbows locked (Figure 6.7).

Thirty compressions can now be given at a rate of 100 per minute, by compressing the chest by 4–5 cm and then releasing to allow the heart to expand and refill with blood.

Once the initial 30 compressions have been administered, two rescue breaths can be given by the lone rescuer, or ideally by a second rescuer.

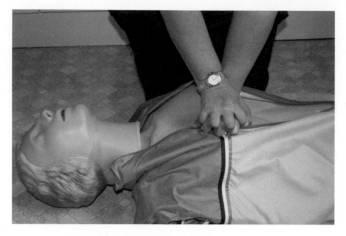

Figure 6.6 Hand lock for chest compressions.

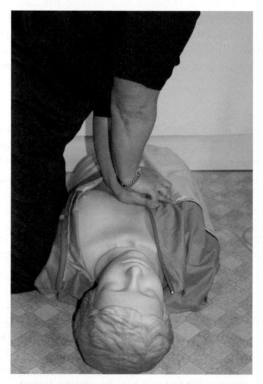

Figure 6.7 Arm lock for chest compressions.

Rescue breathing

Once the first 30 compressions have been administered, any residual oxygen in the blood will have been used up by the body tissues, and especially the brain. To maintain life, the oxygen now has to be regularly replaced before being distributed around the body again by the chest compressions, and this is achieved by artificial ventilation or rescue breathing.

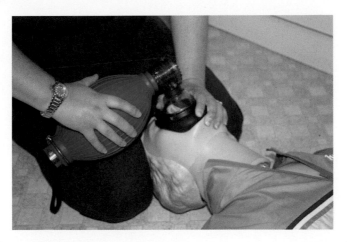

Figure 6.8   Use of the ventilation bag.

The atmosphere contains about 21% oxygen but that expired (breathed out) only contains 16%, as our body tissues use up the 5% difference to produce energy for the cells to work. In an emergency situation, rescue breaths are usually given by breathing expired air into the casualty in a mouth-to-mouth technique. If they have facial injuries affecting the mouth, it may be necessary to use a mouth-to-nose technique instead, and with small children or babies the rescuer will breathe into the casualty's mouth and nose together.

The use of emergency oxygen supplies, such as that held by all dental practices, will increase the amount of available oxygen for rescue breathing when given using a pocket mask or an Ambu-bag, but the technique can only be successfully used by those trained to do so (Figure 6.8).

The airway will already have been cleared of obstructions during the DRSABC procedure, but will need to be held open now to administer rescue breaths, again using the head tilt/chin lift or jaw thrust technique. Two rescue breaths are then given as follows.

- Maintain the head tilt to keep the airway open.
- Pinch the nostrils closed with the fingers of the hand being used to press onto the forehead.
- Support the chin with the other hand while holding the mouth open.
- Take a deep breath, then seal the mouth over that of the individual to ensure no air escapes (Figure 6.9).
- Breathe with normal force into their open mouth for about 2 sec, watching from the corner of the eye to ensure that the chest rises.
- With the airway still held open, move away from their mouth and watch the chest fall as the air comes out.
- Repeat the rescue breath.
- If given successfully, follow with another 30 chest compressions as a BLS cycle.

Sometimes problems will be experienced while attempting rescue breathing, the most common one being that the chest does not rise. In the absence of an obstruction, this is usually due to the airway not being fully opened, and the head tilt procedure should be repeated until successful. Otherwise, ensure that the nostrils are fully closed and that a good mouth-to-mouth seal is being achieved.

If the abdomen is seen to rise while the breath is being given, air is being blown into the stomach rather than the lungs, by being too forceful or too prolonged. The rescue breath should stop once the chest stops rising, usually after just 2 sec at a normal breath force.

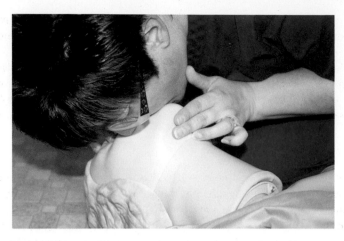

Figure 6.9   Rescue breathing mouth to mouth.

Basic Life Support modifications

The BLS protocols described are to be used for adults and children over the age of 8 years. Babies and young children require less force to be used while carrying out both chest compressions and rescue breathing, to avoid injuring their bodies.

The weight of the foetus in a pregnant woman will also hinder BLS attempts if she is lying on her back, and the usual technique has to be modified for these groups of casualties.

Babies and young children

Anatomically these age groups are different from adults in the following ways.

- They have narrower air passages in the respiratory system.
- These air passages are more prone to blockages.
- The trachea is more flexible, and so it is easily blocked if airway opening attempts are too severe.
- They have a relatively larger tongue than an adult, which is more likely to obstruct the airway when the baby or young child is unconscious.

Cardiac arrest in these younger casualties is rarely due to heart problems, as in an adult, but is far more likely to be caused by lack of oxygen to the brain due to airway obstruction.

As the DRSABC code is being followed, it will soon become apparent if the young casualty is unresponsive and having breathing difficulties or not breathing at all, and it is imperative that rescue breathing is commenced *before* starting chest compressions. This is because the likely cause of their collapse will be a shortage of oxygen to their vital organs, and any reserves will have been quickly used up by their young bodies and must be replenished as soon as possible.

So the full modified BLS sequence of events in cases involving a baby or a young child is as follows.

- **Danger** – check for dangers as usual.
- **Response** – less reliable in younger casualties, so merely determine whether they are unresponsive only.
- **Shout** – summon help from anyone in the vicinity, without leaving the casualty.

- **Airway** – check the airway for obstruction, especially the tongue, then carefully open the airway, taking care not to overextend the head tilt and so block the trachea.
- **Breathing** – look, listen and feel for signs of spontaneous breathing for 10 sec, and if they are absent, *give five rescue breaths using the mouth-to-mouth and nose technique.*
- **Circulation** – give 30 chest compressions, using two fingers for a baby or one hand for a young child, aiming to compress the chest by one-third of its depth at a rate of 100 per minute.
- The lone rescuer must continue BLS for a full minute before going for specialist help.

Pregnant women

Any premenopausal woman who collapses and requires BLS could potentially be pregnant. In some cases it will be known or obvious that they are so, but otherwise it should always be considered a possibility, especially if BLS attempts are failing for no other obvious reason.

In a heavily pregnant woman lying on her back, the uterus (womb) tends to lie over the major blood vessels (the inferior venae cavae) that return blood from the lower body to the right side of the heart. If this casualty collapses and requires BLS, the rescuer has the added difficulty of forcing blood through these squashed blood vessels during chest compressions, and the rescue attempt is likely to fail.

Instead, the pregnant casualty should be laid slightly on the left side with some form of support under the right buttock so that these major blood vessels are not squashed by the uterus. BLS can then be carried out in the normal way, while maintaining this angled position of the woman throughout.

Monitoring and evaluating Basic Life Support

Once the DRSABC code has been followed correctly, the need for BLS established, and rescue attempts are under way, the situation and condition of the casualty must be carefully monitored by the rescuer, to determine if rescue efforts should continue or be stopped.

There are four instances in which BLS attempts should be stopped.

- The casualty recovers and is able to circulate oxygenated blood and breathe without assistance.
- Their life support is handed over to specialists (paramedics).
- The rescuer is too physically exhausted to continue BLS.
- The death of the casualty is confirmed by an authorised practitioner (a doctor at the scene).

Recovery

It is unlikely that spontaneous recovery will occur, as once the heart has stopped beating it usually requires the specialist techniques of either drug administration or defibrillation to start functioning again. The purpose of BLS is to maintain an oxygenated blood flow to the brain to prevent death until specialist help arrives.

However, in the rare event that the casualty does regain airway and circulation control, the rescuer must be able to recognise their improved condition and act accordingly until specialist help arrives. In other emergency situations, they may have stopped breathing but still have a circulation, in which case chest compressions should not be attempted.

It is not advisable for the rescuer to waste valuable time attempting to find a pulse to determine if circulation has been re-established; it can be notoriously difficult to do and should be left to specialists to determine. Indeed, a casualty can die through lack of BLS provision if a rescuer mistakenly identifies a non-existent pulse.

Other more obvious signs that indicate a functioning circulatory system are:

- movement of the individual
- coughing or signs of attempts to breathe
- change in skin and lip colour, from grey or blue to pink, although this will be more difficult to determine in a casualty with darker skin tones.

Once signs of a functioning circulation are recognised, the rescuer must continue giving rescue breaths until either the casualty begins breathing again themselves or specialist help arrives. The continuation of the circulation should be checked for after every 10 rescue breaths.

Recovery position

If all airway obstructions have been cleared, the airway sufficiently opened and rescue breathing carried out effectively by the rescuer, the casualty may begin spontaneously breathing again. Once breathing has begun, or if the casualty has been found unconscious but still breathing, their airway has to be maintained by the rescuer until specialist help arrives. If left lying on their back, the tongue may well fall back towards their throat and close off the airway, causing an obstruction to the oxygen flow in the respiratory system and precipitating a more serious emergency – an event that lay persons often refer to as 'swallowing the tongue'.

To ensure that this does not happen, the rescuer must place the casualty into the recovery position so that their tongue and any fluids (vomit or blood) can drain out of the mouth rather than obstructing the airway (Figure 6.10).

The recovery position involves rolling the casualty onto their side and bending their limbs so that they are supported in that position, with the airway open and unobstructed. This can only be fully performed when they have no potential injuries to their spine or limbs, otherwise a modified position must be achieved.

For a casualty lying on their back and breathing, with no injuries, the recovery position is achieved as follows.

- Kneel at one side of the casualty.
- Straighten out their arms and legs.
- Move their nearest arm out at a right angle and bend up at the elbow.

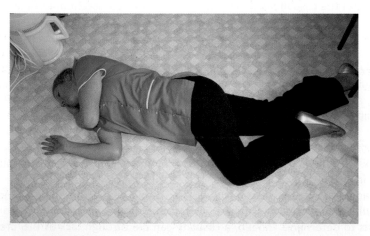

Figure 6.10   Recovery position.

- Gently pull their other arm and furthest leg towards you, so that the casualty begins to roll towards you.
- Place the furthest hand against the side of their face.
- Continue to roll them towards you by pulling the furthest leg, until their knee touches the ground.
- Keep their hand against the face so that their head rolls onto it.
- Once the roll is completed, ensure the airway is open by tilting the head back as necessary.
- Adjust the bent leg to stabilise the recovery position.

The technique is the same for all age groups except babies. A baby will be unstable if placed in the conventional recovery position, and it is much easier to place them in a safe position while holding them. If breathing but unconscious, the baby should be picked up and held on their side, towards the rescuer, with one hand under the baby's head and the other under their side and bottom. They should be tilted down slightly so that the head is lower than their body, allowing the tongue and any fluids to fall forwards away from the airway.

Modified recovery position

If a spinal injury is suspected, such as if the casualty has fallen onto their back from a height, perfoming the full recovery position manoeuvre may cause permanent spinal injury and should not be attempted.

Ideally the casualty should be left in the position in which they were found until specialist help arrives, but this may not be advisable if there is a possibility that their airway could become obstructed. In this situation, they must be rolled onto their side and supported in that position using anything available, such as rolled-up coats or other rescuers. While rolling them, their head and spine must be kept in alignment at all times (the 'log roll'), so the manoeuvre can only be carried out when more than one rescuer is present.

Similarly, if any limb injuries are suspected, the individual must be rolled without pulling on their limbs, and supported by coats, etc. rather than by bending the limbs to achieve stability.

The most important point is that the airway is opened and remains unobstructed, so that life is preserved. The rescuer will need to monitor the breathing and ensure that it continues to be unobstructed until specialist help arrives.

Handing over to specialists

The likely first responders to an emergency call will be paramedics, complete with specialised equipment and drugs to take over the advanced life support of the individual. However, they will require an accurate report of the emergency from all rescuers present to determine how best to proceed, and specifically the following points will require verification.

- **What happened?** Did anyone witness the actual emergency event (trip and fall, road traffic accident, convulsion, heart attack, choking, etc.)?
- **What time?** How long ago did the event occur, and how quickly were rescuers on the scene?
- **Condition?** Was AVPU gone through by the rescuers, and if so, what was the casualty's initial level of responsiveness?
- **BLS?** Was BLS required, how long was it carried out for, were there any problems in maintaining life before the specialists arrived?
- **Background knowledge?** Are any relatives or friends present with further information on the casualty (including their name), are any Medic-Alert identifiers present?

- **Personal items?** Hand over all of the casualty's personal items to the specialists; they will be able to check identity and medical status, and this is especially important in discovering if any medications are taken, such as an asthma inhaler.
- **Remain at the scene** – do not leave until the specialists are happy that they have all the information they require, including your personal and contact details in case the casualty dies, as a statement to the police may be required.

After the emergency

If the emergency occurred in the workplace, it is likely that all other workplace activities will have been postponed. However, the area will be littered with various used items and equipment that may have been abandoned while all minds focused on the rescue attempt.

The area must be cleaned and closed down in accordance with the local infection control policy, paying particular attention to the following.

- Wear full personal protective equipment.
- All sharps should be carefully discarded in the usual sharps container.
- All blood spillages should be covered with sodium hypochlorite (bleach) before being cleaned up.
- All non-sharp items contaminated with body fluids should be disposed of in the infectious hazardous waste sack.
- All dental equipment should be wiped down and switched off as usual.
- All dental instruments should be disposed of, or debrided and autoclaved in the usual manner.
- Any opened and unused dental materials should be disposed of in the non-infectious hazardous waste sack.
- All work surfaces should be wiped down once cleared, with the usual disinfectant.
- All records should be collated and filed in the usual place, those of the emergency casualty having been written up in full beforehand.

Causes of collapse

The various causes of the collapse of a casualty must be known and understood by the dental nurse, so that they can assist usefully in the emergency treatment of these individuals should the need arise. While knowing and understanding the functions of the emergency equipment that all dental surgeries must hold, the dental nurse would not be expected to administer any of the drugs available, except as a last resort where they are the only rescuer and the casualty is likely to die otherwise, before specialist help arrives.

Knowledge of the various signs and symptoms of the medical emergencies, and their correct treatment, is therefore imperative for students to learn thoroughly, so that on qualification they could deal with a medical emergency effectively. Consequently, medical emergencies are a topic that will always appear in the final Diploma examination, in both the written and practical sections.

The following medical emergencies are all potentially life-threatening events, and are covered below.

- Asthma attack.
- Anaphylaxis.

Table 6.1 Emergency drugs information

Emergency	Drug and dose	Route given
Asthma attack	Salbutamol metered dose 0.1 mg Oxygen	Inhaler Facemask
Anaphylaxis	Adrenaline 1:1000 Oxygen Hydrocortisone 100 mg Chlorphenamine 10 mg/mL	IM injection Facemask IM injection IM injection
Epileptic fit	Oxygen if possible Midazolam buccal gel if fit is prolonged	Facemask Oral
Hypoglycaemia	Conscious – Glucogel Unconscious – glucagon 1 mg	Oral IM injection
Angina	GTN metered dose 0.4 mg Oxygen	Sublingual Facemask
Myocardial infarction	Aspirin 300 mg Oxygen	Oral Facemask

GTN, glyceryl trinitrate; IM, intramuscular.

- Epileptic seizure.
- Diabetic hypoglycaemia or coma.
- Angina attack that may lead to myocardial infarction.
- Choking.

In addition, the simple faint (vasovagal syncope) is such a common occurrence in the dental workplace that it is important the dental nurse can recognise and treat this event successfully and it is therefore included in the following text.

All the medical emergencies listed above, except choking, may require the administration of specific emergency drugs to enable the casualty to survive the episode, and the dental nurse must be able to recognise and draw up these drugs ready for the dentist to administer. The details of the emergency drugs that should be present in all dental workplaces, their doses and routes of administration are shown in Table 6.1.

The first column details the medical emergency under discussion, while the second column itemises the drug(s) used and their dosages. The drugs relevant for each emergency are required knowledge for the dental nurse, but not the individual doses to be administered; in fact, the majority of them are supplied in dose increments within the phials, so that they can be drawn up and ready for use immediately. The third column states the administration route for each drug and it should be noted that all are delivered orally or as an intramuscular injection, as some skill is required to administer drugs by the alternative intravenous route, especially in an emergency situation. Oxygen is inspired with the use of a facemask connected to the oxygen cylinder, and can safely be given in all the emergencies listed.

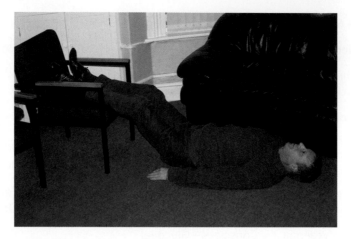

Figure 6.11   Faint recovery position.

Faint

This is a brief loss of consciousness due to a temporary reduction in oxygenated blood to the brain (**hypoxia**), and is the likeliest medical emergency to be encountered in the dental surgery.

- **Signs** – pale and clammy skin, weak and thready pulse, loss of consciousness.
- **Symptoms** – dizziness, tunnel vision, nausea.

Treatment

- If unconscious – lay casualty flat with their legs raised above the head to restore blood flow to the brain (Figure 6.11).
- Maintain airway and loosen tight clothing.
- Provide fresh air flow or oxygen.
- If conscious – sit casualty with head down, loosen tight clothing, provide fresh air.
- Give Glucogel or dextrose tablet when consciousness returns to restore the blood sugar levels.

Asthma attack

Asthma is a prediagnosed hypersensitivity condition affecting the respiratory airways. They narrow in response to exposure to inhaled particles, so that exhaled air has to be forced out of the respiratory system and the casualty has difficulty breathing. The same response can occur in stressful or fearful situations, or with exercise, especially if the casualty has a respiratory tract infection.

- **Signs** – breathless with wheezing on expiration, cyanosis (blueness of lips), restlessness.
- **Symptoms** – difficulty in breathing, sensation of suffocating or drowning.

Treatment

- Administer **salbutamol inhaler** from emergency drug box (Figure 6.12).
- Give **oxygen**.
- Calm and reassure the casualty.
- Call 999 if the casualty does not make a rapid recovery.

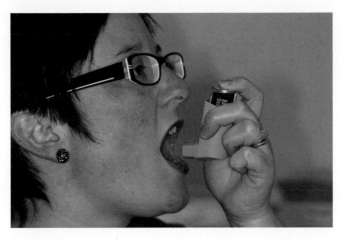

Figure 6.12   Inhaler administration.

Anaphylaxis

This is a severe allergic reaction by the casualty's immune system to an allergen, such as with an allergy to penicillin, latex or food products such as nuts. The immune system over-reacts to the allergen, causing severe swelling of the head and neck in particular, and a sudden fall in blood pressure (*hypotension*), causing collapse.

- **Signs** – rapid facial swelling, formation of a rash, gasping, collapse.
- **Symptoms** – sudden-onset breathing difficulties, becoming severe, tingling of extremities.

Treatment

- Call 999 urgently.
- Trained rescuer to administer **adrenaline** from emergency drug box. Also **steroid** and **antihistamine** if necessary.
- Maintain airway and give **oxygen** (Figure 6.13).
- Perform **BLS** if necessary until specialist help arrives.

Epileptic fit

This is a prediagnosed condition, in which there is a brief disruption of the normal electrical activity within the brain, causing a fit. The fits can occur mildly (*petit mal*) and the casualty may appear as though they are just daydreaming, or they may occur in a major form (*grand mal*).

- **Signs** – sudden loss of consciousness, followed by '**tonic-clonic**' seizure, possible incontinence. Tonic phase – casualty becomes rigid, clonic phase – casualty convulses.
- **Symptoms** – casualty may experience an altered mood (**aura**) just before the fit begins, dazed on recovery, with no memory of the fit.

Treatment

- Protect the casualty from injury, but make no attempt to move them.
- Remove onlookers from the area and maintain the casualty's dignity.

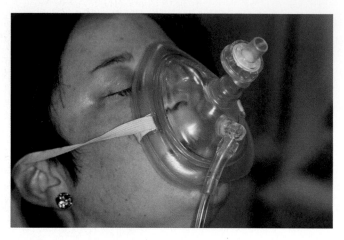

Figure 6.13   Giving oxygen using a mask.

- Allow their recovery, then ensure they are escorted home.
- If no recovery within 7 min, call 999.
- Trained rescuer to administer **diazepam** from emergency drug box, with great caution.

Hypoglycaemia and diabetic coma

These two conditions may occur in patients with prediagnosed diabetes who have either not followed their insulin regime correctly or have not eaten at the correct times. The resulting drop in their blood glucose levels can be catastrophic and cause collapse. The timing of dental appointments involving local anaesthesia is crucial for these patients, as they will be unable to eat without traumatising their oral soft tissues until the anaesthetic has worn off. The dental team must therefore ensure that appointment times fit around the patient's normal insulin and meal regimes.

- **Signs** – trembling, cold and clammy skin, becoming irritable to the point of being aggressive, drowsy, slurred speech, may appear to be drunk.
- **Symptoms** – confusion, disorientated, blurred or double vision.

Treatment

- If conscious, give **Glucogel tube** orally from emergency drug box (Figure 6.14).
- If unconscious, trained rescuer to administer **glucagon** from emergency drug box.
- Maintain airway and give **oxygen**.
- Call 999 if no recovery.

Angina

This usually occurs in prediagnosed patients suffering from coronary artery disease, where these blood vessels supplying the heart are narrowed due to the presence of cholesterol or a thrombus (blood clot). During times of stress or anxiety or while exercising, the reduced oxygenated blood supply to the heart is insufficient to allow full functioning, and the casualty will experience chest pains ranging in severity from indigestion to a heart attack.

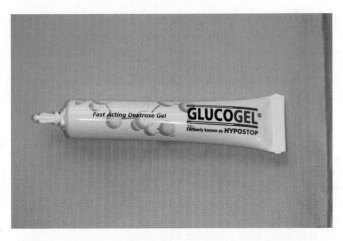

Figure 6.14 Glucogel tube from emergency kit.

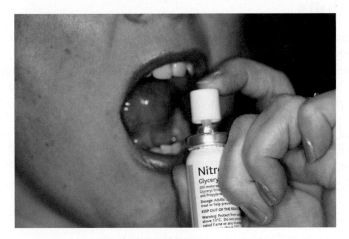

Figure 6.15 GTN spray administration sublingually.

- **Signs** – congested facial appearance, casualty clutching chest or left arm, irregular pulse, shallow breathing.
- **Symptoms** – crushing chest pain that may travel into left arm or jaw, nausea, breathlessness.

Treatment

- Administer **glyceryl trinitrate (GTN) spray** under tongue, from emergency drug box (Figure 6.15).
- Give **oxygen**.
- Keep the casualty sitting upright, but maintain airway.
- Calm and reassure the casualty.
- Call 999 urgently if no recovery or consciousness is lost – suspect cardiac arrest.

Myocardial infarction

This usually occurs in patients with a history of heart disease, especially angina, where either their drug regime has not been followed correctly or they have been exposed to anxiety or stress. During an angina attack, the turbulence caused by the increased coronary artery blood flow may be sufficient to dislodge any blood clots present, and these may lodge and completely obstruct the blood vessel. This will prevent oxygenated blood from supplying that section of the heart muscle, which will then die.

- **Signs** – sudden clutching of chest, grey appearance, possible collapse.
- **Symptoms** – sudden crushing chest pain that is not relieved by GTN spray.

Treatment

- Call 999 urgently.
- Administer **aspirin** from emergency drug box.
- Give **oxygen** and keep the casualty sitting upright.
- Maintain airway.
- Calm and reassure casualty.
- Perform **BLS** if necessary until specialist help arrives.

Choking in adults

Like the simple faint, choking is an emergency that may occur in the dental surgery from time to time, due to the nature of dental treatment. However, unlike the simple faint, choking is a very serious situation that could result in the death of the casualty if not dealt with promptly. It can occur in both the conscious or unconscious casualty, by the partial or full blockage of the respiratory tract causing lack of blood oxygenation. The body tissues will become *hypoxic*, and this can be catastrophic when the brain or heart is affected.

- **Signs** – sudden coughing or wheezing, laboured breathing, inability to speak, blue lips.
- **Symptoms** – aware of respiratory obstruction, breathing difficulties, dizziness.

Treatment

- Calm and reassure the casualty.
- Support them leaning forward and encourage coughing.
- Give five **back slaps** between the shoulder blades to dislodge the obstruction (Figure 6.16).

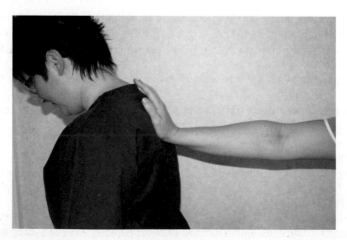

Figure 6.16   Back slaps between shoulder blades.

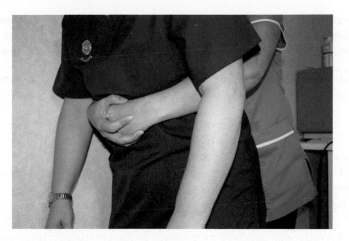

Figure 6.17   Abdominal thrusts.

- Begin **abdominal thrusts (Heimlich manoeuvre)** to cause artificial coughing if the obstruction is still present (Figure 6.17).
- If the casualty becomes unconscious, clear and open the airway as for **BLS**.
- Call 999 if this is unsuccessful.

The technique of giving abdominal thrusts is as follows.

- Stand behind the casualty.
- Rescuer wraps their arms around the casualty, just below their ribcage.
- A fist is formed with one hand and grasped by the other, positioning both in the upper abdomen.
- Both hands are pulled in sharply, to cause an artificial cough.
- Air will whoosh out at each thrust, hopefully dislodging the obstruction.

Choking in young children

The signs and symptoms of choking in a young child will be as for an adult casualty, and they are more likely to experience this emergency due to their lack of awareness of danger and their tendency to put objects into their mouths without realising the consequences.

The procedure to follow is very similar to that for an adult but with less force, and depends on whether the young child is conscious or not. The important point is that rescue breathing should only be carried out on an unconscious child, as their airway often becomes clear as their muscles relax during their loss of consciousness, and rescue breaths may not be necessary.

The procedure in a choking *conscious* child is as follows.

- Keep calm and keep the casualty (and any attending parent) calm.
- Get the child to cough to try and expel the obstruction.
- If unsuccessful, give five back slaps and recheck their mouth.
- If unsuccessful, give five chest thrusts from behind against their breastbone, then recheck their mouth.
- If unsuccessful, send for help then repeat the back slaps and recheck their mouth.
- If unsuccessful, give up to five abdominal thrusts but with less force than that used for an adult, then recheck the mouth.

- Continue alternating all three techniques until the obstruction is cleared, the child loses consciousness or specialist help arrives.
- If successful, have the child medically checked for any signs of respiratory system damage.

If the choking episode is severe and prolonged, or the obstruction is complete, the child will collapse and become unconscious. The rescue procedure is then as follows.

- Check the mouth for any obstruction and remove, then open the airway.
- Try five times to give two rescue breaths; if the chest rises successfully then carry out chest compressions to circulate the oxygen around the body.
- If the chest fails to rise, give five back slaps followed by five chest compressions if the child is still choking.
- Recheck the mouth and open the airway, then give another five rescue breaths.
- If unsuccessful, give another five back slaps followed by five abdominal thrusts.
- Continue the cycle until specialist help arrives or the obstruction is removed.

Choking in babies

Babies are easier for the rescuer to handle during a choking episode, as they can be held face down for back slaps and carried towards help while still being aided, rather than having to be left. Obviously, the force used to attempt to dislodge an obstruction must be significantly less than that used for a young child. Also, under no circumstances should abdominal thrusts be attempted on a baby, as their internal organs would be easily damaged by this technique.

Again, as with a young child, rescue breathing should not be attempted unless the baby is unconscious. If the baby is conscious and choking, the procedure is as follows.

- Check the mouth for any obvious obstruction and remove it.
- With the baby held face down along the rescuer's arm, give five back slaps using fingers only (Figure 6.18).
- Turn the baby face up and remove any obstruction.
- If unsuccessful, give five sharp chest compressions (as for BLS).

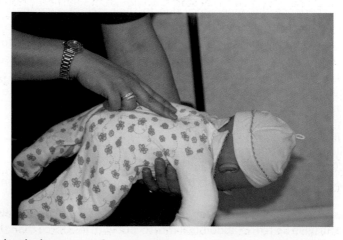

Figure 6.18 Baby back slaps using fingers.

- If unsuccessful, call for specialist help and continue the cycle until the obstruction is removed or the baby becomes unconscious.

If the baby becomes unconscious:

- recheck the mouth and open the airway
- try five times to give two rescue breaths
- if the chest rises, continue chest compressions to circulate the oxygen
- if not, give five back slaps followed by five chest compressions
- recheck the mouth for any obstruction and open the airway, then repeat the cycle until specialist help arrives.

179

Preparation of the dental team for medical emergencies

Besides the legal obligation of complying with the GDC *Standards Guidance* regulations, ensuring that all team members not only have current BLS certificates but that they are updated regularly, the dental team can do much to prepare for a medical emergency event. In particular, the team can have regular 'in-house' emergency training practice sessions that are carried out and recorded accurately.

Although it is not currently a legal requirement for dental workplaces to have an automatic external defibrillator (AED) on the premises, evidence shows that their use by experienced staff in a medical emergency significantly increases the chances of survival for the casualty. Their acquisition and thorough training in their use by all staff should therefore be encouraged. In addition, a policy must be in place to lay out all of the following points.

- Designation of the team leader (usually the senior dentist).
- All staff must stop work and be available to assist with the emergency immediately.
- The location of the emergency drugs box and oxygen cylinders must be known by all staff.
- Duties will be delegated by the team leader and must be carried out correctly by those involved, in particular duties to collect the emergency drugs box and the oxygen, to call 999, to clear other patients away, to direct the specialist emergency personnel to the casualty.
- No duties should be undertaken that staff have not been specifically trained for.
- All staff must be competent in BLS techniques and able to assist as necessary.
- Commands from the team leader must be followed immediately and accurately.
- Duty of care to the casualty must be upheld at all times.

The dental team is also well advised to familiarise themselves with the emergency equipment, and to practise the use of it on a regular basis. In particular:

- the use of the resuscitation masks and Ambu-bags
- the use of the portable suction unit for clearing the airway
- the use of artificial airways
- switching on the oxygen supply, and connecting the tubing and masks correctly
- opening drug phials and correctly drawing up their contents.

If a medical emergency does occur, accurate written records must be kept of the whole event for legal reasons. Any failure to do so, or any altering of the record contents, would cause the offender to be liable to GDC proceedings or even prosecution in serious cases. The dental nurse would be personally responsible for their own actions, and can no longer assume that the senior dentist would be vicariously liable and held to account for everyone else's performance.

The importance of a full written account, then, cannot be overstressed, not only for the protection of the public but also for that of all staff. If it is shown that everything possible was done to avoid an emergency, and that the full and correct actions were taken by all when one occurred, no-one can be held to account for what is then an unfortunate and unavoidable accident.

 Further resources are available for this book, including interactive multiple choice questions and extended matching questions. Visit the companion website at:

www.levisonstextbookfordentalnurses.com

7

Microbiology and Pathology

Key learning points

A **factual knowledge** of
- pathogenic micro-organisms

A **working knowledge** of
- disease processes
- pathology relevant to oral health

A **factual awareness** of
- drugs used to combat oral diseases

Pathology is the study of disease, and disease is the condition of suffering from an illness. Many diseases are caused by contamination of the body cells by microscopic living organisms, collectively called *micro-organisms*. The study of these different micro-organisms, how they live and function, and how they cause disease within the body is called microbiology.

Micro-organisms that have the capability of producing a disease are referred to as *pathogenic organisms*, or *pathogens*, as opposed to those that cannot cause illness or disease which are called *non-pathogens*.

The three main groups of pathogenic micro-organisms are as follows.

- **Bacteria** – microscopic single cell organisms that survive as inactive *spores* when conditions are not favourable for them to grow and reproduce.
- **Viruses** – ultramicroscopic organisms that live within the cells of other organisms.
- **Fungi** – a type of microscopic plant organism that grows across cells and tissues as an extensive branching network of fungal tissue.

Levison's Textbook for Dental Nurses, Eleventh Edition. By Carole Hollins.
© 2013 John Wiley & Sons, Ltd. Published 2013 by John Wiley & Sons, Ltd. Companion website: www.levisonstextbookfordentalnurses.com

A fourth type of micro-organism, called *protozoa*, also exists but has no relevance to dentistry, as protozoa do not cause any diseases within the oral cavity.

In addition, recent research has uncovered the existence of *prions*, which are not a living micro-organism but rather a type of special protein that is capable of causing disease. Those diseases caused by prions that have been discovered so far include 'mad cow disease' and the human variation of it which is called Creutzfeldt–Jakob disease (CJD).

The transmission of CJD is becoming more of a concern in dentistry as prions are not killed by the usual decontamination and sterilisation techniques used in the dental surgery environment. This means that an infected patient could pass on CJD to another patient when supposedly sterile instruments are reused. As the prions are known to specifically affect nerve tissue, all endodontic instruments (those used for root canal treatment, such as barbed broaches and files) now have to be considered as single-use disposable items in dentistry, as they will come into contact with the nerve tissue found within the pulp of the teeth during normal use. These instruments must all be safely discarded in sharps boxes after being used on just one patient, and then new instruments are used on the next patient. This avoids the possibility of passing prions from the first patient to the second.

The new instruments will have been sterilised at the manufacturing stage, using an industrial sterilisation technique such as gamma irradiation. The topics of decontamination, sterilisation and infection control are discussed in detail in Chapter 8.

The oral cavity provides the ideal conditions for micro-organisms to live, especially bacteria, being warm and well oxygenated and providing many sheltered areas for them to lodge without being disturbed and removed. A healthy oral cavity normally contains many different bacteria, many of which are harmless, but others cause disease within the oral cavity when their numbers increase. Other micro-organisms not normally present in health can be transferred to the oral cavity and cause disease, such as by using contaminated crockery or cutlery, or by sharing a toothbrush between individuals. The pathogenic micro-organisms relevant to dentistry are described below.

Bacteria

These single-cell micro-organisms have rigid outer walls which determine their shape, and help to categorise them into named groups (Figure 7.1).

- **Cocci** – are circular micro-organisms; colonies living in clusters are *staphylococci*, while those living in chains are *streptococci*.
- **Bacilli** – are rod-shaped with pointed ends; round-ended ones are *lactobacilli*.
- **Spirochaetes** – are spiral shaped, like a helix.

When their living conditions are not ideal for the colony to grow and expand, bacteria survive as *spores*, in a similar way that plants produce seeds to survive the winter while the parent plant dies from the cold. The spores have a very hard outer coating that protects the bacteria within from chemicals, from drought, and from a wide variation in temperature. Many can therefore survive the action of disinfecting chemicals used in dentistry (such as bleach), and the only sure way of removing the risk of bacterial contamination on dental instruments is to either sterilise them or to only use them once before they are discarded (single-use items). Dental instruments are expensive to buy, so wherever possible they are manufactured to withstand the sterilisation process and can then be reused safely.

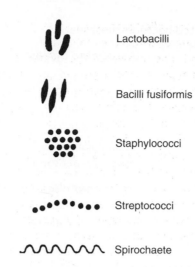

Figure 7.1   Types of bacteria by microscopic shape.

Some bacteria found in the oral cavity have adapted to exist in areas of low oxygen levels, such as deep within a carious lesion or a periodontal pocket. They are referred to as *anaerobic bacteria* and are particularly harmful because they often require different treatment methods to those used against the more usual *aerobic bacteria*.

Although the body's natural defence mechanisms will help to protect it to some extent from attack by micro-organisms, by the existence of its *natural immunity*, drugs have also been developed to fight against them, and for bacteria the important drug groups are the following.

- **Antibiotics** – taken to kill bacteria causing a severe illness, but can also kill some of the helpful bacteria naturally found within the body, especially those in the digestive system. Treatment with antibiotics is therefore often associated with stomach pain or diarrhoea. Different types are required when treating infections caused by either aerobic or anaerobic bacteria.
- **Bactericidal agents** – chemicals used to clean externally (such as surgery work surfaces) that act to kill bacteria.
- **Bacteriostatic agents** – chemicals used to clean externally that do not kill bacteria, but prevent them reproducing and multiplying.

Some of the more important bacteria associated with dentistry are shown in Table 7.1. The specific micro-organisms associated with causing certain bacterial diseases are listed in the first column and the actual disease in the second column. So, for example, there are four micro-organisms listed as being associated with periodontal disease, and two with dental caries – the initial infective agent as well as the micro-organism found in established dental cavities. The names of some of these micro-organisms should be familiar to the dental nurse.

Both dental caries and periodontal disease are caused by bacterial infection of the dental hard tissues, or the supporting structures of the teeth, respectively. Prevention of these diseases and their treatment when present in a patient are the mainstay of the work carried out by the dental team on a daily basis.

Table 7.1   Dentally related bacterial diseases

Bacteria name	Associated disease
Streptococcus mutans	Initial infective bacteria found in dental caries, as a cavity first forms, and the micro-organism responsible for most of the production of the weak organic acids that cause enamel demineralisation
Lactobacillus	Later colonisation of an established carious lesion, as the deeper tooth tissues become infected
Actinomyces Porphyromonas gingivalis Prevotella intermedia Treponema denticola	Periodontal disease, the bacterial infection of the supporting structures of the teeth (gingivae, periodontal ligament, cementum, alveolar bone)
Staphylococci	Skin boils and gingival boils
Bacillus fusiformis Borellia vincenti	Acute necrotising ulcerative gingivitis, a specific periodontal infection often seen in young adults when their oral hygiene is particularly poor

Viruses

These micro-organisms are far smaller than bacteria, being visible only with an electron microscope. They live within the cells of other organisms, including human tissue cells, existing as a protein capsule that contains all the chemicals the virus needs to reproduce within the cells of its host (Figure 7.2). The protein capsule is unique for every virus and causes the body cells to react against it (as an *immune response*) while trying to fight off the disease that the virus has produced.

Viral diseases are more difficult to cure than those caused by other micro-organisms because very few drugs have been developed against them, although some antiviral agents do exist. One such agent of relevance to the dental team is the drug aciclovir, which is used in a topical cream to treat 'cold sore' lesions of the lip. Others are being developed in the ongoing battle against AIDS.

Fortunately, *vaccinations* have been developed to prevent many (but not all) viral diseases instead. They consist of a harmless dose of the dead virus or its protein capsule which is injected into the individual or given orally. The presence of the dead virus or capsules causes the body's immune system to fight against them by making *antibodies*, although the disease itself cannot develop fully and make the person unwell. If the individual is then exposed to the same viral disease again in the future, these antibodies already present in their body will fight off the viral attack and prevent the person from becoming ill. This is called *acquired immunity*.

Viruses are also more difficult to kill than bacteria, and either the process of sterilisation or the use of specialised viricidal chemicals is required to do so. Unless stated on the labelling as viricidal, routine disinfectants are not usually active against viruses.

Some of the more important viral infections of relevance to the dental team are shown in Table 7.2.

There are relatively more viral diseases of importance to the dental team than there are bacterial diseases, although none affect the teeth or their supporting structures and are therefore not associated with caries or periodontal disease. The viral diseases are important from an infection

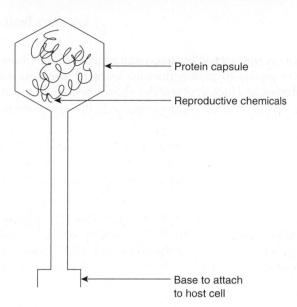

Figure 7.2 Structure of a virus.

Table 7.2 Dentally related viral diseases

Virus name	Associated disease
Hepatitis A, B, C, etc.	Various inflammatory liver diseases, some of which are fatal Hepatitis B vaccinations are an occupational health requirement for all clinical dental personnel
Herpes varicella	Chicken pox, which usually occurs in childhood (but not always) and which affects the area supplied by the trigeminal nerve (fifth cranial nerve) as well as the torso
Human immunodeficiency virus (HIV)	Acquired immune deficiency syndrome (AIDS), a bloodborne and fatal viral infection which was initially only found in certain patient groups (such as intravenous drug users and homosexuals), but has now spread beyond them and can be found in the wider population
Herpes zoster	Shingles, a very painful blistering skin rash which can involve the area supplied by the trigeminal nerve (fifth cranial nerve) as well as the torso
Herpes simplex type I	'Cold sores' which are blister lesions occurring on the lips, and are highly infectious in their initial stages if touched
Epstein–Barr	Glandular fever, a debilitating viral infection which results in painfully swollen lymph glands, including those found in the neck
Paramyxovirus	Mumps, a viral infection of the parotid salivary glands (either one or both), but which seems not to affect any other salivary glands
Coxsackievirus	Hand-foot-and-mouth disease, a common infection seen in young children, which presents as painful blistering in the oral cavity, on the palms of the hands and the soles of the feet

control point of view, as staff should be vaccinated against several of them and their infectivity is usually greater from person to person than for bacterial diseases. Indeed, when a patient is suffering from viral infections such as cold sores, mumps or chicken pox, it is best if their treatment is delayed to avoid the risk of spreading the infection to the workplace personnel.

Fungi

These are plant-like organisms similar to microscopic colonies of mushrooms or toadstools. They grow as an extensive network of branches lying across the body tissues (called *hyphae*) and reproduce by budding out from the ends of the hyphae, or by the production of spores from fruiting bodies (like microscopic mushrooms). They tend to live on the outer surface of the body; such as on the skin, the oral cavity lining, the nails and the surface of the eye, rather than growing within the body tissues.

The only fungal infection of dental importance is that caused by *Candida albicans*, which is responsible for the following oral lesions and diseases.

- **Oral thrush** – appearing as a removable white film with underlying red, sore patches occurring on the soft tissues of the oral cavity, and associated with general ill health, especially in the elderly or those suffering from other serious diseases such as AIDS. When present in an otherwise healthy individual, oral thrush will have developed because of a disruption in the usual oral bacteria colony, usually following a course of antibiotics.
- **Denture stomatitis** – also known as 'denture sore mouth', which occurs in healthy patients beneath both dentures and removable orthodontic appliances, as a reddened but painless area lying exactly beneath the palatal section of the appliance. It is associated with poor appliance hygiene and raised moisture levels beneath the appliance, allowing the fungus to colonise the underlying oral tissues.
- **Angular cheilitis** – a *Candida* infection that specifically involves the angles of the mouth, appearing as a localised area of inflamed and cracked skin which is often crusted over. Wide mouth opening will split the lesion and cause bleeding and further splitting. It is associated with constant saliva leakage into the angle areas, allowing the fungal infection to occur – patients usually have deep tissue folds here or have a 'crumpled face' appearance due to loss of their occlusal face height. This may be due to edentulousness, worn dentures or tooth surface loss with age or in severe cases of attrition.

Fungal infections are treated with antifungal agents, usually provided as oral gels, oral solutions or as a pastille to be sucked and dissolved in the mouth. Antifungal agents in current use include nystatin pastilles or solution, amphotericin lozenges, miconazole gel and fluconazole tablets.

Any suspected underlying illnesses also need diagnosing and treating, and appliance hygiene needs to be reinforced by the dental team in cases of denture stomatitis. Patients suffering from angular cheilitis will require treatment to restore their occlusal face height to an acceptable size so that the folds of tissue at the angles of their mouth are eliminated. This may involve the provision of new or replacement dentures, or the rehabilitation of their dentition to replace the tooth tissue lost by attrition.

General effects of disease on the body

So, the body cells may be attacked by one of many pathogenic micro-organisms to produce an infection which results in a disease or illness. In addition, tissue damage, illness and disease may occur due to other (non-infective) occurrences such as trauma, body cell/tissue malfunction and genetic mutation or predisposition. Whatever the cause, the effects on the body will occur as one of the following.

- **Infection** – the actual invasion of the body cells by the pathogens, resulting in an *inflammatory response* of the cells which produces the five signs of inflammation: *heat, swelling, pain, redness, loss of function*. Examples of dentally relevant infections include:
  - dental caries
  - periodontal disease
  - denture stomatitis
  - herpes simplex.
- **Ulcer** – a shallow break in the skin or mucous membrane, leaving a raw and painful circular base that may bleed when touched. Examples of dentally relevant ulcers are:
  - aphthous ulcers (often associated with stress, vitamin deficiency, poor nutrition)
  - traumatic ulcers (often caused by dental appliances or vigorous tooth brushing).
- **Cyst** – an abnormal sac of fluid that develops within the body tissues over a period of time. Examples of dentally relevant cysts are:
  - dentigerous cyst (develops around an impacted, unerupted tooth)
  - periapical cyst (develops around the tooth apex)
  - trauma to minor salivary glands, producing a cyst called a 'mucocele' (usually occurs on the lower lip).
- **Tumour** – a swelling within any body tissue due to an uncontrolled and abnormal overgrowth of the body cells. When the swelling causes no harm other than to displace any surrounding structures it is called *benign* but when the swelling invades and damages the surrounding structures it is called malignant and is usually referred to as *cancer*. Examples of dentally relevant tumours are:
  - squamous cell carcinoma of the oral epithelium
  - osteosarcoma of the mandible or maxilla
  - salivary gland tumours (benign or malignant)
  - lymphoma affecting the lymph glands of the neck.
- **Congenital/developmental defect** – either an inherited condition or a genetic mutation which produces an illness or condition that is present at birth. Examples of dentally relevant defects are:
  - cleft lip or palate
  - congenital absence of some teeth – hypodontia
  - defect of tooth formation, such as amelogenesis imperfect.

187

Response of the body to pathogen attack

For the dental nurse, the most relevant potential cause of illness and disease in a patient is that due to attack by pathogenic micro-organisms, as an infection. An understanding of the way that the body responds to the pathogen attack, and either fights off the invaders or succumbs to illness and disease, is important for the dental nurse to grasp when considering their role in infection control.

The body has three natural lines of defence against attack by pathogens which, in fit and healthy individuals, are often enough to prevent a serious illness developing.

- Intact skin and mucous membranes which act as physical barriers against the pathogens.
- Surface secretions onto the skin or mucous membranes that help to dilute and neutralise the pathogens and their poisons (*toxins*), such as saliva in the mouth, gastric juice in the stomach, sweat on the skin and tears in the eyes.
- Inflammatory response if the skin or mucous membranes are breached.

Problems may occur in individuals who are not fit and healthy when their body is attacked by pathogens, as they may be unable to defend themselves so that a disease takes hold and they become ill. Those most likely to suffer are the following.

- **Elderly** – the functioning of the body cells in older patients is not as efficient as when they were younger, as cells and tissues wear out with age and cannot be replaced as easily, and other age-related disorders may be present that affect the ability of the body to repair itself.
- **Young children** – including babies, whose natural immune systems will not be functioning fully for some time, so they are more prone to developing diseases after attacks by pathogens, as well as not having received their full vaccination programme.
- **Debilitated** – those patients of any age who are said to be *immuno-compromised* because they have an underlying illness that affects the ability of their immune system to fight off pathogens; this includes those with diabetes, those suffering from a range of illnesses such as leukaemia, kidney failure, AIDS and various cancers, and those taking drugs that suppress their immune systems, due to organ transplant or cancer treatment.

Infection occurs when the pathogenic micro-organisms actually gain entry to the body tissues. In the dental workplace, this can happen in a variety of ways.

- **Direct contact** – with body fluids, such as saliva, blood or vomit.
- **Airborne droplets** – of body fluids, due to the infected host sneezing, coughing or spitting.
- **Aerosol spray** – created during the use of dental handpieces and water sprays, spraying blood and saliva into the atmosphere.
- **Direct entry** – through damaged skin or oral epithelium, from cuts, grazes, piercing of the cornea of the eye.
- **Inoculation injury** – piercing of the skin or oral epithelium with a contaminated instrument, as occurs with a dirty needlestick injury.

Inflammatory response

If the body tissues are breached by the pathogen, then an inflammatory response occurs. This is the normal reaction of the body to exposure to an irritant such as an infective micro-organism, but it may also occur when exposed to physical and chemical irritants such as cuts, fire burns or chemical burns. Microscopically, the reaction of the body is the same, irrespective of the cause.

- Huge increase in the blood flow to the affected area, so that many leucocytes (white blood cells) can be transported there to fight the pathogens.
- This sudden increase in blood volume in the area will cause the tissues to appear *red* and *swollen*, and feel *hot to touch*.
- The swollen tissues will also press against the surrounding nerve cells, causing *pain*, and the affected area will then become too painful to use, resulting in *loss of function*.
- Leucocytes pass out of the capillaries and into the invaded body tissues to fight the pathogens by surrounding and eating them. They are helped to destroy the pathogens by the movement of blood plasma into the tissues, which contains antibodies and antitoxins and acts to neutralise the poisons produced by the pathogens.
- Toxin production by the pathogens may be severe enough to cause a rise in body temperature from the normal 37°C, indicating an intense infection – this rise in body temperature is called *pyrexia*.
- During the battle, both leucocytes and pathogens are killed, and their debris collects to form *pus* in the body tissues.
- If the pus remains contained in the area of invasion, it forms an *abscess*, but if it manages to spread into the surrounding tissues, it is called *cellulitis*.

- When the inflammatory process occurs as above, it is described as *acute infection* but when it occurs over a long period of time with few of the symptoms (especially pain) being evident, it is described as *chronic infection*.
- If the infecting micro-organism is very powerful and difficult for the inflammatory response to control, it is described as *virulent*.
- The elderly, the young and the debilitated may be unable to fight off an infection without the use of drugs such as *antibiotics*, *antivirals* or *antifungals*, and these may also have to be used in healthy individuals when a virulent organism is involved.

So to reiterate, the five classic signs of inflammation are *heat, swelling, redness, pain, loss of function*.

When the inflammatory response occurs in the absence of micro-organisms, no infection will occur, nor pus form, and the body tissues will repair any damage caused by the irritant.

Tissue repair

Once the inflammatory response has overcome the infecting micro-organisms, or the physical or chemical irritant has been removed, the body will repair itself. New leucocytes will travel to the area and remove any damaged or dead tissue, and they will then lay down a temporary layer of repair cells called *granulation tissue*. This consists of basic tissue cells and capillaries which form a fibrous framework for the more specialised tissue cells to grow and develop onto. So if the damage occurred in skin, skin cells will be formed; if in bone, bone cells will be formed, and so on.

If a chronic infection is persistently present, the body's attempts to repair the damage will only be partially successful, and a state will exist where tissue is being repaired at the same time as chronic infection is still present. This is the usual case with infections such as chronic periodontal disease. The infecting micro-organisms are never completely eradicated, the chronic infection is always present and its severity swings between low grade and held at bay, with intermittent acute episodes that require treatment and drug therapy to overcome.

Immune response

During the inflammatory response, certain leucocytes are not involved in fighting the micro-organisms, but are stimulated to release *antibodies* and *antitoxins* into the blood plasma instead. The stimulation occurs because these leucocytes recognise the invaders as being foreign to the normal body tissues; they are identified as *antigens*. Other antigens that will cause a similar response are transplanted organs, foreign bodies, toxins from plant and animal tissues, and incompatible blood transfusions.

The antibodies and antitoxins released are quite specific for an invading micro-organism, and their presence in the body provides *immunity* against that specific disease. The types of immunity that may be present are listed below.

- **Natural immunity** – present from birth by being randomly inherited.
- **Passive immunity** – present from birth and specifically inherited directly from the mother's own pool of antibodies and antitoxins.
- **Acquired immunity** – creation of the necessary antibodies and antitoxins by the leucocytes during a pathogen attack, so that the disease is overcome. These new antibodies and antitoxins then remain in the body for life and prevent a recurrence of the same infection.

- **Vaccination to produce acquired immunity** – by giving a harmless dose of a pathogen (often by injection) to stimulate the leucocytes to develop the antibodies and antitoxins, but without actually causing the disease to develop.

Unfortunately, acquired immunity does not occur for every micro-organism and in addition, many of them (especially viruses) can go through a process called *mutation*, by which they change their chemical make-up slightly and effectively produce a new variation of a disease. The individual will then have to be exposed to this new variant before suitable antibodies and antitoxins can be made by their leucocytes. This is why, for example, influenza vaccinations are necessary on an annual basis, as the virus mutates easily and creates new strains of the micro-organism every year. New vaccines then have to be developed, and the population vaccinated each autumn before the variant disease becomes widespread.

With the use of vaccines, individuals can be protected against serious and fatal infections without having to be exposed to, and survive, the actual attack. Because of the close-up and hands-on nature of dental treatment, the team are exposed to many infections daily and are at risk of catching any of them. Consequently, all must be vaccinated against the following.

- Hepatitis B.
- MMR – measles, mumps and rubella (German measles).
- Tuberculosis and whooping cough (pertussis).
- Poliomyelitis.
- Diphtheria and tetanus.
- Chicken pox (if not already naturally immune).
- Meningitis.

Some serious and fatal diseases have no vaccination available at present, and one of the most important ones in relation to the dental team is AIDS because this is transmitted mainly by blood and many dental procedures produce bleeding. Avoidance of infection by any micro-organism can only occur if procedures are in place with regard to the following factors.

- Staff vaccination.
- Use of personal protective equipment (PPE) during treatment and cleaning procedures.
- Use of single-use disposables where possible.
- Correct decontamination and sterilisation of reusable instruments and equipment.
- Correct cleaning of the clinical area.
- Thorough hand washing.

Allergy

Occasionally the normal immune response goes into overdrive after exposure to some substances, and the body completely over-reacts to the presence of an antigen. An *allergic reaction* occurs, and results in sudden swelling of the tissues and the production of copious fluids from the body tissues. The substance that stimulated the over-reaction is called an *allergen*. The effects of the allergen on the individual can range in severity from hayfever-like symptoms, to a mild rash, to a full anaphylactic shock episode, which is potentially fatal (see Chapter 6).

Often, individuals prone to an allergic reaction will already suffer from disorders such as asthma, eczema or hayfever, so they should be identified from their medical history and treated with caution. Particular precautions to be taken during dental treatment include the avoidance of known allergens, such as *latex products* (gloves, rubber dam sheets, local anaesthetic cartridge bungs) and certain drugs such as the antibiotic *penicillin* and its derivatives.

There is also an increased incidence of a condition called *contact dermatitis* amongst dental and medical staff nowadays, possibly due to the increased use of hand-cleaning agents in the workplace. In addition, the increased use and variety of surface cleaning sprays and wipes that are necessary to comply with current infection control legislation are thought to be linked to an increase in staff numbers experiencing upper respiratory tract allergic reactions. It is hoped that as new products are developed, their effects on the staff exposed to their increased use will be taken into consideration by the manufacturers.

Dentally related pathology

191

With an understanding of the various types of micro-organisms that may cause disease and illness in the body, a summary of the lesions and conditions that may occur in the oral cavity and be seen by the dental nurse is given below. Oral cancer will be discussed in detail.

- **Dental caries** – bacterial infection of the hard tissues of the tooth.
- **Periodontal disease** – bacterial infection of the gingivae and periodontal supporting tissues.
- **Oral thrush** – fungal infection of the oral soft tissues.
- **Periapical abscess** – bacterial infection of the tooth pulp causing abscess formation at the apex (can be acute or chronic – Figure 7.3).
- **Periodontal abscess** – bacterial infection within a periodontal pocket causing abscess formation.
- **Aphthous ulcers** – ulceration of the oral soft tissues that is not related to infection.
- **Herpetic ulceration** – viral infection of the oral soft tissues causing ulceration.
- **Acute necrotising ulcerative gingivitis** – acute bacterial infection of the gingivae causing ulceration.
- **Dental cyst** – cyst formation associated with a tooth, either erupted or unerupted.
- **Alveolar bone cyst** – cyst formation within the jaw bone.
- **Pericoronitis** – acute bacterial infection of the soft tissues (operculum) associated with a partially erupted tooth.
- **Localised osteitis** – bacterial infection of the bony walls of an extraction socket (also called 'dry socket').
- **Cellulitis** –bacterial infection spreading from a tooth into the surrounding deep soft tissue structures.

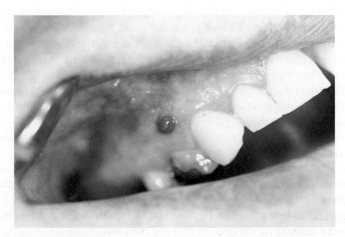

Figure 7.3   Chronic abscess with sinus.

- **Cleft palate** – developmental defect of the palate (roof of the mouth) where the two bony halves fail to join together completely.
- **Oral cancer** – malignant tumour usually affecting the oral soft tissues initially, and then spreading into the underlying tissues if not treated.

Oral cancer

Oral cancer can affect various areas of the mouth: the soft tissues, the salivary glands or the jaw bones. Ninety percent of oral cancers affect the soft tissues initially, as a lesion called *squamous cell carcinoma* (SCC). The suggested causative factors are listed below.

- **Tobacco habits** – all tobacco products contain chemicals capable of causing cancer (*carcinogens*).
- **High alcohol consumption** – alcohol acts as a solvent for the carcinogens, and allows their easier entry into the soft tissues.
- **Both together** – smokers who also drink to excess are at most risk of SCC.
- **Sunlight** – in fair-skinned people, sunlight is associated with SCC affecting the lower lip.
- **Diet** – research is ongoing into links between SCC and diets high in fats and red meat, or low in vitamin A and iron intake.
- **Genetics** – some people are genetically predisposed to developing SCC.

The signs and symptoms of SCC may be any of the following, and will be specifically looked for during routine dental examinations by the dentist.

- Painless ulcer that has no obvious cause, and fails to heal fully within 2–3 weeks.
- In particular, an ulcer occurring beneath or on the side of the tongue or in the floor of the mouth.
- Presence of a white or red patch associated with the ulcer.

The risk factors mentioned previously make the occurrence of the signs and symptoms far more serious in certain individuals, and any suspicious lesions must be referred to an oral surgery hospital department for immediate investigation. Even then, the 5-year survival rate from SCC is only around 55%, and is very dependent on early detection and aggressive treatment.

Years ago, the typical oral cancer sufferer was a 60 plus male patient, usually from a lower socio-economic background, who was a life-long smoker and drinker. In recent years, this has changed and those being diagnosed with oral cancer are more likely to be much younger patients (even in their 20s), both male and female, usually smokers and especially binge drinkers, and also those who use sunbeds or sunbathe with little ultraviolet protection for their lips. Obviously this last group will also be at much greater risk of developing skin cancer (melanoma).

The dental team has a vital role to play not only in early detection of SCC but also in patient education about the risk factors, especially in these high-risk patients. This is especially important with smoking and tobacco usage, whether with cigarettes, cigars or pipes, and including the habitual chewing of betel nuts and tobacco paan by some Asian societies.

In addition, the effects of smoking on dental and general health should also be discussed with suitable patients, and should cover all of the following topics.

- Oral health effects
  - Oral cancer
  - Development of oral precancerous lesions (especially white patches in the mouth)
  - Periodontal disease

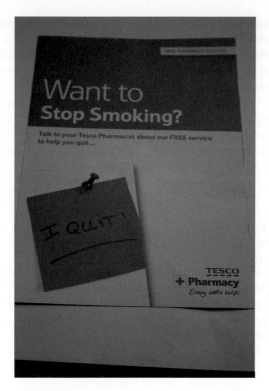

193

Figure 7.4   'Quit smoking' leaflet.

- ○ Poor wound healing, especially after extraction
- ○ Tendency to develop 'dry socket' after extraction
- ○ Stained teeth
- ○ Halitosis (bad breath)
- General health effects
  - ○ Heart disease – in particular, hypertension and coronary artery disease
  - ○ Stroke
  - ○ Respiratory disease – in particular, chronic bronchitis and emphysema
  - ○ Other cancers – in particular, throat, lung and stomach cancer

In the last few years, and in recognition of the alarming increasing incidence of smoking-related cancers and illness in the population, the Department of Health has developed an excellent national 'Quit Smoking' scheme that is freely accessible to anyone wishing to stop smoking, and information on local help and support is widely available (Figure 7.4).

The dental team has a valuable role to play in advising their patients of this scheme, referring them for help and treatment whenever possible, and supporting them as they undergo any treatment.

Relevant drugs used in dentistry

All drugs available by prescription from the dentist to a patient (prescription-only medicines – POM) or available to buy 'over the counter' without prescription are detailed in the Dental Practitioners' Formulary (DPF) section of the *British National Formulary* (BNF), and this is issued to all practising dentists by the Department of Health (see Figure 5.7). It is an invaluable guide to the drugs available, as well as giving details of their actions, dosages, contraindications and side-effects. The dentist may prescribe any other drugs on a private basis to a patient,although special rules and regulations apply to those categorised as controlled drugs (pethidine, midazolam, etc.).

The drugs discussed in this section are those used in dentistry to fight disease, specifically those used against micro-organisms. Many other drugs are used for other purposes by the dentist while providing treatment, and they will be discussed in their relevant chapters.

Drugs are classified into groups with a specific action, although some may have more than one use. Those of relevance here are:

- antibiotics
- antivirals
- antifungals
- analgesics.

Drugs may be applied externally, such as ointments and creams, or taken internally, such as tablets, capsules and oral solutions. When applied externally, their strength tends to be recorded as a percentage, while those used internally are recorded as milligrams for solids or millilitres for liquids. The drugs used more frequently to fight micro-organisms and alleviate the symptoms of infection are discussed below.

Antibiotics

These are drugs used specifically to fight against infection by bacteria. Many different bacteria exist that can cause dental problems, including dental caries, periodontal disease, dental abscesses and pericoronitis. Some bacteria thrive in the oxygen-rich environment of the mouth and are referred to as aerobic bacteria but others prefer to live in oxygen-poor areas such as deep within the periodontal pockets of a patient with periodontal disease. These bacteria are called anaerobes and they often require the use of different antibiotics for their eradication.

The bacteria can become immune to the antibiotics if used over a prolonged period or inappropriately, so their use must always be justified.

Typical antibiotics used in dentistry are shown in Figure 7.5 and are described below.

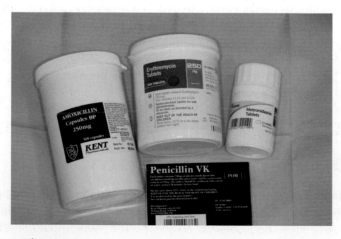

Figure 7.5   Various antibiotics.

- **Penicillin** – used against the spread of infection in pericoronitis and cellulitis, and to prevent secondary infection after oral surgery procedures. Typical dose is 250 mg taken four times daily for 3–5 days. Can cause allergic reaction in some patients (even anaphylaxis), and reacts with the drug methotrexate.
- **Amoxicillin** – type of penicillin with a wider range of action (referred to as a 'broad-spectrum antibiotic'); typical dose may be increased to 500 mg taken three times daily for up to 5 days in severe infections. Also used to be given as a prophylaxis against infective endocarditis in susceptible patients, as a single 3 g liquid dose taken 1 h before dental treatment, but this is no longer considered necessary for the majority of these patients.
- **Erythromycin** – as an alternative for penicillin and its derivatives, in patients who are allergic to them.
- **Clindamycin** – as a prophylactic alternative against infective endocarditis in patients allergic to amoxicillin, given as a single 600 mg dose 1 h before dental treatment; again, this is no longer considered necessary for these previously susceptible patients.
- **Metronidazole** – used against anaerobic bacteria often associated with pericoronitis, periodontal disease and acute ulcerative necrotising gingivitis. Typical dose is 200–400 mg taken three times daily for 3 days, depending on the severity of the infection. Has a severe reaction with alcohol, so patients must be suitably warned.

195

Antivirals

These are drugs used specifically against infections caused by a virus, but the only infection of dental relevance is the 'cold sore' produced on the lip after infection with the herpes simplex type I virus. Aciclovir antiviral cream applied to the lesion several times a day may prevent the full development and blistering of the cold sore infection. The lesions are highly infective while present, and the dental team must protect themselves by wearing full PPE during treatment. Ideally, the patient should not be treated while a cold sore is present, unless they require emergency treatment.

Antifungals

These are drugs used specifically against fungal infections, and the relevant dental lesion is in cases of infection causing oral thrush. This may appear as denture stomatitis beneath removable appliances or as sores at the angle of the mouth called angular cheilitis. Both are due to infection with the fungus *Candida albicans*. When present within the mouth, patients are prescribed antifungal lozenges or pastilles to suck, or oral gels or solutions to apply while their appliance is out. Other antifungals may be prescribed as capsules to be taken internally, and all of the following presentations are available.

- **Fluconazole** – used in difficult fungal infections as a once-daily 50 mg capsule dose for between 7 and 14 days.
- **Nystatin** – as an oral suspension or as lozenges to be used four times daily after food for 7 days.
- **Amphotericin** – as 10 mg lozenges to be slowly dissolved in the mouth four times daily for between 10 and 15 days.
- **Miconazole** – as an oral gel to be swilled around the mouth four times daily.

Analgesics

These are drugs used primarily to relieve pain, although some have other effects too. They are invaluable to dental patients experiencing pain (especially toothache) although dental treatment is often required to solve the problem and eliminate the pain completely. All analgesics should be avoided during pregnancy.

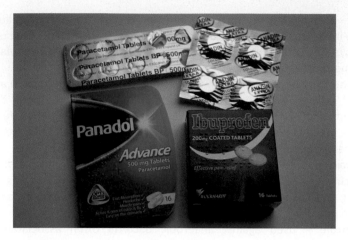

Figure 7.6 Various analgesics.

Frequently used analgesics are shown in Figure 7.6 and are all available as 'over-the-counter' analgesics, or they can be prescribed by the dentist.

- **Paracetamol** – is an analgesic and has *antipyretic* properties – it reduces body temperature when fever is present. It has no anti-inflammatory effect. Causes serious liver damage if the recommended dose is exceeded, and this may be fatal.
- **Ibuprofen** – a non-steroidal anti-inflammatory and analgesic which is safer than paracetamol but can cause stomach ulcers if used to excess. It should not be given to asthmatics.
- **Aspirin** – an analgesic with anti-inflammatory properties. It has several contraindications that limit its use: it acts as an anticoagulant so must not be given after surgical procedures (including tooth extraction), and can cause stomach ulcers. It should be avoided in asthmatics and must not be prescribed to children under 16 years of age because of the rare complication of *Reye's syndrome* (an often fatal brain disease).

 Further resources are available for this book, including interactive multiple choice questions and extended matching questions. Visit the companion website at:

www.levisonstextbookfordentalnurses.com

8

Infection Control and Cleanliness

Key learning points

A **factual knowledge** of
- the basic principles of infection control

A **working knowledge** of
- decontamination, disinfection, and sterilisation techniques
- personal protective equipment and its correct usage in the dental workplace

A **factual awareness** of
- cross infection and inoculation injury and their avoidance in the dental workplace

The maintenance of a high standard of cleanliness and the control of infection are topics of fundamental importance in the dental workplace, as they are in any clinical environment. All members of the dental team (including trainee dental nurses) have a duty of care to protect their patients and themselves from coming to harm while on the premises, and one potential area of vulnerability is to become contaminated by, or to acquire an infection from another patient or a member of staff, or from a dirty instrument. This is called *cross-infection*.

The methods used to avoid this are the foundations of good infection control, and of the principles of maintaining an adequate standard of cleanliness.

Levison's Textbook for Dental Nurses, Eleventh Edition. By Carole Hollins.
© 2013 John Wiley & Sons, Ltd. Published 2013 by John Wiley & Sons, Ltd. Companion website: www.levisonstextbookfordentalnurses.com

Legislation and national variation

Over the last few years, many changes and updates in the safe running of the dental workplace have occurred throughout the UK, including in the area of infection control. Unfortunately, the four countries of the UK (England, Wales, Scotland and Northern Ireland) have produced slightly different guidelines and are answerable to different regulators when following those guidelines. This has resulted in a complicated set of work practices in the dental environment that still must be understood and followed by dental staff, irrespective of where they work in the British Isles – and this is particularly so in the area of infection control.

For the purposes of this text, the legislation and guidelines applicable in England will be described in detail, and further information is available at www.dh.gov.uk. Students working in Northern Ireland are advised to access further specific information at www.dhsspsni.gov.uk.

Those areas of general knowledge common to all countries (definitions, basic principles, standard precautions, etc.) will form the bulk of the text.

In England, the guidelines applicable to decontamination in general dental practice (primary care dental practices) are covered by the Department of Health document *Health Technical Memorandum* 01-05 (HTM 01-05, Figure 8.1). Northern Ireland and Wales have their own modified versions of this document, while Scotland has not adopted it but instead has a number of organisations which provide guidance on compliance with decontamination standards. HTM 01-05

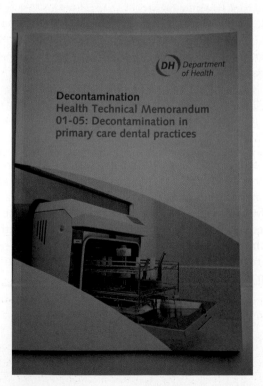

Figure 8.1   HTM 01-05 guidance booklet.

is produced as a guide on decontamination techniques for use in the dental workplace itself, and is a 'working document' in that it may be updated as evidence of better techniques and systems becomes available. It is intended to help dental workplaces establish a programme of continuous improvement in their decontamination techniques. Those currently included are listed in two categories.

- **Essential quality requirements** – the basic level of decontamination standards that all workplaces will achieve within the first year of implementation of the guidance.
- **Best practice** – the 'gold standard' to be aimed at in the future (no timescale has currently been set); the additional improvements required to achieve best practice cover the following main points.
    - Use of a washer-disinfector to clean instruments
    - Separate facility for decontamination tasks, away from the clinical treatment area
    - Separate storage area for sterilised items, away from the clinical treatment area (a 'clean zone' within the decontamination room would be adequate).

Although it is accepted that many dental workplaces will be unable to achieve full 'best practice' status due to the limitations of their building layout, all will need to assess the improvements they can make and have a plan in place to implement what is achievable.

Throughout this chapter, the impact of HTM 01-05 on decontamination techniques will be highlighted.

Recently, registration for healthcare providers, including all dental practices in England (private, NHS or mixed practice), has been introduced and is overseen by the Care Quality Commission (CQC). Compliance with the *essential quality requirements* of HTM 01-05 will ensure that each dental workplace satisfies the registration requirements of the CQC in the areas of patient safety and decontamination. Initially, and in line with clinical governance requirements (see Chapter 3), the registration system will rely on self-audit and effective management within the dental workplace, although practice inspections by the CQC will occur at some point in the future.

Full registration with the CQC is provisional on each dental workplace showing that it meets essential standards of quality and patient safety in all its regulated activities, not just decontamination. This topic is discussed in more detail in Chapter 3.

The CQC acts only in England, and is not recognised in the other countries of the UK.

Need for infection control

As discussed in Chapter 7, the mouth is full of micro-organisms, some of which are harmful to the patient and to others. Consequently instruments and equipment used in dental treatment become contaminated with these micro-organisms whenever they are used, whether they are drilled into teeth, used to cut into soft tissues or are simply placed in the contaminated oral cavity. If no action were taken to clean these items after use, this micro-organism contamination would be passed on from patient to patient, from patient to dental staff, and from staff to patient. In addition, the use of dental air turbines (high-speed drills) creates an aerosol in the surgery, which falls onto the working surfaces and contaminates them too. If staff are not personally clean while taking part in chairside dental procedures, they can also contaminate patients and other staff.

The transfer of infection from person to person is called *direct cross-infection*, and that from person to equipment and onto a second person is called *indirect cross-infection*. The techniques,

199

policies and safeguards in place to prevent the occurrence of cross-infection form the basic principles of infection control procedures.

Basic principles of infection control

A system of *standard precautions* (previously referred to as 'universal precautions') has been adopted in healthcare work, which is designed to protect staff from inoculation and contamination risks, and to protect patients from being exposed to the risk of cross-infection.

The basic principle is to assume that any patient may be infected with any micro-organism at any time, and therefore they pose an infection risk to all dental staff and to other patients. A detailed medical history questionnaire, completed at the patient's initial attendance and updated at every appointment thereafter, will identify the majority of problems.

However, a patient may be infected with a micro-organism without showing any signs of disease, and therefore be unaware of the risk they pose to others – these are called *carriers*. Also, a patient may choose not to disclose their full medical history to the dental staff, and would then mistakenly be assumed to be 'safe' to treat.

So, if all patients are considered to be a possible source of infection and treated as such, the infection control techniques used in the dental environment will be good enough to reduce all cross-infection risks to a minimum. The other general basic principles of infection control to be adopted are summarised below.

- Apply good basic personal hygiene with regular appropriate hand washing.
- Cover existing wounds with waterproof dressings.
- Do not undertake invasive procedures if suffering from chronic skin lesions on the hands, such as eczema or dermatitis.
- Wear non-latex clinical gloves at all times when assisting in the surgery, and discard after single use.
- Avoid contamination with body fluids by wearing appropriate protective clothing, safety spectacles and masks – referred to as *personal protective equipment* (PPE).
- Institute approved procedures for decontamination of instruments and equipment.
- Apply good basic environmental cleaning procedures.
- Clear up blood and other body fluid spillages promptly.
- Follow the correct procedure for safe disposal of contaminated waste and sharps.
- Ensure all staff are aware of, understand and follow infection control policies and procedures.
- Ensure all staff are fully vaccinated against hepatitis B (this is now a legal requirement for all who work in the clinical environment) and that all childhood immunisations are up to date (see Chapter 7).

In the dental surgery environment itself, special methods of infection control are now routinely practised, as well as following the general points listed above. Best practice dictates that good general infection control is achieved by the following.

- Correct cleaning of the hands.
- Use of personal protective equipment.
- Correct cleaning of the clinical area.
- Correct cleaning and/or disposal of dental equipment, handpieces and instruments.
- Correct and safe disposal of hazardous waste.

Each point is discussed in detail later in this chapter.

HTM 01-05 implications – infection control policy

Under clinical governance requirements, all dental workplaces have had to have a written infection control policy in place for some time. Under HTM 01-05 guidance, the policy must now specifically cover the following points.

- Policy of action following an inoculation (sharps) injury, including occupational health contact details.
- Decontamination and storage policy for dental instruments, indicating full compliance with essential quality requirements and plans in place to achieve best practice.
- Details of procedures in use for decontamination of reusable items.
- Details of the correct management of instruments and equipment in the workplace to avoid cross-infection.
- Hazardous waste disposal policy.
- Hand hygiene policy.
- Details of required use of personal protective equipment.
- Details of recommended disinfectants and their correct use.
- Chemical spillage procedure, in line with Control of Substances Hazardous to Health (COSHH) requirements.

The infection control policy is subject to update in line with the requirements of the Health and Social Care Act 2008 – Code of Practice, or at 2-yearly intervals if shorter.

General definitions

The terms 'cleaning' and 'cleanliness' in a clinical context are quite different from a lay person's concept of them, and the relevant terms used here are defined below.

- **Social cleanliness** – clean to a socially acceptable standard for personal hygiene purposes but not disinfected nor sterilised.
- **Disinfection** – the killing/destruction of bacteria and fungi, but not spores nor some viruses (the technique usually involves the use of special chemicals).
- **Sterilisation** – the process of killing all micro-organisms and spores to produce asepsis (involves the use of autoclaves, which produce high temperatures and pressure within the sterilising chamber).
- **Asepsis** – the absence of all living pathogenic micro-organisms.
- **Decontamination** – the process used to remove contamination from reusable items, so that they are safe for further use on patients and for staff to handle. This may also be referred to as 'reprocessing' and involves the following four stages.
  - Cleaning
  - Disinfection
  - Inspection
  - Sterilisation.

All areas of the dental workplace should be socially clean, as a minimum standard. All clinical areas of the dental workplace must be cleaned to a higher standard still, by disinfection of the contaminated work surfaces using specific cleaning agents. Equipment and instruments that are not used in the patient's mouth but are contaminated by aerosol or splatter must also be decontaminated by disinfection. Some items may be protected by coverage with disposable plastic barrier sheets. All instruments that are used directly in the patient's mouth and that are not single-use disposable must be sterilised before being safe to reuse on another patient.

Cleaning of the hands and general appearance

Hand washing is the most important method of preventing cross-infection, and the technique used should be that stipulated by the Health and Safety Council. Recent studies have suggested that many instances of hospital-based infection of patients with micro-organisms such as methicillin-resistant *Staphylococcus aureus* (MRSA) are due to poor hand hygiene amongst hospital staff and visitors.

When working in the clinical area, nails should be kept short and wounds covered with a waterproof dressing to reduce the number of areas for micro-organisms to contaminate. False nails should never be worn when working at the chair side. The minimum amount of jewellery (earrings, rings, bracelets and watches) should be worn by those working in a clinical environment, for the same reason. Professionally, facial piercings and tattoos should be kept to an absolute minimum, and preferably are removed or discretely covered wherever possible.

HTM 01-05 implications – hand hygiene

Hand hygiene covers the topics of the different methods of hand washing as well as the recommended use of hand gels for disinfection purposes, as an alternative or in addition to washing, depending on the circumstances. Hand hygiene is a required topic of coverage in staff induction training, under the essential quality requirements.

Dedicated hand-washing sinks must be available in the dental workplace, and marked as such. They should have taps that can be operated either by the elbow or by foot, to avoid contamination from dirty hands.

The three levels of hand hygiene recognised are as follows.

- **Social** – to become physically clean from socially acquired micro-organisms, using general-purpose liquid soap.
- **Hygienic** – to destroy micro-organisms, maintain cleanliness and avoid direct cross-infection, using an approved antibacterial hand cleanser.
- **Surgical** – to significantly reduce the numbers of micro-organisms normally resident on the hands, before an invasive surgical procedure is carried out, using an approved antibacterial hand cleanser.

Social hand washing provides a general level of cleanliness, and should be carried out at the start and end of each session, before preparing food or eating, and especially after using the toilet facilities. It follows a similar technique to that used for hygienic hand cleansing as described below, but should take just 10–15 sec as it need not include the wrists or forearms.

The correct procedure for *hygienic hand washing* should be displayed in poster form at each dedicated sink, and the instructions are as follows (Figure 8.2).

- Turn on the tap using the foot or elbow control, to prevent contaminating the tap.
- Wet both hands under running water of a suitable temperature.
- Apply a suitable antibacterial liquid soap from the specially operated dispenser, and wash all areas of both hands and wrists thoroughly – this should take up to 30 sec to carry out correctly.
- Nailbrushes are not advised unless they are autoclavable, as they can become contaminated with repeated use.

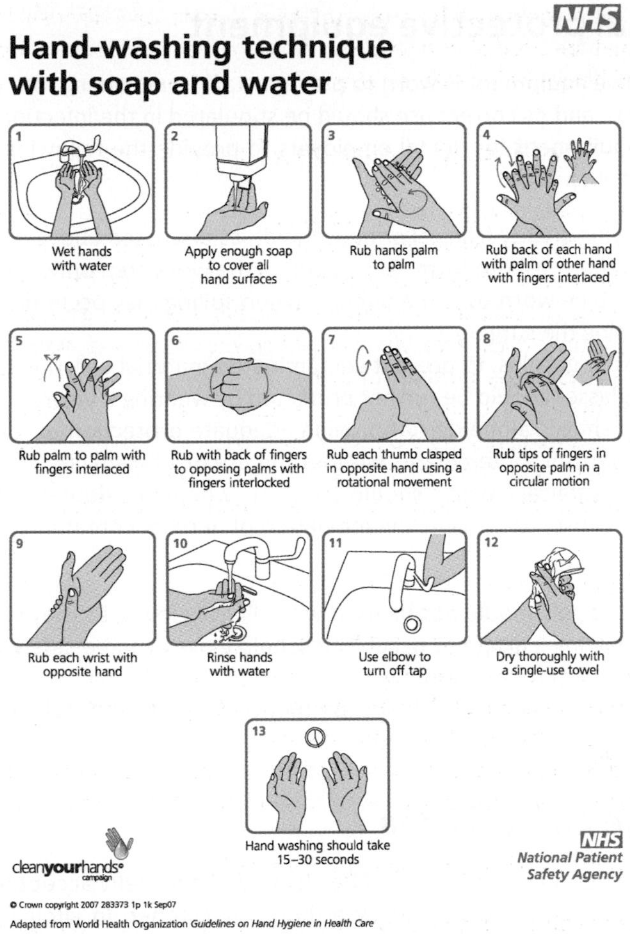

Figure 8.2 Hand wash poster. © Crown copyright. Contains public sector information licensed under the Open Government Licence v1.0.

- Rinse both hands under running water, holding them up so that the water does not flow back over the fingers.
- Dry the hands thoroughly, using single-use disposable paper towels.
- Heavy-duty gloves must be worn when the cleaning of dirty instruments is being carried out.
- Clinical gloves must be worn whenever patients are being treated, and discarded between patients. These should be non-powdered and of a non-latex material, such as nitrile or vinyl, to avoid the development of skin sensitisation conditions.

Whenever an invasive surgical procedure is to be carried out (oral, periodontal or implant surgery), the hand-washing procedure described above should be extended to include the forearms and should be carried out for a minimum of 2 min to be completed effectively. Special surgical-grade hand wash should be used, with a sterile, single-use scrubbing brush.

At the end of the cleaning, the hands should be held up during rinsing to allow the water to drain off the elbows, and then the hands and forearms should be dried with sterile paper towels. Sterile gloves should then be placed on both hands. This 'scrubbing-up' procedure is known as the *surgical (aseptic) technique* of hand washing.

Use of personal protective equipment

Personal protective equipment is worn to prevent staff from coming into contact with blood and other bodily fluids, and its correct use should be stipulated in the infection control policy.

It is a legal requirement for dental employers to provide the following protective clothing for their staff (Figure 8.3).

- **Gloves** of varying quality (clinical or household), as discussed above.
- High-temperature wash **uniform**, to be worn in the work area only.
- **Plastic apron** to be worn over the uniform when soiling may occur during surgical procedures or while cleaning the surgery.
- **Safety glasses** or goggles, to prevent contaminated material entering the eyes.
- Prescription glasses should be further protected by wearing a **visor** or face shield.
- Visors or face shields alone do not provide adequate protection to the eyes, nor prevent the inhalation of aerosol contaminants without the use of a facemask.
- **Facemasks** of surgical quality should be worn whenever dental handpieces or ultrasonic equipment is in use, to prevent the inhalation of aerosol contamination and pieces of flying debris.

Alcohol-based hand gels should not be used with clinical gloves, as they can damage the nitrile or vinyl material, allowing leakage to occur. Household gloves can be safely washed with detergent and hot water, then left to dry naturally.

There has been no change in the recommended use of PPE following the publication of HTM 01-05.

Cleaning of the clinical area

The whole of the dental practice should be cleaned to a socially acceptable standard on a daily basis, and this is usually carried out by a domestic cleaner. In clinical areas, however, a far higher standard of cleaning is necessary because these are the areas where contamination of the environment by body fluids is greatest, and where the highest chance of cross-infection is likely to occur.

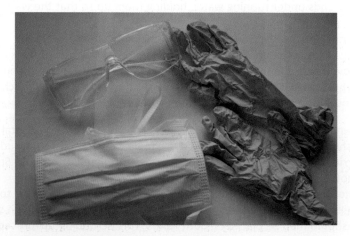

Figure 8.3   Personal protective equipment – examples.

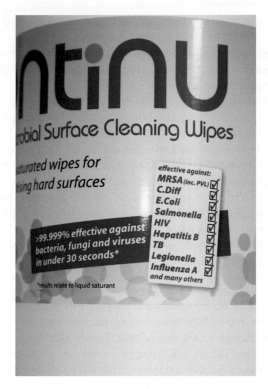

Figure 8.4   Disinfectant cleaning product.

The standard to be achieved in the clinical environment is that of *disinfection*. This involves the use of various chemicals to inhibit the growth of, or ideally kill, bacteria and fungi (Figure 8.4). However, most are not effective against bacterial spores or some viruses.

Those in common use in the dental workplace include the following.

- **Bleach-based cleaners** – containing sodium hypochlorite and used to disinfect all non-metallic and non-textile surfaces, and to soak laboratory items.
- **Aldehyde-based cleaners** – can be used on metallic surfaces and to soak laboratory items.
- **Isopropyl alcohol wipes** – to disinfect items such as exposed x-ray film packets for safe handling during processing.
- **Chlorhexidene gluconate** – as an irrigating disinfectant during root canal treatments, and as a skin cleanser.

The practice as a whole should be kept clean, dry and well ventilated. Some workplaces have air conditioning installed, but care should be taken that the system does not recirculate the contaminated surgery air. In addition, special precautions are required to ensure that the air conditioning unit does not become contaminated with the waterborne micro-organism *Legionella*.

A written protocol for surgery cleaning should be available in all dental workplaces, which lays out the correct procedure in a logical manner and details how each item should be dealt with. In general, it should include the following.

- All work surfaces should have the minimum items of equipment out for each procedure, and when these items are not in use they should be stored in drawers or cupboards to prevent aerosol contamination.

- Areas should be designated as 'clean' and 'dirty' so that dirty used instruments are not placed where clean items should be – this is called *zoning*.
- Equipment likely to be contaminated, such as chair and light controls, and headrests, should be covered with impervious plastic sheets (such as 'Clingfilm') and changed between patients – this is called using *protective barriers*.
- Dental aspirators which exhaust outside the surgery area will reduce the risk of aerosol contamination; they should be used routinely and flushed through daily with a recommended non-foaming disinfectant.
- Clinical records and computer keyboards should not be handled while gloves are being worn.
- All non-metallic equipment can be wiped down with a bleach-based preparation, which is particularly effective against viruses, at the end of each day.
- Bleach-based disinfectants cannot be used on metallic items as they will corrode the metal.
- All intraoral radiographs should be wiped with an isopropyl alcohol (IPA) wipe before being handled with clean gloves and taken for processing.
- Reusable digital devices must be decontaminated in accordance with manufacturers' instructions and then sterilised.

Most of these disinfectant products are sold as convenient sprays or presoaked wipes, but bleach products have to be made up on a daily basis as a fresh solution. This is because the chlorine content is lost over the day so that the resulting solution becomes weaker, and cannot then be assumed to be strong enough to act as a viricide. Bleach also has to be used with caution on any fabrics as it will remove the colour, and it has an unpleasant smell and taste.

The uses of bleach-based disinfectants are as follows.

- 1% fresh solution to disinfect all non-metallic, non-fabric surfaces within the surgery.
- 1% fresh solution to disinfect impressions and removable prostheses before transferring between the patient and the laboratory.
- Up to 10% fresh solution to clean blood spillages within the surgery.

As all disinfectants are poisonous if ingested, their manufacture and usage are strictly controlled by the COSHH legislation, which is discussed in detail in Chapter 4.

HTM 01-05 implications – clinical area decontamination

The key issue of reducing the risk of cross-infection has brought about the following updates.

- The protocol in use for cleaning of the clinical areas should be written down and should clearly outline the steps to be taken by staff for the decontamination procedure.
- All surfaces and equipment should be impervious (resistant to fluids) and easily cleanable.
- Work surfaces and floor coverings should be continuous so no joints should occur between sections of the surface and with the walls of the room (Figure 8.5).
- The clinical area should be cleaned after each session using:
  - disposable cloths or clean microfibre material
  - water to wet cloths
  - detergent.
- Commercially available bactericidal cleaning wipes and sprays can also be used to reduce any viral contamination of work surfaces, between patients (Figure 8.6).
- Alcohol wipes, although active against viral contamination, should be used as the sole cleaning agent with caution, as they may actually seal protein-based contaminants onto the surface.

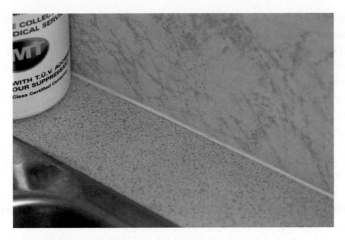

Figure 8.5   Sealed work surface detail.

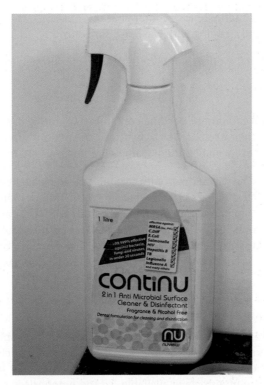

Figure 8.6   Example of surface cleaning spray.

- Alcohol is not a suitable cleaning agent for use on stainless steel surfaces, for the above reason.
- Wherever possible, covers should be used on as many chairside items as possible, as an effective barrier against contamination. In particular, computer keyboards *must* be covered during clinical sessions.

- Cleaning of all the following should occur at the end of each patient treatment, or have barrier covers changed after single use.
  - Work surfaces in close proximity to the dental chair
  - Dental chair and control panel
  - Bracket table/trolley/delivery unit
  - Aspirator unit and spittoon
  - Inspection light and handles
  - X-ray unit if in close proximity to the dental chair.

Wherever possible, items not in use should be stored inside cupboards and drawers, and only placed on work surfaces when their use is likely on a patient.

Cleaning of equipment, handpieces and instruments

The three main techniques currently available for cleaning reusable dental equipment, handpieces and instruments are:

- manual cleaning
- manual cleaning with ultrasonic decontamination
- decontamination and cleaning with washer-disinfector.

Wherever possible, items should then be subjected to sterilisation in an autoclave.

Equipment

Various items of dental equipment become contaminated during use, often because of their close position to the dental chair itself as well as by use in the patient's mouth. They are not likely to be sterilisable, and their cost prohibits them from being single-use items.

- **Curing light** – should be wiped down with a suitable cleaning agent after each use; the fibre-optic tip should be protected with a single-use barrier cover – follow manufacturers' instructions.
- **Aspirator tubing** – should be wiped down externally with a suitable cleaning agent after use, or protected with a single-use barrier cover (see later for inner tube cleaning).
- **X-ray unit tube** – should only come into contact with the outside of a positioning device, rather than the patient's skin or oral tissues, so should be wiped down with a suitable cleaning agent after use.

Handpieces

Various different makes of air turbine and slow handpiece are available nowadays, and the manufacturers' instructions should always be followed in relation to their cleaning, lubrication and sterilisation, to prolong the life of the item. Currently, it is accepted that full sterility of the handpiece is unlikely with any type of autoclave available, so the emphasis is more on reducing the risk of cross-infection rather than completely eliminating it.

However, all handpieces should be able to undergo the following processes.

- External cleaning using a suitable cleaning agent.
- Lubrication of bearings before and/or after cleaning and sterilisation, according to the manufacturers' instructions.
- Sterilisation in an autoclave.

Handpieces should never be immersed in an ultrasonic bath (the bearings which drive the burr rotation will be irreparably damaged), but some are suitable for decontamination in washer-disinfectors where indicated by the manufacturer. The point at which burr removal should occur may also vary between makes, and again, the manufacturers' instructions should be consulted for the correct procedure.

Dental instruments

These are all those instruments that are used directly in the patient's mouth, including items such as triple syringe tips and aspirating tips (high and low speed). These two items in particular should be single use disposable wherever possible, as successful sterilisation of their inner hollow surfaces (lumens) is only achieved with some types of autoclave, not with all of them.

Dental hand instruments which are used to assess patients and provide dental treatment tend to be made of high-quality metals, especially stainless steel. Some are also available with ceramic coatings, for use with composite restorative materials. Their metallic content reduces the likelihood of surface corrosion, so wire brushes should not be used to remove hardened debris as this scratches the surface and allows corrosion to occur. Microscopically, the scratches and corroded areas will harbour micro-organisms very easily.

Of the three techniques available for cleaning reusable instruments before sterilisation, manual cleaning alone is only suitable where items have been available for use but were not actually used in the patient's mouth during the dental procedure; such as when a full conservation tray is provided but only one or two items were used.

However, if some used items have to be decontaminated in an ultrasonic bath or washer-disinfector, then all items may as well go through the process together.

HTM 01-05 implications – equipment, handpieces and instrument cleaning

Essential quality requirements allow the use of manual cleaning alone before sterilisation of items that cannot be processed using an ultrasonic bath or washer-disinfector first. The use of automated processes (ultrasonic bath or washer-disinfector) is not compulsory under the essential quality requirements, but the use of either and especially a washer-disinfector is necessary under best practice guidelines.

The procedure to be followed in each dental workplace for cleaning of all items should be written down and included in the infection control policy document, and evidence of staff training in the various techniques should also be recorded.

Dedicated sinks must be available (and marked as such) for manual cleaning procedures where immersion is required. Likewise, separate dedicated sinks or bowls must be available for rinsing items after both manual cleaning and ultrasonic bath usage, and contain either distilled water or reverse osmosis water – tap water is not acceptable.

Both types of special water can be bought from dental suppliers, or they can be produced from tap water on the dental premises – this is by far the cheaper option. As the name suggests, distilled water is made from the distillation of tap water in a special kettle-like machine (Figure 8.7).

The reverse osmosis technique takes tap water through a series of finer and finer filters, so that any impurities are removed by osmosis and just pure water remains. The equipment can be plumbed directly into a source of tap water on the premises so that a supply of pure water is always available (Figure 8.8).

209

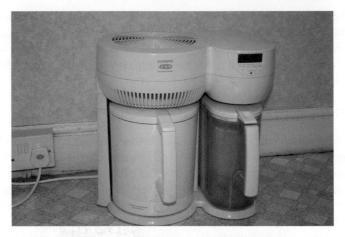

Figure 8.7 Water distillation unit.

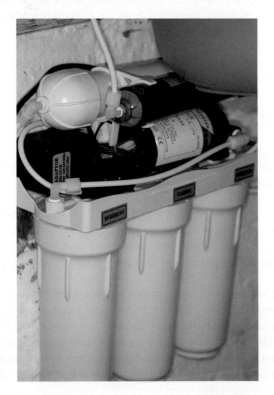

Figure 8.8 Reverse osmosis water unit.

Cleaning techniques for reusable items

Manual cleaning

This is the simplest method of cleaning reusable items before sterilisation, but is the most difficult to validate; that is, to prove that it has been effective, as it depends entirely on the thoroughness

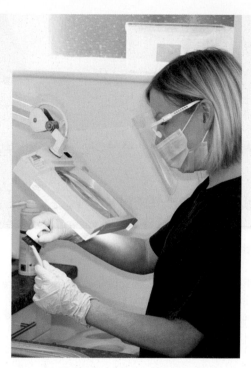

Figure 8.9   Magnifier in use.

of cleaning by the staff member at the time. Because of its 'hands-on' nature, it is also the technique most likely to result in an inoculation injury to the staff member.

Under essential quality requirements, manual cleaning is an acceptable method to use (as long as plans are clearly in place to introduce automated cleaning at some point in the future), but under best practice guidance it should only ever be used on items where the manufacturer states that automated cleaning is unsuitable.

The basic procedure to manually clean items safely and effectively is as follows.

- Wear suitable PPE – to avoid inoculation injury, thick household gloves should be worn whenever any items are cleaned manually, as well as face and eye protection.
- Always clean the items as soon as possible after use, to avoid contamination drying onto their surfaces – this is far more difficult to remove than wet contamination.
- Use cold water and a suitable detergent in a dedicated instrument cleaning sink/bowl – hot water 'fixes' contaminants such as blood onto the item surface and makes it far more difficult to remove.
- Use nylon-bristled, autoclavable scrubbing brushes to remove difficult contaminants, as wire bristles will scratch the metal surfaces and allow corrosion and rusting to occur.
- The items should be scrubbed while under the water surface, to avoid spraying contaminants into the immediate vicinity.
- A separate sink/bowl of distilled or reverse osmosis water should be used to rinse the items after cleaning, to remove any detergent and loose contamination.
- The items should be visibly inspected (ideally using an illuminated magnifier – Figure 8.9), to ensure that all contamination has been removed; if any is found the item should be recleaned and rinsed again.

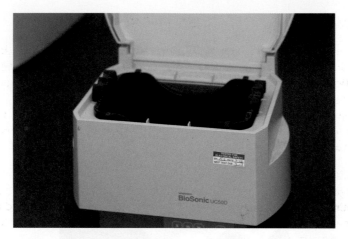

Figure 8.10   Ultrasonic bath.

- The items should then be autoclaved as soon as possible before they can dry in the air – this can result in corrosion or recontamination.
- Those that are to be bagged before vacuum sterilising should be dried thoroughly first.

Ultrasonic bath

These devices remove debris from items by vibrating at an ultrasonic frequency and transmitting that vibration onto the instruments loaded into the bath on the tray (Figure 8.10). They require the use of special detergents diluted in distilled/reverse osmosis water within the bath to be effective, and the solution should be replaced at the end of each clinical session or when it is obviously heavily contaminated with particles of debris.

Ultrasonic baths should not be used to debride handpieces, as the bearings will become damaged. Manufacturers' instructions should be consulted for any particular operating advice relevant to each machine used in the dental workplace.

The basic procedure to decontaminate items using the ultrasonic bath is as follows.

- Heavy soiling with blood and other visible contaminants should be reduced by briefly soaking the items in cold detergent solution beforehand, and then rinsing.
- Hinged items (such as extraction forceps) should be opened and assembled items (such as amalgam carriers) should be disassembled.
- All items should be placed on the bath tray and fully immersed beneath the solution, to allow debridement to occur effectively.
- The bath should not be overloaded with items, as debridement will not be effective.
- The timer should be set according to the manufacturer's instructions, the lid closed on the machine and the programme started – the lid must be closed to prevent aerosol contamination of the vicinity.
- When the timer ends, the basket and its contents should be lifted and allowed to drain, then the items should be rinsed in a dedicated sink/bowl of distilled or reverse osmosis water.
- The items should be visibly inspected to ensure debridement has occurred, and put through the process again if debris remains.
- Items should be sterilised as soon as possible after being decontaminated, as for manually cleaned items.

Maintenance and testing of ultrasonic bath

As with all electrical items that are used to perform certain tasks in the dental workplace, the ultrasonic bath should be maintained by a service engineer or a delegated person competent in decontamination, on a regular basis. For many units manufacturers recommend that this is carried out annually, as a minimum.

The working efficiency of the bath will be maintained if regular in-house testing is also carried out, and these daily and weekly duties are often delegated to the dental nurse.

Daily duties are as follows.

- **Strainer/filter cleaning** – remove these items from the bath and clean using a suitable detergent solution and brush, to remove the contamination produced during normal operation.
- **Tank draining** – the bath solution should be fully drained out at the end of the day, or at the end of a busy clinical session, so that contaminants are disposed of rather than transferred onto other instruments.
- **Cleaning check** – all instruments placed in the bath should be visibly checked at the end of the cycle, to ensure that all visible debris has been removed – an illuminated magnifier should be available for use during this procedure (see Figure 8.9).

Additional weekly duties are as follows.

- **Safety check** – ensure that the lid of the bath fits adequately and continues to prevent aerosol contamination of the surroundings during use; check for signs of any solution splatter around the unit.
- **Protein residue test** – use of a special test device to ensure that protein residues are being removed effectively during the ultrasonic cycle, so that items are indeed decontaminated before sterilisation (proteins are present in blood, pulp, tooth and soft tissues, and micro-organisms).

One final test that can be carried out in house to test the efficiency of the debridement action of the ultrasonic bath is an *activity test using aluminium foil*. The test should be carried out once every 6 months. Details of the test can be found in the HTM 01-05 document but basically, it involves immersing several strips of aluminium foil into the bath solution and running a normal cycle. On inspection, the aluminium should be eroded off the strips at similar points along their length, indicating that the debridement action occurs similarly throughout the whole tank. Any variation in the position and extent of the aluminium erosion indicates that the tank is not vibrating uniformly, and instrument debridement will therefore be on a 'hit and miss' basis.

Washer-disinfector

These devices (Figure 8.11) are the preferred method of item decontamination under the best practice guidelines of HTM 01-05, although they are under further review with regard to the possibility of 'protein fixing' during the cycle. The washer-disinfector operates in a similar fashion to a specialist dishwasher machine, and some makes are suitable for the safe disinfection of dental handpieces, as well as other dental items and instruments.

Each typical machine cycle goes through five stages during the cleaning and disinfection process.

- **Flush** – an initial pressure rinse to remove gross solid and liquid debris from items. Previously this was using water at high temperatures but now a temperature below 45°C is recommended

213

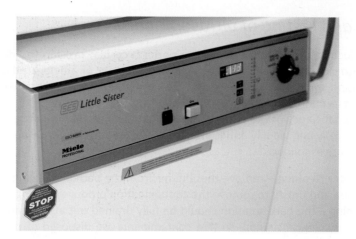

Figure 8.11   Washer-disinfector unit.

to prevent the possibility of protein fixing and the consequent complete failure of the disinfection cycle.

- **Wash** – use of a recommended detergent and/or disinfectant with water to complete the removal of liquid and solid debris, by both chemical and mechanical actions during the wash process (so the detergent/disinfectant breaks down the debris chemically, and the mechanical action of the solution swishing around in the machine mechanically dislodges the debris from the items).
- **Rinse** – using suitable quality mains water (this will vary across the UK and needs to be clarified with the water provider in the area) or reverse osmosis water, to remove all traces of the detergent/disinfectant solution. Any evidence of marking, smearing or spotting on the cleaned items indicates that the water quality is inadequate for use in the machine.
- **Thermal disinfection** – the temperature is preset at the start of the cycle, and can be varied depending on the contents of the load to be disinfected; the chosen temperature is then achieved and held for the required time within the machine.
- **Drying** – heated air is pumped into the disinfection chamber so that any residual moisture is removed from all items before the end of the cycle, as wet items will allow micro-organisms to recolonise their surfaces more readily.

Full training of staff in the correct use of the washer-disinfector is vital in ensuring that every cycle produces clean and disinfected items, ready for sterilisation. Written records of any training received should be kept by the dental workplace, and the full procedure for machine use should be included within the infection control policy documentation.

Maintenance and testing of washer-disinfector

As with the ultrasonic bath and other electrical devices, maintenance and testing of the washer-disinfector must be carried out on a regular basis by a service engineer. Intermediate in-house tests are also advised.

Some washer-disinfectors have automatic data-logging devices incorporated into their design that produce printouts of their operational parameters for each cycle (in a similar way to those

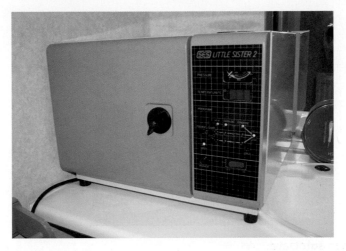

Figure 8.12   Downward displacement autoclave.

produced by some autoclaves). This ensures that a validated record is available to prove that each cycle ran efficiently and had produced clean and disinfected items at its endpoint.

However, daily and weekly in-house efficiency tests should still be carried out, as for the ultrasonic bath. In addition, the following in-house tests should also be carried out on the washer-disinfector once every 6 months.

- **Automatic control test** – to ensure that the cycle parameters set are actually achieved, with regard to temperature, time, drying, etc.
- **Chemical dosing** – test to ensure that the detergent and/or disinfectant is released into the machine correctly during the cycle, and that low levels of either are indicated as necessary.
- **Thermometric disinfection test** – using a heavily soiled load, the temperatures achieved during the cycle are tested to ensure that those reached are suitable to ensure that disinfection has occurred.

Autoclave

Once reusable items have been decontaminated by either manual or automated means, they are ready to be rendered safe for reuse on another patient by undergoing sterilisation. The machines used in the dental workplace to achieve sterilisation are called autoclaves, and there are two basic types – 'N' type and 'B' type. A third type ('S' type) is more frequently seen in the hospital environment. The details of the more usual types are shown below.

'N' type (downward displacement – Figure 8.12) autoclave

- Heats to 134°C and holds for 3 min at 2.25 bar pressure (32 pounds per square inch).
- Steam displaces air downwards in the chamber so that it contacts all items.
- Cycle lasts for 15–20 min, depending on its make and how often it has been in use previously, as it warms up and retains the heat after each use.
- Suitable for unwrapped solid items laid in a single layer on perforated trays.
- Machine can hold several trays at a time, cutting the number of cycles required.
- Cycle can be set to dry instruments before they are removed from the autoclave.
- Door cannot be opened during operation until the cycle is completed.

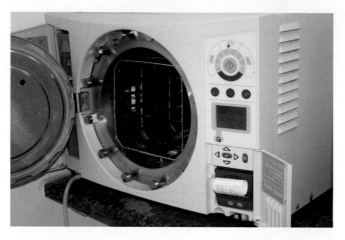

Figure 8.13   Vacuum autoclave.

'B' type (vacuum – Figure 8.13) autoclave

- Heats to 134°C and holds for 3 min at 2.25 bar pressure.
- Air is sucked out of the chamber to create a vacuum so that steam contacts all the items present as it is also sucked through, including the insides of hollow items.
- Various cycles to choose from, depending on the requirements of the loaded items for each cycle.
- Cycle can last for up to 45 min if a vacuum programme is required.
- Vacuum cycle is suitable for wrapped items and those with a hollow lumen, such as handpieces and triple syringe tips.
- Machine often has a data-logging device so that the operating parameters for each cycle are recorded and can be checked (Figure 8.14).
- Machine can hold several trays at a time, cutting the number of cycles required.
- Cycle can be set to dry instruments before they are removed from the autoclave.
- Door cannot be opened during operation until the cycle has been completed.
- More expensive than the 'N' type autoclave.

However, neither type of autoclave will sterilise items thoroughly unless they have been suitably processed beforehand, and this is one of the most important duties for the dental nurse to complete on a daily basis, as detailed previously.

Handling and storage of sterilised items

The correct handling and storage of items once they leave the autoclave are imperative in ensuring that their sterility is maintained until they are required for use again. The obvious ways of achieving this are as follows.

- Removed from the autoclave and handled while wearing clean PPE.
- Dried using single-use cloth or towel.
- Placed within a device to act as a barrier between the items and the general atmosphere to avoid aerosol and micro-organism recontamination, such as:
  - sealed view pouch
  - lidded tray
  - sterilisation bag (for use with vacuum autoclave only).

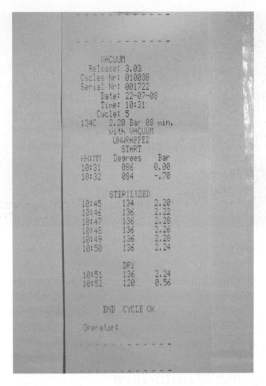

```
                    VACUUM
            Release: 3.03
          Cycles Nr: 010038
          Serial Nr: 001722
               Date: 22-07-08
               Time: 10:31
              Cycle: 5
      134C    2.20 Bar 08 min.
              with VACUUM
               UNWRAPPED
                 START
      HH:MM    Degrees    Bar
      10:31      086      0.00
      10:32      084      -.70

                 STERILIZED
      10:45      134      2.20
      10:46      136      2.22
      10:47      136      2.28
      10:48      136      2.26
      10:49      136      2.28
      10:50      136      2.24

                   DRY
      10:51      136      2.24
      10:52      120      0.56


            END  CYCLE OK

      Operator:
```

Figure 8.14 Cycle sterility printout.

With all autoclaves, the sterilised items must be dry before any further packaging occurs, before storage. Residual moisture makes recontamination of the items with micro-organisms a more likely scenario, so it must be removed by using the drying cycle of the autoclave or by manually drying the items as soon as they are removed from the autoclave.

Similarly, a damp cloth or towel that is repeatedly used to dry the items is also more likely to become contaminated with time, so single-use towels must be available.

For 'N' type autoclaves, all items must be sterilised unwrapped and then dried and wrapped after removal from the machine. As they must therefore be handled to do so, it was previously recommended that the storage packages were date stamped so that the items are used or resterilised after 21 days (Figure 8.15). This has recently been extended to a maximum of one year, in line with requirements for other healthcare settings.

If the items are to be used again during a session, they can be covered only, rather than fully wrapped.

With vacuum autoclaves, items can complete the sterilisation cycle while enclosed in pouches and lidded trays, and then dried and further packaged at the end of the cycle. These items were previously date-stamped to a 60-day future date, but can now be stored for reuse for up to a maximum of one year, in line with requirements for other healthcare settings.

Once all items have been dried and packaged, they should be stored in their designated place within the dental workplace. While it is acceptable under essential quality requirements to store packaged items within the clinical area for ease of access, they must be kept within drawers or cupboards until immediately before use, and as far away from the chair side as possible. However, in the clinical area the potential for recontamination is greater than for other areas of the workplace due to the aerosol scatter created during dental treatment, as well as due to the throughput of the patients.

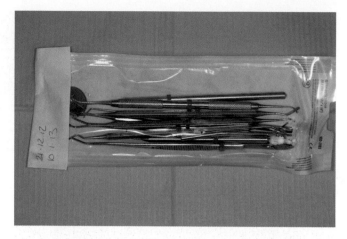

Figure 8.15   Date-stamped pouch.

The least contaminated area of the workplace should be the 'clean zone' of the actual decontamination area itself, where the sterilised items are produced (see later), and where the public have no access. For this reason, best practice guidelines recommend that all sterilised items are stored within the clean zone of the decontamination room, and collected from there by staff when their use is imminent, and taken to the clinical area as required.

Maintenance and testing of autoclave

Autoclaves use pressure to ensure sterilisation of the contained items, and this means that they have to comply with various Health and Safety legalities because of the potential danger they pose to staff and patients if they malfunction. The Health and Safety policy in all dental surgeries must contain written requirements for the correct use of autoclaves, as they are considered to be *pressure vessels*. The requirements are as follows.

- A daily test should be carried out on each autoclave, recording the temperature, pressure and time interval for a full cycle – these details must be kept as a written record in a dated log book.
- An automatic control test should be carried out daily for all types of autoclave, and the test strip retained within the workplace records – the usual technique is to use a 'TST' strip (Figure 8.16) or something similar.
- A steam penetration test should also be carried out for vacuum autoclaves, to ensure that steam does indeed penetrate to the inside of any packaging used during the sterilisation cycle – these are usually a Helix or Bowie-Dick test (Figure 8.17).
- Only purified or reverse osmosis water should be used within the autoclave, never tap water.
- Water should be drained from the reservoir and replaced daily.
- Door seal and safety devices used to prevent door opening during the cycle must be visually checked on a weekly basis by designated staff.
- An authorised engineer must carry out an annual inspection to ensure each autoclave operates correctly, and issue a certificate to that effect.
- Each autoclave must also be checked for its conformation with the Pressure Systems Safety Regulations on a regular basis.
- Practice insurance policy must include third party liability cover for the use of autoclaves, in case of their explosion and resultant injury to any staff or patients.

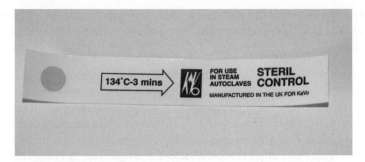

Figure 8.16   TST strip – unused.

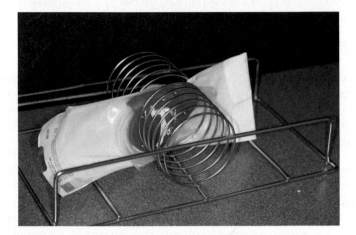

Figure 8.17   Helix test holder.

- Any serious accident involving an autoclave, including its explosion, must be reported to the Health and Safety Executive under the Reporting of Injuries, Diseases and Dangerous Occurrences Regulations (RIDDOR).

The first six points are often delegated to a dental nurse, following suitable training.

Some single-use products are provided by manufacturers as prepackaged sterile items, such as syringes and needles, local anaesthetic cartridges, scalpel blades, swabs and other cotton products, gutta percha and paper points used in endodontic treatments, and more recently the endodontic hand instruments themselves. These are industrially sterilised within sealed packages after production, by exposure to *gamma rays*, a type of radiation similar to x-rays. As gamma radiation is highly dangerous, it must be used under strict regulation and in specialised control zones, so it is not suitable for use in dental practice.

Decontamination room layout

Although the provision of a decontamination room is a requirement only under best practice guidelines, the need for a separate area in which to process reusable items away from the clinical area is an obvious one, and many dental workplaces have operated with separate facilities for some time.

However, some older dental workplaces may still have a system of cleaning reusable items within the clinical area, and if so the following points should be incorporated into the procedure as soon as possible.

- Reprocessing should be carried out between patients, and not while patients are present.
- The reprocessing area should be as far away from the chair side as physically possible.
- Ultrasonic baths and autoclaves must not be in use while the patient is present.
- Manual washing of items should not be carried out while the patient is present.
- Strict zoning of clean and dirty areas must be followed at all times, to avoid cross-contamination.
- Thorough surface decontamination should be carried out between patients, and after each reprocessing activity.

Ideally, all reprocessing activities should be carried out in a designated decontamination room, physically separated from the clinical area.

HTM 01-05 implications – decontamination room

Under best practice guidelines, the crucial points of the decontamination room layout and operating procedures are as follows.

- The decontamination room must be separated physically from all clinical areas (so a separate room is required).
- Ideally, the dirty zone where items are received for reprocessing and the clean zone where the sterilised items are produced should be separate rooms – this allows for the maximum possible separation of dirty and clean items, and therefore the minimum possibility of recontamination.
- There should be a clean to dirty airflow within the decontamination room(s) – this should be an active air flow system provided by an extractor fan sucking air out of the dirty zone to the exterior of the premises, thereby causing clean air to be passively pulled in to the clean zone and across to the dirty zone in a one-way flow system (Figure 8.18).
- A single worktop area should run the length of the room, with enough length to allow the autoclave to be well away from the cleaning/decontamination area.
- The worktop should be sealed along its length and be made of an easily cleanable surface (so smooth rather than indented).
- The areas should then be set out in the following order.
  - Set-down area for dirty items ↓
  - Hand-washing sink ↓
  - Instrument washing sink ↓
  - Ultrasonic bath (if required) ↓
  - Rinsing sink ↓
  - Washer-disinfector ↓
  - Illuminated magnifier for inspection ↓
  - Autoclave ↓
  - Packaging and storage
- The dirty and clean zones should be clearly labelled as such, to avoid cross-contamination of the two areas.

It is accepted that some older dental premises may not be able to achieve a full best practice decontamination room layout without major building alterations or even a rebuild – essential quality requirements must be achieved as a minimum then.

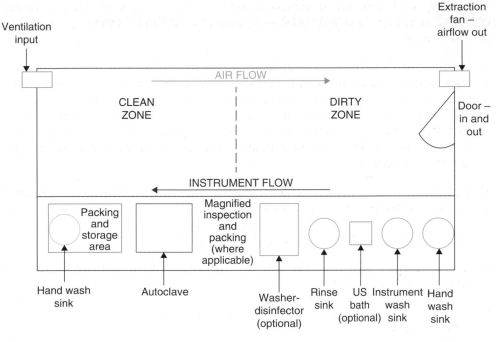

Figure 8.18 Decontamination room layout.

Safe disposal of hazardous waste

This topic is covered in detail in Chapter 4, and the current classification of waste is shown in Figure 4.13.

The hazardous waste produced in the dental workplace is divided into four broad categories – non-hazardous waste, offensive waste, trade waste and hazardous waste. The last category is the most important when aiming to avoid cross-infection, as the items segregated here are those which have the potential to harm members of the dental team, patients or waste contractors if not handled and stored correctly while on the premises. The hazardous waste category is further subdivided into infectious (clinical) and non-infectious (chemical) streams, and each subdivision requires specific handling skills and storage vessels to be used for the items included. The flowchart in Figure 4.13 gives examples of the typical types of waste produced in the dental workplace.

Offensive waste is defined as 'wastes which are non-infectious, do not require specialist treatment or disposal but may cause offence to those coming into contact with it'. In the dental workplace this will include any PPE, cleaning towels, x-ray films and other similar items that have not been contaminated with body fluids, medicines, chemicals or amalgam, as well as toilet hygiene waste.

Trade waste includes items such as dental equipment (dental chairs, curing lights, portable suction units, etc.), as well as commercial electronic waste like computer screens, televisions, fluorescent lighting tubes and batteries.

The main change in the update of this area of infection is the renaming of the previous 'special waste' category to that of 'non-infectious hazardous waste'. The exception is the lead foil waste from x-ray film packets which is now classed as non-hazardous waste, because the lead is only toxic when present in solution (dissolved in water).

The addition of the offensive waste category has occurred in all workplaces.

221

Occupational hazards – cross-infection and inoculation injury

There are three major occupational hazards in dentistry: radiation, mercury poisoning and cross-infection. All three concern dental nurses, and they must be trained to be aware of the dangers and know how to avoid them. The former two are described in Chapter 4, but cross-infection is covered here as its prevention is the purpose of good infection control.

The close nature of dental treatment exposes all surgery staff to a variety of micro-organisms on a daily basis, as dental treatment often involves the shedding of blood. Even the most minute blood-stained droplets may contain viruses, and such bloodborne viruses can be sprayed over a wide area of the surgery when using high-speed handpieces and ultrasonic scalers, as an aerosol, and by three-in-one syringes as spatter. So not only instruments but work surfaces, surgery equipment and surgery staff are exposed to potential contamination in this way.

Those pathogenic micro-organisms of particular concern to the dental team are the following.

- **Human immunodeficiency virus (HIV)** – a viral infection that destroys the body's leucocytes, weakening the patient's immune system and leaving them unable to fight off diseases naturally. They eventually go on to develop acquired immune deficiency syndrome (AIDS), a fatal condition for which there is no vaccine currently available.
- **Hepatitis B** – a viral infection causing liver inflammation, which is often fatal. All dental staff must be immunised against the virus before working in the clinical environment.
- **Hepatitis C** – a similar virus to that causing hepatitis B, but much more likely to prove fatal. There is no current vaccination against the virus.
- **Herpes simplex type I** – a viral infection affecting particularly the lips and oral cavity. It is not fatal but is highly contagious when 'cold sore' lesions are present on the lips of the sufferer.

By always following standard precautions to control infection within the clinical environment, the risk to staff and other patients of being cross-infected from sufferers of these diseases should be minimal. However, it is good practice to take additional precautions when treating patients known to be suffering from any of the first three, more serious, of these infections.

Any patient attending with an active cold sore should not be dentally treated except in an emergency. The lesion will diminish within 10 days, so their appointment can be rebooked as necessary.

In addition, dental staff may come into contact with other diseases during a normal working day, or even be the source of an infection to colleagues or patients if not appropriately vaccinated themselves. It is therefore of great importance that all dental staff receive the following immunisation programme before working at the chair side.

- **Diphtheria** – normally received routinely during childhood.
- **Pertussis** – whooping cough, normally received routinely during infancy.
- **Poliomyelitis** – normally received routinely during childhood.
- **MMR** – measles, mumps and rubella (German measles), normally received during infancy.
- **Tetanus** – normally received routinely during childhood, and can be boosted as required.
- **Tuberculosis** – received routinely after giving a negative Heaf test, but may need boosting after 15 years.
- **Hepatitis B** – received as an occupationally required vaccine before working in any clinical area; a blood test is required to prove seroconversion and ensure immunity but boosters are currently not considered necessary.

- **Chicken pox** – if not naturally immune due to childhood exposure.
- **Meningitis** – normally received routinely as a teenager.
- **Influenza and swine influenza** – received as an adult when winter outbreaks are expected.

Special care should be taken if child patients have been in contact with viral infections such as measles, mumps or rubella (German measles). The virus is present in saliva before any signs of illness are apparent, and surgery staff may become infected in this way from an apparently fit child. If there is any evidence of contact, appropriate questioning of parents will allow the dentist to assess the risk of infection and decide whether to postpone treatment. Although such infections are usually trivial in children, they can cause serious complications in susceptible adults.

If rubella occurs in the first 3 months of pregnancy it can affect the unborn child – and this may happen before pregnancy is confirmed. Such a child is likely to have serious physical defects and in such cases there are strong medical grounds for advising termination of the pregnancy.

Adult males are most at risk from mumps as it may cause sterility. All surgical staff should therefore check their own medical history and vaccination records. They should be immune from common childhood infections previously contracted and are only at risk from any which are not included in these records.

Even such a trivial viral infection as the common cold is infectious. If surgery staff or their patients have a cold, transmission to others can be prevented by wearing protective clothing. Although the effects of a cold are not serious, they often necessitate time off work with the resultant inconvenience caused by staff shortage.

Hepatitis B

Hepatitis B is an inflammation of the liver caused by a virus. Its effect varies from a mild attack of jaundice to a severe or fatal illness. Over 50% of cases are undiagnosed as their symptoms are too mild to indicate the disease. On the other hand, 80% of primary liver cancers are as a result of hepatitis B.

The hepatitis B virus (HBV) is always present in the blood of people suffering from the disease. It may also be present in people who have no symptoms of the disease. Such people are called *carriers*; they may or may not have had any symptoms before, and most of them are unaware that they are carriers. About one person in every 1000 of the population is an HBV carrier, so all dentists are likely to treat carriers at some point in their career.

Hepatitis B is highly infective and is very resistant to destruction. It can survive boiling for up to half an hour, and immersion in chlorhexidine disinfectant, and can live outside the body for some weeks. Disinfectants capable of killing HBV include those based on hypochlorite.

Hepatitis B virus has been found in all body fluids, including blood, saliva and breast milk. It is transmitted by people suffering from the disease, and by carriers who have no symptoms at all and are unaware of their condition. Diagnosis is by blood test.

In dental practice the main source of infection is by direct contact with blood containing HBV. This is most likely to occur from an inoculation injury, i.e. accidentally pricking oneself with a syringe needle used on an HBV carrier. One in three of such accidents results in HBV infection.

Staff are also at risk from the use of high-speed equipment, such as an air turbine handpiece with water spray, an ultrasonic scaler or a three-in-one syringe. These release a cloud of water and saliva particles into the air which, if contaminated with a carrier's blood, may infect the dentist or dental nurse via the nose, eyes or skin abrasions. Furthermore, adjacent working surfaces become infected too, while inadequate sterilisation procedures may cause infection of other patients.

Infection of staff from non-sharp causes may be prevented by protective clothing, as described previously.

Although the risks may seem alarming, all dental nurses and other chairside staff are required to be vaccinated against HBV and should therefore be immune to danger.

High-risk groups

Among the general population the main modes of transmission of HBV are childbirth, the sharing of needles by drug addicts and sexual contact. Thus certain groups of people are much more likely to be carriers.

- Drug addicts.
- The sexually promiscuous.
- Those who have received long-term regular blood transfusions, such as haemophiliacs, dialysis and transplant patients.
- Special needs patients living in institutions, and staff in close contact with them.
- Those working or living in institutions such as prisons or rehabilitation centres for drug addicts and alcoholics.
- Partners and close relatives of carriers, not necessarily with sexual contact.

Prevention of cross-infection

As the majority of HBV carriers are unaware of their condition, it has been estimated that 400 are treated daily in dental practice. But provided the sterilisation and surgery hygiene procedures in this chapter are adopted, there need be no cause for alarm. However, the existence of high-risk groups emphasises the importance of obtaining an adequate medical history before treatment.

Fortunately, all dental staff can obtain protection against hepatitis B by vaccination. This will also protect their patients against HBV infection from dental staff. Vaccination is available under the NHS. It involves a series of three injections, followed by a blood test to check its success. A booster injection may be required at a later date. As vaccination is a requirement for chairside employment, documentary evidence of successful immunisation must be kept. Although vaccination is completely safe, special arrangements are necessary for staff who are pregnant, or become pregnant, during the course of injections.

Treatment of known carriers

The basic principle of preventing infection with HBV is to avoid contact with the patient's blood. In addition to the sterilisation and surgery hygiene procedures already detailed, the following extra precautions have been recommended for general practice.

- For operations involving extensive loss of blood, such as multiple extractions and minor oral surgery, or if the disease is in an active state, refer the patient to hospital where full sterile surgical facilities are available.
- Reserve the last appointment of the day for treatment of known carriers. This allows more time for infection control procedures before any more patients are seen but does not excuse non-compliance with the full infection control procedures at other times.

- Move all unnecessary equipment and materials away from the chair side. Protect essential working surfaces and equipment controls, such as switches, operating light handle and three-in-one syringe, with plastic bags or Clingfilm.
- Take great care to avoid inoculation injuries.
- Regard steel burs and matrix bands as disposable. After treatment, flush the aspirator with hypochlorite and leave the solution in a collection jar overnight.
- Items which cannot be sterilised by heat or hypochlorite should be immersed in a suitable disinfectant for the manufacturer's recommended time.
- Launder linen and towelling in a hot wash of 90 °C for 10 min.
- Pregnant staff or those who have not been vaccinated against HBV should not have any contact with known carriers.

Hepatitis C

This disease is similar to hepatitis B in the way that it is contracted, transmitted and diagnosed. However, it is a far more dangerous disease with a much higher mortality rate, and there is no vaccine for it. In the past cases were caused by blood transfusion, but this has not happened since 1993, when screening of donors began.

Nowadays the main sources of infection are drug addiction, tattooing, body piercing and other modes of infected blood-to-blood contact but sexual transmission is uncommon. The pathogenic micro-organism involved is the hepatitis C virus (HCV).

The greatest risk to dental staff is from an inoculation injury but provided that the safety precautions to prevent this are followed, there is no danger of HCV infection. However, it should be understood that if such a situation does arise, there is a one in 30 chance of transmission of the disease.

Acquired immunodeficiency syndrome

In acquired immunodeficiency syndrome (AIDS), the body's natural defence mechanism against infection is seriously impaired. Consequently AIDS patients succumb to infections which are not normally serious or which are not normally experienced. The outcome of AIDS is usually fatal as there is no cure, no vaccination and no resistance to infection. However, progress of the disease can be delayed, and life prolonged, by the use of antiviral and other drugs which boost the immune system. The apparent success of these treatments is, unfortunately, having the perverse effect of increasing the number of people contracting the disease. The reason for this is that many people are now ignoring the safety measures that were followed in the past, when AIDS was rapidly fatal.

The acquired immunodeficiency syndrome is caused by infection with a virus called the human immunodeficiency virus (HIV). There are no particular symptoms of AIDS as they depend solely upon whichever chance infection affects the sufferer. Like hepatitis B, the AIDS virus has been found in most body fluids but is transmitted mainly by contact with blood containing the virus. HIV is present in the blood of all infected persons but it usually takes years before they suffer any effects. Furthermore, as there are no specific symptoms, many of those infected with HIV are unaware that they have AIDS. Diagnosis is by blood test.

Infectivity

Unlike HBV, the AIDS virus is not very infective and is not resistant to heat or disinfectants. Although every infected person is potentially infectious, repeated exposure to HIV in blood or body fluids is usually required for transmission of AIDS. Among the general population, the usual modes of transmission are sexual promiscuity, the sharing of needles by drug addicts, childbirth and repeated transfusions with contaminated blood.

In dental practice the main hazard is an inoculation injury, but the infectivity of HIV is so low that a single such accident would only result in a one in 300 chance of contracting AIDS. However, no chances can be taken as AIDS is a fatal disease for which there is no cure and no vaccine.

High-risk groups

Those most at risk of being carriers are:

- the sexually promiscuous
- drug addicts
- haemophiliacs and other patients who have received long-term regular blood transfusions
- sexual partners of these groups
- infants born to infected mothers.

Prevention

Although no preventive treatment by drugs or vaccination is possible, AIDS is easily avoided. All that is required as far as the general population is concerned is to avoid any form of sexual promiscuity or the sharing of needles between drug addicts.

In dental practice, prevention is the same as for hepatitis B, by correct sterilisation and surgery hygiene procedures.

Dentists may be the first healthcare workers to see the early signs of AIDS as some very unusual mouth conditions may occur for no apparent reason. As in the case of oral cancer, early referral to a specialist may be a life-saving measure.

Treatment of known carriers

This is the same as for hepatitis carriers. Fortunately, HIV has a very low infectivity and is easily destroyed by routine sterilisation procedures. Nevertheless, no chances can be taken as AIDS is fatal and no vaccination is available.

Known carriers of HIV and hepatitis viruses are those who are aware of their condition and have informed the dentist when their medical history is taken. The requirement of confidentiality mentioned in Chapter 2 is of paramount importance in such cases. Most carriers are either unaware of their condition or unwilling to disclose it in case their affliction is revealed to unauthorised people. Some are also afraid of being denied dental treatment if they admit to being carriers. When any medical history is taken, it is ethically and legally essential to ensure that it cannot be overheard anywhere else in the practice, and takes place under conditions that give patients the confidence to provide a complete relevant history without embarrassment.

As only a minority of carriers are known to be such, most are treated without the dentist being aware of their condition. This emphasises the importance of strict adherence to correct procedures for the prevention of cross-infection by all staff within the dental workplace.

New-variant Creutzfeldt–Jakob disease (vCJD)

New-variant Creutzfeldt–Jakob disease (vCJD) is one of a group of rare but fatal related diseases (similar to 'mad cow disease') caused by infection with a unique non-microbial source of disease called a *prion protein*. The infection occurs within nerve tissue, affecting both the brain and all nerve tissues throughout the body, including that found within the pulp of the teeth. Its importance is entirely due to the fact that prions cannot be destroyed by normal methods of sterilisation.

Consequently, current recommendations are to consider all endodontic instruments that come into contact with the tooth pulp as single-use items, to prevent the transmission of the disease by indirect cross-infection, although the risk is considered to be only theoretical. Therefore broaches, files, reamers and handpiece-driven endodontic instruments must be safely disposed of as infectious hazardous waste (sharps) after a single use.

227

Inoculation injury

Nearly all dental procedures involve the use of sharp items including local anaesthetic needles, sharp instruments and scalpel blades. All must be handled with great care to avoid an inoculation injury.

Every dental workplace must have a policy in place to avoid a sharps injury, and it should ideally include all of the following points.

- The dentist using a local anaesthetic needle should be the person responsible for its resheathing and safe placement in a sharps bin, so that injury to others does not occur as there is no transference of the sharp item from one person to another.
- Needle guards should be used when resheathing needles, so that they can be placed within their plastic sheath without being held in the fingers.
- Heavy-duty rubber gloves and full PPE should be worn by any staff responsible for instrument cleaning and debridement before sterilisation.

Although a sharps injury from a sterile, unused instrument may be momentarily painful, it is of no consequence save to reconsider the level of care taken by the staff member involved. However, if a contaminated inoculation injury occurs, the following actions must be carried out.

- Stop all treatment immediately and attend to the wound.
- Squeeze the wound to encourage bleeding, but do not suck the wound.
- Wash the area with soap and running water, then dry and cover the wound with a waterproof dressing.
- Note the name, address and contact details of the source patient if a contaminated item is involved, so that their medical history can be checked immediately.
- Complete the accident book.
- Report the incident to the senior dentist/line manager.
- The consultant microbiologist at the local hospital must be contacted immediately if the source patient is a known or suspected HIV or hepatitis C carrier, as emergency antiviral treatment must commence within 1 h of the injury.

The contact details for the consultant microbiologist should be readily available within the infection control policy documentation, and updated whenever necessary.

 Further resources are available for this book, including interactive multiple choice questions and extended matching questions. Visit the companion website at:

www.levisonstextbookfordentalnurses.com

9

Head and Neck Anatomy and Physiology

Key learning points

A **factual knowledge** of
- the gross anatomy of the skull
- the head and neck musculature
- the nerve supply to the head and neck, including the dentally relevant cranial nerves
- the blood supply to the head and neck

A **factual awareness** of
- disorders of the dentally relevant cranial nerves

The anatomy of the head and neck region of the human body is of relevance to the dental nurse in providing the underpinning knowledge required to understand their role within the dental team, as well as knowledge of the full range of topics covered in their dental nurse training programme. Dental nurses are often asked for information and advice from patients with regard to their oral health, and within the bounds of their profession, they will be able to give more accurate and useful information when it is based on the head and neck area in full, rather than just on teeth. For instance, a full understanding of the subject of local anaesthesia requires knowledge of the skull and oral anatomy, as well as of the drugs used.

Levison's Textbook for Dental Nurses, Eleventh Edition. By Carole Hollins.
© 2013 John Wiley & Sons, Ltd. Published 2013 by John Wiley & Sons, Ltd. Companion website: www.levisonstextbookfordentalnurses.com

Anatomy of the skull

The skull is the topmost part of the bony skeleton of the body, the head, and is made up of three main areas.

- **Cranium** – the hollow cavity which surrounds the brain.
- **Face** – the front vertical part of the skull, containing the orbital cavities of the eyes and the nasal cavity of the nose.
- **Jaws** – the upper and lower jaws of the oral cavity, supporting the teeth and the tongue, and providing the openings for the respiratory tract and the digestive tract.

All the bones of the skull except the lower jaw, the *mandible*, are fixed to each other by immovable joints called *sutures*.

The base (underside) of the cranium articulates with the topmost bone of the vertebral column, the *atlas*, and allows nodding movements of the head.

Like most bones in the body, the skull develops in the fetus as cartilage, which is gradually converted to bone during the growth of the body into adulthood.

The outer layer of all bone is called *compact bone*, and is perforated by many natural bony openings (*foramina*) to allow the passage of nerve and blood vessels. The inner layer is called *cancellous bone* and is quite sponge-like in appearance, because if it was a solid structure it would make the bone too heavy for the muscles to be able to lift. Nerves and blood vessels run freely within the spongy structure of the cancellous layer, and pass into and out of it through the foramina.

Cranium

At birth and during infancy, the bony plates making up the cranium are separated from each other by two natural membrane-covered spaces called *fontanelles*, which allow growth of the brain without any bony restriction. During growth, the spaces gradually become filled with bone and close together to provide a protective helmet surrounding the brain. The bony plates join together like a jigsaw puzzle at the *coronoid sutures*. By the age of 18 months the fontanelles should have closed completely, following the natural growth together of the bony plates making up the cranium.

The cranium is composed of eight bones which are separated by the coronoid sutures – these are visible on a dry skull as the zig-zagged joints between the bony plates. The bones themselves are as follows.

- **Frontal bone** – single plate at the front of the cranium above the eyes, forming the forehead.
- **Parietal bones** – pair of plates forming the top and the greater area of the sides of the cranium.
- **Temporal bones** – pair of fan-shaped plates in the temple region of the lower sides of the cranium, in front of the ears.
- **Occipital bone** – single plate at the back and partial underside of the cranium.
- **Sphenoid bone** – single plate forming the majority of the base (underside) of the cranium.
- **Ethmoid bone** – single plate at the front base section of the cranium, immediately behind the nose.

The skull and cranial bones are illustrated in Figure 9.1.

All the sensory nerve cells running from the body to the brain and all the motor nerves running from the brain to the body have to pass in and out of this bony cavity, and they do so through the

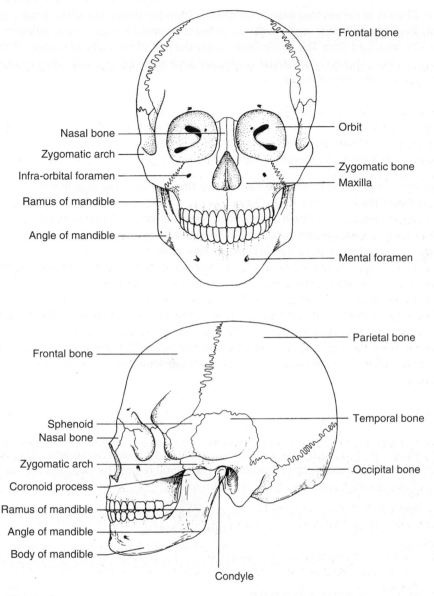

Figure 9.1   The skull.

many natural foramina on the underside of the cranium. Similarly, all the blood vessels supplying the head and neck structures pass through these same foramina or between natural spaces between adjacent bones, called *fissures*.

In addition to these bony openings, some cranial bones also have various bony projections and plates on their outer surfaces, which serve as attachments for ligaments and muscles associated with head and jaw movements or which form part of various facial structures.

The largest foramen of all in the cranium is the *foramen magnum*, which opens through the occipital bone and allows the exit of the spinal cord from the base of the brain and into the vertebral column of the spine.

The 12 pairs of nerves that branch off directly from the underside of the brain itself, and which supply the head and neck region only, are called the *cranial nerves* – those relevant to the dental nurse are discussed later. The nerves that supply the rest of the body all branch off the spinal cord at various points down the vertebral column, and are referred to as the *systemic nerves*. They are not relevant to the dental nurse.

Face

The face is composed of 11 bones which are separated from each other by sutures, as in the cranium. The main bones themselves are as follows.

- **Vomer** – single bone behind the nasal cavity, that connects the cranial and facial regions of the skull together.
- **Lacrimal bones** – pair of fragile bony plates forming the inner wall of the orbital cavities (eye sockets).
- **Nasal bones** – pair of bones forming the bridge of the nose.
- **Nasal turbinates** – pair of fragile curled bones projecting into the nasal cavity, which increase the contact of inspired air with the nasal mucosa; this aids debris removal before inhalation to the lungs, and warms the air as it passes over the capillary beds covering the bones. They are separated in the midline by the nasal septum.
- **Palatine bones** – pair of bony plates forming the posterior section of the hard palate, and the side wall of the nasal cavity.
- **Zygomatic bones** – pair of facial bones that articulate with the cranium posteriorly and extend anteriorly into the zygomatic arch (cheek bone) to articulate with the maxilla.

The skull and facial bones are shown in Figure 9.1.

Jaws

Although strictly speaking the jaw bones are actually part of the facial skeleton, they are considered separately as they are of such importance to the dental team. The two jaws are each made up of a pair of bones which are fixed solidly in their midlines.

- **Maxilla** – pair of bones forming the upper jaw, the lower border of the orbital cavities, the base of the nose and the anterior portion of the hard palate.
- **Mandible** – appears as a single horseshoe-shaped bone forming the lower jaw, with its posterior vertical bony struts articulating with the cranium at the temporomandibular joint (TMJ).

Maxilla and palatine bones

The maxilla effectively forms the middle third of the face and as with various other cranial bones, it has several foramina and bony projections which are dentally relevant.

The maxilla is made up of two bones which are separated above by the nasal cavity. They join together below the nose as the front section of the *hard palate*. The back section of the hard palate is formed by the palatine bones, and the whole palate forms the floor of the nose and the roof of the oral cavity, or mouth (Figure 9.2).

Each side of the maxilla forms part of the eye socket, the nose and the front of the cheekbone. The two maxilla bones themselves are hollow within, because if they were solid they would be too heavy to allow the head to be lifted up. Each hollow space is called the *maxillary antrum* or *sinus*, and lies just above the root apices of the upper molar and second premolar teeth (Figure 9.3). This

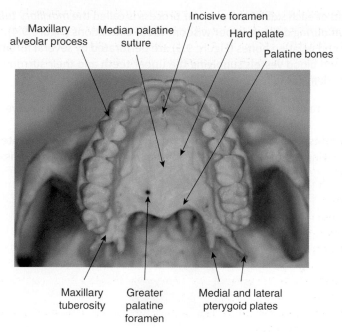

Figure 9.2   Palate – anatomical landmarks.

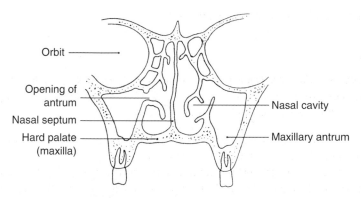

Figure 9.3   Facial bones and air spaces (cross-section).

hollow space can be easily perforated during the extraction of these teeth, causing an unwanted connection between the mouth and the antrum called an *oroantral fistula*. A natural connection between the nasal cavity and the antra exists, to allow drainage of the sinuses to occur, and to give resonance to the voice.

Inflammation of these air spaces (sinusitis) due to a respiratory infection often mimics dental pain in these teeth, or conversely a dental infection can be mistaken for sinusitis.

The two maxilla bones join together in the centre-line of the face at the intermaxillary suture and the lowest portions of these two sections form the alveolar process. This horseshoe-shaped structure is where both sets of upper teeth develop before birth, and later erupt as the upper primary and then secondary dentition.

The back end of each side of the alveolar process is called the *maxillary tuberosity*, and this can be fractured off during difficult upper wisdom tooth extractions (Figure 9.4).

The maxilla and palatine bones (Figure 9.5) are perforated by several foramina to allow passage of the nerves and blood vessels supplying the upper teeth and their surrounding soft tissues, the four main ones being as follows.

- **Infraorbital foramen** – beneath the eye sockets, through which the nerves supplying the upper teeth and their labial soft tissues pass.
- **Greater and lesser palatine foramina** – at the back of the hard palate, through which the nerves supplying the palatal soft tissues of the upper posterior teeth pass.

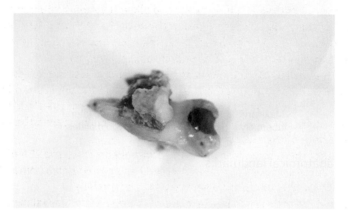

Figure 9.4   Extracted upper tooth with fractured tuberosity.

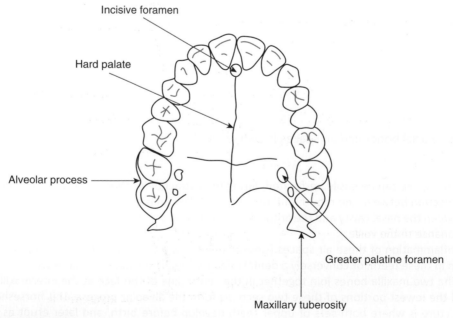

Figure 9.5   Palate and maxillary teeth.

- **Incisive foramen** – at the front centre of the hard palate, through which the nerves supplying the palatal soft tissues of the upper anterior teeth pass.

Mandible

The mandible is also made up of two bones, joined together in the centre-line at the *mental symphysis* to create a single horseshoe-shaped structure, and with its two back ends bent up vertically to the horseshoe. The vertical section is called the *ramus of the mandible*, the horizontal section is called the *body of the mandible*, and the point at which they join is the *angle of the mandible* (Figure 9.6).

The mandible's only connection with the rest of the skull is at the two *temporomandibular joints* (TMJ), where the bone moves as a hinge joint and allow the mouth to open and close. The point at which the mandible connects with the temporal bone at the TMJ is the *head of condyle* (Figure 9.7). The muscles of mastication, which allow jaw-closing and chewing movements, all connect between the cranium and various points on the mandible, as discussed later.

The mandible also has an *alveolar process* running around it, which supports all the lower teeth. Below this process, on the inner side of the body of the mandible lies a ridge of bone called the *mylohyoid ridge*, where the mylohyoid muscle attaches to form the floor of the mouth. A bony ridge also lies on the outer surface of the ramus of the mandible, called the *external oblique ridge*, which marks the base of the alveolar process in this area.

The front edge of the ramus rises up to the *coronoid process*, and the dip between it and the head of condyle at the back of the ramus is called the *sigmoid notch*. When the mouth is closed, the coronoid process slots under the zygomatic arch of the face.

The two foramina in the mandible which are of interest to the dental nurse are as follows.

235

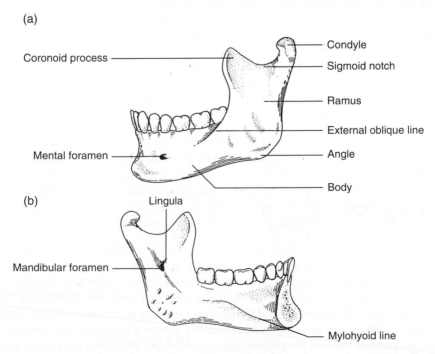

(a)

Coronoid process —
Condyle
Sigmoid notch
Ramus
External oblique line
Mental foramen —
Angle
Body

(b)   Lingula

Mandibular foramen —

Mylohyoid line

Figure 9.6 The mandible. (a) Outer side. (b) Inner side.

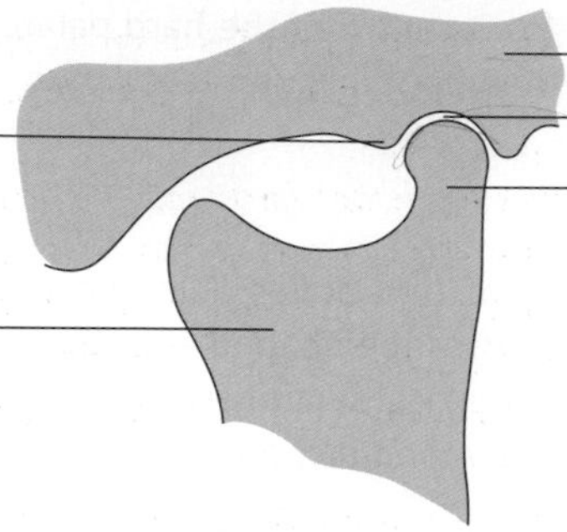

Figure 9.7 Temporomandibular joint.

- **Mandibular foramen** – halfway up the inner surface of the ramus and protected by the bony lingula, through which the nerve supplying the lower teeth and some of their surrounding soft tissues enters the mandible.
- **Mental foramen** – on the outer surface of the body of the mandible, between the positions of the premolar teeth, through which the same nerve exits the mandible.

Temporomandibular joint and chewing action

This joint is formed between the condyle of the mandible and the temporal bone at the base of the skull. When the mouth is shut the condyle rests in a hollow region of the temporal bone called the *glenoid fossa*. The front edge of the glenoid fossa is formed into a ridge called the *articular eminence*. So the mandibular surface of the joint consists of the condyle, and the temporal surface consists of the glenoid fossa and articular eminence. Between these two surfaces there is a disc of fibrous tissue called the *meniscus*, which prevents the two bones from grating against each other during jaw movements. When the meniscus slips in front or behind its normal position during opening and closing of the mouth, the patient experiences the effect as 'jaw clicking'. This disarrangement of the joint is called *subluxation*.

During normal jaw movements, the joint allows three basic types of mandibular movement to occur.

- **Gliding movement** – mainly occurs when the disc and the condyle together slide up and down the articular eminence, allowing the mandible to move forwards and backwards.
- **Rotational movement** – occurs when the condyle rotates anteriorly and posteriorly over the surface of the disc itself, which remains static, allowing the mandible to move down and up.
- **Lateral movement** – this occurs when one joint glides alone, so that the other condyle rotates sideways over its disc, swinging the mandible on the side opposite from the gliding action.

As already described, the first stage of opening the mouth is a hinge-like opening of the mandible to separate the incisors. The condyle remains in the glenoid fossa during this stage. As the mouth opens further, the condyle slides downwards and forwards from the glenoid fossa along the slope of the articular eminence. When the condyle reaches the crest of the articular eminence, the mouth is open to its fullest extent and the incisors can grasp food between their cutting edges.

For the closing movement, which produces the shearing action of the incisors, the condyle returns to its rest position in the glenoid fossa, as the mandible moves backwards and closes. This produces a shearing action of the incisors which thereby cut the food into smaller pieces ready for chewing. It is similar to the cutting action of a pair of scissors. Chewing is brought about by rotational movements of the mandible which swings from side to side, crushing food between the cusps of opposing molars and premolars.

Sometimes the condyle slips too far forward and gets stuck in front of the articular eminence. When this happens, it cannot move back and the joint is said to be *dislocated*, recognised by an inability to close the mouth. It can be resolved by pressing down on the lower molars to force the condyle downwards and backwards into the glenoid fossa but sedation or a general anaesthetic may be necessary to allow the muscles of mastication to relax fully and treatment to be carried out.

The opening movements of the mandible are due to the actions of the *suprahyoid muscles* which lie in the floor of the mouth and in the throat. The closing and chewing actions of the mandible are due to the actions of the *muscles of mastication* which run between the mandible and the cranium or facial bones. Both are discussed later.

237

Disorders of the temporomandibular joint

The TMJ and muscles of mastication may be subjected to excessive strain from seemingly trivial causes and these can produce a variety of effects, ranging from spasm of the muscles of mastication to degenerative changes in the joint. They result in a wide range of symptoms but the most common are pain or tenderness over the joint, clicking noises and restricted movement of the mandible.

As with any joint, the TMJ can also be affected by osteoarthritis and require the use of anti-inflammatories or steroids to relieve the painful symptoms. In extreme cases involving younger patients, the joints can even be replaced by artificial prostheses, such as with hip and knee replacements.

Abnormal or parafunctional habits of the patient, especially habitual clenching and grinding of the teeth over long periods, are common findings by the dental team. These habits tend to exhaust the joint musculature and cause pain and discomfort, and the parafunctional action is called *bruxism*. Most patients are unaware that they perform these habitual movements, often doing so in their sleep. Sufferers will experience any or all of the following symptoms.

- **Trismus** – involuntary painful contracture of the joint musculature, resulting in the inability to open the mouth fully.
- **Face and/or neck pain** – often worse in the morning following a night of bruxing, and eased by relaxation and the use of anti-inflammatories.
- **Attrition** – enamel wear facets on the teeth, due to the constant grinding of the occlusal and incisal surfaces of each arch against the other.
- **Restorative failure** – repetitive fracture and loss of dental restorations, with or without tooth fracture, due to the excessive and prolonged occlusal forces produced.
- **Sore mouth** – especially the tongue and cheeks, where cheek ridges and tongue scalloping develop as the tongue is thrust against the teeth and the cheeks are bitten (Figure 9.8).

Similar symptoms are often seen in patients who use chewing gum excessively.

Following diagnosis and advice on the particular cause of the bruxism, which can often be in relation to stress, treatment involves counselling, use of anti-inflammatories and muscle relaxants, muscle exercises and physiotherapy, and sometimes the provision of nightguards or splints to wear as necessary. While not preventing the bruxing action, these devices will hold the jaws open slightly and relieve the tension put on the joint musculature. In some cases involving stress as the causative factor, life changes may be necessary.

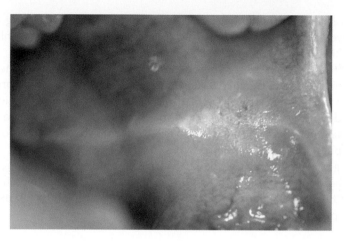

Figure 9.8   Cheek biting.

Trismus may also occur when a patient is suffering from pericoronitis (acute inflammation of the operculum of an erupting lower wisdom tooth), following the surgical extraction of these teeth, or during a bout of the viral disease mumps (acute infection of the parotid salivary glands).

Muscles of the head and neck

Muscles of mastication

These are the four sets of muscles connected between the mandible and the base of the cranium or the face, which allow chewing movements and mouth closing to occur.

- **Temporalis**
- **Masseter**
- **Lateral pterygoid** ('p' is silent, so pronounced 'terygoid')
- **Medial pterygoid**

They all receive nerve impulses from the fifth cranial nerve (trigeminal nerve) which cause them to contract so that the length of the muscle shortens. This then causes the various movements of the mandible associated with mouth closing, jaw clenching and chewing, as described previously. The muscles of mastication do not cause mouth opening – this is controlled by a different group of muscles called the suprahyoid muscles. Each set of the muscles of mastication is connected to the cranium or the face at one end – called their *point of origin* – and at their other end to the mandible – called their *point of insertion*. The contraction of individual sets of muscles, or of just one of the lateral pterygoid muscles alone, shortens their length between these two points. As the mandible is the only movable bone of the TMJ, this muscle shortening causes the movement of the mandible into various positions to allow closing and chewing actions to occur.

The muscles of mastication are summarised below.

Temporalis

Point of origin – **temporal bone** of the cranium
Point of insertion – **coronoid process** of the mandible, passing under the zygomatic arch
Action – **pulls the mandible backwards and closed**

Masseter

Point of origin – outer surface of **zygomatic arch**
Point of insertion – outer surface of **mandibular ramus and angle**
Action – **closes the mandible**

Lateral pterygoid

Point of origin – **lateral pterygoid plate** at the base of the cranium
Point of insertion – **head of the mandibular condyle** and into the TMJ meniscus
Action – **both contracting brings the mandible forwards** to bite the anterior teeth tip to tip, **one contracting pulls the mandible to the opposite side**

Medial pterygoid

Point of origin – **medial pterygoid plate** at the base of the cranium
Point of insertion – inner surface of **mandibular ramus and angle**
Action – **closes the mandible**

When the teeth are clenched together, the temporalis and masseter muscles can be felt by placing a hand on the side of the head and face respectively. They form the superficial layer of the muscles of mastication, while the medial and lateral pterygoid muscles form the deep layer. The superficial muscles are shown in Figure 9.9, along with some of the suprahyoid muscles and the muscles of facial expression.

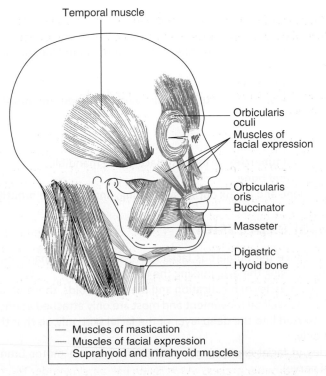

Figure 9.9   Oral musculature.

Suprahyoid muscles

As their name suggests, one end of all these muscles is attached to the horseshoe-shaped hyoid bone which lies suspended in soft tissue beneath the mandible, in the throat. They then all lie above this bone, as opposed to a separate group of muscles lying beneath the bone called the *infrahyoid muscles*.

The suprahyoid muscles are responsible for mouth opening and swallowing actions. One group of these muscles lies in front of the hyoid bone and the others behind, producing anterior and posterior groups respectively. The anterior group is of some relevance to the dental nurse. They are listed below.

- **Anterior belly of digastric**
- **Mylohyoid**
- **Geniohyoid**

The anterior digastric and mylohyoid muscles are innervated by the motor branch of the trigeminal nerve (fifth cranial nerve), and the geniohyoid is innervated by the hypoglossal nerve (12th cranial nerve).

Anterior digastric

Point of origin – **hyoid bone**
Point of insertion – inner surface of **mental symphysis** of the mandible
Action – helps to lift the hyoid bone and larynx during swallowing, pulls the mandible down to **open the mouth**

Mylohyoid

Point of origin – mylohyoid line of the inner surface of the mandible, fusing in the midline to form the **floor of the mouth**
Point of insertion – **hyoid bone**
Action – lift hyoid bone and larynx during swallowing, and **open the mouth**

Geniohyoid

Point of origin – **genial tubercles** on inner surface of the mandible
Point of insertion – **hyoid bone**
Action – lift hyoid bone and larynx during swallowing, and **open the mouth**

Muscles of facial expression

These muscles produce the numerous facial expressions that humans are capable of showing – smiling, frowning, winking the eye, pursing the lips, and so on.

In contrast to the muscles of mastication and the suprahyoids, those of facial expression are not involved in producing skeletal movement and most are only attached at one end to the skull. Their other ends are inserted into the deep layer of the facial skin only, so that their contraction causes skin movement only.

All the muscles of facial expression are innervated by the motor branch of the facial nerve (seventh cranial nerve).

For the sake of simplicity, they can be grouped according to the facial region that their actions involve.

- The scalp
- The eyes and surrounding area
- The mouth and surrounding area

Only the last group are of relevance to the dental nurse.

The main muscle of the eye is a ring of tissue called *orbicularis oculi* and that of the mouth is *orbicularis oris*. Thin straps of muscle run between these rings and into the surrounding tissues, to allow movement of the eyelids, lips, mouth and nostrils.

The cheek muscle is called *buccinator* and is attached above and below to the outer surface of the alveolar process of each jaw. It connects to the muscular wall of the throat behind and to orbicularis oris in front. Buccinator helps with chewing movements by helping to keep ingested food within the confines of the teeth, while the jaw actions cause the teeth to cut and shred the food before swallowing.

The three sets of muscle relevant to the dental nurse are shown in Figure 9.9.

Nerve supply of the head and neck

The head is supplied by 12 pairs of *cranial nerves*. They all branch off from the brain, one from each pair supplying the left side, while the other supplies the right.

The nerves which make muscles and glands work are called *motor* nerves and they carry electrical impulses from the brain to effect contraction of the muscles or secretion from the glands. Those nerves which convey pain and other sensation are called *sensory* nerves and they carry electrical stimulation from the body tissues (including teeth) to the brain. Cranial nerves are either motor or sensory, or a combination of the two types, and those relevant to dental nurses are as follows.

- **Trigeminal nerve** – the fifth (V) cranial nerve, supplying the teeth and surrounding soft tissues and the muscles of mastication.
- **Facial nerve** – the seventh (VII) cranial nerve, supplying some taste sensations, some salivary glands and the muscles of facial expression.
- **Glossopharyngeal nerve** – the ninth (IX) cranial nerve, supplying some taste sensations, the parotid salivary glands and the muscles of the pharynx.
- **Hypoglossal nerve** – the 12th (XII) cranial nerve, supplying the muscles of the anterior two-thirds of the tongue.

The nomenclature used to name the various nerves follows that used in other areas of anatomy, so *anterior* and *posterior* refer to front and back, respectively, and *superior* and *inferior* refer to upper and lower, respectively. The areas of supply in relation to the teeth and their surrounding soft tissues follow the dental terminology used in naming tooth surfaces, as discussed in Chapter 10.

Trigeminal nerve

The name of this nerve indicates that it splits into three divisions, each of which has several branches.

- **Ophthalmic division** – sensory supply of the soft tissues around the eye and the upper face.
- **Maxillary division** – sensory supply of the upper teeth, the maxilla and the middle area of the face.

241

● **Mandibular division** – sensory supply of the lower teeth, the mandible and the lower area of the face, and motor supply to the muscles of mastication and some of the suprahyoids.

The maxillary and mandibular branches of the trigeminal nerve are of most importance to the dental nurse, as together they relay sensory information from the whole of the oral cavity to the brain, and provide the motor supply to the muscles of mastication, to effect jaw closing and chewing movements, and to some of the suprahyoid muscles to effect jaw opening.

Maxillary division

The maxillary division of the trigeminal nerve splits further into five branches, all of which are sensory (Figure 9.10). By definition, then, they transmit sensations (such as heat, cold, pressure and pain) from this area to the brain, including from the upper teeth. It is these branches that have

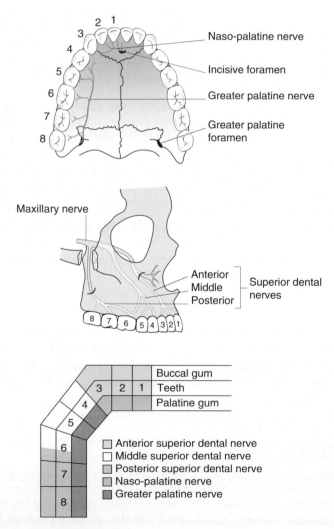

Figure 9.10   Nerve supply of the upper teeth.

to be anaesthetised before painless dental treatment can be carried out on the upper teeth. The five branches are as follows, and their general anatomical paths are described below.

- **Anterior superior dental (alveolar) nerve** – supplies sensation from the upper incisor and canine teeth, and their labial gingivae. In addition, it supplies sensation from the soft tissues of the upper lip and around the nostrils of the nose.
- **Middle superior dental (alveolar) nerve** – supplies sensation from the upper premolar and the anterior half of the upper first molar teeth, and their buccal gingivae.
- **Posterior superior dental (alveolar) nerve** – supplies sensation from the posterior half of the upper first molar and the second and third molar teeth, and their buccal gingivae.
- **Greater palatine nerve** – supplies sensation from the palatal gingivae of the upper molar, premolar and posterior half of the canine teeth.
- **Nasopalatine nerve** – previously called the **long sphenopalatine nerve**, this supplies sensation from the palatal gingivae of the upper incisor and anterior half of the canine teeth.

The maxillary nerve emerges from the base of the brain, leaves the skull through the *foramen rotundum* and passes forward through the floor of the eye socket (orbit). Before entering the orbit, it gives off its posterior superior dental and palatine branches. Within the orbit, it gives off the middle and anterior superior dental nerves. It emerges from the orbit through the *infraorbital foramen* on the front of the maxilla to supply the skin and mucous membrane of the lower eyelid, cheek and upper lip.

The posterior superior dental nerve enters the back of the maxilla to reach its destination, while the greater palatine nerve also passes through the back of the maxilla and reaches the surface of the hard palate through the *greater palatine foramen*, opposite the third molar tooth.

The nasopalatine nerve passes through the floor of the nasal cavity to reach the surface of the palate through the *incisive foramen* behind the central incisors, and the anterior and middle superior dental nerves branch off from the maxillary nerve in the floor of the orbit. They pass down inside the maxilla, in the walls of the maxillary sinus, to reach the teeth. The sensory nerve impulses from the upper teeth and their surrounding soft tissue structures pass from the nerve endings back along these nerve pathways to the maxillary nerve trunk, and then enter the skull and join the other two divisions to form the trigeminal nerve trunk, which then enters the brain itself.

Mandibular nerve

The mandibular division of the trigeminal nerve emerges from the skull through the foramen ovale and splits into four branches which carry both sensory and motor components (Figure 9.11). The sensory branches of this nerve require anaesthetising before painless dental treatment can be carried out on the lower teeth. The four branches are as follows, and their general anatomical paths are described below.

- **Inferior dental (alveolar) nerve** – supplies sensation from all the lower teeth, and from the buccal or labial gingivae of all *except* the molar teeth. In addition, it supplies sensation from the soft tissues of the lower lip and the chin.
- **Lingual nerve** – supplies sensation from the lingual gingivae of all the lower teeth, the floor of the mouth, and touch sensation from the anterior two-thirds of the tongue.
- **Long buccal nerve** – supplies sensation from the buccal gingivae of the lower molar teeth.
- **Motor branch** – supplies stimulation to the muscles of mastication, to effect jaw closing and chewing movements.

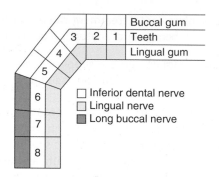

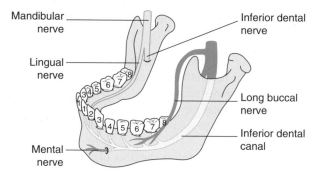

Figure 9.11   Nerve supply of the lower teeth.

The mandibular nerve passes down from the base of the skull on the inner side of the ramus of the mandible, between the medial and lateral pterygoid muscles, and divides into the above branches.

The *inferior dental nerve* supplies all the lower teeth and enters the mandible through the *mandibular foramen*. This is situated at the centre of the inner surface of the ramus and is guarded on its front edge by a small bony projection called the *lingula*. After entering the mandibular foramen, the nerve passes through a canal running inside the mandible, below the apices of the teeth. The end branch of the inferior dental nerve emerges on the outer surface of the mandible through the *mental foramen* which is situated below the apices of the premolars. From this point, it is called the *mental nerve* and supplies the buccal gum of the incisors, canines and premolars, plus the lower lip and chin.

The *long buccal nerve* supplies the buccal gum of the molars. It passes into the gum on the outer surface of the mandible, over the external oblique ridge.

The *lingual nerve* supplies the lingual gum of all the lower teeth. It passes along the floor of the mouth on the inner surface of the mandible, above the mylohyoid muscle, where it also supplies the anterior two-thirds of the tongue and the floor of the mouth.

The full distribution of the trigeminal nerve is shown in Figure 9.12.

Trigeminal neuralgia

This is a condition affecting the sensory nerves of either the maxillary or mandibular divisions only of the trigeminal nerve, with no known cause. The sufferer experiences sudden-onset, severe pain in various facial trigger zones, accompanied by muscle spasms in the area. The neuralgia can be initiated by touch, chewing movements or even speaking, and is usually of short duration.

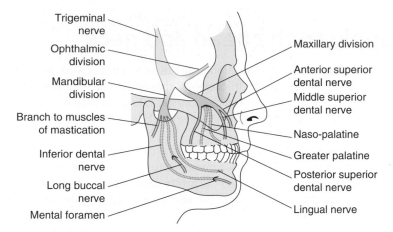

Figure 9.12   Trigeminal nerve distribution.

Treatment is difficult without a known cause, and often drastic measures such as the surgical or chemical destruction of the sensory section of the nerve is undertaken, to relieve the debilitating symptoms.

Facial nerve

This is a combination nerve, carrying both sensory and motor fibres. Its sensory component carries taste sensation from the anterior two-thirds (front part) of the tongue, while its motor components supply the muscles of facial expression and the saliva secretions of both the submandibular and sublingual salivary glands. Temporary paralysis of this nerve (left or right) gives rise to the condition of *Bell's palsy*.

Glossopharyngeal nerve

Again, this is a combination nerve. Its sensory component carries taste sensation from the posterior one-third of the tongue, while its motor component supplies the muscles of the pharynx and the saliva secretions of the parotid salivary gland.

Hypoglossal nerve

This nerve has a motor component only and supplies the muscles of the tongue, to effect its complicated movements during speech, mastication and swallowing.

As with all the cranial nerves, the electrical transmissions of these dentally relevant four can be affected by many disorders involving the brain, including tumours. Dental patients who complain of altered taste sensations or the sudden loss of facial sensations with no obvious cause require rapid neurological investigations to rule out any sinister causes. The dental team has a significant role to play in detecting these aberrations, and in referring patients for more specialist investigation and diagnosis.

Blood supply to the head and neck

The blood vessels involved tend to run alongside the nerves of the area, as *neurovascular bundles*. This arrangement tends to occur throughout the body and, conveniently for the medical professions, ensures that the vessels can be more easily located than if they all ran along their own courses. Similarly, they may also enter and leave the bony cavities of the skull through the same foramina and fissures as do the nerves.

The names of the various blood vessels of the oral cavity are not required knowledge for dental nurses, but they tend to follow the nerve nomenclature covered previously by being named after their area of supply, as a general rule. So the artery supplying the maxillary portion of the face is, unsurprisingly, the maxillary artery, while the vein associated with the same area is the maxillary vein, and so on.

The major arteries carrying oxygenated blood to the head and neck region are the *common carotid arteries*, which are direct branches from the arch of the aorta as it leaves the left ventricle. These travel up the left and right sides of the neck and are palpable against either side of the larynx as the carotid pulse, often taken by professional resuscitation personnel during medical emergencies. Around this position of palpation, the common carotids divide into the following major arteries.

- **External carotid artery** – supplying all the head outside the cranium, including the face and the oral cavity.
- **Internal carotid artery** – supplying all the inner cranial structures, including the brain, and the eyes.

Once the usual gaseous exchange has occurred in the capillary beds of the head and neck region, deoxygenated blood tends to flow from small venules into gradually widening veins, until they reach the main venous vessels of the area.

- **External jugular vein** – draining a small area of extracranial tissues only.
- **Internal jugular vein** – draining the brain and the majority of the head and neck tissues.

These veins run on and eventually join the superior vena cava and enter the right side of the heart, where the deoxygenated blood that they carry is pumped to the lungs for reoxygenation.

The flow of deoxygenated blood from the head and neck region is not always in one direction, as occurs in other areas of the body. This is because the veins of this area usually do not contain the one-way valve system present in the majority of these vessels, so blood can flow forwards and backwards depending on changes affecting the local pressure.

Generally, then, it is easier for localised infections to spread in the head and neck regions than elsewhere in the body. The seriousness of this statement is compounded further by the fact that the blood travels through the most important organ of the body, the brain, and that pathogens may enter the area in a variety of ways.

- Inhaled through the nose or mouth.
- Ingested through the oral cavity.
- Carried by the circulatory or lymph systems.
- Traumatically deposited through the soft tissues, such as during dental treatment, local anaesthetic injection or following head and neck injury.

The maintenance of high standards of infection control in the field of dentistry is therefore of paramount importance, and of great concern to the whole oral healthcare team.

 Further resources are available for this book, including interactive multiple choice questions and extended matching questions. Visit the companion website at:

www.levisonstextbookfordentalnurses.com

10

Oral Anatomy and Physiology

Key learning points

A **factual knowledge** of
- the gross anatomy of the tissues and structures of the oral cavity
- the microscopic anatomy of teeth and their supporting structures

A **working knowledge** of
- the functions of the tissues and structures of the oral cavity
- the morphology and functions of teeth
- the salivary glands

The oral cavity contains many anatomical structures besides the teeth, and to gain a full understanding of the topics of oral health and disease, the dental nurse must have knowledge of all these structures. The bones, muscles, nerves and blood supply to this region are discussed in Chapter 9; this chapter will focus on the following specific anatomical structures and their physiology.

- Oral soft tissues and soft palate.
- Tongue.
- Teeth.
- Supporting structures of the periodontium.
- Salivary glands.

Levison's Textbook for Dental Nurses, Eleventh Edition. By Carole Hollins.
© 2013 John Wiley & Sons, Ltd. Published 2013 by John Wiley & Sons, Ltd. Companion website: www.levisonstextbookfordentalnurses.com

Soft tissues of the mouth

Epithelial membrane

The whole of the mouth is lined with epithelial mucosal tissue as a type of mucous membrane, which is continuous with that lining the digestive tract. Throughout the oral cavity there are three types of this membrane, each with its own particular features.

- Lining membrane.
- Masticatory membrane.
- Specialised membrane.

Their details are shown in Table 10.1. The first row identifies the area of the oral cavity where each type of epithelial membrane is normally found, while the second row describes its appearance in each case. The final row explains the function(s) of the membrane in relation to its appearance – so the ridged nature of the masticatory membrane, for example, and its firm underlying attachment are explained by its function of providing a hard-wearing surface that can withstand the regular abrasive contact it has with food.

   Within the oral cavity, the space between the posterior teeth and the mucous membrane lining the cheeks is called the *buccal sulcus* whilst that between the anterior teeth and lips is the *labial sulcus*. The upper lip is attached to the centre of the gingiva above the central incisors by a band of fibrous tissue called a *frenum*, and when this attachment is thicker than usual, there is often a space created between the two incisor teeth, called a *median diastema*.

Table 10.1   Oral mucous membranes

Lining membrane	Masticatory membrane	Specialised membrane
Covers inner surfaces of the cheeks and lips, floor of the mouth, underside of the tongue, soft palate	Covers gingivae, topside and edges of the tongue, hard palate	Interspersed throughout the masticatory membrane covering of the topside and edges of the tongue
Appears as red, smooth and moist membrane, which can be squashed and stretched Contains minor salivary glands	Appears as red, moist membrane, often ridged or stippled, firmly attached to underlying structures – forms the **mucoperiosteum** where it lies over the alveolar processes	Appear as discrete papillary structures of the taste buds, in a visible pattern over the tongue
Provides a physical barrier between anything entering the mouth and the deep structures of the oral cavity, acts as a cushion, provides lubrication and cleansing	Provides a hard-wearing surface that prevents traumatic damage from food, chemicals, oral hygiene products, etc.	Provides taste sensation

249

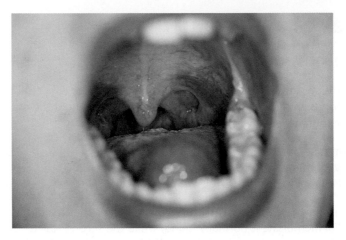

Figure 10.1   Tonsils and oropharynx.

Soft palate

The soft palate is a flap of soft tissue attached to the back of the hard palate. Its function is to seal off the oral cavity from the nasal cavity during swallowing, in order to prevent food passing up into the nose. The free edge of the soft palate has a central prolongation called the *uvula*. You can see this for yourself by looking in a mirror with your mouth wide open. To either side of this area at the back of the mouth, called the *oropharynx*, lie the tonsils which appear as small ball-like structures with a pitted surface (Figure 10.1). They are most noticeable when inflamed during a throat infection, such as *tonsillitis*.

Tongue

The floor of the mouth lies within the arch of the mandible and is occupied by the tongue, which is a muscular organ situated in the oral cavity and also the throat. The posterior one-third section, the base of the tongue, lies in the throat and attaches to the floor of the mouth. It is relatively firmly attached and is mainly concerned with swallowing movements. The correct term for swallowing is *deglutition*.

The remaining anterior two-thirds of the tongue, the body, lie within the oral cavity and this section is relatively moveable, being able to perform numerous convoluted movements, as it is composed of many bands of muscle lying in various directions. It is attached to the floor of the mouth by a thin band of fibrous tissue called the *lingual frenum*. Where excess of this fibrous tissue occurs, the tongue is held more rigidly than normal so that its movements are restricted, and the person affected is often described as 'short-tongued' or 'tongue-tied', due to the lisp created as they speak.

The body of the tongue is concerned with taste, chewing activities and speech.

All the muscles of the tongue are innervated by the hypoglossal nerve (12th cranial nerve).

The functions of the tongue are as follows.

- **Speech** – by allowing certain sounds to be created by touching the tongue to the upper anterior teeth or the palate (such as 's', 't', 'n', 'the').
- **Taste** – the tongue is covered by various different types of taste buds (including *filiform papillae*, *fungiform papillae* and *vallate papillae* – Figure 10.2) that allow recognition of the four basic tastes – sweet, sour, salt and bitter.

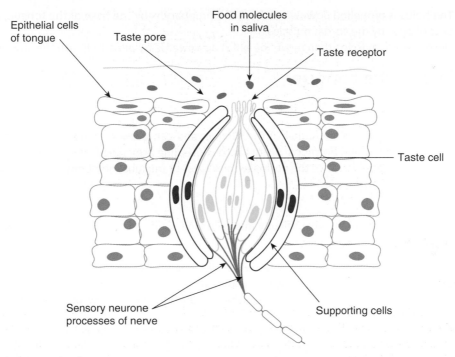

Figure 10.2   Taste bud.

- **Aids mastication** – by assisting the buccinator muscles to package ingested food into a parcel, or *bolus*, for easier chewing before swallowing.
- **Aids swallowing** – by guiding the bolus to the back of the mouth, the oropharynx.
- **Cleansing** – by moving around the oral cavity and the smooth surfaces of the teeth to dislodge food particles.

The lining epithelium of mucous membrane covering the underside of the tongue is so thin that it allows the very rapid absorption of drugs placed here into the underlying capillaries of the tongue. Patients given glyceryl trinitrate (GTN) tablets or spray for the treatment of angina pectoris use their medications in this way.

Swallowing

Swallowing is a complex muscular action which aims to direct the food bolus into the oesophagus while also preventing it from entering the nasal cavity or the larynx. The bolus is mixed with saliva to lubricate it, and then propelled by the tongue from the mouth to the oropharynx, and then into the oesophagus. The sequence of events in the swallowing process is as follows (see Figure 5.11).

- The lubricated ball of food is propelled backwards to the oropharynx by the actions of the body of the tongue.
- The soft palate rises up and seals off the nasopharynx from the oropharynx, to prevent the bolus from passing upwards into the nose.
- At the same time, the larynx lifts up and is sealed by the epiglottis to prevent the bolus passing into the trachea and being inhaled into the lungs.

- The bolus is propelled downwards from the oropharynx by the base of the tongue, and to the oesophagus by the throat muscles.
- Oesophageal muscles then move the bolus downwards by peristalsis into the stomach.

Disorders of the tongue

Glossitis

This is soreness and inflammation of the tongue, and can occur in conditions such as anaemia, vitamin B deficiency and hormonal disturbances (including pregnancy). It is associated with a thin, smooth glazed appearance of the normally thick layer of mucous membrane on its upper surface.

Dysphagia

This is the condition of having difficulty in swallowing, which occurs relatively frequently and has several causes.

- **Psychological** – an inability to swallow (usually) medication in tablet form, although food and drink can be swallowed normally by the patient.
- **Xerostomia** – dry mouth syndrome, where reduced salivary flow prevents adequate bolus lubrication.
- **Oesophagitis** – inflammation of the oesophagus, often due to acid reflux.
- Other conditions affecting pharyngeal or oesophageal function, including cancers.
- Central nervous system disorders preventing correct muscle innervation, such as stroke and multiple sclerosis.

Teeth

The teeth are the anatomical structures within the oral cavity that are of the greatest relevance to the dental team, as their development, health, disease and restoration are the fundamentals of dentistry. The teeth have the following functions.

- To cut up and masticate food into suitable sized portions before swallowing.
- To expose the food surfaces to enzymes and allow digestion to begin.
- To support the oral soft tissues of the cheeks and tongue, and therefore enable clear speech.

Humans have two sets of teeth – the primary (deciduous) teeth of childhood and the secondary (permanent) teeth of adulthood. The number and type of teeth in each set differ, although the shape of the common ones is the same.

The detailed anatomical shape of each tooth, and its function, is called *tooth morphology*.

The four types present in the secondary dentition, from the midline of the mouth posteriorly, are as follows.

- **Central and lateral incisors**
- **Canine**
- **First and second premolars**
- **First, second and third molars**

The primary dentition has just two molars and is made up of just three different types of teeth – there are no premolars present.

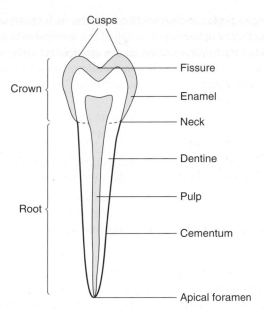

Figure 10.3 Structure of a tooth.

Each tooth of all types, and in both sets, has three sections – the crown, the neck and the root(s). The *crown* is the section of the tooth visible in the oral cavity, following its eruption from the underlying alveolar bone. The *neck* is the section where the tooth and the gingival tissues are in contact with each other at the point where the tooth emerges through the gums, and the *root* is the (usually) non-visible section that holds the tooth in its bony socket.

All teeth are composed of the same four tissues.

- **Enamel** – a highly calcified tissue covering the whole crown of the tooth.
- **Dentine** – a less calcified tissue than enamel, which forms the inner bulk of the crown and root.
- **Cementum** – a thin calcified covering of the root dentine only.
- **Pulp** – the inner neurovascular tissue of the tooth, within the central pulp chamber.

The structure of a typical tooth is shown in Figure 10.3.

Microscopic structure of the teeth

The differences in the microscopic structure of the four layers of the teeth are what determine how they function, how they develop disease, how they are treated for that disease, and how they are restored or extracted by the dental team.

Enamel

This is the highly calcified, protective outer covering of the crown and is the hardest substance in the body. Its properties and microscopic structure are as follows.

- It is made up of 96% mineral crystals (inorganic) arranged as **prisms** in an organic matrix called the **interprismatic substance**.
- The main mineral crystals are **calcium hydroxyapatite**.

- The prisms lie at right angles to the junction with the next tooth layer, the **dentine**.
- The junction between these two layers is called the **amelodentinal junction** (ADJ).
- Enamel is formed before tooth eruption by the **ameloblast cells**, which lie at the ADJ.
- It contains no nerves nor blood vessels and therefore cannot experience any sensation.
- It is a non-living tissue which cannot grow and repair itself, so progressive damage caused by injury or tooth decay is permanent.
- It can, however, remineralise its surface after an acid attack, by taking in minerals from saliva and from oral health products such as toothpaste and mouthwash.
- The crystal structure can also be altered without undergoing acid attack, by the exchange of hydroxyl ions in the hydroxyapatite with **fluoride**, to form **fluorapatite crystals** – these make the enamel surface harder and more resistant to acid attack.
- The enamel layer is thickest over the biting surface of the tooth (the occlusal surface or the incisal edge) and thinnest at the neck of the tooth (the cervical margin).
- It is translucent, so the shade of a tooth is determined by the colour of the underlying dentine.

Dentine

This tissue forms the main bulk of a tooth and occupies the interior of the crown and root. It is also mineralised, but to a lesser extent than enamel, and is covered by enamel in the crown of the tooth and by cementum in the root of the tooth. Its properties and microscopic structure are as follows.

- It consists of up to 80% inorganic tissue, mainly **calcium hydroxyapatite** crystals.
- It is composed of **hollow tubes** which originally surrounded the cells within the dentine structure as it was first being formed.
- In a fully formed tooth, these **odontoblast** cells lie along the inner edge of the pulp chamber only, but are present throughout life and can lay down more dentine as required.
- In this way, it can repair itself by laying down secondary dentine.
- This type of dentine is also formed as part of the natural ageing process, and its formation gradually narrows the pulp chamber.
- The hollow tubes contain sensory nerve endings called **fibrils**, which run from the nerve tissue within the pulp chamber.
- Dentine is therefore a living tissue and can transmit sensations of pain and thermal changes to the brain.
- Its hollow structure allows it a degree of elasticity so that it can absorb normal chewing forces without breaking.
- However, it also allows tooth decay (**caries**) to spread more rapidly through its hollow structure.
- Dentine is a yellowish colour, and gives teeth their individual shade.

Cementum

This is the calcified protective outer covering of the root and is similar in structure to bone. Cementum meets enamel at the neck of the tooth, and normally lies beneath the gingivae. Its properties and microscopic structure are as follows.

- Around 65% mineralised, with calcium hydroxyapatite crystals.
- The crystals lie within a matrix of fibrous tissue, with the ends of collagen fibres from the periodontal ligament inserted into the outer layer of the cementum.
- This allows the attachment of the root to the periodontal ligament, and therefore to the walls of the tooth socket.

- The cementum is formed by cells called **cementoblasts** and they can continue laying down more tissue layers when required.
- The thickness of cementum may vary at different parts of the root, and changes throughout life, depending on the forces exerted on individual teeth.
- The cementum contains no nerves nor blood vessels itself, so it receives nutrients from the periodontal ligament.

Pulp

Unlike enamel, dentine and cementum, the pulp contains no mineral crystals and is composed purely of soft tissue. It lies within the very centre of every tooth, from the crown as the coronal pulp and into each root as the radicular pulp. The radicular pulp is often referred to as the 'root canal' of the tooth. The properties and microscopic structure of the pulp are as follows.

- The pulp contains sensory nerves and blood vessels.
- The sensory nerves are end sections of the trigeminal nerve (fifth cranial nerve), either as the inferior dental nerve for the lower teeth or one of the superior dental nerves for the upper teeth.
- They allow the tooth to feel hot, cold, touch and pain by the stimulation of its sensory nerve endings which run as fibrils in the hollow dentine tubules.
- These pulp tissues enter the tooth through the **apical foramen**, lying at the root apex of every tooth.
- The pulp chamber itself is lined by the odontoblast cells which form dentine.
- The chamber gradually narrows with age, so that it can become completely obliterated in older patients, making endodontic treatment very difficult.
- It can also become blocked by **pulp stones** which are formed by lumps of calcium-containing crystals.
- The point where the cementum and the root dentine are in contact with each other is called the **dentinocemental junction**.
- Some teeth have additional contact between the pulp and the surrounding periodontal ligament via accessory canals, whose presence can make successful endodontic treatment of the tooth very difficult to achieve.

Tooth morphology

All people have two sets of teeth: the first or *deciduous* teeth, and the second or *permanent* teeth. All have different appearances or morphology, which depends on the set and the individual teeth themselves. Their morphology enables each tooth to be individually identified by any trained member of the dental team, this identification being based on the tooth shape and size, the number of cusps present, and the number of roots present. Curvature of the roots will also help to indicate whether a tooth is from the right or the left side of the dental arch.

Deciduous teeth

The deciduous teeth are the first set and are also known as milk, temporary or primary teeth (Figure 10.4).

- Total set of **20 teeth**, 10 in each jaw.
- They begin developing in the jaws of the early embryo, around 6 weeks after conception.
- They are referred to in dentistry by letter – **A, B, C, D** and **E** – starting from the midline of the jaw.

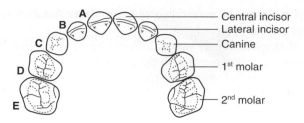

Figure 10.4   Deciduous teeth.

Table 10.2   Primary dentition: tooth and root morphology

Tooth	Letter	Number of roots	Number of cusps (where applicable)
Uppers			
Central incisor	A	One	N/A
Lateral incisor	B	One	N/A
Canine	C	One	N/A
First molar	D	Three	Four
Second molar	E	Three	Five
Lowers			
Central incisor	A	One	N/A
Lateral incisor	B	One	N/A
Canine	C	One	N/A
First molar	D	Two	Four
Second molar	E	Two	Five

- They are **smaller** than permanent teeth, and **whiter** in colour.
- Their roots are **resorbed** by the underlying permanent teeth, as the deciduous teeth gradually loosen and fall out – this is called **exfoliation**.
- The roots of the deciduous molars are splayed out to accommodate the presence of the underlying permanent premolar teeth, so the roots are described as **divergent**.
- They have a **larger pulp chamber** than the permanent teeth, with **thinner enamel**, which makes them more prone to the development of dental caries.
- They begin erupting at around 6 months of age, and are usually all present by about 29 months, although individual variation does occur.

The five deciduous teeth present in each quadrant of the oral cavity are the *central and lateral incisors*, the *canine*, and the *first and second molars*. There are no premolar teeth in the primary dentition. Their tooth and root morphology is summarised in Table 10.2.

Table 10.3   Average eruption dates of the deciduous teeth

Tooth	Letter	Uppers in months	Lowers in months
Central incisor	A	10	8
Lateral incisor	B	11	13
Canine	C	19	20
First molar	D	16	16
Second molar	E	29	27

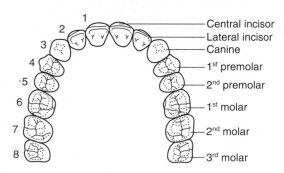

Figure 10.5   Permanent teeth.

The three roots of the upper molars are arranged as a tripod, with the developing permanent premolar teeth lying within this area, while the two roots of the lower molars lie one in front of the other in the alveolar bone of the mandible. The average eruption dates of the deciduous teeth, in months, are shown in Table 10.3.

The usual eruption pattern of the deciduous dentition is the lower central incisors first, followed by the other incisors, then the first molars followed by the canines, and finally the second molars.

The dentition begins changing again at about 6 years of age, when the permanent teeth begin to erupt by resorbing the roots of their deciduous predecessors and causing their exfoliation.

Permanent teeth

Permanent teeth are the second and final set, and are also called the adult teeth (Figure 10.5).

- Total set of **32 teeth**, 16 in each jaw.
- They begin developing in the jaws just before birth, and continue for many years afterwards.
- They are referred to in dentistry by number – **1, 2, 3, 4, 5, 6, 7** and **8** – starting from the midline of the jaw.
- They are of very similar morphology to the deciduous teeth, with eight extra teeth called **premolars** present, two in each quadrant.
- They are **larger** in size and **darker** in colour than deciduous teeth, with relatively **smaller pulp chambers**.
- The three permanent molar teeth in each quadrant develop behind the deciduous teeth, using the space created as the jaws grow during childhood and the teenage years.

Table 10.4   Permanent teeth: tooth and root morphology

Tooth	Number	Number of roots	Number of cusps (where applicable)
Uppers			
Central incisor	1	One	N/A
Lateral incisor	2	One	N/A
Canine	3	One	N/A
First premolar	4	Two	Two
Second premolar	5	One	Two
First molar	6	Three	Five
Second molar	7	Three	Four
Third molar	8	Three	Four
Lowers			
Central incisor	1	One	N/A
Lateral incisor	2	One	N/A
Canine	3	One	N/A
First premolar	4	One	Two
Second premolar	5	One	Two
First molar	6	Two	Five
Second molar	7	Two	Four
Third molar	8	Two	Four

- So the **deciduous molar teeth** are succeeded by the **permanent premolar teeth**.
- It is relatively common for some adult teeth to be **congenitally missing** from the dentition, especially the third molars.
- They begin erupting at around 6 years of age, and all except the third molars are usually present by the age of 13 years.
- The third molars may be congenitally missing, present but unerupted due to lack of jaw space, or they may erupt from the age of 18 years onwards.

The eight permanent teeth present in each quadrant of the oral cavity are the *central and lateral incisors*, the *canine*, the *first and second premolars*, and the *first, second and third molars*. Their tooth and root morphology is summarised in Table 10.4.

Again, the three roots of the upper molars are arranged as a tripod, and the two roots of the lower molars lie one in front of the other in the alveolar bone of the mandible. The two roots of

Table 10.5　Average eruption dates of the permanent teeth

Tooth	Number	Uppers in years	Lowers in years
Central incisor	1	7–8	6–7
Lateral incisor	2	8–9	7–8
Canine	3	10–12	9–10
First premolar	4	9–11	9–11
Second premolar	5	10–11	9–11
First molar	6	6–7	6–7
Second molar	7	12–13	11–12
Third molar	8	18–25	18–25

the upper first premolar teeth lie across the maxillary alveolar bone. The average eruption dates of the permanent teeth, in years, are shown in Table 10.5.

Permanent teeth erupt before their roots are fully grown. About two-thirds of their root length has formed when permanent teeth erupt and the apex is still wide open. It takes another 3 years before root growth is complete and the apex closes. The only exceptions are canines and third molars which do not erupt until root growth is complete.

Surfaces of the teeth

To enable the dental team to describe and discuss individual teeth and the treatment they may require, each surface of every tooth has its own name in relation to the midline of each jaw, and the anatomical structures that they sit against. It is this *tooth surface nomenclature* that allows the charting of every patient to be recorded accurately – a key task of the dental nurse.

Charting is discussed in detail in Chapter 12, as it forms an important part of oral health assessment techniques.

The general terminology used for describing the tooth surfaces is summarised below.

- **Labial** – surface adjacent to the lips, applies in both arches and relates to incisor and canine teeth.
- **Buccal** – surface adjacent to the buccinator muscle of the cheeks, applies in both arches and relates to premolars and molars.
- **Palatal** – surface adjacent to the palate, applies to all maxillary teeth.
- **Lingual** –surface adjacent to the tongue, applies to all mandibular teeth.
- The sharply raised points of these surfaces are called **cusps**, and the crevices between them are the **fissures**.
- **Incisal** – biting edge of anterior teeth, applies to both arches and relates to incisors (canines have a cusp rather than an edge).
- **Mesial** – interdental surface of all teeth closest to the midline of each arch, so the front interdental surface (Figure 10.6).
- **Occlusal** – biting surface of posterior teeth, applies to both arches and relates to premolars and molars (Figure 10.7).

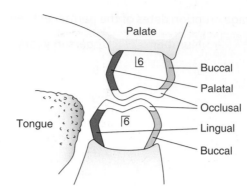

Figure 10.6 Surfaces of the teeth – mesial aspect.

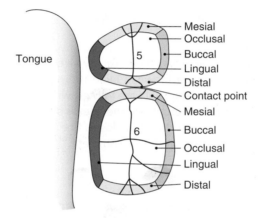

Figure 10.7 Surfaces of the teeth – occlusal aspect.

- **Distal** – interdental surface of all teeth furthest from the midline of each arch.
- **Contact point** – the point where the mesial and distal surfaces of adjacent teeth are in contact with each other.
- **Cervical** – the neck region of any tooth, on the buccal, labial, palatal or lingual surface.

Using these named surfaces, the anatomy of individual teeth can be described in detail.

Anatomy of individual teeth

A collection of extracted teeth in good condition is a great help in learning dental anatomy and tooth morphology, but they are more difficult to acquire nowadays due to infection control issues. The secondary dentition is shown diagrammatically for clarity in Figure 10.8, and various extracted teeth are shown in Figure 10.9.

In the primary dentition there are five teeth in each quadrant of the mouth: central and lateral incisors, a canine, and first and second molars.

In the secondary dentition there are eight teeth in each quadrant: central and lateral incisors, a canine, first and second premolars, first, second and third molars. The morphology and function of the similar teeth in each dentition are the same.

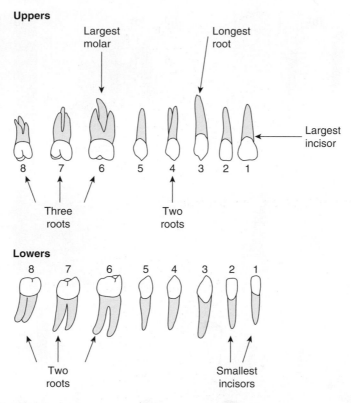

Figure 10.8   Tooth anatomy.

Central incisor

- Chisel-shaped crown with an incisal biting edge.
- Single root.
- Palatal or lingual surface has a raised area called the **cingulum**.
- Upper permanent central incisor is the **largest** of all incisors.
- Lower central incisor is the **smallest tooth**.
- Functions are to:
  - cut into food and separate bite-size chunks from the food product
  - assist tongue in making certain speech sounds ('th')
  - assist lips in making certain speech sounds ('f').

Lateral incisor

- Narrow, chisel-shaped crown with an incisal biting edge.
- Single root.
- Lower lateral incisor sometimes has a second (lingual) root canal, especially if the root has split into two.
- Palatal or lingual surface has a cingulum.
- Function is to bite in a scissor action with the upper incisors, and break off separate bite-size portions.
- Uppers can be congenitally absent or develop as abnormally small teeth – often called **peg laterals**.

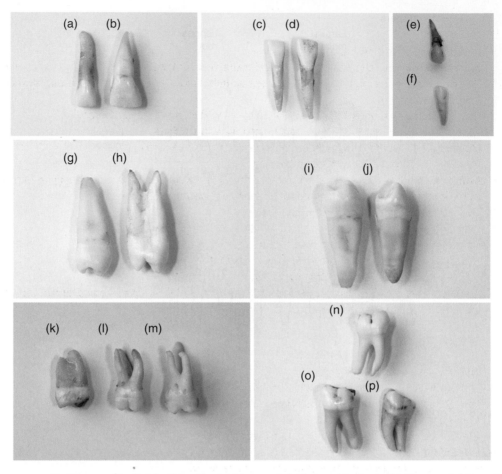

Figure 10.9 Features of individual teeth. (a) Upper right lateral incisor. (b) Upper right central incisor. (c) Lower left central incisor. (d) Lower left lateral incisor. (e) Upper right canine. (f) Lower left canine. (g) Upper right second premolar. (h) Upper right first premolar. (i) Lower left second premolar. (j) Lower left first premolar. (k) Upper right third molar. (l) Upper right second molar. (m) Upper right first molar. (n) Lower right first molar. (o) Lower left second molar. (p) Lower left third molar.

Canine

- Robust tooth forming the 'corner' of each dental quadrant.
- Incisal edge is sloped to a sharp cusp tip that lies more mesially than distally.
- Single root and the **longest** of all teeth.
- Root apex sometimes curves distally slightly.
- Upper and lower canines have a cingulum, the upper is joined to the cusp tip by a palatal ridge.
- Functions are to:
  - pierce food and tear into it
  - support the oral soft tissues at the 'corners' of the oral cavity
  - provide 'guidance' for normal occlusion, especially when the mandible is moved sideways.

First premolar

- Not present in primary dentition.
- Are the permanent successors to the deciduous first molars.
- Has occlusal surface arranged as two cusps lying bucally and palatally, or buccally and lingually (upper or lower).
- Cusps are of equal height in uppers, but lingual is always smaller in lowers.
- Mesial and distal edges of all are raised into **marginal ridges**.
- Upper has two roots lying in the same orientation as the cusps.
- Root apices sometimes curve distally.
- Concavity between the roots mesially is called the **canine fossa**, and can be a harbour for micro-organisms and calculus in patients with periodontal disease.
- Lower first premolar has one root.
- Functions are to:
    - assist canine to pierce and tear food (cusps)
    - assist molars to grind food (occlusal surface)
    - help maintain the shape of the mouth.
- Usual tooth to be extracted for orthodontic reasons, as it lies midway along the dental arch and can therefore relieve either anterior or posterior crowding.

Second premolar

- Not present in primary dentition.
- Is the permanent successor to the deciduous second molar.
- Has occlusal surface arranged as two cusps, like the first premolars.
- Cusps are of equal height in all.
- Mesial and distal edges are raised as marginal ridges.
- Upper is usually slightly smaller than the first premolar.
- Lower is usually slightly larger than the first premolar.
- Single root, apex sometimes curves distally.
- Root apex of uppers can lie very close to the floor of the maxillary antrum.
- Functions as for first premolars.
- Lowers are sometimes congenitally absent.
- Can become impacted in either arch, following the early loss of deciduous predecessor and the eruption of the permanent first molars, so that the arch space for the second premolars is lost.

First molar

- Primary first molars are succeeded by the first premolars, and are the smaller of the deciduous molars.
- Widely divergent roots present in deciduous molars, with the crown of the developing first premolar lying contained by them.
- Permanent first molars are the **largest** of all teeth.
- Upper has occlusal surface arranged as four cusps – two buccally and two palatally.
- Fifth palatal cusp of uppers may develop as the **cusp of Carabelli**.
- Lower has five cusps – three buccal and two lingual.
- Mesial and distal edges are raised as marginal ridges.
- Uppers have three roots arranged as a tripod – large palatal, shorter mesiobuccal and distobuccal – apices of latter two are sometimes curved distally.

- Lowers have two roots arranged as mesial and distal, apices are sometimes curved distally.
- Junction of the roots beneath the crown is called the **furcation area** and can be a harbour for micro-organisms when periodontal disease is present.
- Function is to grind and masticate food chunks so that they can be swallowed.
- Root apices of uppers can lie close to, or even penetrate, the floor of the maxillary antrum.

Second molar

- Primary second molars are succeeded by the second premolars, and are the larger of the deciduous molars.
- Widely divergent roots present in deciduous molars, with the crown of the developing second premolar lying contained by them.
- Crown of both upper and lower is smaller than that of the first molar.
- Has occlusal surface arranged as four cusps.
- Mesial and distal edges are raised as marginal ridges.
- Uppers have three roots, arranged as for the first molar and sometimes curved distally.
- Lower has two roots, arranged as for the first molar and sometimes curved distally.
- Furcation area present in both.
- Function as for the first molar.
- Root apices of the upper can also lie in close proximity to the floor of the maxillary antrum.

Third molar

- Not present in the primary dentition.
- Not always present in the secondary dentition.
- Referred to as **wisdom teeth**.
- Morphology varies widely.
- Smaller crown size than the second molar usually.
- Has occlusal surface arranged as three or four cusps, with marginal ridges present.
- Uppers usually have three roots, but not always.
- Lowers usually have two roots, but not always.
- Furcation area present unless the roots are fused together.
- Function as for the first and second molars.
- Often extracted if involved with recurrent bouts of disease, or if impacted and associated with pericoronitis.

Occlusion of the teeth

When the upper and lower teeth are closed together, they are said to be in *occlusion*. The arch of the upper teeth is larger than the lower so upper teeth overlap the lower on the buccal side. Lower buccal cusps accordingly bite into the fissure between upper buccal and palatal cusps (Figure 10.10).

The mesial edges of upper and lower central incisors form one straight vertical line. This is called the midline. As lower central incisors are much narrower than uppers, all the remaining lower teeth occlude with two upper teeth – their corresponding upper tooth and the one in front.

From this explanation of *normal occlusion* it is clear that:

- the mesial cusp of the upper first molar bites into the fissure between the mesial and distal cusps of the lower first molar
- the lower canine bites in front of the upper canine
- the mesial edges of the upper and lower central incisors form one straight vertical midline.

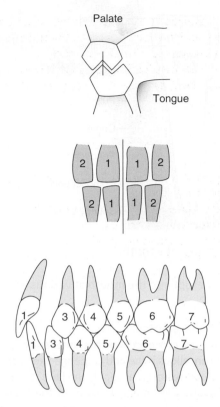

Figure 10.10   Normal occlusion.

Supporting structures of the periodontium

The supporting structures are collectively referred to as the periodontium, and are those lying around the roots of the teeth which hold them in their sockets (Figure 10.11). Their hold on the teeth is not a rigid one; rather, it allows the teeth to 'bounce' in their sockets so that there is some shock absorption effect when the teeth are used for chewing. This prevents fracture of the tooth under normal occlusal forces.

The four supporting structures are as follows.

- **Alveolar bone**– specialised ridge of bone over the bony arch of each jaw, where the teeth sit in their sockets.
- **Gingiva** – specialised soft tissue covering of the alveolar processes, that are also in attachment with the teeth at their necks.
- **Periodontal ligament** – connective tissue attachment between the tooth and the alveolar bone.
- **Cementum** – hard tissue covering of the root that anchors the periodontal ligament to the tooth (discussed previously).

Alveolar bone

The maxilla and the mandible both contain a horseshoe-shaped ridge of bone called the alveolar process. It is here that the teeth form during the growth of the fetus and then the

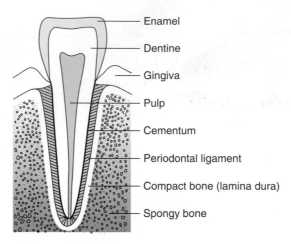

Figure 10.11   Supporting structures of a tooth.

child, and from where they erupt into the mouth at various ages. The properties of the alveolar bone are as follows.

- It is a specialised bone found only in the jaws.
- Its outer layer is made of hard, **compact bone** the outer surface of which is called the **lamina dura**.
- The inner layer is called **cancellous bone** and is sponge-like in appearance, to allow the passage of the various nerves and blood vessels that supply the jaws, teeth and surrounding oral soft tissues.
- The sole purpose of the alveolar bone is to support the teeth, and it is gradually lost when a tooth is extracted as the bone slowly resorbs away.
- The teeth lie within individual **sockets** in the alveolar bone, each one being lined by lamina dura which shows on dental radiographs as a continuous white line – its absence indicates the presence of dental disease.
- The outer surface of the alveolar bone is covered in specialised **alveolar mucosa**, which forms the **gingivae** (gums) around the necks of the teeth.
- Destruction of the alveolar bone occurs in **periodontal disease**.

Gingiva

This is the correct anatomical term for the gums (plural – gingivae). It is a continuous layer of specialised epithelium found only in the oral cavity, which is firmly attached to the underlying alveolar bone as a **mucoperiosteal layer** of tissue. This layer is raised as a flap during oral surgical procedures, to expose the bone below.

There are three distinct areas of gingival coverage (Figure 10.12).

- **Attached gingiva** – that covering the majority of the alveolar process, which is firmly attached to the underlying bone as the **mucoperiosteum**.
- **Marginal gingiva** – that forming the gingival margin of the teeth, which is free from the underlying bone and follows the shape of each tooth in the arch, as well as extending between the teeth in the contact areas. The level at which these two areas meet is called the **free gingival groove**.
- **Junctional tissues** – the specialised gingival tissue lying within the gingival crevice and forming the anatomical junction between the teeth and the oral epithelium – this point is called the **junctional attachment**, and the tissues are called the junctional epithelium.

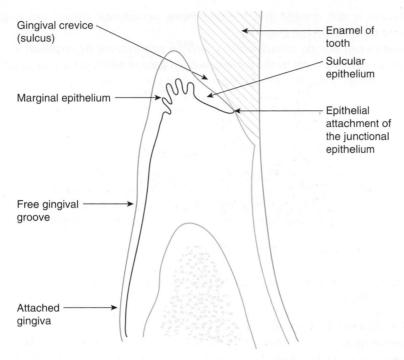

Gingival crevice
(sulcus)

Enamel of
tooth

Sulcular
epithelium

Marginal epithelium

Epithelial
attachment of
the junctional
epithelium

Free gingival
groove

Attached
gingiva

Figure 10.12   The three gingival areas.

The junctional attachment is the point where the integrity of the periodontium has to be main-tained in order to avoid the devastation of periodontal disease, and the resultant tooth loss that can occur. It provides a mechanical barrier between the oral cavity and the deeper periodontal tissues, preventing micro-organisms from gaining entry and causing disease. The main method of maintaining the health and functionality of the whole gingival area is to carry out good levels of oral hygiene on a daily basis.

During a periodontal examination, the gingival crevice should be less than 3 mm deep when probed, with the periodontal probe contacting the junctional attachment at its deepest point.

The properties of the gingiva are as follows.

- The gingivae fit around the neck of every tooth like a tight cuff, when healthy.
- The **gingival crevice** exists as a shallow space of less than 3 mm between the tooth surface and the gingival margin, and contains the junctional epithelium.
- A natural mound of gingival tissue occurs between each tooth and is called the **interdental papilla**.
- In health, the gingivae are pink in colour with a stippled surface, like orange peel.
- Inflammation of the gingivae is called **gingivitis**; it affects the marginal gingivae and occurs in the presence of **dental plaque** due to poor oral hygiene control.
- Gingivitis appears as red and shiny gingivae that are swollen due to their inflammation, and they bleed easily on touching – either during tooth brushing or during dental examination.
- The swollen appearance of the inflamed gingivae presents as '**false pockets**' when probed, giving the impression that the gingival crevice is deeper than 3 mm – in fact, the junctional

attachment is still present and the underlying periodontal tissues are unaffected by the inflamed condition of the gingivae.

- The gingiva can also be stimulated to overgrow and become **hyperplastic** as a side-effect of various drugs being taken by the patient, including some antihypertensives (such as nifedipine) and some drugs used to control epilepsy (such as phenytoin).

Oral diseases, including gingivitis and periodontitis, are discussed in detail in Chapter 11.

Periodontal ligament

The periodontal ligament is a specialised fibrous tissue which attaches the teeth to the alveolar bone and the surrounding gingivae. It acts as a shock absorber to the teeth during chewing, and its main fibres run between the alveolar bone and the cementum covering the root of the tooth. Other fibres run between the necks of the teeth, and from the cementum into the surrounding gingivae.

The various periodontal ligament fibre groups and their functions are summarised below, and illustrated in Figure 10.13.

- **Alveolar crest fibres** – run from the alveolar bone crest to the cementum at the neck of the tooth; prevent tooth movements in (intrusion) and out (extrusion) of the socket, as well as resisting tilting and rotation.
- **Horizontal fibres** – run horizontally from the alveolar bone to the cementum, just below the crest fibres; resist tilting and rotation of the tooth.
- **Oblique fibres** – run at an angle from the alveolar bone down to the cementum; prevent intrusion and rotation of the tooth.
- **Apical fibres** – occur at the root apex and run between the bone and cementum; prevent extrusion and rotation of the tooth.

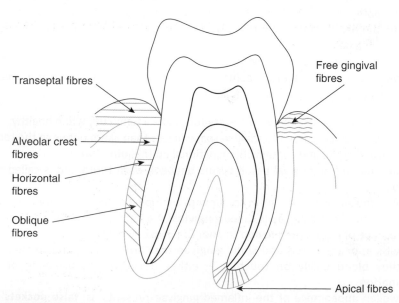

Figure 10.13   Fibre groups of the periodontal ligament.

- **Transeptal fibres** – run between the cementum of adjacent teeth through the interdental region; maintain the gingival attachments between the teeth and therefore their positions in the dental arch.
- **Free gingival fibres** – run from the cervical cementum into the gingival papillae; maintain the gingival cuff around each tooth.

The properties of the periodontal ligament are as follows.

- Its fibres are made up of a protein called **collagen**.
- They run in various directions, the end result being that the teeth are held in their sockets but can 'bounce' under normal chewing forces.
- This prevents tooth fracture and pain during normal occlusal loading and chewing actions.
- When excessive occlusal forces are applied, the resultant pain experienced by the patient tends to stop further overuse from occurring.
- The ligament has a sensory nerve supply which transmits pressure, pain, touch and temperature changes; the ability of the tooth to detect and transmit these sensations is called **proprioception**.
- Inflammation of the ligament is called **periodontitis** and occurs during periodontal disease.

Salivary glands

The salivary glands are present in the oral cavity as either numerous minor glands dotted throughout the lining membrane of the oral mucosa, or as one of the three pairs of major salivary glands (Figure 10.14).

- **Parotid salivary glands** – located between the ramus of the mandible and the ear, and deep to the muscles in that area.
- **Submandibular salivary glands** – located in the posterior area of the floor of the mouth, beneath the mylohyoid muscle.
- **Sublingual salivary glands** – located in the anterior area of the floor of the mouth, above the mylohyoid muscle.

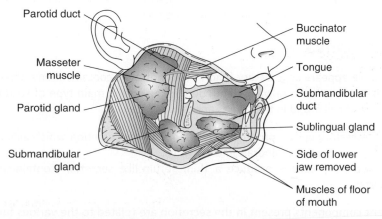

Figure 10.14   Floor of the mouth (cross-section).

The function of all the salivary glands is to produce the secretion *saliva*, which is deposited from the glands into the oral cavity only – it occurs nowhere else in the body. The saliva is transported to the oral cavity through tube-like structures called ducts, so the salivary glands are classed as *exocrine glands*. Other structures elsewhere in the body are classed as *endocrine glands* – their secretions pass directly into the adjacent blood vessels (without travelling through ducts) and are transported by the circulatory system to their area of action. Examples are certain glands within the pancreas, the stomach, the liver and the adrenal glands that lie over the kidneys.

Both types of glands have their secretions controlled by the effects of motor nerve transmission, via the autonomic nervous system.

Parotid gland

The parotid gland lies partly over the outside and partly behind the ramus of the mandible, in front of the ear. It is the largest of the three major salivary glands, and the only one to be affected by the viral infection *mumps*, which is caused by a paramyxovirus.

The tube connecting the gland to the oral cavity, the *Stenson duct*, passes forwards across the surface of the masseter muscle and then inwards through the cheek to open into the buccal sulcus opposite the upper second molar. The parotid gland is innervated by the glossopharyngeal nerve (ninth cranial nerve) and is the salivary gland most commonly associated with both benign and malignant tumours.

Submandibular gland

The submandibular gland lies in the posterior region of the floor of the mouth below the mylohyoid line, against the inner and lower surface of the body of the mandible and near the angle. The submandibular duct (*Wharton duct*) passes forward in the floor of the mouth to open at the midline, beside the lingual frenum. It is the longest of the salivary ducts, and the most likely to become blocked by salivary stones (calculi). The submandibular gland is innervated by the facial nerve (seventh cranial nerve).

Sublingual gland

The sublingual gland also lies in the floor of the mouth, but above the mylohyoid line and much further forward than the submandibular gland. There are several sublingual ducts, and these open into the floor of the mouth just behind the orifice of the submandibular duct (Figure 10.15). The sublingual gland is also innervated by the facial nerve.

Functions of saliva

Although saliva appears as a watery fluid in the mouth, it contains many different components which differ between each salivary gland, depending on the main type of secretory cell present. The two types of cell found in the glands are as follows.

- **Mucous secretory cells** – produce a thick, mucus-like secretion which aids lubrication in the oral cavity, and contains minerals and enzymes.
- **Serous secretory cells** – produce a thin, serum-like secretion containing antibodies and electrolytes.

The different components present in the secretion are related to the various functions and roles of saliva, as shown in Table 10.6. The seven components of saliva are individually identified in the

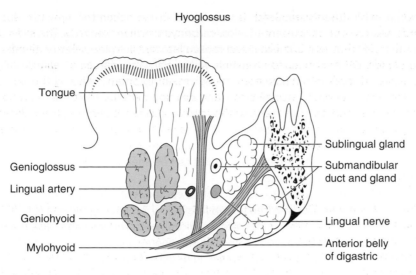

Figure 10.15   Salivary glands.

Table 10.6   Components of saliva and their functions

Component	Function or role
Minerals – sodium, calcium, potassium, and their electrolytes – such as phosphates	Neutralise dietary acids Buffering to maintain stable pH in the oral cavity Also allow mineralisation of plaque to form supragingival calculus
Salivary amylase	Digestive enzyme that begins starch digestion, before food is swallowed. Also called ptyalin
Antibodies	Immunoglobulins (especially IgA) present to fight infections, such as periodontal disease Promote wound healing IgA is the most common antibody of the immune system
Leucocytes	White blood cells, as a defence mechanism against oral infection and disease
Mucus	From the mucous secretory cells, to aid lubrication and allow speech and swallowing to occur
Other enzymes	Antibacterial enzymes, to aid in the defence of the oral cavity against disease Promote wound healing
Water	Carrying agent for other components Aids with lubrication for speech and swallowing Dissolves food particles to allow taste sensation Cleansing action by dislodging food particles from around the teeth

first column, while their function(s) are explained in the second column. So, for example, the enzyme salivary amylase is present to allow carbohydrate digestion to begin in the oral cavity, and acts on the food bolus as it is chewed and broken into smaller pieces before being swallowed.

Patients with low mineral content, mainly watery saliva tend to develop little calculus but have a higher caries incidence than patients with high mineral content saliva. Those with a high mineral content tend to have thick, stringy saliva and develop calculus more readily, in the absence of adequate oral hygiene. They also tend to have a lower incidence of caries, often despite inadequate dietary sugar control.

The position of the salivary ducts against the upper molars and the lower incisors allows dental calculus to build up easily in these areas, and it can be seen as particularly heavy deposits when patients attend for scaling treatment.

Saliva is slightly alkaline, due to its electrolyte components, but maintains the oral cavity at a neutral pH of 7 between meals. When the pH falls below 7 following the intake of food, the mineral content of saliva acts to neutralise the acidic environment produced and raise the pH again. If the pH of the oral cavity falls to the critical level of 5.5, enamel demineralisation will occur.

The role of saliva in oral health is discussed in detail in Chapter 11.

Disorders of the salivary glands

Xerostomia

This is the uncomfortable condition of having a constantly dry mouth due to the decreased production of saliva. It is relatively common, and has several causes.

- **Irradiation** – of the head and neck area, usually as radiotherapy treatment for cancer in this area.
- **Medications** – any that affect the nerve supply to the salivary glands to reduce their salivary flow, or that act as a diuretic and stimulate fluid loss, as well as certain drugs such as tricyclic antidepressants which cause dry mouth as a side-effect.
- **Sjögren's syndrome** – a syndrome that occurs in conjunction with an autoimmune disorder, such as rheumatoid arthritis, where the body's defence system attacks itself and destroys its own glandular tissues, including the salivary glands and the lacrimal glands in the eye.

As all dental professionals know, saliva has many functions in the oral cavity and any reduction in its production will have serious oral consequences.

- Increased incidence of **dental caries**, as the self-cleansing ability is lost.
- Increased risk of **oral infections**, as the defence capability is reduced.
- Increased risk of **oral soft tissue trauma**, as the protective mechanism is reduced.
- **Problems with speech, swallowing and chewing**, as the lubrication effect is reduced.
- **Poor taste sensation** and lack of food enjoyment, as the taste buds cannot function correctly in a dry field.

Other than to change the patient's drug regime where possible, there is little else that can be done to ease this condition. The use of salivary stimulants and artificial saliva sprays may help in some cases, and research is currently ongoing into salivary gland tissue transplant.

Dental patients suffering from xerostomia should be advised by the dental team as follows.

- Frequent recall attendance to monitor for the onset of caries and other oral problems.
- Use of artificial saliva sprays or constant sipping of plain water.

- High standard of oral hygiene, and especially the use of topical fluoride products to strengthen teeth against caries.
- Dietary advice to avoid cariogenic products.
- Avoidance of oral health products containing alcohol, as these tend to worsen the drying effect.

Ptyalism

Excessive salivation, or ptyalism, is a symptom associated with an underlying disease rather than a disorder in its own right. It can occur due to any of the following disorders.

- Periodontal disease.
- Oral soft tissue injury or trauma, including that caused by sharp-edged dental appliances.
- Oesophagitis and other conditions causing acid reflux.
- Disorders affecting the nervous system, including Parkinson's disease and mercury poisoning.

Treatment is focused on the causative disease and the relief of its symptoms, although some drugs may be used to directly reduce the salivary gland secretions. In particular, the drug *atropine* may be used during oral and maxillofacial surgery to significantly reduce saliva flow and provide a clear, dry operating field for the surgeons.

273

 Further resources are available for this book, including interactive multiple choice questions and extended matching questions. Visit the companion website at:

www.levisonstextbookfordentalnurses.com

11

Oral Disease

Key learning points

A **working knowledge** of
- the causes and risk factors involved in dental caries
- the process of cavity formation, and its progress ultimately to an alveolar abscess
- non-carious tooth surface loss
- the causes and risk factors involved in periodontal disease
- the onset of gingivitis and its progress to periodontitis
- the non-surgical treatment of periodontal disease

A **factual awareness** of
- other periodontal conditions
- the risk factors associated with oral cancer

The two main oral diseases of concern to the dental team are dental caries and chronic periodontal disease, and the prevalence of both throughout the human race provides the vast majority of the day-to-day work of dental team members. Other periodontal conditions that may be seen from time to time are also mentioned.

Dental caries and chronic periodontal disease are discussed in detail within this chapter, while full details of oral health assessment and diagnosis techniques, and oral disease prevention are covered elsewhere.

Although oral cancer was discussed in Chapter 7, it is included again here as a worryingly increasing disease condition that may be seen from time to time in the dental workplace, and the importance of the dental team in its early diagnosis and prevention cannot be overestimated.

Levison's Textbook for Dental Nurses, Eleventh Edition. By Carole Hollins.
© 2013 John Wiley & Sons, Ltd. Published 2013 by John Wiley & Sons, Ltd. Companion website: www.levisonstextbookfordentalnurses.com

Dental caries

Dental caries (tooth decay) is a bacterial disease of the mineralised tissues of the tooth, where the strong crystal structure found in both enamel and dentine is *demineralised* (dissolved) by the action of acids. This allows the softer organic component of the tooth structure to be broken down to form cavities.

The acids involved are created as a waste product by oral bacteria, as they digest the foods we eat for their own nutrition. Although the acids are relatively weak organic ones, such as *lactic acid* or *citric acid*, they are strong enough to attack enamel and dentine. Not all the bacteria found in the oral cavity are associated with the production of these acids – the usual ones are:

- *Streptococcus mutans* (initial stages of cavity formation)
- *Streptococcus sanguis*
- Some lactobacilli (later stages of cavity formation).

Not all the foods that we eat can be broken down into acids either, but those foods that can easily be formed into these damaging organic acids contain carbohydrates. Foods that consist of protein or fats are not relevant to the onset of dental caries. So in summary, the relevant factors in the development of dental caries are:

- the presence of certain types of **bacteria**
- **carbohydrate foods**
- the production of **weak organic acids** by these bacteria
- adequate **time or frequency** for the acids to attack the tooth.

The bacteria need to become attached to the tooth surface to be able to digest food debris and initiate dental caries, and they do this by forming themselves into a sticky layer called *bacterial plaque*.

Bacterial plaque

Millions of bacteria live in our mouths, flourishing on the food that we eat. Some of this food sticks to our teeth and attracts colonies of bacteria to the tooth surfaces. This combination of bacteria and food debris on a tooth surface forms a thin, transparent, protein-containing, soft and sticky film called *plaque*. It tends to form and stick most readily in areas where it cannot be easily dislodged, such as at the *gingival margins* of the teeth, in the *fissures* of teeth, and around the edges of *dental restorations*. These are called *stagnation areas*.

The build-up of plaque at the gingival margins of the teeth is directly associated with the onset of *gingivitis* and *periodontal disease*.

The plaque that sticks to the tooth surfaces allows the bacteria living within it to turn sugar into weak acids, which in turn dissolve enamel to produce *dental caries*.

The main micro-organism which initiates the process of caries is *Streptococcus mutans*. Large numbers of *lactobacilli* are then able to thrive in the acid environment, and the presence of these two micro-organisms is put to practical use as a test for caries activity. By periodically counting the number of streptococci or lactobacilli in a patient's saliva, the level of caries activity and the effect of preventive measures can be monitored.

Sugars

As referred to in Chapter 5, all types of food are classified into three distinct groups.

- **Protein** – such as meats, fish and various dairy products and pulses.
- **Fat** – such as animal fats and vegetable oils.
- **Carbohydrate** – natural sugars and starches from fruit and vegetables, and artificial sugars from processed foods.

Of these, only carbohydrates can be turned into acid by bacteria and thereby cause caries – so they are described as *cariogenic foods* because they are capable of causing caries. The most acid-producing carbohydrates are those which are artificially added during food preparation, and which therefore tend to be based on *non-milk extrinsic sugars* (NMEs).

As their name suggests, these types of sugar are not derived from milk and have been added artificially during the manufacturing process, rather than being found naturally in the food product itself. The most damaging ones of all are the refined sugars *sucrose* and *glucose* (also called dextrose).

Naturally occurring sugars that produce so little organic acid that they are considered harmless to teeth include the following.

- **Intrinsic sugars** – found naturally in foods, such as **fructose** in fruits.
- **Milk extrinsic sugars** – especially lactose.

Refined sugars can be instantaneously turned into acid by the bacteria concerned and available types include table sugar, sugar used in cooking, and sugar added to anything else taken by mouth, whether liquid or solid. Any food containing added sugar can cause caries and some obvious ones are:

- cake, biscuits, jam and sweets
- breakfast cereals
- pastry, desserts, canned fruit, syrups and ice cream
- soft drinks
- hot beverages sweetened with sugar.

Sugar is widely added to many savoury foods too, in order to flavour or preserve them but without making its taste apparent. Such foods can include soups, sauces, canned vegetables and breakfast cereals which are accordingly sources of *hidden sugar*. Medicines may also contain hidden sugar and can be a significant cause of caries in chronically sick children.

Sugar occurring naturally in milk, fruit and vegetables is *not* a significant cause of caries. Naturally starchy and fibrous vegetables such as potatoes, carrots, peas and beans are rich in carbohydrate but may be regarded as insignificant causes of caries as long as no sugar is added by producers or during cooking. The prime cause of dental caries is refined sugar (sucrose), processed from sugar beet and sugar cane, and commercial glucose, which together constitute such a large proportion of the manufactured and sweetened food in our diet. Unfortunately, foods containing these NMEs tend to be cheap and readily available in most First World countries, along with acidic drinks such as carbonated fizzy 'pops'.

Acid formation

As soon as the carbohydrate source is eaten, the oral bacteria take the sugar component into the plaque structure and begin to digest it themselves. Within just a minute or two, it is turned into acid by the plaque bacteria and then attacks the enamel surface beneath the plaque. Enough acid is produced to last for about 20 min and in this initial acid attack, a microscopic layer of enamel is dissolved away. This phase is called *demineralisation*.

At the end of the meal or snack, when the intake of sugar is over, the acid persists for a period of time ranging from 20 min to 2 h before it is neutralised by the buffering action of saliva.

Saliva is the fluid bathing the oral cavity that is secreted from the salivary glands (see Chapter 10). Amongst its many roles, it maintains the mouth at a *neutral level*, being neither acidic nor alkaline. The measure of acidity/alkalinity of a solution is called its *pH level* and the neutral level maintained by saliva is *pH 7*. When the weak organic acids are produced by the oral bacteria, the pH level starts to fall and once it passes the critical pH 5.5, the environment is acidic enough to attack the enamel and dentine of teeth, and produce cavities.

Once neutralisation has occurred, no further demineralisation can take place until such time as more sugar is consumed. In this phase where no more sugar is present in the plaque, some natural healing takes place; mineral constituents naturally present in saliva enter demineralised enamel and restore the part lost by the initial acid attack. This healing phase is called *remineralisation*.

What happens next is entirely dependent on the frequency of sugar intake. If it is confined to mealtimes only, for example, at breakfast, midday and early evening, there can only be three acid attacks a day on the teeth. The amount of time available for remineralisation will greatly exceed that of demineralisation and the initial phase of caries will be arrested. But if a series of snacks is eaten between meals throughout the day, the reverse will occur. Most processed snacks contain some added sugar and the result is a rapid succession of acid attacks, with insufficient respite between them for saliva to neutralise the acid and allow the healing process of remineralisation to become dominant. Caries can then spread rapidly through affected teeth, as described later.

The longer the sugar stays on the teeth, the longer the duration of acid production. Thus sweet fluids, such as tea or coffee with sugar, which are rapidly washed off the teeth by saliva, are not normally a major cause of caries unless many drinks are taken throughout the day, whereas the much more frequent consumption of very sweet soft drinks by children is far more serious. But, overall, the most dangerous sources of sugar are those which have a sticky consistency when chewed, as it is far more difficult for the natural saliva flow to wash them away. The adherent nature of such foods allows them to cling to the teeth for a very long time, throughout which they are supplying plaque bacteria with the raw materials for prolonged acid formation and demineralisation.

Foremost among these sticky forms of sugar which cause caries are:

- toffee and other sweets
- cakes, biscuits, white bread and jam
- puddings with syrup or treacle.

With our modern diet, added sugar is consumed nearly every time something is eaten, and the teeth are attacked by acid on each of these occasions. If snacks containing such sugar are frequently taken between meals, there will be a corresponding increase in the number of acid attacks on the teeth. The delicate balance between the forces of destruction (demineralisation) and those of repair (remineralisation) will then be completely upset in favour of tooth destruction and *irreversible* damage will occur.

Thus it is evident that the prime cause of caries is the frequent and unrestricted consumption of sweet snacks *between* meals. It is not the amount of sugar eaten but the *frequency* with which it is eaten that is all-important. This fundamental fact forms the basis of personal caries prevention and good dental health education.

Sites of caries

The parts of a tooth most prone to caries are those where food tends to collect and plaque bacteria can flourish. Such sites are known as *stagnation areas*. Occlusal fissures and the spaces between the mesial and distal surfaces of adjoining teeth (the interproximal areas, or contact points) are the most common stagnation areas. That is why caries occurs most often on occlusal and proximal surfaces. However, anywhere food debris can accumulate is a stagnation area where plaque will proliferate and caries is likely to occur. Such food traps are the necks of teeth covered by ill-fitting partial dentures, irregular teeth and unopposed teeth.

Minimal harm is caused by partial dentures which fit perfectly, but those which do not are a menace to dental health. They leave spaces between the necks of the teeth and the acrylic plate, or between any metal clasps and the teeth, which are dangerous stagnation areas.

During mastication, the movement of saliva and the food bolus over the tooth surfaces as it is chewed actually helps to clean teeth which are in good occlusion. This does not prevent plaque formation, but does reduce the amount of retained food debris which is responsible for the harmful effects of plaque. Teeth which are not in good occlusion, such as irregularly positioned and unopposed teeth, are not so exposed to this beneficial cleansing effect. Consequently food collects around these instanding or outstanding irregular teeth. It also covers the crown of any tooth which has lost its opposite number, and remains unopposed because the space has not been replaced artificially. To make the situation even worse, the sticky sweet food most likely to produce caries needs the minimum amount of mastication anyway, and therefore has a negligible cleansing effect – even on teeth in good occlusion.

Caries and cavity formation

Unrestricted consumption of carbohydrates and their sugar content produces an abundance of acid-forming bacteria in the plaque which collects in stagnation areas. The resultant series of continual acid attacks prevents remineralisation and allows acid to eat through the enamel until it reaches dentine, whereupon the caries spreads more rapidly through the more open structure of this inner tooth layer (Figure 11.1).

Microscopically, the process of cavity formation is as follows.

- Very early acid attacks will show as 'white spot lesions' on the enamel surface.
- Continued and frequent acid attacks will follow the prism structure of the enamel, and eat into any exposed cementum on the tooth root.
- **Demineralisation** occurs, followed by episodes of **remineralisation** if the acid attacks are not too frequent – these areas of repair often appear as brown lesions on the teeth, especially at contact points (Figure 11.2).
- With frequent or prolonged acid attacks, the mineral structure of the enamel is eventually destroyed and caries enters the tooth.
- Caries extends deep into the enamel and eventually reaches the **amelodentinal junction (ADJ)**.
- Up to this point, the patient will feel no pain as enamel contains no nerve tissue.
- Once past the ADJ, the caries enters dentine and can spread more rapidly because of the hollow structure of this tooth layer and its lower mineral content compared to enamel.
- This undermines the overlying enamel, and normal occlusal forces are able to fracture off pieces of the tooth surface, leaving a hole in the tooth structure – this is called a **cavity** (Figure 11.3).
- Odontoblast cells at the ADJ react to the bacterial attack by laying down **secondary dentine** in an attempt to protect the underlying pulp tissue.

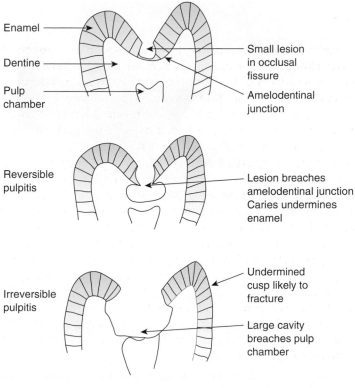

Enamel

Dentine

Pulp
chamber

Small lesion
in occlusal
fissure

Amelodentinal
junction

Reversible
pulpitis

Lesion breaches
amelodentinal junction
Caries undermines
enamel

Irreversible
pulpitis

Undermined
cusp likely to
fracture

Large cavity
breaches pulp
chamber

Figure 11.1   Cavity formation.

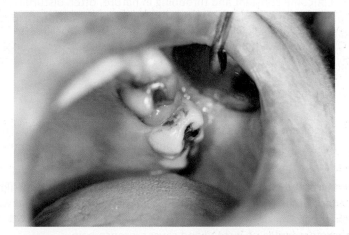

Figure 11.2   Brown spot lesion.

- The nerve fibrils lying within the dentine tubules will be stimulated as the caries progresses, and the patient will begin to feel sensitivity to temperature changes and to sweet foods.
- The pulp tissue will also become irritated and inflamed – this is called **pulpitis**.
- At this point, the caries can be removed by the dentist and the cavity restored with a **filling** (see Chapter 15), the inflamed pulp will settle and the tooth will be restored to its normal function – the inflammation is better described then as **reversible pulpitis**.

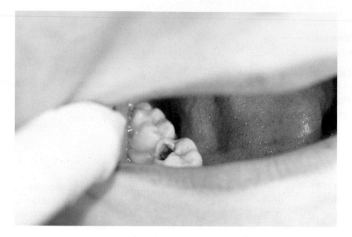

280

Figure 11.3   Cavity.

- Otherwise, the cavity will continue to enlarge and the caries will progress towards the pulp chamber, as the production of secondary dentine is overrun by the speed of the bacterial attack.
- The patient will be experiencing more severe pain of longer duration, and will eventually be unable to bite with the affected tooth.
- When the carious attack reaches the immediate surroundings of the pulp chamber, the level of inflammation is too great to be resolved simply by removing the caries – this is called **irreversible pulpitis**.
- The pain will become constant and throbbing in nature, often disturbing the patient's sleep.
- Once the pulp chamber itself is breached by the caries, a **carious exposure** of the contents occurs and the pulp will eventually die.
- The tooth can now only be treated by undergoing an endodontic procedure (see Chapter 15) or by extraction (see Chapter 17).

Irreversible pulpitis

Pulpitis occurs when caries extends through the dentine to reach the pulp. The pulp is then said to be *cariously exposed* and the sequence of events described under inflammation (see Chapter 7) follows.

- There is an increased blood flow through the apical foramen into the pulp.
- Swelling cannot occur, however, as the pulp is confined within the rigid walls of the root canal and pulp chamber.
- Pressure therefore builds up instead and causes intense pain.
- A much more important result of this pressure, however, is the compression of blood vessels passing through the tiny apical foramen – this cuts off the blood supply and causes death of the pulp.
- When the pulp dies, its nerves die too, and the severe toothache stops abruptly.
- The respite is short, however, as pulp death leads to another very painful condition called **alveolar abscess**.

Pulpitis may be acute or chronic. It has many causes, apart from caries, but almost always ends in pulp death. Other causes of pulpitis are covered in Chapter 15.

Alveolar abscess

When pulpitis occurs, the pulp eventually dies as its blood supply is cut off by inflammatory pressure. The dead pulp decomposes and infected material passes out of the tooth through the apical foramen and into the alveolar bone at the apex of the tooth. These irritant products give rise to another inflammatory reaction in the tissues surrounding the apex. Pus formation occurs and an *acute alveolar abscess* develops.

- This is an extremely painful condition.
- The affected tooth becomes loose and very tender to the slightest pressure.
- There is a continual throbbing pain and the surrounding gum is red and swollen.
- Frequently the whole side of the face is involved in inflammatory swelling and the patient may have a raised temperature.
- Looseness is caused by swelling of the periodontal ligament.
- Pain is caused by the increased pressure of blood within the rigid confines of the periodontal ligament and alveolar bone. The tooth is so tender that it cannot be used for eating.
- Thus an acute alveolar abscess may show all the cardinal signs of acute inflammation:
  - pain
  - swelling
  - redness
  - heat
  - loss of function
  - raised body temperature.

Pulp death is sometimes followed by the development of a *chronic alveolar abscess* instead of an acute one. This usually gives rise to very little pain and most patients are quite unaware of its presence. It may often be detected by the presence of a small hole in the gum called a *sinus*, which is a track leading from the abscess cavity in the alveolar bone to the surface of the gum. Pus drains from the abscess through the sinus into the mouth. This outlet prevents a build-up of pressure inside the bone and explains the lack of pain. Patients often refer to this lesion as a 'gum boil'.

If an acute abscess is not treated, it eventually turns into a chronic abscess by the drainage of pus through a sinus (see Figure 7.3). This relieves the pain and the features of acute inflammation largely disappear. The relative freedom from pain does not last indefinitely, however, as a chronic alveolar abscess is liable to revert into an acute abscess at any time.

It should now be clear that pulpitis is followed by pulp death, and this eventually leads to an acute alveolar abscess, either directly or via a chronic abscess.

It was formerly taught that all carious dentine should be removed, but this is now considered unnecessary. Adequate preparation, filling and sealing of a cavity cuts it off from further plaque and acid formation, and allows a vital pulp to remineralise the deeper underlying dentine. Removal of carious dentine should therefore stop short of exposing the pulp when possible.

Role of saliva in oral health

The oral soft tissues in health are constantly bathed in saliva, the watery secretion from the three pairs of major salivary glands as well as from the numerous minor salivary glands present in the cheeks and lips (see Chapter 10).

Saliva contains the following components.

- **Water**, as a transport agent for all the other constituents.
- **Inorganic ions and minerals**, such as calcium ions and phosphate.

- **Ptyalin**, a digestive enzyme which acts on carbohydrates (also called **salivary amylase**).
- **Antibodies**, as part of the defensive immune system, and known as **immunoglobulins**.
- **Leucocytes** or white blood cells, also part of the body's defence system.

These constituents all have important functions in the maintenance of a healthy oral environment.

- The **inorganic ions** and **minerals** are released as required to act as **buffering agents** to help control the pH of the oral environment, by neutralising the organic acids produced by bacteria.
- A high inorganic ion/mineral content produces thick, stringy saliva which gives the teeth good protection against caries, but allows **dental calculus** (tartar) to form easily and in large amounts.
- A low inorganic ion/mineral content produces watery saliva, which offers little protection against caries to the teeth, but prevents large amounts of calculus from forming.
- Calculus formation is associated with **periodontal disease**.
- **Water** forms the carrying agent for the other salivary constituents, and allows self-cleansing of the oral environment to occur by dislodging food debris from the teeth before being swallowed.
- The water also moistens the food bolus and the soft tissues, allowing **swallowing** (deglutition) and **speech** to occur.
- It also **dissolves** food particles, so that the sensation of **taste** is produced – the taste buds on the tongue can only detect the taste of food when it is in solution.
- Both **antibodies** and **leucocytes** help to protect and defend the oral environment from infection by micro-organisms.

Reduced salivary flow

The condition of reduced salivary flow is called *xerostomia* or dry mouth. There are many reasons why a patient can suffer from this, apart from it being the result of normal age-related changes of the salivary glands themselves.

- Normal age-related changes to the salivary glands and their ability to function.
- Low fluid intake over a period of time, or even dehydration.
- Some autoimmune disorders, especially **Sjögren's syndrome** which specifically affects the salivary glands and the lacrimal glands of the eyes, which produce tears.
- Several routinely prescribed drugs, including **diuretics** (prescribed to alleviate water retention in patients with heart failure), some **antidepressants** (prescribed to alleviate anxiety), and **beta-blockers** (prescribed to slow down the heart rate, especially in angina sufferers).

Reduced salivary flow has several important consequences for the patient and for the oral health team.

- Reduced self-cleansing allows more food debris to accumulate around the teeth, increasing plaque production and the likelihood of caries and periodontal disease developing.
- It will also allow food debris to stagnate in the mouth, causing **halitosis** (bad breath).
- Reduced buffering of the oral environment allows longer and more frequent acid attacks, increasing the likelihood of caries developing.
- Poor lubrication of the oral soft tissues makes speech and swallowing more difficult.
- Reduced amounts of water in the saliva affects the sensation of taste.
- Reduced flow and amounts of saliva in the mouth will make the retention of dentures more difficult.

The opposite condition to xerostomia, that of excessive saliva production, is called *ptyalism*, which is often seen in patients with periodontal disease. It can also occur in Parkinson's disease and in pregnancy.

Diagnosis of caries

Before caries is treated, it must first be detected. Early diagnosis is very important in controlling the extent of the damage done, as well as the level of discomfort experienced by the patient. The earlier a cavity is detected, the better the chance of saving the tooth. This is why regular dental examinations are recommended, and the frequency of attendance should be determined by the caries experience of the patient – those with a high caries incidence need to be examined more frequently than others. Unfortunately, these are often the very patients who do not attend regularly for dental examination, for whatever reason.

Large cavities are obvious to the naked eye but it is easier to treat caries before cavities reach such a size. The dentist has various methods available for detecting smaller carious lesions.

- Close visible inspection under magnification (Figure 11.4), with the help of a bright examination light and a mouth mirror to reflect the light onto less visible areas.
- The use of various **blunt dental probes** to detect any stickiness in suspicious areas – particularly a **sickle probe** or **right-angle probe** for occlusal surfaces, and a special double-ended **Briault probe** for interproximal areas (Figure 11.5).
- **Transillumination** of anterior teeth, using the curing light to shine through their contact points and viewed from behind with a mouth mirror to detect any shadowing (Figure 11.6).
- **Caries dyes** wiped into prepared cavities to stain any residual bacteria and allow their removal.
- Periodical **horizontal bite-wing radiographs** (Chapter 12) to detect interproximal caries in posterior teeth.
- These can also detect **recurrent caries** beneath existing restorations, as well as early caries beneath occlusal fissures.

Although probes have traditionally been manufactured as sharp instruments, it is now realised that they may damage the enamel in the earliest stages of caries. For early detection of occlusal caries, current advice is to thoroughly clean and dry the surface, and carefully examine it with the

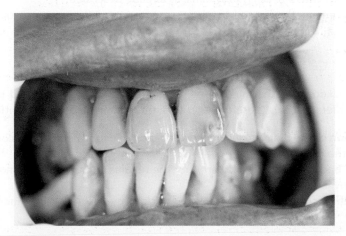

Figure 11.4   Enamel undermined by caries.

283

(a)   (b)   (c)

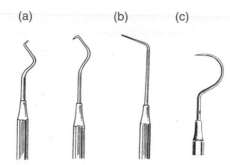

Figure 11.5   Probes. (a) The two ends of a Briault probe. (b) Right angle probe. (c) Sickle probe.

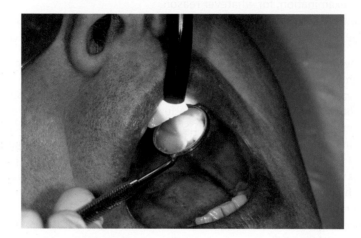

Figure 11.6   Transillumination technique.

aid of a very bright light and magnification. Early caries will then be indicated by loss of the normal shiny enamel surface, and its transition to a dull white matt appearance. Early mesial and distal caries is detected with bite-wing x-ray films, as already described.

The assessment methods used to diagnose and record the presence of carious lesions are discussed in detail in Chapter 12.

Prevention of caries

Caries is a breakdown of the mineralised tooth structure, caused by acid produced by plaque bacteria from dietary sugar. Therefore, there are three main areas of prevention available.

- **Modification of the diet** – to include fewer cariogenic foods and drinks containing sugars, and to reduce the frequency of their intake.
- **Control of bacterial plaque** – to carry out the regular and thorough removal of plaque, using good oral hygiene techniques.
- **Increase the tooth resistance to acid attack** – by incorporating fluoride into its crystal structure.

All these methods are discussed in detail in Chapter 13.

Non-carious tooth surface loss

The enamel surface of the tooth can be lost due to causes other than dental caries, specifically by the following processes.

- Erosion.
- Abrasion.
- Attrition.
- Abfraction.

Erosion occurs due to the action of extrinsic acid on the enamel. This is dietary acid that has been ingested in foods or drinks by the patient. The usual dietary sources of these extrinsic acids are as follows.

- Carbonated fizzy drinks – whether labelled as 'diet' types or not.
- Acidic fruits such as lemons, oranges, limes and grapefruit which are eaten raw in large quantities.
- Pure fruit juice of the above, especially when consumed in large quantities and between meals.
- Wines.
- Excessive vinegar consumption.

In a similar way, there are some medical conditions and eating disorders that involve the regular regurgitation, or actual vomiting, of the stomach contents into the mouth. As described in Chapter 5, the gastric juices of the stomach are very acidic (pH 2), and have a similar erosive effect on the tooth enamel as extrinsic acids. Some likely conditions and disorders are listed below.

- Bulimia.
- Reflux oesophagitis.
- Hiatus hernia.
- Stomach ulcers.
- Some chemotherapy treatments for cancer.

In contrast to tooth surface loss due to dental caries, no bacteria are involved in the enamel loss caused by erosion. The tooth surface appears pitted and worn but shiny and clean, with no plaque present. Erosion particularly affects the labial or palatal surfaces of the upper incisors, and the occlusal surfaces of the lower molars (Figure 11.7). The teeth affected are often hypersensitive to hot, cold and sweet stimulation as the underlying dentine is exposed. This therefore mimics the symptoms of caries, but no cavity is present.

Treatment of erosion does not necessarily involve restoration, but does involve all of the following.

- Dietary and/or medical advice.
- Desensitisation of the dentine.
- The use of high-concentration fluoride toothpastes and mouthwashes to help restore the pH balance of the oral cavity.

Abrasion occurs when patients scrub their teeth using excessive side-to-side sawing forces, rather than brushing them correctly to remove plaque. The condition is especially seen in smokers with significant tar staining on their teeth, who either brush with a sawing action or use abrasive smokers' toothpastes to remove the stains.

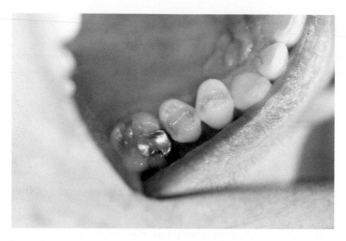

Figure 11.7   Enamel erosion.

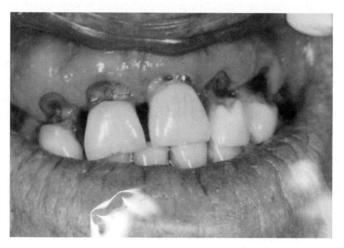

Figure 11.8   Extensive abrasion cavities.

Abrasion is seen at the cervical necks of the teeth, as a deep ridge on the buccal or labial surfaces (Figure 11.8). The surface is shiny rather than carious, and sometimes the ridge is deep enough to see the pulp chamber within the tooth itself. Again, no bacteria are involved in the production of these lesions, and the patient often experiences hypersensitivity with temperature changes. As the ridges can be so deep, they are often restored with glass ionomer cements or composites (Chapter 15). In extreme cases the pulp can be exposed, and endodontic treatment will be required to save the tooth from extraction.

Attrition is the loss of enamel specifically from the biting surfaces of the teeth, and is caused by any of the following.

- Normal 'wear and tear' of chewing, especially in older patients (Figure 11.9).
- Occlusion of natural teeth onto ceramic restorations, such as crowns and bridges (Chapter 16).
- **Bruxing** – the abnormal, and often subconscious, action of clenching and grinding the teeth.

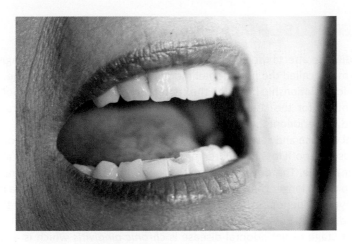

Figure 11.9   Tooth attrition.

287

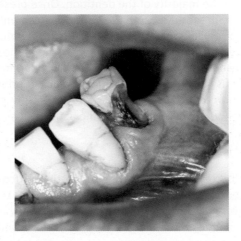

Figure 11.10   Abfraction with caries.

Bruxing is a very common condition, seen in many patients but especially those under stress. It can also occur habitually while undertaking repetitive tasks, such as while exercising. Besides the obvious enamel loss and tooth fracture that occur due to bruxing, patients often experience face pain and disruption of the temporomandibular joint (TMJ). The joint and the muscles of mastication go into spasm in severe cases, and can cause jaw clicks or even jaw locking. Various muscle relaxants, anti-inflammatory drugs and occlusal splints can be used to alleviate these symptoms, but the reason for the bruxing must also be investigated and reduced or removed.

Abfraction is the specific loss of tooth in the cervical (neck) region, due to the shearing forces that occur by overloading single standing teeth. It appears visibly as an abrasion cavity but can affect the buccal, lingual or palatal surfaces of a tooth and will occur suddenly rather than as a gradual loss of tooth structure, as happens with abrasion.

The teeth affected are usually single standing premolars, especially where the molars have been lost in the same jaw (Figure 11.10). Treatment involves not only restoration of the affected tooth but also replacement of any missing teeth to reduce the occlusal loading of the affected tooth and prevent a recurrence of the tooth loss.

Periodontal disease

Periodontal disease affects the supporting structures of the teeth – the gingivae, the periodontal ligament (formerly called the periodontal membrane) and the alveolar bone. In addition, the intimate anatomical relationship between the cementum covering the tooth root and the periodontal ligament accounts for the cementum being included as a supporting structure, and therefore being affected by periodontal disease too.

Periodontal disease and caries are amongst the most common diseases of civilisation. Caries is the major cause of tooth loss in children and young adults, while periodontal disease is the major cause in older people. This does not mean that periodontal disease starts much later in life – only that it takes so much longer than caries to cause tooth loss. Indeed, there is a relatively uncommon but specific type of periodontal disease that begins in childhood rather than in adults, called *juvenile periodontitis*.

The earliest stage of periodontal disease is *chronic gingivitis* which is a chronic inflammation involving the gingivae alone. This can occur in a localised area and affect only a few teeth, or it can occur generally and affect the majority of the dentition. Once present and if allowed to continue, the chronic inflammation spreads deep into the underlying cementum and periodontal ligament, and eventually to the alveolar bone. These structures are gradually destroyed and the teeth become very loose as their supporting tissues are lost. The name given to this late stage of the disease is *chronic periodontitis*. There is no obvious dividing line between the two stages, as untreated chronic gingivitis usually progresses into chronic periodontitis.

Although the disease process occurs gradually, there are usually intermittent episodes of disease activity occurring throughout quiescent phases of no activity, in a sporadic manner.

Causes of periodontal disease

Periodontal disease is a bacterial infection of the supporting structures of the tooth, caused by an initial accumulation of *bacterial plaque* at the gingival margin of the tooth. Plaque is a tenacious transparent film of saliva, micro-organisms and oral debris on the tooth surface (Figure 11.11). Food debris adheres to plaque and the resultant paste of saliva and food remnants attracts more micro-organisms which feed and multiply on it.

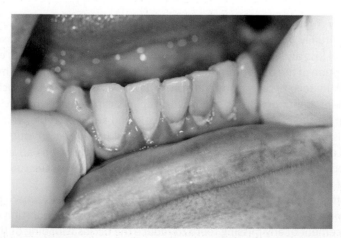

Figure 11.11   Gingival plaque.

It is the same plaque as that involved in the onset of dental caries. However, whereas caries can only occur when sugar is present in the plaque to form the acids that cause enamel demineralisation, the presence of sugar is not necessary for periodontal disease to occur. Any sort of food debris will allow plaque microbes to proliferate and cause periodontal disease.

Plaque can be removed by adequate tooth brushing but in the absence of this counter-measure, it thickens as its microbial population flourishes amid a permanent food supply. Toxic by-products of the plaque micro-organisms then act as a continual source of bacterial irritation which causes chronic inflammation of the gum margin (chronic gingivitis). The plaque extends above and below the gum margin, and wherever it is present *calculus* (tartar) formation can occur.

Calculus is the hard rock-like deposit commonly seen on the lingual surface of lower incisors. Two factors are necessary for its formation: plaque and saliva. Their interaction allows mineralisation to occur within the plaque and produce a deposition of calculus, which may be defined as solidified plaque. It is most easily seen opposite the orifices of salivary gland ducts – on the lingual surface of lower incisors and the buccal surface of upper molars. This visible calculus on the crowns of teeth has a yellowish colour and is called *supragingival calculus* as it forms above the gum margin. However, it also occurs in plaque beneath the gum margin on all teeth and in that situation it is known as *subgingival calculus*. This is harder and darker than supragingival calculus and its surface is covered with a layer of the soft microbial plaque from which it was formed.

Calculus plays only a *passive* mechanical role in periodontal disease. Its' rough surface and ledges create food traps which are inaccessible to a toothbrush and thus allow even more food debris to fertilise the plaque. The *active* role in periodontal disease belongs to plaque micro-organisms.

This description shows that supragingival plaque and calculus are associated with bad oral hygiene. If teeth are cleaned properly they are less able to accumulate. But if they are allowed to do so, they spread subgingivally and become inaccessible to tooth brushing.

Furthermore, there are some additional reasons for plaque formation which are not the patient's fault. These are caused by imperfect dentistry and are known as *iatrogenic factors*, such as:

- fillings or crowns which have an overhanging edge at their cervical margin
- fillings or crowns with loose contact points
- ill-fitting or poorly designed partial dentures.

These defects are food traps which act as stagnation areas that the patient cannot keep clean. Plaque and calculus proliferate there and periodontal disease follows at these sites, even though the rest of the mouth may be perfectly healthy. Food stagnation also occurs on unopposed and irregular teeth, with consequent susceptibility to periodontal disease as well as caries. The full microscopic sequence of events leading to periodontal disease will be described later in this chapter.

Periodontal tissues in health

To be able to recognise the presence of periodontal disease, the appearance of these tissues in health must first be identified. This is illustrated in Figure 11.12 and anatomically is as follows.

- The tooth sits in its socket within the alveolar bone.
- It is attached to the bone by the fibres of the periodontal ligament, which run from the cementum of the root into the alveolar bone.
- Other periodontal ligament fibres run from the alveolar bone crest to the neck of the tooth, and from the neck of the tooth into the gingival papilla.
- The bone and the periodontal ligament are covered by the mucous membrane of the gingiva which lines the alveolar ridges.

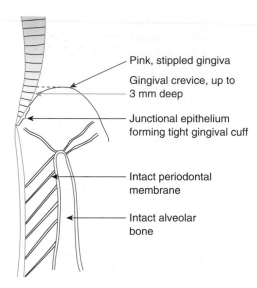

Figure 11.12   Periodontium in health.

- The gingiva is attached directly to the neck of the tooth itself at a specialised site called the **junctional epithelium**.
- In health, a gingival crevice of up to 3 mm deep runs as a 'gutter' around each tooth, the deepest part of which is the attachment of the junctional epithelium. Looking at the tissues in the mouth, then, the gingiva is pink with a stippled appearance like orange peel (ethnic colour variations will occur).
- There is a tight gingival cuff around each tooth, with a gingival crevice no deeper than 3 mm.
- The interdental papillae between the teeth are sharp, with a knife-edge appearance.
- No bleeding occurs when the gingival crevice is gently probed during the dental examination.
- Subgingivally, the periodontal ligament and alveolar bone are intact – this will only be visible on x-ray.

If plaque is allowed to accumulate around the gingival margins of the teeth, the gingiva will become inflamed and the first stage of periodontal disease, *gingivitis*, will develop. When this is a generalised condition affecting the oral cavity as a whole because of poor oral hygiene, it is called *chronic gingivitis*.

Chronic gingivitis

The sequence of events that occur microscopically and lead to chronic gingivitis is illustrated in Figure 11.13.

- The bacteria within the plaque at the gingival margins use food debris to nourish themselves, so that the colony grows in size.
- They produce **toxins** (poisons) as a by-product during their own food digestion.
- These toxins tend to accumulate in the gingival crevice, as they are not removed by oral hygiene measures, nor washed away by the normal cleansing action of saliva.
- The gingiva in direct contact with the toxins becomes irritated, causing inflammation and the early signs of **chronic gingivitis**.

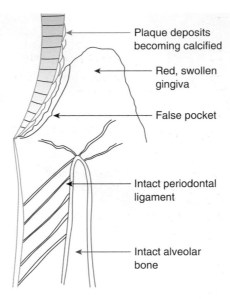

Plaque deposits
becoming calcified

Red, swollen
gingiva

False pocket

Intact periodontal
ligament

Intact alveolar
bone

Figure 11.13   Chronic gingivitis.

- The inflamed gingiva becomes red in colour, and the swelling associated with the inflammation creates **false pockets** around the necks of the teeth – there appears to be a deepening of the gingival crevice but it is due to the swelling only, not to a loss of attachment between the junctional epithelium and the tooth.
- The presence of these pockets allows more plaque to accumulate, as cleansing becomes even more difficult, and the plaque now begins to extend below the gingival margin.
- In this environment, there is little oxygen available for the initial bacteria to use, and the plaque becomes colonised by specialised bacteria that are able to survive without oxygen – these are called **anaerobic bacteria**.
- Examples of these are **Actinomyces** and *Porphyromonas gingivalis*, bacteria specifically associated with periodontal disease.
- In the meantime, the inorganic ions within saliva are incorporated into the structure of the plaque so that it hardens and mineralises as **dental calculus** develops.
- Calculus forming above the gingival margin is called **supragingival calculus** and is **yellow** in colour (Figure 11.14).
- That forming below the gingival margin is called **subgingival calculus** and is **brown** in colour, due to the blood pigments incorporated into it from the bleeding gingival tissues.
- The rough surface of the calculus irritates the gingiva further, and allows more plaque to develop on it.
- The rough calculus and the irritation of the bacterial toxins cause painless **micro-ulcers** to develop within the gingiva, so that they **bleed** on touch or gentle probing.
- The red swollen gingiva and the presence of bleeding on probing are the classic visible signs of **chronic gingivitis**.

Chronic gingivitis is fully reversible if the plaque and calculus are completely removed from above and below the gingival margins. This requires the intervention of the dental team, and then the patient must maintain a good standard of oral hygiene.

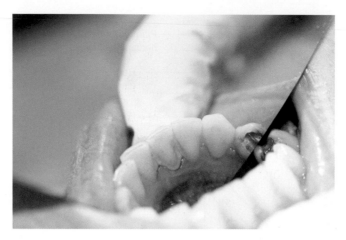

Figure 11.14   Lingual supragingival tartar.

Chronic periodontitis

If chronic gingivitis is not treated, microbial poisons from the plaque soak through the micro-ulcers in the gingival crevice and penetrate the deeper tissues. These poisons gradually destroy the periodontal ligament and alveolar bone and while this is progressing, the gingival pocket deepens, thus further aggravating the condition. Whereas the false pockets of chronic gingivitis are caused by inflammatory swelling of the gum only, in chronic periodontitis they are *true pockets* caused by destruction of the base of the gingival crevice and its attachment to the tooth. In other words, the attachment between the junctional epithelium and the tooth surface is lost.

At the same time the gingival margin may recede, exposing the root to view. This *gingival recession* is commonly known as being *long in the tooth*. If no treatment is provided, so much bone is lost that the teeth eventually become too loose to be of any functional value.

The sequence of events that occur microscopically in the development of chronic periodontitis is illustrated in Figure 11.15.

- The bacterial toxins build up within the false pockets and eventually begin soaking into the gingival tissue itself, through the micro-ulcerated areas.
- Here, they gradually destroy the periodontal ligament and the attachment of the tooth to its supporting tissues, and a **true pocket** forms.
- The loss of attachment gradually moves down the tooth root, creating deeper pockets which allow more plaque and calculus to develop within them.
- The toxins eventually begin attacking the alveolar bone itself, destroying the walls of the tooth socket so that the tooth becomes loose.
- This is often the first indication that the patient has of the presence of their disease, as it is usually painless and often takes several years to reach this point.
- Periodontitis also tends to have intermittent active phases where much tissue destruction occurs, interspersed with quiet phases of little bacterial activity, rather than occurring as a gradually progressive condition.

This description of periodontal disease follows a slowly progressive but painless course of several years but, during that time, pus and micro-organisms in the pockets cause bad breath (*halitosis*) and may affect the patient's general health.

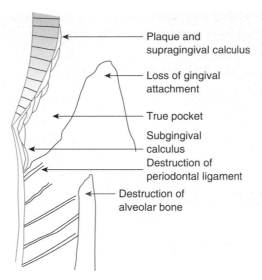

Figure 11.15   Chronic periodontitis.

Once periodontal disease is actually established it can be made worse by certain other factors, which do not in themselves cause the disease alone.

- Smoking.
- Unbalanced or excessive masticatory stress.
- Natural hormonal changes such as puberty and pregnancy.
- Open lip posture (such as occurs during mouth breathing).

Certain medical conditions and drugs may also have the same effect.

- Diabetes, AIDS, leukaemia,and other blood disorders or diseases where resistance to infection is poor – these patients are referred to as being **immune-compromised**.
- Epilepsy treated with phenytoin (Epanutin).
- Vitamin C deficiency.
- Treatment with immune-suppressant drugs such as ciclosporin and cytotoxic agents (used to fight cancers).

Dental plaque forms in everyone's mouth in a short space of time after tooth brushing, but some factors exacerbate its accumulation in certain areas and in some patients' mouths. These are called *plaque retention factors*, some of which have already been mentioned.

- Poor oral hygiene due to patient apathy.
- Poorly aligned teeth, which increases the number of stagnation areas available for plaque to accumulate.
- Incompetent lip seal, which allows the oral soft tissues to dry out and prevents the self-cleansing action of saliva to occur.
- Small oral aperture, making effective tooth brushing difficult for the patient to achieve.
- Iatrogenic causes (poor dentistry).

The rate of progress of periodontal disease depends on the balance between the patient's individual resistance to the bacterial attack and the toxic effects of plaque bacteria. Both these

293

factors vary from time to time and in different parts of the mouth, and the predominant one will determine whether the disease appears dormant or progressive.

Diagnosis of periodontal disease

The diagnosis of periodontal disease is based on the medical history, appearance and recession of the gums, depth of gingival pockets, amount of bone loss, tooth mobility and the distribution of plaque.

Medical history

Periodontal disease affects the vast majority of the population, but most people are otherwise healthy and curable if they exercise adequate plaque control. However, patients with certain conditions are more at risk of severe periodontal disease and less likely to respond so favourably to treatment.

A regularly updated medical history is an essential feature of all patients' records, whatever their reason for attendance or the treatment required. As far as periodontal disease is concerned, the dentist will be particularly interested in:

- past and present illnesses
- drugs prescribed
- hormonal changes, e.g. pregnancy
- smoking habits.

Relevant illnesses are those where resistance to infection is low.

- Diabetes, leukaemia and other blood disorders.
- Vitamin deficiencies.
- AIDS.
- Treatment with immune-supressant drugs, e.g. ciclosporin, used for some types of cancer, and for organ transplant patients.
- Patients at risk of infective endocarditis require antibiotic cover prior to scaling and periodontal surgery.

Certain drugs can cause a severe, non-inflammatory enlargement of the gums called *gingival hyperplasia*, which requires surgical correction.

- Phenytoin (Epanutin) used to control epilepsy.
- Nifedipine (Adalat) used to control angina pectoris and reduce high blood pressure.
- Ciclosporin used to prevent organ rejection after transplant.

There are many clinical signs that the dentist will look for at a routine dental examination to determine if periodontal disease is present. The signs of early-onset chronic gingivitis are as follows.

- The gingiva bleed on brushing or on gentle probing.
- They appear visibly red and swollen.
- Plaque is visible at the gingival margins of the teeth, or can be shown using disclosing solution (see Chapter 12).
- The patient has halitosis.

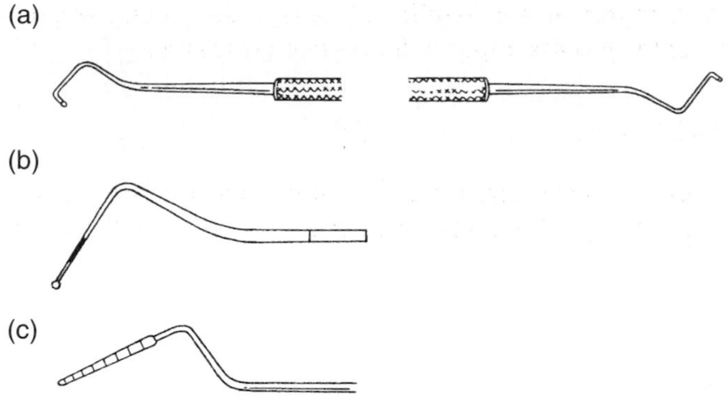

(a)

(b)

(c)

Figure 11.16   Periodontal probes. (a) Calculus probe. (b) WHO (CPITN) probe. (c) Pocket measuring probe.

With established gingivitis, pus can be expressed from the gingival crevice when the gingiva is gently pressed.

The clinical signs of the presence of chronic periodontitis are as follows.

- Periodontal probing detects pockets greater than 3 mm.
- Both supragingival and subgingival calculus will be present.
- Some teeth may be mobile.
- Radiographs will show destruction of the alveolar bone in long-standing cases, with associated deep periodontal pockets present.

It can be seen that one of the early diagnostic signs of periodontal problems is bleeding of the gingiva. The nicotine from tobacco smoking acts on the gingival blood vessels to constrict them, causing less bleeding, if any. The resultant lack of bleeding on brushing or probing masks the presence of periodontal disease in smokers, so that the disease is not evident to either the patient or the dentist without other clinical signs being present.

The easiest assessment carried out by the dentist is to determine the presence of periodontal pockets, by using special *periodontal probes* (Figure 11.16).

Basic periodontal examination (BPE)

Normal healthy gums are firm and pink (ethnically variable) and do not bleed. They have a stippled surface, and the gingival crevice is no deeper than 3 mm. In chronic gingivitis the gums have a soft, smooth surface, are darker in colour and swollen, they bleed on pressure, and have a deeper gingival crevice which may contain subgingival calculus. In chronic periodontitis these gingival changes may not be so obvious, as pockets are deeper and the active disease processes are occurring out of sight at that deeper level.

Tooth mobility and the appearance of the gums are easily checked. Detection of plaque and subgingival calculus, and the assessment of pocket depth, gingival recession and bone loss require examination with periodontal probes and the use of special charts, such as the example shown in Figure 11.17. Dental nurses are advised to study the definitive format and accepted notation of the current periodontal charts in the current version of the National Examining Board for Dental Nurses charting booklet.

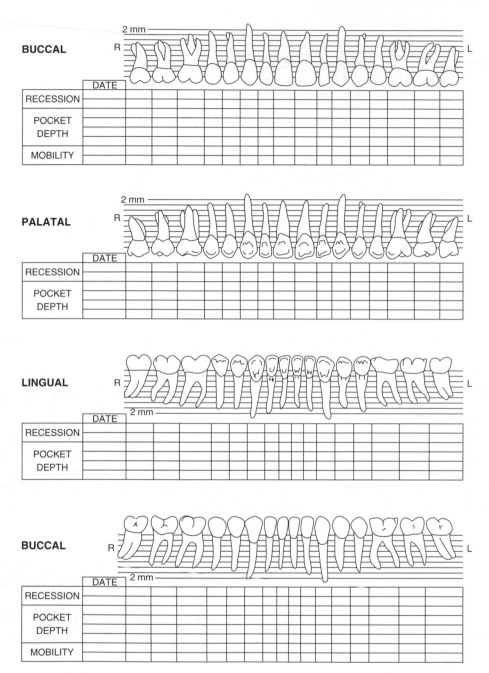

Figure 11.17　Periodontal diagnosis and treatment plan.

A World Health Organization (WHO) probe, also known as a Community Periodontal Index of Treatment Needs or BPE probe, is used for initial screening and charting. This has a coloured band which assesses pocket depth by the amount of band showing (if any) after insertion into the gingival crevice, and a tiny ball on the end which detects subgingival calculus and prevents any bleeding that might be caused by a sharp point.

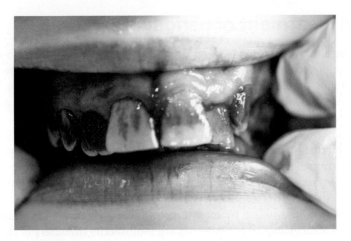

Figure 11.18   Disclosed teeth.

A *pocket measuring probe* may also be used for charting. This has a blunt flat end (rather like that of a flat plastic instrument) with a millimetre scale marked on it. When inserted into the gingival crevice, the pocket depth is read off from the scale.

Subgingival calculus is detected with a *calculus probe*. This resembles a Briault probe but has blunt ends which catch on the scales of calculus in the gingival crevice.

Bone loss can be assessed from pocket depth and dental radiographs (Chapter 12). As true pockets extend almost to the bone margin, a pocket measuring probe will indicate the amount of bone loss. X-rays show this as well, together with subgingival calculus and the cervical edges of restorations.

Plaque is normally invisible as a thin, transparent film, or visible to the trained eye as a creamy white deposit on the gingival margin of the tooth but if a coloured dye is painted on the teeth, supragingival plaque becomes stained and shows up clearly. Dyes used for this purpose are called *disclosing agents* (Figure 11.18). This part of the examination is left until last as the coloured dyes can mask any gingival colour changes that are already present.

Periodontal charting

Full details of the assessment methods used to detect periodontal disease are discussed in Chapter 12, while oral disease prevention is discussed in Chapter 13. A brief summary of periodontal charting is given here.

Whereas the mouth is divided into quarters (quadrants) for tooth charting (Chapter 12), sixths (sextants) are used for periodontal charting. The sextants are upper and lower, left, centre and right:

- molar sextant (876)
- premolar and canine (543)
- incisor (21).

A typical periodontal chart has a 2 mm interval grid to record pocket depths and boxes for the numerical scores of pocket depth, gingival recession, bone loss, tooth mobility, plaque distribution and other factors such as imperfect fillings, dentures or other sources of plaque accumulation.

A similar sextant system is used by orthodontists for descriptive purposes.

Non-surgical treatment of periodontal disease

The prevention of periodontal disease is far more desirable than having to cure it, so good oral hygiene instruction from the dental team from an early age is the best course of action. Obviously, this is not possible for patients who are seen initially as adults, especially if they already have periodontal disease. Oral hygiene instruction and methods of achieving a good standard of oral hygiene are discussed in Chapter 13.

The oral health messages given by the dental team will need to be reinforced regularly if problems persist, and the advice given will vary for the different age groups. Removal of all plaque and its subsequent control by the patient will bring about a complete resolution of chronic gingivitis. Failure to achieve this will allow calculus to form, and the dental team will then have to intervene to remove it.

Accessible plaque is removed by *tooth brushing* and *interdental cleaning*. Subgingival plaque and calculus are inaccessible to patients and are removed by members of the dental team during *scaling*. Once these aims have been achieved and then routinely maintained, the causal sources of irritation which produce the disease are lost.

In chronic gingivitis, bleeding ceases, swollen gums return to their normal healthy condition and false pockets are thereby eliminated. The patient is then cured but strict oral hygiene and regular dental checks are required thereafter to prevent recurrence of plaque and calculus formation.

In chronic periodontitis there is no regeneration of lost bone, but mild cases can be cured in the same way as chronic gingivitis. In the advanced stages of the disease, scaling alone cannot eliminate true pockets if they are too deep to be accessible. In such cases they are treated surgically by repositioning and/or recontouring the gingival margin as described in Chapter 17.

In this way, even advanced periodontal disease can be arrested but a return of the condition is inevitable unless the patient follows the advice given and the instructions on supragingival plaque control, and also attends regularly for the team to check progress and continue subgingival plaque control.

Apart from scaling and gingival surgery, appropriate treatment is given for any other conditions facilitating plaque retention, for example, unsatisfactory fillings, crowns and dentures, unopposed and irregular teeth.

As periodontal disease is an infection by plaque bacteria and other micro-organisms, one approach to treatment is the application of antimicrobial drugs directly into the gingival crevice and pockets, such as with *Periochip, Dentomycin gel* and *Gengigel* applications. The establishment of their long-term success in the battle against periodontal disease is an ongoing and exciting area of clinical research.

Supragingival plaque control

Supragingival calculus and any overhanging cervical margins of restorations are removed in the surgery. At home, thorough, twice-daily tooth brushing by the patient will then keep accessible plaque under control. Appropriate instruction in the surgery, and the use of disclosing agents at home, will show patients how well they are performing and indicate where improvement is required.

Areas of the oral cavity which are inaccessible to an ordinary toothbrush are the interdental spaces above or below the contact points of adjacent teeth (interproximal areas). They can be cleaned with dental floss, wood sticks and an interspace brush. The dentist or hygienist must give the patient special instruction in these methods as they can do more harm than good if used incorrectly or unnecessarily.

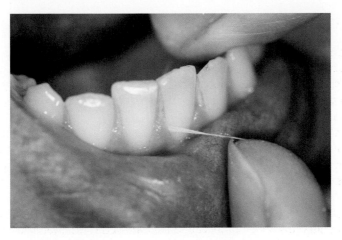

Figure 11.19   Flossing.

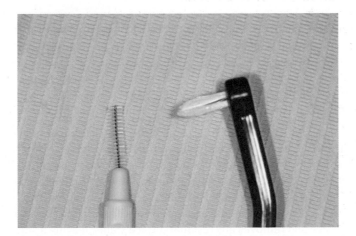

Figure 11.20   TePe® and interspace brushes.

Dental floss is thread or tape which is worked between the teeth to keep their contact areas clean (Figure 11.19). Where recession of the gum has occurred or gingival surgery has been performed, the resulting interdental spaces may be too large for flossing.

Wood sticks (also called interspace sticks) are used for these large spaces. They are soft wooden sticks which are passed through the spaces to keep them clear of food debris and reduce plaque formation.

Interspace brushes and *interdental brushes* are special types of toothbrush designed to clean interdental spaces and the interproximal tooth surfaces in the same way as floss and wood sticks. The former have only one tuft of bristles, while the latter appear similar to a bottle brush (Figure 11.20).

Any calculus present cannot be removed by the patient as it is hardened onto the tooth surface, and instead must be treated by regular scaling. This is done by a dentist, therapist or hygienist and the patient's own efforts at supragingival plaque control are checked at the same time. Supragingival scaling removes plaque and calculus deposits from the enamel surface of the teeth down to the gingival crevice.

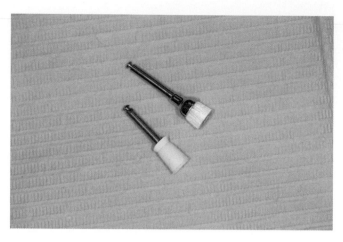

Figure 11.21   Polishing cup and brush.

Scaling hand instruments are made in various designs appropriate for the removal of calculus from any part of a tooth, and those used for supragingival calculus removal include the following.

- Sickle scaler.
- Cushing's push scaler.
- Jaquette scaler.

Hand scaling is tiring for the operator to carry out but gives excellent tactile sensation, so specks of residual calculus are easily detectable and can be fully removed. Alternatively, an ultrasonic scaler may be used which is much faster and less tiring. However, its action depends on the water spray produced during use, and this can be uncomfortable for patients with sensitive teeth unless performed under local anaesthesia. Once scaling has been completed, the teeth are polished with prophylactic polishing paste using a rubber cup or bristle brush in the slow handpiece (Figure 11.21). The paste is abrasive and removes any residual surface stains, leaving a smooth tooth surface that slows down the reaccumulation of plaque.

Subgingival plaque control

With chronic periodontitis any alveolar bone loss is permanent, although research is ongoing into the use of synthetic bone in both humans and other animal species, to replace that lost due to natural resorption or periodontal disease. In the meantime, if subgingival calculus is thoroughly and regularly removed by the dental team, and a good standard of oral hygiene is maintained by the patient, there is every chance that the periodontal ligament will reattach and any periodontal pockets will heal.

The instruments used to remove subgingival calculus have to be long enough to reach the base of any periodontal pockets, and thin enough to do so without tearing the gingival tissues. In addition, they are used to scrape the tooth root surfaces and dislodge any contaminated cementum, which is then removed from the pockets by both aspiration and irrigation. This technique is called subgingival debridement. The instruments used for subgingival scaling include the following (Figure 11.22).

- Gracey curette.
- Other subgingival curettes.

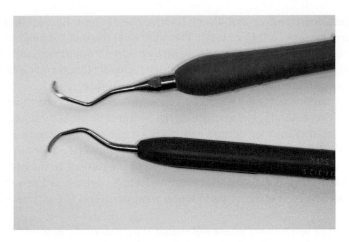

Figure 11.22   Curettes.

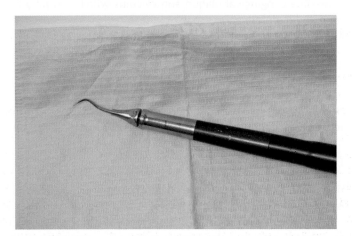

Figure 11.23   Ultrasonic scaler.

- Periodontal hoe.
- Ultrasonic scaler.

Once subgingival debridement is complete, the periodontal tissues can heal and the junctional epithelium can reattach to the tooth surface. In doing so, the periodontal pockets are eliminated.

Subgingival scaling entails much instrumentation within the gingival crevice and pockets. This, in addition to the gingivitis already present, produces considerable bleeding and trauma, and requires the use of local anaesthesia. Scaling with hand instruments is a tedious procedure for operator and patient, but may be done more easily and quickly with an *ultrasonic scaler* (Figure 11.23). This produces ultrasonic vibrations which are transmitted through a cable to a special scaling instrument. When it is applied to a tooth, the vibrations help loosen the plaque and calculus and they are flushed away by a water-cooling spray which is part of the apparatus. The scaling instrument consists of a special handpiece with a range of detachable scaling tips of various shapes. Use of a chlorhexidine mouthwash by the patient, before scaling, reduces any risk of cross-infection of staff. Patients are advised to take analgesic tablets, if required, as the area may feel rather sore for a day or two afterwards.

Scaling, as just described, cannot always remove the deepest, hardest and most adherent layer of calculus from the root surface of teeth. The additional stage of *subgingival debridement* is then carried out, using Gracey curettes. These are distinguished from other curettes by having only one cutting surface. Their planing action eliminates any residual plaque and calculus as it scrapes away some of the root cementum, to provide a smooth root surface.

Provided the patient achieves adequate supragingival plaque control while the dentist deals with any restoration overhangs, imperfect partial dentures or other hindrances to plaque removal, and the hygienist/therapist or dentist can maintain subgingival plaque control, most cases of straightforward chronic periodontitis can be cured. Continued periodontal health is dependent to a large degree on the co-operation and motivation of the patient to maintain a consistently good standard of oral hygiene. Of all the exacerbating factors that can worsen the situation, smoking plays a large part in the failure of periodontal treatment and the ultimate loss of teeth by the patient.

Also, some cases will remain where non-surgical periodontal treatment alone cannot succeed. Patients with very deep pockets, especially those involving multi-rooted teeth, may present a problem of inaccessible subgingival plaque and calculus which can only be removed by surgical procedures to gain and maintain access to it.

These and other surgical techniques are described in Chapter 17.

Other periodontal conditions

Several other interesting periodontal conditions exist, which may present from time to time in the dental workplace, although they are not as common as chronic gingivitis and periodontitis.

Subacute pericoronitis

This is an infection of the gingival flap that lies over a partially erupted tooth, called the *operculum*, and sometimes affects the surrounding soft tissues too (Figure 11.24). It especially affects the lower third molars as they erupt, because these teeth are not only difficult to clean, allowing plaque bacteria to proliferate, but the operculum is often traumatised by the opposing tooth during normal mouth closure. The combination of infection and trauma produces inflammation of

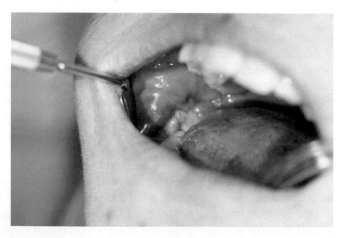

Figure 11.24   Pericoronitis around lower right third molar.

the operculum, which then swells and becomes more traumatised. It is treated in a number of ways, depending on the severity of the infection and the regularity of its occurrence.

- Irrigation of any food debris from under the operculum, ideally using a chlorhexidine-based disinfectant.
- Oral hygiene instruction for the area, especially the use of hot salt water or disinfectant mouth-washes, or an oxygen-releasing mouthwash to remove the ideal conditions for the bacteria involved.
- Antibiotics if the patient has a raised temperature (anaerobic bacteria are usually involved, so metronidazole is often prescribed).
- Operculectomy if the condition recurs (the surgical removal of the operculum from over the tooth).
- Alternatively, the extraction of the opposing tooth to break the cycle of trauma and inflammation.

Acute herpetic gingivitis

This condition is caused by the herpes simplex virus and most commonly affects infants. All the signs of acute inflammation are present and the rest of the oral mucous membrane may also be involved in the form of tiny blisters which leave painful ulcers (*acute herpetic gingivo-stomatitis*). The condition is short-lived but uncomfortable; the patient feels unwell and may be unable to eat solids, but it resolves without treatment and the gingival condition returns to normal.

However, the virus remains dormant in the body and can be reactivated later by a common cold to produce a cold sore (herpes labialis) on the lip (Figure 11.25). During the acute phase or the presence of a cold sore, the condition is highly infectious and dental treatment is best deferred until the condition has resolved.

Acute necrotising ulcerative gingivitis

This is abbreviated to ANUG and was formerly called acute ulcerative gingivitis (AUG) or Vincent's disease. It is an acute gingivitis characterised by pain and halitosis (bad breath). The affected gingiva appears bright red, with a covering layer of yellow/grey sloughing membrane where the

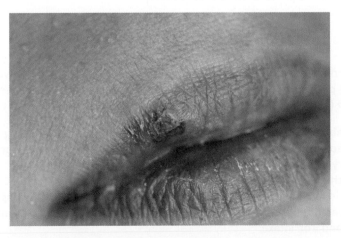

Figure 11.25   'Cold sore' on upper lip.

303

gum margin has been destroyed by bacterial action. The bacteria involved include *Bacillus fusiformis* and *Treponema vincenti*.

All the features of acute inflammation are present: red, swollen, painful gums; loss of function, because it is too painful to chew hard food; and the patient often has a raised temperature.

It usually affects young adults and usually occurs in areas already affected by chronic gingivitis. In many cases stress, heavy smoking and a lowered general resistance precipitate an attack; thus it is more common in winter when colds, influenza and other infections are rife but more importantly in AIDS, and perhaps as its first sign. It is treated as follows.

- Antibiotic treatment that is specific for anaerobic bacteria, usually **metronidazole**.
- If the patient is pregnant, this cannot be used so penicillin is substituted.
- Use of a disinfectant mouthwash, such as those containing chlorhexidine while the area is too painful to clean by brushing.
- Thorough scaling and polishing once the symptoms have settled, followed by oral hygiene instruction.
- Smoking cessation advice, where relevant.
- Long-term use of mouthwash and an adequate brushing technique.

Acute lateral periodontal abscess

This is an occasional complication of chronic periodontitis in which pus formation in a deep pocket is unable to drain through the gingival crevice. The pus accumulates instead at the base of the pocket to form an abscess. This condition must not be confused with an acute alveolar abscess, which follows pulp death and occurs at the root apex. Acute lateral periodontal abscess occurs on a *vital* tooth at the side of the root (the lateral region of the root).

Treatment depends on the depth of the pocket and the probability of curing the underlying periodontal disease. The options are as follows.

- Drainage of the pus present.
- Thorough subgingival scaling of the affected tooth.
- Local administration of antibiotic into the pocket itself, especially metronidazole.
- Oral hygiene instruction.
- If all else fails, extraction of the affected tooth.

Oral cancer

Oral cancer can affect various areas of the mouth, the soft tissues, the salivary glands or the jaw bones. Ninety percent of oral cancers affect the soft tissues initially, as a lesion called *squamous cell carcinoma* (SCC). The suggested causative factors are as follows.

- **Tobacco habits** – all tobacco products contain chemicals capable of causing cancer (**carcinogens**).
- **High alcohol consumption** – alcohol acts as a solvent for the carcinogens, and allows their easier entry into the soft tissues.
- **Both together** – smokers who also drink to excess are at most risk of SCC.
- **Sunlight** – in fair-skinned people, sunlight is associated with SCC affecting the lower lip.
- **Diet** – research is ongoing into links between SCC and diets high in fats and red meat, or low in vitamin A and iron intake.
- **Genetics** – some people are genetically predisposed to developing SCC.

The signs and symptoms of SCC may be any of the following, and will be specifically looked for during routine dental examinations by the dentist.

- Painless ulcer that has no obvious cause, and fails to heal fully within 2–3 weeks; obvious causes are trauma from denture flanges, chipped restorations or vigorous tooth brushing, or even burns from hot foods and drinks.
- In particular, an ulcer occurring beneath or on the side of the tongue, or in the floor of the mouth, as these are the oral areas where more sinister lesions develop.
- Presence of a white or red patch of oral mucous membrane that is associated with the ulcer (these are called leucoplakia and erythroplakia, respectively).

The risk factors shown previously make the occurrence of the signs and symptoms far more serious in certain individuals, and any suspicious lesions must be referred to an oral surgery hospital department for investigation immediately. Even then, the 5-year survival rate for SCC is only around 55%, which is very dependent on early detection and aggressive treatment.

The aggressive surgical treatment will be carried out by maxillofacial surgeons, and often involves the removal of large sections of the jaw and facial bones and their surrounding soft tissues, depending on the position of the cancer and the depth and area of its spread.

Years ago, the typical oral cancer sufferer was a 60-plus male patient, usually from a lower socio-economic background, who was a life-long smoker and drinker. In recent years, this has changed and those being diagnosed with oral cancer are more likely to be much younger patients (even in their 20s), both male and female, usually smokers and especially binge drinkers, and also those who use sunbeds or sunbathe with little ultraviolet protection for their lips. Obviously this last group will also be at much greater risk of developing skin cancer (melanoma).

The dental team has a vital role to play not only in early detection of SCC but also in patient education of the risk factors, especially in these high-risk patients. This is especially important with smoking and tobacco usage, whether with cigarettes, cigars or pipes, and including the habitual chewing of betel nuts and tobacco paan by some Asian societies.

In addition, the effects of smoking on dental and general health should also be discussed with suitable patients, and should cover all of the following topics.

- Oral health effects.
  - Oral cancer
  - Development of oral precancerous lesions (especially white patches in the mouth)
  - Periodontal disease
  - Poor wound healing, especially after extraction
  - Tendency to develop 'dry socket' after extraction
  - Stained teeth
  - Halitosis (bad breath)
- General health effects.
  - Heart disease – in particular, hypertension and coronary artery disease
  - Stroke
  - Respiratory disease – in particular, chronic bronchitis and emphysema
  - Other cancers – in particular, throat, lung and stomach cancer

In the last few years, and in recognition of the alarming increasing incidence of smoking-related cancers and illness in the population, the Department of Health has developed an excellent national 'Quit Smoking' scheme that is freely accessible to anyone wishing to stop smoking (see Figure 7.4). The dental team has a valuable role to play in advising patients of this scheme, referring them for help and treatment whenever possible, and supporting them as they undergo any treatment.

Further resources are available for this book, including interactive multiple choice questions and extended matching questions. Visit the companion website at:

www.levisonstextbookfordentalnurses.com

12

Oral Health Assessment and Diagnosis

Key learning points

A **working knowledge** of
- the assessment methods used to examine the oral tissues and structures
- the methods used to chart teeth
- the methods used to record malocclusion
- the methods used to assess the periodontal tissues
- processing techniques

A **factual knowledge** of
- ionising radiation and the principles of its use in dentistry

A **factual awareness** of
- determining radiographic faults

Oral health assessments are carried out each time that a patient attends the dental workplace, usually for an examination.

Some patients attend more or less frequently than others by their own personal choice, and some require more frequent attendance than others, in the dentist's professional opinion. The dentist's opinion is based on the known risk factors of various oral diseases, and the patient's frequency of exposure to these risk factors.

The two main purposes of carrying out the oral health assessment are:

- prevention of disease by regular opportunities to reinforce oral health education messages
- early detection and diagnosis when disease is already present.

Levison's Textbook for Dental Nurses, Eleventh Edition. By Carole Hollins.
© 2013 John Wiley & Sons, Ltd. Published 2013 by John Wiley & Sons, Ltd. Companion website: www.levisonstextbookfordentalnurses.com

If disease is already present, regular oral assessment will detect it at an earlier stage and allow the necessary treatment to be carried out so that a full recovery is more likely. If a serious and potentially life-threatening disease is present, such as oral cancer, regular inspection will identify it earlier and allow the patient to be referred for urgent specialist care, with a better chance of successful treatment and recovery.

Although the oral health assessment should detect an abnormality in any of the areas assessed, the obvious oral diseases that are particularly looked for are dental caries, chronic gingivitis and chronic periodontal disease.

The whole dental team has an important role to play in this assessment and prevention process.

- **Dentist** – makes the initial diagnosis, formulates a treatment plan and carries out all treatments restricted to the dentist only.
- **Hygienist** – works under the prescription of the dentist to carry out scaling and oral hygiene instruction.
- **Therapist** – works under the prescription of the dentist to carry out suitable treatments as necessary.
- **Dental nurse** – assists the dentist during the assessment by accurately recording all the information as necessary, assists the other dental team members while treating the patient, reinforces all the oral hygiene messages given to the patient.

Assessment of oral health is carried out in the following areas.

- Extraoral soft tissues.
- Intraoral soft tissues.
- Deciduous and mixed dentition of children.
- Permanent dentition.
- Occlusion.
- Periodontal tissues.

Methods used to carry out assessment

The main methods available to carry out oral health assessments are the following.

- Use of **vitality tests** to determine if an individual tooth is alive, dying or dead (non-vital).
- Use of **study models** to record the occlusion of the teeth, and the individual appearance and position of each tooth.
- Use of **photographs** to record the visible appearance of a structure at that time, and for comparison with earlier or later views.
- **Visual inspection** to detect visible abnormalities, such as size and colour changes.
- **Manual inspection** to feel abnormalities, such as a lump where none should be present.
- Use of **mouth mirrors** for intraoral soft tissue and tooth charting assessments.
- Use of various **dental probes** for tooth inspections and charting.
- Use of **transillumination** of anterior teeth to detect interproximal cavities (bright light such as that from the curing lamp is shone through the tooth, and cavities show as dark lesions).
- Use of **periodontal probe** for periodontal assessment.
- Use of various **radiograph** views, to determine both the presence or absence of various structures or pathology.

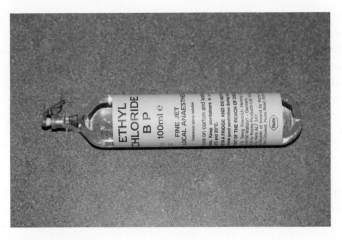

Figure 12.1   Ethyl chloride container.

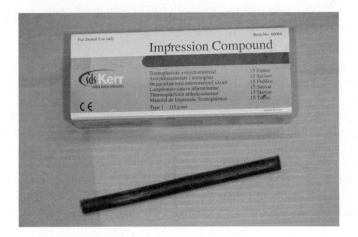

Figure 12.2   Greenstick compound.

Vitality tests

These are sometimes necessary to help in determining whether a tooth is vital (alive) or non-vital (dead).

- Cold stimulus with **ethyl chloride** (Figure 12.1).
- Hot stimulus with warmed **gutta percha** (Figure 12.2).
- Electrical test with **electric pulp tester**.

The first two techniques are used to diagnose toothache where the symptoms include pain with cold or heat, whereas electric pulp testers are more accurate in determining the 'degree' of vitality of a tooth, as follows.

- Normal response – healthy pulp.
- Increased response – early pulpitis present.

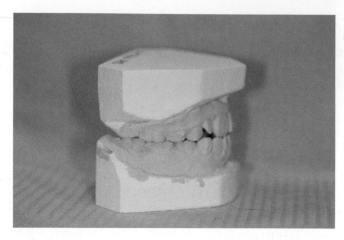

Figure 12.3   Study model set.

- Reduced response – pulp is dying, or tooth has heavily lined deep restoration present so the voltage cannot be adequately transmitted to the pulp.
- No response – pulp tissue is dead.

Patients will vary in their response to electric pulp testers, so it is always advisable to test several apparently healthy teeth to establish what their 'normal' response is, before testing the suspect tooth.

Electric pulp testers are either battery operated or mains operated, and they work by sending an increasing voltage into the tooth until the patient is aware of a tingling sensation in that tooth. The point at which the patient indicates a sensation is recorded numerically on a scale, so that the 'degree' of vitality can be determined in relation to 'test' teeth.

Ethyl chloride is a liquid that vaporises quickly at room temperature, leaving ice crystals which provide a cold stimulus when touched by the skin or onto a tooth. This cold sensation is detected particularly well by a hypersensitive tooth, and can help to indicate which one requires dental treatment.

Gutta percha is a natural rubber-like product with several uses in dentistry. As a compound of greenstick (see Figure 12.2), it can be warmed in a flame and placed on a pulpitic tooth to determine a hypersensitivity reaction to heat, indicating which one requires dental treatment. The teeth to be tested should be dried in both cases first, and a thin smear of Vaseline placed before applying the warm greenstick compound to avoid the substance sticking to the tooth and causing pain to the patient.

Study models

In some situations, it is necessary for the dentist to consider the patient's occlusion before being able to decide on any treatment necessary, for example when providing partial dentures or orthodontic treatment. Impressions are taken of both dental arches using alginate impression material (see Chapter 16) and then cast up to produce a set of study models (Figure 12.3).

Study models are useful in the following cases.

- Occlusal analysis in complicated crown or bridge cases.
- Orthodontic cases, to determine if extractions are required and which type of appliance is necessary.

- Occlusal analysis where full mouth treatment may be necessary, to determine the functioning of the dentition.
- Where tooth surface loss is evident, either by erosion from acidic foods and drinks or by attrition due to tooth grinding, so that the progression of the tooth wear can be monitored and treatment determined.

Photographs

These can be taken to record various aspects of the dentition or soft tissues, for future reference. They can be produced using conventional cameras (especially 'Instamatic' types), digital cameras with 'macro' lenses for close-up shots, or by using specialist intraoral digital cameras. Specialised computers and equipment are required for this last technique.

Photographs are useful to record:

- soft tissue lesions to aid diagnosis
- the extent of injury following trauma
- before-and-after views of dental treatment.

Extraoral soft tissue assessment

The dentist will often be visibly assessing the extraoral soft tissues (those outside the mouth) of the patient while greeting them into the surgery area, and chatting to them before beginning the intraoral assessments. In particular, they will be looking at and palpating the following structures for any signs of abnormality.

- **External facial signs** – checking for skin colour, facial symmetry, the presence of any blemishes, especially moles and 'cold sores'.
- **The lips** – checking for any change in colour or size, the presence of any blemishes, and palpating for any abnormalities.
- **The lymph nodes** – lying under the mandible and in the neck, these are palpated to detect any swellings or abnormalities, the presence of which may indicate an infection or a more sinister lesion.

Variations in skin colour do occur, especially in different ethnic groups. Some patients are naturally pale and others are naturally ruddy. However, an unusual facial appearance can sometimes indicate problems, such as nervous patients becoming pale and clammy as they are about to faint or the unnatural ruddiness of a patient with hypertension.

Facial asymmetry (where one side of the face is shaped differently from the other) could indicate the presence of a swelling, or problems with the nerve supply or muscular control of that area, all of which require further investigation.

The sudden appearance of unusual skin blemishes, especially moles, may indicate the presence of an early skin cancer (*melanoma*), which will need urgent referral for treatment.

Similarly, the lips are examined and details recorded of blemishes, such as the presence of a 'cold sore' indicating infection with the herpes simplex type 1 virus, or the presence of minor salivary gland cysts (*mucoceles*).

Lips that are generally tinged bluish-purple indicate some degree of chronic heart failure, which needs noting before local anaesthesia and traumatic dental procedures are carried out.

Lymph nodes are part of the body's immune system and are present in certain areas throughout the body. Any enlargement of those accessible to the dentist in the head and neck region indicates that the body is fighting infection or some other disease process, and requires further investigation.

311

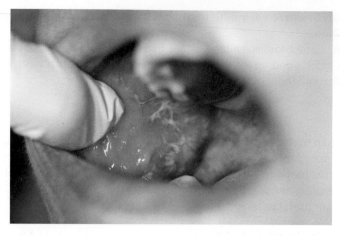

Figure 12.4   Leucoplakia of buccal mucosa.

Intraoral soft tissue assessment

This is carried out at each dental examination and in a systematic manner, so that no areas or lesions are missed out.

- **Labial, buccal and sulcus mucosa** – checked for their colour and texture, the presence of any white patches (especially the buccal mucosa – Figure 12.4), and the moisture level is noted.
- **Palatal mucosa** – both the hard and soft palates, the oropharynx and the tonsils (if present).
- **Tongue** – checked for colour and texture, symmetry of shape and movement, the level of mobility; all surfaces are checked, especially beneath the tongue, as this is one of the most common sites for oral carcinoma to develop.
- **Floor of mouth** – checked for colour and texture, the presence of any white or red patches, and the presence of any swellings.

Low moisture levels in the mouth can indicate problems with the functioning of the salivary glands, such as *Sjögren's syndrome*, or *xerostomia* (dry mouth) due to age-related changes to the glands or as a side-effect in those taking certain medications. Saliva has important functions with regard to defence, cleansing and dental disease initiation, and any indication of reduced flow levels is of great importance to the dental team, with regard to maintaining a healthy oral environment for the patient.

The more likely areas for oral cancers to develop are on the borders of, or beneath, the tongue and in the floor of the mouth, and these areas will be particularly well examined in patients with known risk factors, such as smoking and excessive alcohol consumption. All findings can then be recorded on a suitable assessment sheet (Figure 12.5). In addition, photographs can be taken at the time and retained for comparison at a later date, while any benign lesions are kept under observation.

Tooth charting

Accurate tooth charting is one of the most important skills acquired by a dental nurse in their role as an assistant to the dentist, both during oral health assessments and during the provision of dental treatment.

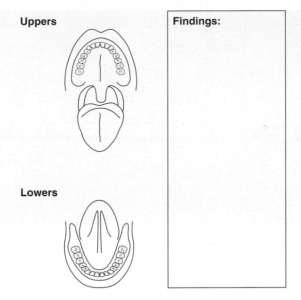

Uppers

Lowers

Findings:

Figure 12.5   Soft tissue assessment sheet.

Inaccuracies in the charting can result in catastrophic consequences for the patient, such as the wrong classification or type of restoration being provided or even the wrong tooth being extracted. It is a fundamental skill of all members of the dental team to record and follow a tooth chart correctly.

Charting is used as a style of 'dental shorthand' to quickly and accurately record a patient's dentition, as it appears at the time of the oral health assessment. Dental nurses are referred to the definitive charting booklet produced by the National Examining Board for Dental Nurses (NEBDN). This describes the approved current charting notations used both for teeth and for periodontal conditions, following the three styles currently in use.

- **Palmer notation** – for tooth charting.
- **International Dental Federation (FDI) notation** – for tooth charting.
- **Basic periodontal examination (BPE)** – for periodontal charting.

Although many dental workplaces are now computerised, the software systems in use for tooth charting vary enormously (Figure 12.6) and very often cannot actually distinguish the finer points of the written notation, which may lead to errors. Therefore, it is necessary for trainee dental nurses to be taught tooth charting using written records, so that they are standardised upon qualification.

With tooth charting, a two-grid system is used (forensic notation) which separates the current dental status from any treatment required. Each anterior tooth charted diagrammatically is shown with four surfaces and an incisal edge or canine cusp, and each posterior tooth with five surfaces, as shown in Figure 12.7.

The teeth are recorded from the centreline backwards for both the deciduous and the permanent dentition, and the charting grid is arranged as follows.

- Inner grid – shows current dental status and dental treatment already present in the mouth.
- Outer grid – records all dental treatment that needs to be carried out.

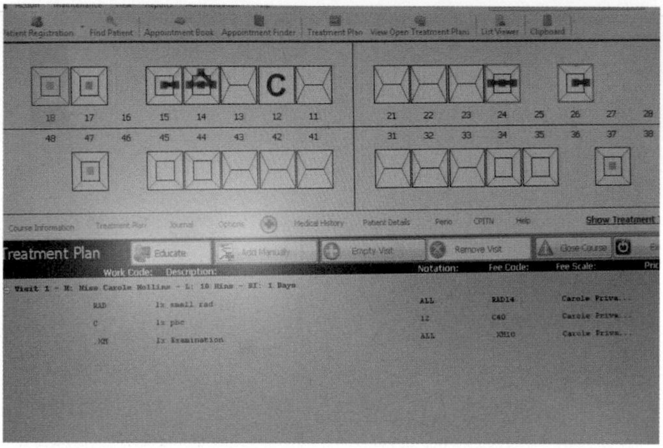

Figure 12.6   Computer chart example.

For the purpose of tooth charting, current dental status refers to the following notations only.

- The presence or absence of a tooth.
- The presence of a root.
- The notation of any tooth that is stated as unerupted, and charted as 'UE'.
- The notation of any tooth that is stated as partially erupted, and charted as 'PE'.
- The position of a tooth in relation to the normal dental arch, and may be stated as 'instanding' or 'buccal to the arch', for example.

The condition of the teeth and the presence of any restorations can then be charted in a code form on the inner grid, and work to be carried out is recorded in the outer grid. Examples of some of the recognised charting notations are shown in Figure 12.8, but readers are again advised to consult the charting booklet produced by NEBDN for the full range of current definitive notations.

The notable exception to the usual rules of inner grid versus outer grid is the charting of a fracture to a tooth. A fracture can range from a minimal incisal edge chip to a tooth, which requires no treatment (and is therefore charted on the inner grid as it represents 'current dental status'), or it can be a full fracture of the crown of the tooth from its root at gingival level (and is therefore charted on the outer grid as it represents 'dental treatment that needs to be carried out').

The charting symbol in both these instances of a fracture is '#', so the dental nurse must be careful to determine if an indication is made as to whether the tooth is to be restored or not, as this will determine which grid should be used for the notation.

Palmer notation

This is based on the division of the dentition into four quadrants when looking at the patient from the front: upper right and left, and lower left and right. Using either the letters representing the deciduous dentition or the numbers representing the permanent dentition (see Chapter 10), each tooth can then be written and identified individually. With the increased use of computers to record the patient's dental records, including tooth chartings, the use of the quadrant symbol has been superseded by the use of the following.

- UR for upper right.
- UL for upper left.

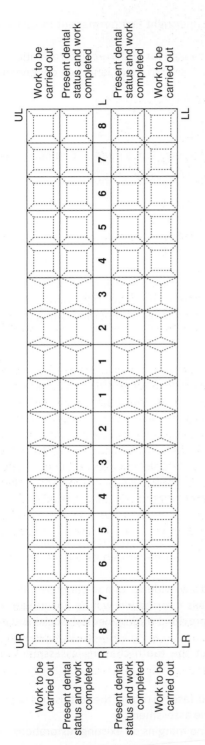

Figure 12.7 Manual charting grid.

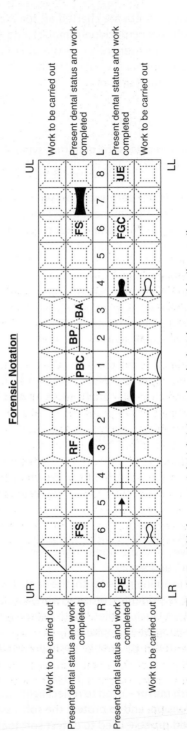

Forensic Notation

The inner grid is for present dental status and work already present in the mouth.
The outer grid is for work to be carried out.

Figure 12.8 Completed charting grid.

- LL for lower left.
- LR for lower right.

So, individual teeth are charted as, for example, UR6 (upper right first permanent molar) and LLE (lower left second deciduous molar), and so on.

The Palmer system relies on the use of the English language for its correct interpretation, and a more international system of tooth charting is also available that is not language dependent, but is based on numbers only.

Two-digit FDI notation

This system replaces the quadrant symbol or use of UR, UL, etc. with a quadrant number as well as a tooth number.

- Upper right – permanent quadrant 1, deciduous quadrant 5.
- Upper left – permanent quadrant 2, deciduous quadrant 6.
- Lower left – permanent quadrant 3, deciduous quadrant 7.
- Lower right – permanent quadrant 4, deciduous quadrant 8.

The quadrant number forms the first digit while the second identifies an individual tooth as 1–8 in the same way as the Palmer system. Reading clockwise from the upper right third molar, all 32 permanent teeth and 20 deciduous teeth have their own two-digit number indicating their quadrant (first digit) and identity (second digit).

For permanent teeth:

18 17 16 15 14 13 12 11	21 22 23 24 25 26 27 28
48 47 46 45 44 43 42 41	31 32 33 34 35 36 37 38

And for deciduous teeth:

55 54 53 52 51	61 62 63 64 65
85 84 83 82 81	71 72 73 74 75

The lower left second premolar, for example, is written as 35 and pronounced 'three-five', not 'thirty-five', and the upper right deciduous first molar would be written as 54 and pronounced 'five-four', and so on.

While examining the teeth, the dentist will also record any evidence of non-carious tooth surface loss that is evident – erosion, abrasion or attrition. This information will be linked with other information (such as diet, tooth brushing habits, etc.) provided during medical, social and dental history taking (see Chapter 13).

The dental instruments normally used to carry out the tooth charting assessment are as follows.

- **Mouth mirror** – used to reflect light onto the tooth surface, to retract the soft tissues to provide clear vision, and to protect the soft tissues during the assessment.
- **Angled probe** – used to detect soft tooth surfaces and margins on existing restorations.

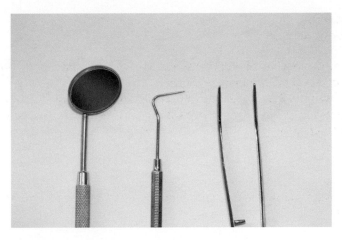

Figure 12.9   Mirror, probe and tweezers.

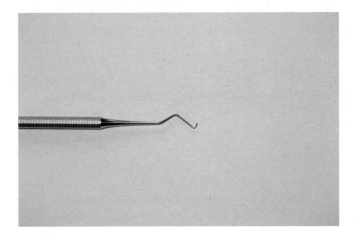

Figure 12.10   Briault probe.

- **Tweezers** – used to hold cotton wool pledgets to wipe tooth surfaces dry, or to place cotton wool rolls (Figure 12.9).
- **Briault probe** – two-ended probe specially designed to detect interproximal caries, either mesially or distally (Figure 12.10).

Occlusion

Occlusion is the term used to describe the situation when the mouth is closed and the teeth of both jaws interlock together so that their occlusal surfaces are in contact. When each jaw is of a normal size in relation to the other, and they have developed during childhood in the correct relationship to each other, the cusps of the teeth in one arch should interdigitate with the fissures and interproximal areas of the other (Figure 12.11).

In normal occlusion, all the teeth are well aligned and there is no crowding, no protruding teeth and no undue prominence of the chin. Upper incisors slightly overlap the lowers vertically and

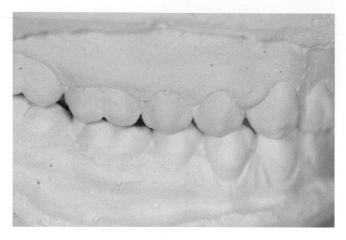

Figure 12.11   Buccal occlusion.

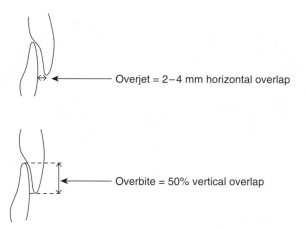

Figure 12.12   Overjet and overbite.

horizontally and special names are given to this overlap; vertical overlap is called *overbite* and horizontal overlap is called *overjet* (Figure 12.12). With the mouth closed and the teeth touching together in occlusion, the position of the first molars and the canines in each jaw determines ideal occlusion and malocclusion. This is called *Angle's classification*.

Ideal *class I occlusion* occurs where the mesiobuccal cusp of the upper first molar lies in the buccal groove of the lower first molar (Figure 12.13). The ideal overjet is 2–4 mm and the ideal overbite is 50%.

For teeth to erupt into normal occlusion, the jaws must be in correct horizontal and vertical relationship to each other, and of sufficient size to accommodate their full complement of teeth. The teeth can then erupt into a normal position of balance between the pressures exerted by the lips and cheeks on their outer side, and the tongue on the inner side of the dental arches.

When normal occlusion is not present, the patient is described as having a *malocclusion*.

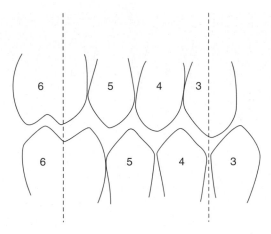

Figure 12.13   Class I molar and canine relationship.

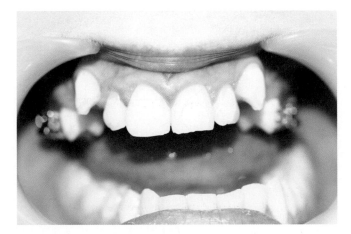

Figure 12.14   Buccally displaced upper canines.

Types of malocclusion

The basic types of malocclusion are caused by a combination of any of the following.

- Crowding.
- Protruding upper incisors.
- Prominent lower jaw.

Crowding

Crowding is caused by insufficient room for all of the teeth to erupt in line and occurs in jaws which are too small to accommodate 32 permanent teeth. The teeth become crooked and overlapping as the permanent dentition erupts, and those which are normally last to erupt cannot take up their proper position in the dental arch as there is insufficient room left. Thus, the upper canines are usually displaced buccally (Figure 12.14), the lower second premolars lingually and the lower third molars are impacted within the bone of the mandible at the ramus.

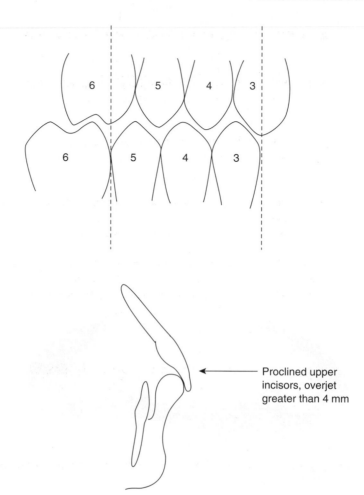

Proclined upper incisors, overjet greater than 4 mm

Figure 12.15   Class II division 1 malocclusion.

Early extraction of carious deciduous molars also contributes to the crowding in these cases. The gap left by an extraction soon closes, as the remaining posterior tooth drifts forward and takes up some of the space required for the permanent successor.

Protruding upper incisors

Many children attend for orthodontic treatment because their upper front teeth protrude (procline) between their lips. This condition usually arises from a jaw relationship in which the upper teeth are too far forward relative to the lowers. It is commonly associated with an open lip posture and is called a *class II division 1 malocclusion* (Figure 12.15).

This tends to occur because the mandible is too far behind its normal position, and not because the maxilla is too far forwards, as may be thought. The maxilla is a fixed bone of the facial skeleton and cannot alter its position during growth, whereas the mandible is the only moveable bone of the skull and its position can alter markedly as it grows and develops.

When the mandible is not so far posterior to its normal position, so that the jaw relationship is not quite so severe, the upper incisors become trapped behind the tightened lower lip and

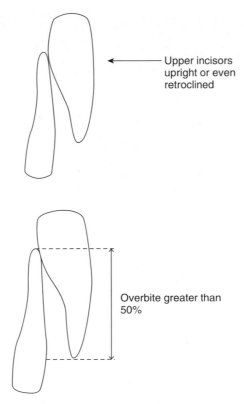

Upper incisors
upright or even
retroclined

Overbite greater than
50%

Figure 12.16 Class II division 2 incisors.

erupt upright, or even pulled back (retroclined). This is called a *class II division 2 malocclusion* (Figure 12.16).

Prominent lower jaw

This condition, in which the chin is unduly prominent, is caused by a jaw relationship in which the mandible and the lower teeth are too far forward relative to the maxilla and the upper teeth. It usually results in the incisors biting edge to edge or with the lowers in front of the uppers, instead of behind them. This is called a *class III malocclusion* (Figure 12.17).

Causes of malocclusion

Most kinds of malocclusion are genetic in origin (so, inherited from a family member); far fewer are acquired. The most common are inheritance of an abnormal jaw relationship or jaw size. Other genetic factors include supernumerary teeth and missing teeth. The most common acquired causes of malocclusion are early loss of teeth and thumb-sucking habits.

Jaw relationship

With a normal (ideal) jaw relationship, the teeth should occlude in a class I relationship as shown in Figures 12.12 and 12.13. This is the most attractive type of occlusion and is accordingly regarded as normal. Other jaw relationships give rise to either a class II or a class III malocclusion.

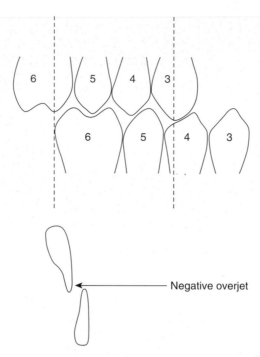

Figure 12.17   Class III malocclusion.

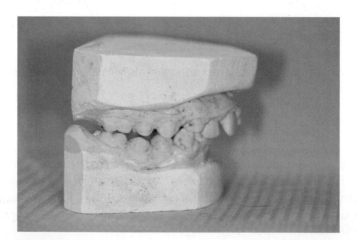

Figure 12.18   Class II division 1 study models.

A jaw relationship in which the lower jaw is too far back causes two different types of class II malocclusion.

- Class II division 1 in which the upper incisors protrude, the overjet is increased and the lower lip is trapped inside the overjet (Figure 12.18).
- Class II division 2 in which the upper central incisors tilt backwards into contact with the lowers, giving a decreased overjet and increased overbite (Figure 12.19), maintained by a strap-like action of the lower lip across the labial surface of the upper incisors.

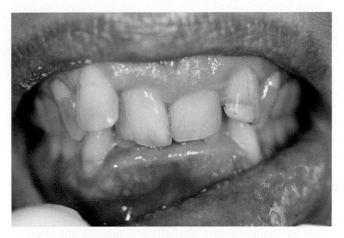

Figure 12.19   Class II division 2 with increased overbite.

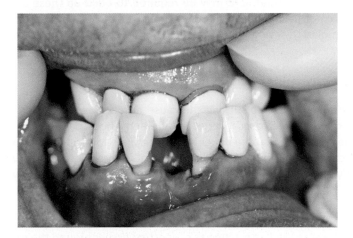

Figure 12.20   Class III with reverse overjet.

A relationship in which the lower jaw is too far forward causes a class III malocclusion. The chin appears prominent and the overjet is reversed, with lower incisors occluding in front of the uppers (Figure 12.20) or, in milder cases, edge to edge.

Angle's classification is based on the relationship of the first molars to each other, as described previously, but this is no longer suitable as the early loss of teeth may cause changes in the position of the first molars. It is more convenient to use the incisor relationship as the determination of classification.

Jaw size

Among the most common abnormalities of all jaw size discrepancies are those jaws which are too small to accommodate all the teeth. This is a genetic cause of crowding which is usually localised to the front teeth whereas the effect of premature loss, described previously, is an acquired cause and is usually localised to the premolar region. Unfortunately, all causes of crowding often occur together, thus producing an even worse malocclusion.

Jaws which are too large cause spacing of the teeth but this type of malocclusion is not so common.

Supernumerary teeth

A supernumerary tooth is an extra one, in addition to the normal complement of 32 teeth. It occurs most commonly in the upper incisor region as a *mesiodens* and may either prevent a central incisor from erupting or cause it to erupt in an abnormal position.

Congenitally missing teeth

This is the opposite condition to supernumerary teeth where a patient is born with an absence of one or more of their permanent teeth. Upper lateral incisors are often missing and orthodontic treatment may be necessary to close the resultant gaps. Sometimes, instead of being absent, upper lateral incisors develop as tiny conical teeth, called *peg laterals*. Again, the appearance is unsightly and restorative treatment may be required to build up these abnormally small lateral incisors to a more normal size. The other teeth which are most commonly missing are third molars and second premolars. If several teeth are missing, the condition is called *hypodontia*, but this is a rare occurrence.

Sucking habits

Habits such as finger or thumb sucking can cause displacement of anterior teeth resulting in a decreased overbite and increased overjet. In addition, the sucking action tends to exert excess pressure on the cheeks, so that the upper buccal teeth are forced to develop inside the arch of the lowers. This is called a *cross-bite*. These displacements may correct themselves if the sucking habit is stopped early enough, otherwise orthodontic treatment will be necessary.

Periodontal tissue assessment

The periodontal tissues are those acting as *supporting tissues* around the tooth – the gingivae, the periodontal ligament and the underlying alveolar bone forming the tooth socket. These tissues can undergo disease processes to varying degrees, and in the worst case scenario healthy teeth can be lost due to periodontal disease. Periodontal disease is the most common dental disease found in adult patients, and its presence can easily be missed or remain undetected for many years due to its slow onset and painless nature.

As with tooth charting, a system has been developed whereby the presence of periodontal disease can be quickly recorded during routine oral assessment, by dividing the mouth into sextants and recording the presence and depth of any unnatural spaces down the side of the teeth – these are called *periodontal pockets*.

This recording technique is called a *BPE assessment* and is noted as shown in Figure 12.21.

Healthy periodontal tissues appear pink, firmly attached to the necks of the teeth with a gingival crevice no deeper than 3 mm, and they do not bleed when touched. Teeth are firmly held in their sockets by the periodontal supporting tissues, and no plaque is present on the tooth surfaces.

Specially designed periodontal probes (such as a BPE probe – Figure 12.22) are used to record the presence and depth of any periodontal pockets discovered in each sextant of the dental arches, and the coding system used is as follows.

Upper teeth		
18–14	13–23	24–28
48–44	43–33	34–38

Lower teeth

Figure 12.21   BPE chart.

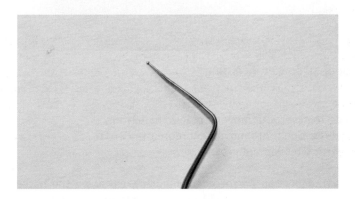

Figure 12.22   BPE probe.

2	0	4
2	1	3

Figure 12.23   Completed BPE chart.

- **Code 0** – healthy gingival tissues with no bleeding on probing.
- **Code 1** – pocket no more than 3.5 mm, bleeding on probing, no calculus nor other plaque retention factor present.
- **Code 2** – pocket no more than 3.5 mm but plaque retention factor detected.
- **Code 3** – pocket present up to 5.5 mm deep.
- **Code 4** – pocket present deeper than 5.5 mm.
- **Code *** – gingival recession or furcation involvement present.

A typical completed BPE chart is shown in Figure 12.23.

Higher codes therefore indicate a more serious periodontal problem, such as that shown in Figure 12.24. Where codes greater than 3 are recorded, a full pocket depth record will be made of each tooth in that sextant so that specific problem areas can be identified, and intensive periodontal treatment can be initiated. In addition, the presence and extent of any plaque found will be recorded, as well as the mobility of any tooth. Tooth mobility is graded as follows.

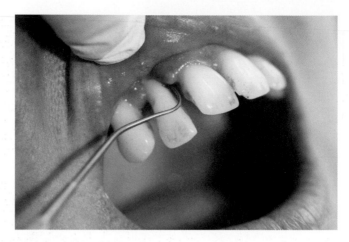

Figure 12.24   Periodontal pocket recording.

- **Grade I** – side-to-side tooth movement less than 2 mm.
- **Grade II** – side-to-side tooth movement more than 2 mm.
- **Grade III** – vertical movement present.

All of these assessments can be recorded manually, either on the patient's record card or on specific pre-printed charts (Figure 12.25), or directly into the relevant files of computerised record systems.

The standard of oral hygiene can be graded as excellent, good, fair or poor, and should be recorded at each oral health assessment so that patient motivation and compliance can be monitored.

Dental radiography

Dental radiography is an important diagnostic tool used in dentistry and medicine to help the clinician to see within the body tissues and help to diagnose the cause of dental and medical problems. In dentistry, radiographs are used to detect and diagnose the following lesions and structures.

- **Dental caries** – this shows up as a dark area of destruction extending inwards from the enamel surface.
- Presence and extent of **periodontal disease** – this shows up as a loss of the lamina dura forming the crest of the alveolar bone, loss of height of the alveolar bone, and a widening of the periodontal ligament space.
- Periodontal and periapical **abscesses** – chronic alveolar abscesses show up as a dark circular area at the apex of an affected tooth, caused by destruction of the apical lamina dura and spongy bone.
- **Cysts** affecting the dental tissues – these can show up as enlarged darker areas surrounding other structures, and can sometimes be seen to be pushing tooth roots out of their normal positions.

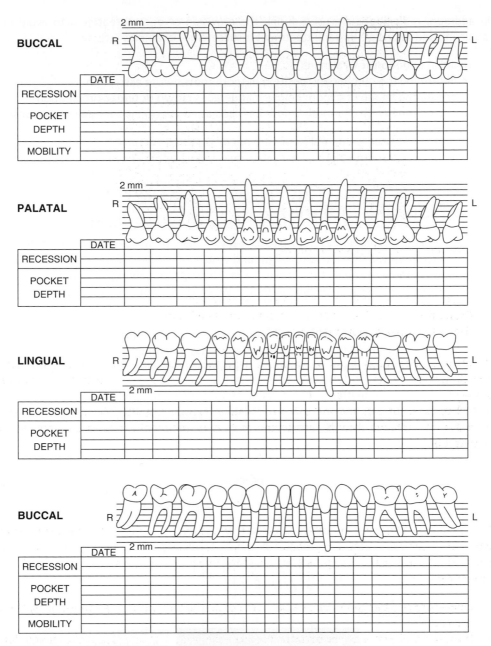

Figure 12.25   Periodontal disease recording chart.

- **Iatrogenic problems** – that is, those caused by the dentist, such as overhanging restorations or tooth perforations by posts.
- To detect **supernumerary** teeth and **unerupted** teeth, or to determine the **congenital absence** of unerupted teeth.
- To diagnose **hard tissue lesions**, such as bone cysts and tumours, salivary calculi and jaw fractures.

In addition, radiographs are used during the provision of dental treatment to avoid problems occurring and to ensure that the treatment is successful – examples include:

- to aid in **endodontic** treatment
- to determine the number and position of tooth roots before **extraction**
- to ensure the health of a tooth before it undergoes **crown or bridge** preparation
- to ensure the health of a tooth before it is used as an abutment during **denture construction**.

For examination purposes, dental nurses are not expected to interpret radiographs but they should be able to describe both normal and abnormal radiographic appearances of common dental conditions.

Nature of ionising radiation

Ionising radiation is commonly referred to as 'x-rays'. X-rays are a type of electromagnetic radiation that possess energy, as are ultraviolet light and visible light. The radiation types differ from each other in the amount of energy they possess, x-rays having more energy so that they are capable of passing through matter such as human tissue. When they do so, one of three events will occur (Figure 12.26).

- X-rays pass cleanly between the atoms of the matter and are **unaltered**.
- X-rays hit the atoms of the matter and are **scattered**, releasing their energy as they do so.
- X-rays hit the atoms of the matter and are **absorbed**, releasing their energy as they do so.

With larger atoms of matter, such as some metals (including calcium), most of the x-rays are absorbed or scattered, and these are *radiopaque* substances. Those which allow the majority of the x-rays to pass through unaffected are called *radiolucent* substances, and include the soft tissues.

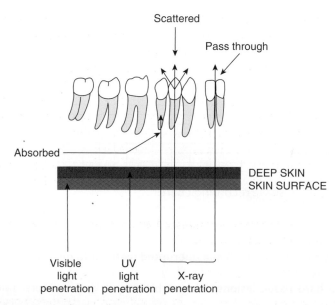

Figure 12.26 Passage of x-rays in human tissue.

As bone and enamel have a high calcium content, and dentine and cementum also contain calcium hydroxyapatite crystals, these tissues are variably radiopaque to x-rays. They show up on processed radiographs as varying shades of white/grey images, the more radiopaque structures being the whitest.

Effect of ionising radiation on the body

The energy released when the x-rays interact with human tissue is capable of causing tissue damage, so it is imperative that x-rays are used only as necessary and at the lowest dose possible, to reduce the amount of energy released and therefore reduce the amount of tissue damage which occurs.

Effects occur when the x-rays hit the atoms of the tissue cells and are either scattered or absorbed, because of the energy that is released during these events. The energy released can cause *tissue damage* to the human tissue cells. The cells contain chromosomes which are made up of our DNA – the building blocks of life that determine exactly the organism that we are, and if the energy hits the chromosomes it can damage them so that they undergo change (*mutation*) or even die.

This ability of x-ray exposure to cause cell death is used in medicine to treat some types of cancer, during radiotherapy treatment. The cancer cells can be accurately targeted to be hit by the ionising radiation beam so that they are killed outright, or so that the cancerous tumour is reduced to a size that can undergo surgical removal. High doses of x-rays are used for this treatment, and tissue cells that divide and grow rapidly, such as skin cells and the body cells of children, are more easily affected.

However, cell death is an undesirable effect during the production of dental images. As there can be no 'safe' level of exposure to ionising radiation (that is, there is always some cell damage caused during x-ray exposure), strict legislation and guidelines have been introduced to ensure that the following occur when x-rays are used in dentistry.

- All use of dental imaging has to be **clinically justified** – so there must be a clinical reason why the patient is being exposed to the x-rays; this will be one of the diagnostic or treatment reasons listed above.
- The dose of x-rays used must be kept **as low as reasonably achievable (ALARA)** – so the minimum dose of x-rays must be used, for the shortest time, and aimed at the smallest area of tissue possible, to produce a functional image.
- This tecnique is now more usually referred to as being **as low as reasonably practicable/ possible (ALARP)**.
- Only the patient should be exposed to the x-ray beam – all staff and family members must be outside the **controlled zone** during the exposure (the only exception being when a parent assists a small child during exposure).
- Machines must be well maintained and serviced regularly.
- No untrained personnel can be involved in radiation exposure procedures.
- **Quality assurance systems** must be operated to ensure that the dental images produced are to a consistently high standard.

The legislation, Health and Safety, and quality assurance aspects of the safe use of dental radiography are all discussed in detail in Chapter 4.

Principles of dental radiography

As stated previously, there are many sound clinical reasons for dental radiographs to be taken in the dental workplace, and their use is particularly invaluable as a diagnostic tool in dentistry.

329

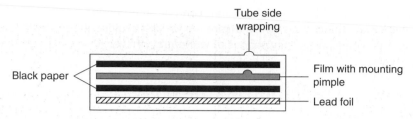

Figure 12.27   Contents of intraoral film packet.

However, to avoid their indiscriminate use, guidelines have been drawn up for the safe prescription of dental radiographs in dental practice, as follows, and must be adhered to by all.

- A history and a clinical examination must be performed before any radiograph is taken.
- Only new patients with clear evidence of some dental disease should have full mouth radiographs taken.
- Regularly attending child patients in the mixed dentition stage who have orthodontic problems developing can be radiographed as necessary.
- Recall patients with a low caries risk should be radiographed no more frequently than every 18 months.
- Those with a moderate caries risk should be radiographed every 12 months.
- Those with a high caries risk should be radiographed at 6-monthly intervals, gradually reducing this rate as the caries is brought under control.
- Patients exhibiting evidence of periodontal disease can have selective radiographs taken of problem areas, as necessary.
- Edentulous patients should only have selective radiographs taken if there are any clinically suspicious areas (such as retained roots or hard tissue lesions).

Types of views used in dental radiography

There are various types of film used in dental radiography, depending on the reason for taking the dental image, but all are either those taken within the oral cavity – *intraoral films* – or those taken outside the oral cavity – *extraoral films*.

    Intraoral films are supplied in child and adult size packets that contain the following (Figure 12.27).

- Plastic envelope to protect the contents from saliva contamination.
- Wrap-around black paper to prevent exposure of the film to light.
- Film, which is exposed to the ionising radiation and produces the dental image once processed or loaded onto the computer (digital imaging).
- Lead foil to prevent scatter of the ionising radiation past the film packet.
- Raised pimple marker on the film and packet side towards the x-ray tube, which is used to correctly determine the left and right side of the image produced (film is mounted with the pimple towards the observer).

The intraoral views that can be produced using these films are as follows.

- **Horizontal bite-wing** (Figure 12.28) – show the posterior teeth in occlusion and are taken to view:
  - ○ interproximal areas and diagnose caries in these regions
  - ○ restoration overhangs in these areas

(a)   (b)

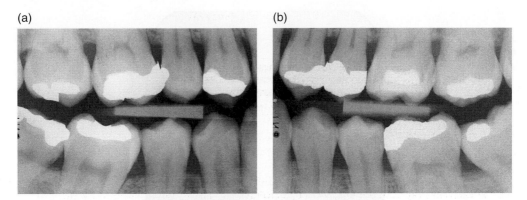

Figure 12.28   Bite-wing radiographs.

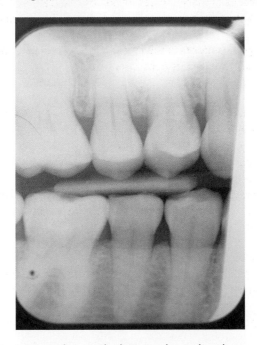

Figure 12.29   Vertical bite-wing radiograph showing bone levels.

- ○ recurrent caries beneath exisiting restorations
- ○ occlusal caries.
- **Vertical bite-wing** (Figure 12.29) – show an extended view of the posterior teeth, from midroot of the uppers to midroot of the lowers as a minimum, and are taken to view:
  - ○ periodontal bone levels of the posterior teeth
  - ○ true periodontal pockets.
- **Periapical** (Figure 12.30) – show one or two teeth in full length with their surrounding bone, and are taken to view the area and the teeth in close detail.
- **Anterior occlusal** (Figure 12.31) – show a plane view of the anterior section of either the mandible or the maxilla, and are used especially to view the area for unerupted teeth, supernumerary teeth and cysts.

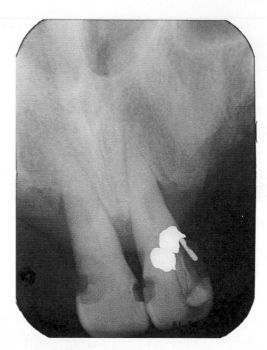

Figure 12.30   Periapical radiograph.

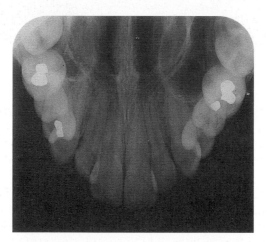

Figure 12.31   Maxillary anterior occlusal radiograph.

Extraoral films are used to produce much larger images showing many structures, and are supplied in cassettes that contain the following (Figure 12.32).

- Cassette case that is loaded into special imaging machines for use.
- Intensifying screens in both sides of the cassette, to reduce the dose of radiation exposure required to produce a dental image.
- Film, of a type compatible with the intensifying screens, to produce the dental image once exposed and processed.
- Marker to correctly determine the left and right side of the image produced.

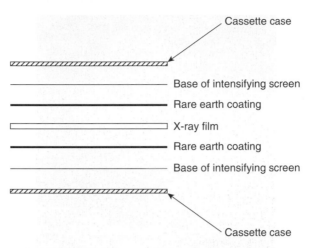

Figure 12.32   Contents of extraoral cassette.

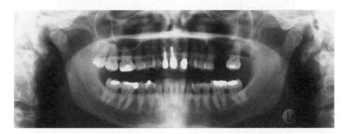

Figure 12.33   Dental panoramic tomograph.

Extraoral films are packed differently from intraoral films. The latter are individually packed in light-proof wrappers but extraoral film is not. Packets of extraoral film only contain unwrapped film and can only be opened in a darkroom. On removal from the packet in the darkroom, a film is placed immediately in the special light-proof container or *cassette*, which is then kept closed ready for use.

A typical cassette opens like a book and the film is placed in the middle. On each inside cover of the cassette there is a white plastic sheet called an *intensifying screen*, and the film is sandwiched between the two screens when the cassette is closed ready for use. The screens *fluoresce* on exposure to x-rays, and the brightness of the fluorescence creates the image on the film itself, rather than being produced by the actual x-ray beam. This allows the use of a reduced exposure time of x-rays to the patient, making the technique safer.

The extraoral views that can be produced using these films are the following.

- **Dental panoramic tomograph (DPT)** (Figure 12.33) – shows both jaws in full and their surrounding bony anatomy, and is taken for orthodontic and wisdom tooth assessments, as well as to help diagnose pathology and jaw fractures.
- **Lateral oblique** – shows the posterior portion of one side of the mandible, including the ramus and angle and the lower molar teeth, and is an alternative to a DPT to view the position of unerupted third molar teeth (it is used infrequently now, as the image produced on a well-aligned DPT is far superior).

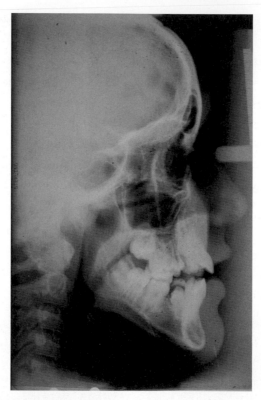

Figure 12.34 Lateral skull radiograph.

- **Lateral skull radiograph** (Figure 12.34) – this is a view of the side of the head, taken in a specialised machine called a *cephalostat* (which may be present as an attachment to a DPT machine or as a 'stand-alone' device), and is used to monitor jaw growth and determine orthognathic surgery techniques in complicated cases of malocclusion.

When DPTs initially became widely available to the dental profession, they were called 'orthopantomographs' and referred to as OPGs or OPTs – these abbreviations are still in current use in some areas.

Radiographic techniques

Any dental image is produced by the correct placing of the film on the far side of the area to be exposed from the x-ray machine. In other words, the radiation beam passes from the machine through the area to be exposed and then hits the film inside either the plastic envelope or the cassette.

Intraoral films are held in the correct position by the use of film holder devices where possible, as shown in Figures 12.35 and 12.36. These are correctly loaded with the film packet and placed inside the oral cavity for the patient to bite upon so that the radiograph can be produced (Figure 12.37). If a digital imaging technique is used, the film is replaced by a special sensor that is positioned in exactly the same way, but instead of an exposed film being produced which is then

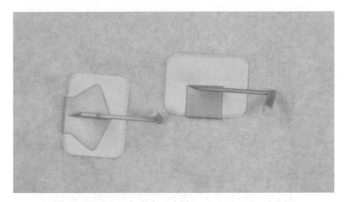

Figure 12.35   Bite-wing holders – loaded.

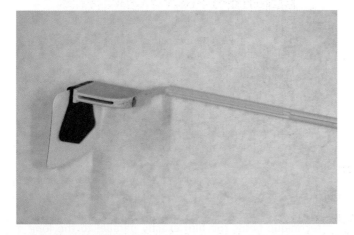

Figure 12.36   Posterior periapical holder – loaded.

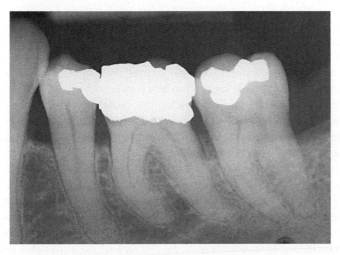

Figure 12.37   Posterior periapical radiograph.

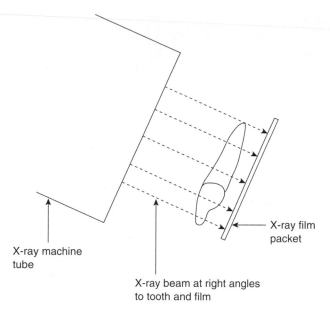

X-ray film
packet

X-ray machine
tube

X-ray beam at right angles
to tooth and film

Figure 12.38   Paralleling technique.

chemically processed, the digital image is transmitted directly to a computer where it can be viewed immediately.

Intraoral films can be exposed in one of two angulations, depending upon which is the best technique for the given clinical situation. They are called the *paralleling* technique and the *bisecting angle* technique.

The paralleling technique holds the film exactly parallel to the long axis of the tooth being exposed, so that the image produced is exactly the same size as the actual tooth. This is especially important during endodontic procedures, when the correct diagnostic length of the tooth has to be determined to ensure accurate root filling of the canal (Figure 12.38).

Sometimes the film cannot be placed parallel to the tooth, because of the size restriction of the patient's mouth. In these situations the bisecting angle technique is used. The film is placed intraorally and the angulation of the long axis of the tooth against the film is determined by the operator. This angle is then halved (bisected) and the collimator of the tube head is angled to be at right angles to it (Figure 12.39), before the film is exposed.

Anterior occlusal views are produced using the bisecting angle technique, with the patient holding the actual film packet between the teeth anteriorly, as illustrated in Figure 12.40.

Lateral oblique cassettes are held in position by the patient's hand, on the far side of the head from the radiation machine, and angled so that the x-ray beam passes up through the angle of the jaw on that side, so that the third molar teeth on that side only are exposed (Figure 12.41).

Extraoral DPT film cassettes are loaded into their special radiation machines, and then the patient is accurately placed within the machine and the cassette is revolved around their head during the exposure process (Figure 12.42). Both types of extraoral film are processed in the same way as intraoral films, either manually or by the use of an automatic processing machine, as described later.

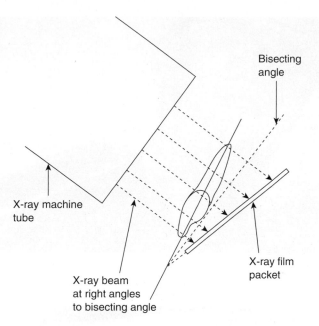

Figure 12.39   Bisecting angle technique.

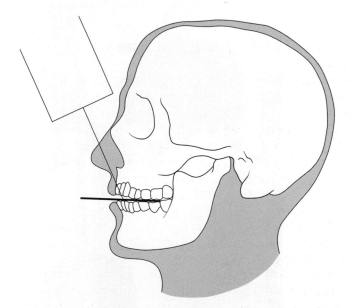

Figure 12.40   Maxillary anterior occlusal positioned. (*Dental Radiography*, 2nd edn, N.J.D. Smith, Blackwell Science Ltd, Oxford. Used with permission).

Digital radiography

Conventional x-ray techniques rely on the use of a chemically coated plastic film being exposed to the x-ray beam, and then processed in a dark room or an automatic processor, using special chemicals to produce the image permanently onto the film.

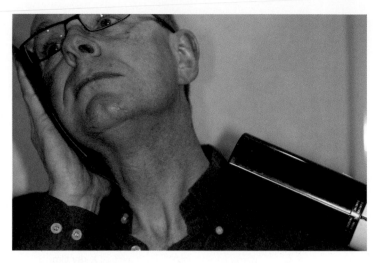

338

Figure 12.41   Lateral oblique position.

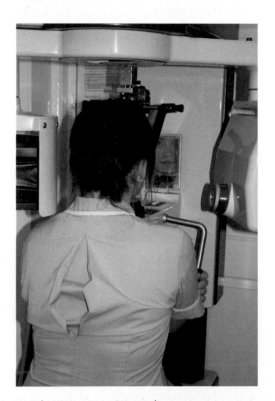

Figure 12.42   DPT machine with patient positioned.

Digital radiography avoids the use of both the chemically coated plastic film and the need for processing it, as the x-ray beam is fired at a special sensor plate instead (Figure 12.43), which then relays the image directly to a computer screen on the surgery worktop (Figure 12.44). The reusable intraoral sensor plate is used instead of film and the radiation dose is far less than

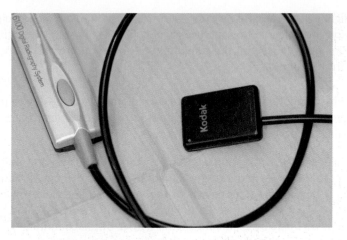

Figure 12.43   Digital sensor plate.

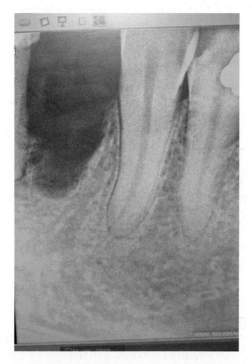

Figure 12.44   Digital image on computer screen.

with ordinary film. It is a technique similar to the use of digital cameras to produce photographic images that can then be loaded onto the computer either from a memory card or from a scanner.

The sensor plate is the same size as whichever intraoral view is being taken – bite-wing, periapical or occlusal. It is positioned exactly the same in the patient's mouth, using holders so that a paralleling technique is possible. The plate is connected directly to the computer via a cable, and the image produced is visible on the screen within seconds.

Extraoral digital views can also be taken with specialised radiography equipment, but their size and cost are considerable and they are usually only found in hospital radiography departments.

The digital image produced on the computer screen can be treated in the same way as digital photographs from a camera.

- Stored on the computer hard drive or transferred onto a storage device (disk or flash drive).
- Printed onto paper and stored as a hard copy in the patient's record card.
- Sent via email to be viewed by other colleagues.

However, as with digital photographs, the image can be adjusted and edited on the computer screen, and this raises issues in dentolegal situations where an image can be enhanced to make a clinical case look better than it actually is or the image can be selectively deleted so that poor-quality treatment is not so apparent. Fortunately, computer experts would be able to detect that alterations had been made by examining the hard drive of the computer.

Digital radiographic techniques are now popular but have not fully superseded conventional techniques in the dental workplace, and many still rely on x-ray films that have been processed either manually or with an automatic processor, such as a Velopex machine. The advantages and disadvantages of digital radiographs are shown below.

Advantages

- Financial savings of not having to buy film packets and processing chemicals and equipment.
- Avoidance of health and safety issues surrounding Control of Substances Hazardous to Health (COSHH) and the handling of the processing chemicals.
- Help towards achieving ALARA/ALARP as the use of the sensor always ensures a lower dose of radiation than if conventional film is used.
- The image is produced in seconds at the chair side, rather than several minutes in the processing area.
- The patient is able to view the magnified image on the computer screen, at the chair side and with the dentist.
- The magnified image can give greater clarity in some instances.
- The same sensor can be used over and over again, as long as adequate infection control techniques are in place to avoid cross-infection.

Disadvantages

- The issue of adequate infection control to avoid cross-infection.
- Financial implications of buying the computer with suitable specifications for use with the digital radiography software, the computer software itself (including any updates), and the sensor plates and their attachments.
- The ability to alter the image without detection raises dentolegal concerns in complaint and fraud cases, unless an expert is employed to examine the computer hard drive.

Formation of the conventional image

An intraoral x-ray film packet contains a celluloid film coated with light-sensitive silver bromide salts in an emulsion, surrounded by black paper to protect it from unwanted light and enclosed in a waterproof plastic packet. On one side of the film is a lead foil which prevents the emulsion coat being exposed twice, by absorbing scattered radiation during the actual exposure to x-rays.

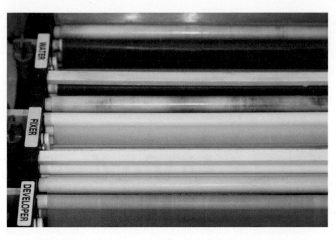

Figure 12.45   Velopex processing machine – internal detail.

The passage of the x-rays through the tissue causes the energy release discussed earlier, and an exact pattern of the tissue is produced within the chemicals on the film itself, as a *latent* (hidden) image, with radiopaque tissues causing the most energy release and therefore a clearer (white) image. Unless a digital imaging technique is used, the latent image can only be seen on the film by the use of special chemicals to make it visible during the processing procedure, in much the same way that conventional photographs from a camera are developed before being able to be viewed as prints.

Film processing

As discussed above, intraoral digital images are transmitted directly to the computer and can be viewed within seconds, on the computer screen. All other films require chemical processing to convert the latent image to a visible image for viewing, and this can be done using an automatic processing machine or by manual processing, with the film being passed through the chemical tanks by hand and in the correct sequence.

Automatic processing

The machine consists of a base containing the chemical and water tanks, with a conveyor belt style of rollers that carry the film through the machine during processing (Figure 12.45). These are all beneath a removable, light-tight lid which has hand entry ports so that the film packet or cassette can be put into the light-tight environment before being opened. If the film is exposed to visible light before being processed, the image will be permanently lost.

The procedure of automatic processing is as follows.

- Observe the warning light system to check that the chemical and water levels are adequate, and that the temperature is correct for processing (Figure 12.46).
- When the temperature is correct, the warning light will go out and the machine is ready for use.
- Intraoral film packets are taken into the machine through the hand ports, while wearing clean gloves.
- Extraoral cassettes are placed into this section by lifting and replacing the lid, and then can be opened and handled via the hand ports.

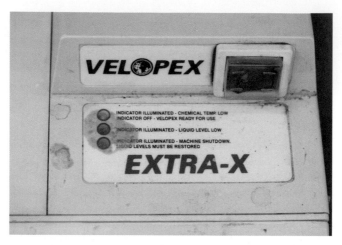

Figure 12.46   Velopex warning lights.

- The rollers become operational once the processing start button is pressed.
- The film packet is carefully opened and the plastic envelope, black paper and lead foil are all dropped to the base of the tank, for removal later.
- The film is then held by its sides only, as finger marks on the surface will damage the image.
- The film is carefully inserted into the entrance to the rollers, and it will be gently tugged into the machine to be processed.
- Once the film has passed through the machine, been processed and dried, it will reappear at the delivery port and can be safely handled and viewed.

Manual processing

Although the vast majority of dental workplaces use automatic processing machines or digital radiography techniques, it is important for the dental nurse know about the manual processing technique, so that it can be carried out safely and effectively whenever necessary.

Manual processing follows the same procedure as that occurring in an automatic processor, but is carried out by hand and in a 'dark room' – a light-tight lockable room containing the processing chemicals and water tanks, sitting in a main water tank that is heated and maintained in the correct temperature range of 18–22 °C.

Four tanks will be present (Figure 12.47).

- **Lidded developing tank** – containing the alkaline developing fluid that produces the initial **latent image**; the lid is only removed during developing as the solution will deteriorate in air.
- The image is still unstable in visible light at this point.
- **First water tank** – to wash off the developing solution after the correct developing time, using tap water.
- **Fixing tank** – containing the acid fixing solution which permanently fixes the image onto the celluloid film, so that it can be viewed in visible light.
- **Second water tank** – to wash off the fixing solution after the suitable fixing time, again using tap water.

Some vision is required within the room, so an orange or red *safe light* will be present under which the processing can be carried out without exposing the film to actual visible light, thereby ruining

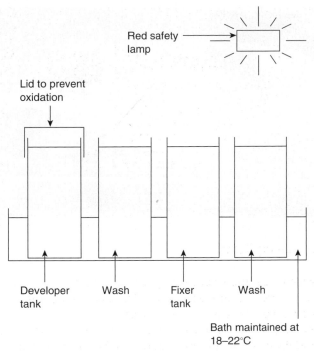

Red safety lamp

Lid to prevent oxidation

Developer tank

Wash

Fixer tank

Wash

Bath maintained at 18–22°C

Figure 12.47   Darkroom layout.

the image. The room must be lockable from within so that the door cannot be opened by anyone else, resulting in the accidental exposure of the film to light and the destruction of the image before it has been fully processed.

The procedure of manual processing is as follows.

- Check that the chemical and water levels are adequate.
- Check the temperature of the solutions, and determine the developing and fixing times required from the chemical manufacturers' guidelines.
- Check that a timing clock and suitable film hangers are available in the room.
- Wipe surfaces dry of any previously spilt chemicals or water, if necessary.
- Lock the door and switch off all lights except the safe light.
- Open the film packet or cassette, locate the film and clip it to one of the hangers available, carefully handling the film by its edges only, to avoid spoiling it with fingerprints.
- Remove the developer lid, immerse the hanger into the solution so that the film is completely covered by the solution, and start the timer.
- When the timer sounds, remove the hanger and film and immerse in the first water tank, agitating the hanger to ensure thorough washing occurs.
- Shake off excess water, then fully immerse the hanger and film into the fixer solution, and start the timer.
- Replace the developer lid to prevent the solution being weakened by exposure to air, which would allow oxidation to occur.
- When the timer sounds, remove the hanger and film and immerse in the second water tank, agitating the hanger to ensure thorough washing occurs.

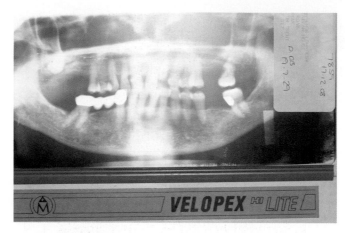

Figure 12.48   Viewing screen.

- Switch on the ordinary light.
- Shake off excess water and dry the film – a slow-running hairdryer is suitable for this, as the radiograph must not be dried too quickly.

Once dry, the films can be correctly mounted as necessary and returned to the dentist for viewing.

Mounting and viewing films

Once the films have been successfully processed, they will be viewed by the dentist so that diagnoses can be made and treatment plans formulated. Ideally, a light box and magnifier will be available for viewing the films (Figure 12.48), but it is imperative that they are mounted and positioned correctly, otherwise the left teeth will be viewed as the right, and vice versa.

Extraoral cassettes are marked with an 'L' to indicate the patient's left side and unless the cassette has been placed upside down in the machine, the film is easily orientated on the viewer so that it is viewed as if looking at the patient from the front (see Figure 12.33).

Various plastic envelope designs are available to mount all types of intraoral films nowadays, but they must be loaded correctly by the dental nurse first. All intraoral films have a raised pimple in one corner which must be facing out to view the film correctly, and not back to front. It is irrelevant which corner of the film the pimple appears in, but it must face out towards the person viewing the radiograph.

Also, the dental nurse should use their knowledge of oral anatomy to check themselves – molar teeth are posterior to all other teeth so correct mounting of bite-wing films, for instance, should result in the molar teeth appearing on the outer side of both films, with their pimples palpable in one corner (see Figure 12.28). Upper periapical films should be mounted with the roots above the crowns of the teeth, as they are in the patient's maxilla (Figure 12.49), and so on.

Dental workplaces are likely to use one of the various different methods of patient identification and storage of the films, and the dental nurse has to be aware of the methods in use in their workplace and use them appropriately. These may include any of the following.

- Digital images will be stored on computer or downloaded onto disks.
- Intraoral films may be mounted in plastic envelopes, with patient identification details written in indelible ink.

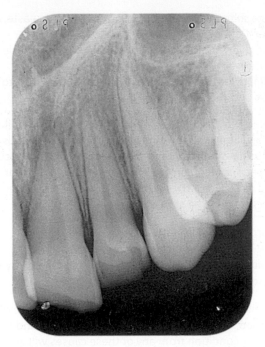

Figure 12.49 Periapical radiograph.

- These may be stored within each patient's record card and filed.
- If clinical notes are computerised, there may be a separate filing system used exclusively for films.
- Extraoral films may be too large to store within the record cards, so may also have their own exclusive filing system.

Whichever system is used, all films must be marked with the patient's identification details (such as name, computer number, etc.), the date the image was taken, and a note of the view used, before being stored or filed.

Care of processing equipment and film packets

One of a dental nurse's many duties will be to care for all processing equipment, once trained adequately to do so. This is a vital role with regard to patient safety; poorly maintained equipment will lead to poor-quality radiographs that may need to be retaken, causing unnecessary x-ray exposure for the patient. And as stated previously, there is no 'safe level' of x-ray exposure – each one could cause cell damage. The following list summarises the points that should be included in any care and maintenance protocol.

- Ensure adequate training in processing techniques has been given.
- Always carry out the pre-processing checks correctly.
- Always wear suitable personal protective equipment (PPE) when handling all processing chemicals, as they are toxic.
- Follow the surgery policy on topping up and changing spent solutions; normally all will require full replacement on a monthly basis.

- Dispose of all waste solutions as **non-infectious hazardous waste**, under the Health and Safety policy (see Chapter 4).
- Follow the training given and the manufacturer's guidelines on cleaning the processing area or the automatic processor, to avoid film contamination.
- This is especially important with regard to the roller system in automatic machines, as films can stick to dirty rollers and their images will be destroyed.

Be aware of the correct functioning of the equipment, so that failures can be recognised, the equipment switched off safely and the matter reported to the necessary person for repair.

In addition, poor-quality or unreadable radiographs will be produced if old film stock is used or if the stock has not been stored correctly. Films can still deteriorate before their expiry date if stored in hot or damp places, or if they are kept too near an x-ray set.

Unexposed film packets must be stored as follows.

- Away from all sources of radiation.
- Away from all heat sources, and ideally at room temperature.
- Away from all liquids that may penetrate the packets and destroy the films before use.
- In stock rotation, so that older films are used first.

If an expiry date is given on a packet of film it should not be used beyond that date. Any remaining films should be discarded, as old film will not expose correctly and the image produced will be of poor quality. Film in poor condition from any of these causes will give a radiograph of poor quality which may have to be retaken.

Exposure faults

Although many practices have abandoned manual processing in favour of automatic methods, it is still necessary for all dental nurses to understand what happens to a film during exposure and processing. This will help to run quality assurance systems that will trace any causes of error and prevent the need for retakes.

Faults that occur during exposure are the responsibility of the operator taking the view.

Any part of a film exposed to x-rays or white light is turned black and opaque by developer. The remaining unexposed part is still sensitive to light and appears green and opaque. Fixer dissolves away the unexposed green part, leaving it completely transparent and no longer sensitive to light. Some common faults that occur during exposure are listed in Table 12.1, some of which are shown in Figure 12.50.

Handling faults

Faults can also occur due to poor handling technique or poor preparation of the processing equipment – these are both the responsibility of the dental nurse tasked with processing the exposed film. All of these faults are avoidable by adequate training and by following procedures accurately. Some common handling faults are listed in Table 12.2, some of which are shown in Figure 12.51.

Processing faults

Poor-quality radiographs can also be produced due to equipment preparation faults, and especially by lack of solution preparation and maintenance of the automatic processor. As the majority of film processing will be undertaken by the dental nurse in the workplace, knowledge of the

Table 12.1   Some common faults that occur during exposure

Fault	Reason
Elongation of image (Figure 12.50a)	Collimator angulation is too shallow, producing a long image
Foreshortening of image (Figure 12.50b)	Collimator angulation is too steep, producing a squat image
Coning (Figure 12.50c)	Collimator angulation is not central to the film, so film is only partly exposed
Blurred image	Patient or collimator moved during exposure
Transparent film or faint image with overlying pattern (Figure 12.50d)	Film placed the wrong way round to the collimator for exposure, with the lead foil pattern superimposed onto the film – this may not always appear as the traditional 'herringbone' pattern
Fogged film	Exposed to light before x-ray exposure (this may occur with extraoral films, as they are being loaded into the cassette)
Blank film	X-ray machine not switched on, although this is unlikely to happen with modern machines, as they have exposure lights and audio signals installed

faults, their occurrence and avoidance, and correct processing techniques should be basic topics of study and understanding for every dental nurse.

Some common processing faults are listed in Table 12.3, some of which are shown in Figure 12.52.

Every radiograph must not only be clinically justified but also of diagnostic value, so that an accurate diagnosis can be made and treatment planned accordingly. There should be no need for retakes because of faulty exposure or handling techniques, or poor processing skills. Retakes mean unnecessary additional exposure of patients and staff to x-rays. To ensure perfect results, the films must be in good condition, exposed correctly, processed carefully and mounted properly.

Quality assurance of films

All the faults described previously are avoidable. However, the dental team may not realise that a recurring problem exists unless radiographs are regularly checked for quality, and this is especially so in large, multi-dentist surgeries. A processing fault may affect the radiographs of several dentists but unless someone is analysing the radiographs from all surgeries, it can easily be overlooked. This is the purpose of a quality assurance system, in which *all* radiographs are analysed and scored according to a universal system of quality so that commonly occurring problems will be identified.

The running of a quality assurance system of radiographs is a very important task that is often allocated to the dental nurse, and it is described in detail in Chapter 4.

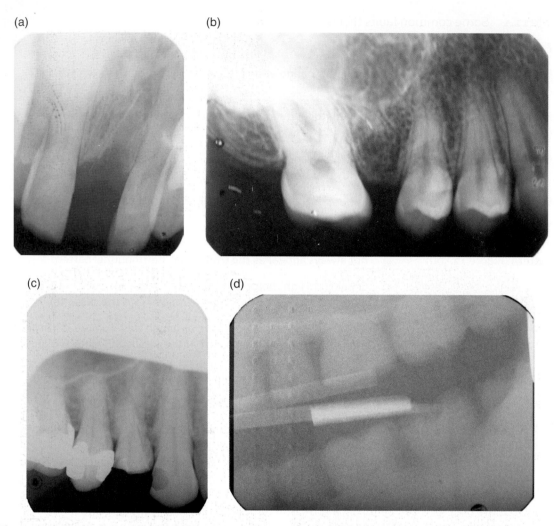

Figure 12.50 Radiograph exposure faults. (a) Elongation. (b) Foreshortening. (c) Coning. (d) Reversed film.

Table 12.2 Some common handling faults

Faults	Reasons
Scratches or fingerprints (Figure 12.51a)	Catching the film on the tank side during immersion Not holding the film by the edges
Blank spots (Figure 12.51b)	Film splashed with fixer before developing
Black line across film	Film bent or folded during processing
Brown or green stains	Inadequate fixing due to old solution
Crazed pattern on film (Figure 12.51c)	Film dried too quickly over a strong heat source
Presence of crystals on film (Figure 12.51d)	Insufficient washing after fixing

349

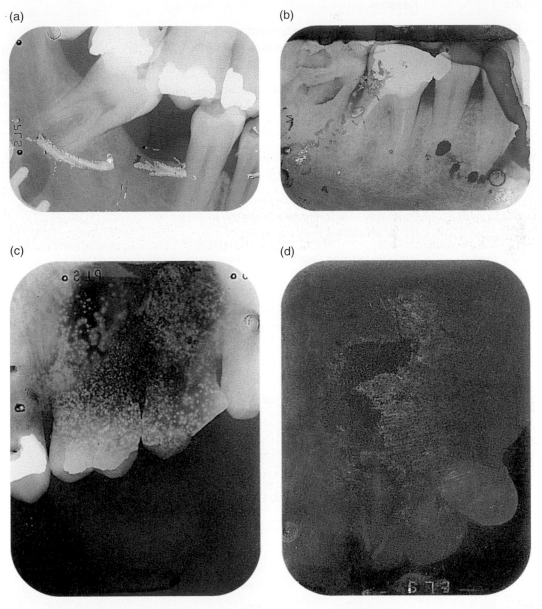

Figure 12.51 Radiograph handling faults. (a) Scratched. (b) Splashed. (c) Crazed. (d) Insufficient washing.

Table 12.3 Some common processing faults

Faults	Reasons
Dark film (Figure 12.52a)	Developer solution too concentrated Developer solution temperature too high Overdeveloped
Blank film (Figure 12.52b)	Film placed in fixer solution before developer solution, so the image is destroyed
Partly blank film	Film partially immersed in developer solution
Fogged film (Figure 12.52c)	Processing room or machine is not light-tight, so the film is exposed to light before processing
Faint image (Figure 12.52d)	Developer solution too weak Developer solution temperature too low Underdeveloped
Fading image	Inadequate fixing time so image is not permanently held on the film
Loss of film	Film stuck in roller system due to poor cleaning and maintenance of automatic processor
Visible artefacts	Film contaminated with solution spillages, in cassettes or on work surfaces

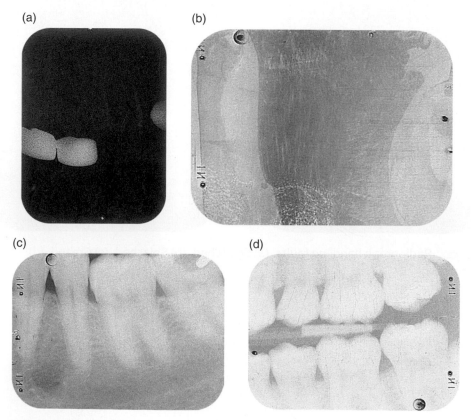

Figure 12.52 Radiograph processing faults. (a) Dark film. (b) Blank film. (c) Fogged film. (d) Faint film.

Conclusion

For each patient who attends the dental workplace, an oral health assessment will guide the dentist towards diagnosing the presence of an oral disease, and help to formulate a treatment plan where necessary or to refer on for specialist tests and treatment in some cases. Not every patient will have to undergo every assessment method described, and the dentist will use their professional knowledge and discretion in each case to determine the assessment, diagnosis and treatment planning required. The role of the dental nurse is to understand the need for the various assessments, and to be able to assist the dentist and patient while they are carried out, as well as to accurately record all the findings in each case.

Further resources are available for this book, including interactive multiple choice questions and extended matching questions. Visit the companion website at:

www.levisonstextbookfordentalnurses.com

13

Oral Health Promotion and Disease Prevention

Key learning points

A **factual knowledge** of
- the role of bacterial plaque in dental disease

A **working knowledge** of
- the methods available to control bacterial plaque
- dietary advice to control caries incidence
- the use of fluoride in caries prevention
- the modification of risk factors to control periodontal disease
- the use of communication skills in oral health evaluation, motivation and promotion
- the effect of general health on oral health

A **factual awareness** of
- the genetic predisposition to periodontal disease

As discussed in Chapter 11, the main oral diseases of concern to the dental team are as follows.

- **Dental caries** – the bacterial infection of the mineralised tissues of the tooth.
- **Gingivitis** – the inflammation of the gingival tissues at the neck of the tooth.
- **Periodontitis** – the inflammation of the supporting structures of the tooth.
- **Oral cancer** – the malignancy specific to the oral cavity that presents as squamous cell carcinoma (this accounts for 90% of oral cancers, although others do occur).

Levison's Textbook for Dental Nurses, Eleventh Edition. By Carole Hollins.
© 2013 John Wiley & Sons, Ltd. Published 2013 by John Wiley & Sons, Ltd. Companion website: www.levisonstextbookfordentalnurses.com

A huge part of the day-to-day work of the dental team is to educate patients in the risk factors of these four diseases, so that they can avoid their initial onset or avoid their recurrence once treatment has resolved any diagnosed disease that was present.

The success of this 'dental education' depends on various factors, listed below, some of which are outside the control of the dental team.

- **Communication skills** – irrespective of how important the advice is to the patient, if it is delivered in a way that the patient cannot understand, it will not be followed.
- **Age group** – the style of communication and the advice to be given will vary between age groups, and these groups are generally divided into:
  - adults
  - young people
  - children.
- **Patient motivation** – despite the best attempts by the dental team, some patients are simply uninterested in their own oral health, and are unwilling to participate in efforts to assist them in achieving good oral health.
- **General health** – some medical and physical conditions (including old age) will affect the likelihood of oral disease development in some patients, while other conditions will affect the patient's ability to carry out effective oral hygiene methods.

All of these factors and their influence on the patient's standard of oral health will be discussed here, but throughout and in following chapters it will be seen that the old adage holds true:'*Prevention is better than cure*'. Self-help by patients, supported by the robust oral health efforts of the dental team, is much easier to achieve and obviously better than suffering the pain, misery and expense of dental disease and its necessary treatment.

Bacterial plaque as a risk factor in dental disease

As discussed in detail in Chapter 11, the presence of bacterial dental plaque is a prerequisite for the development of all three of the main dental diseases (dental caries, gingivitis and periodontitis), in addition to other causative factors as described below.

The causative factors of dental caries are:

- a diet containing a high proportion of non-milk extrinsic sugars (NMEs)
- poor oral hygiene allowing the accumulation of dental plaque and the bacteria it contains
- stagnation areas of the teeth themselves such as occlusal fissures, overhanging restorations and abutments with dentures and orthodontic appliances
- the action of the bacteria on the NMEs to produce acid, which demineralises the tooth structure and allows cavities to develop.

The causative factors of gingivitis and periodontitis are:

- poor oral hygiene which allows the accumulation of dental plaque, specifically in the gingival crevice and periodontal pockets, and on any pre-existing surface of tartar
- the existence of stagnation areas, including the gingival crevice, which allows the plaque to accumulate specifically around the necks of the teeth against the gingiva
- failure to treat and eradicate the subsequent gingivitis allows inflammation of the periodontal supporting structures, leading to periodontitis.

Dental plaque

The full name is bacterial dental plaque but in general usage, and hereafter, it is simply referred to as plaque. As it plays such an important part in dental disease, its origin and effects should be clearly understood by all whose work involves dental treatment or dental health education.

Plaque is a thin transparent layer of saliva, oral debris and normal mouth bacteria which sticks to the tooth surface and can only be removed by cleaning. It is replaced within a few hours by a new deposit of plaque, and its presence in the mouth may be regarded as a natural occurrence. The harm it causes comes from food debris which sticks to the plaque during meals and snacks and provides a plentiful supply of nourishment for its bacteria and other micro-organisms. They accordingly flourish, the plaque grows thicker, and caries and periodontal disease begin.

Which of the two diseases predominates depends on the following factors, but the plaque is the same whichever disease occurs.

- The site of the plaque.
- The diet, and specifically the presence of NMEs.
- The age of the patient.

If the plaque is in contact with a tooth surface, caries will develop there unless the plaque is removed. If the plaque is in contact with the gingiva, gingivitis and then periodontitis will develop unless the plaque is removed.

Caries is mainly a disease of children and young adults whereas periodontal disease predominates in later life. The difference is caused by the rate at which the two diseases progress. Caries can cause loss of teeth within a few years whereas periodontal disease may take decades to have the same effect. By the time periodontal disease has reached an advanced stage, the earlier onslaught of caries has already been overcome and is no longer a problem, as the teeth which were susceptible to caries have already been treated by exposure to fluoride, fissure sealing, filling or other restoration, or extraction.

Another reason explaining which disease predominates in each age group is the diet they tend to follow. Consumption of sweets and sugary food and drinks is probably far greater, and far less controlled, in children and young people, and their teeth are consequently much more vulnerable to caries. However, it must not be assumed that adults and older people are immune to caries. It still occurs if childhood patterns of unrestricted, indiscriminate consumption of sweets persist. A typical example is the adult smoker who continually sucks mints after giving up the habit for health reasons – and then develops rampant caries affecting the buccal tooth surfaces, as the sugary mints dissolve and wash over the teeth.

Likewise, an aggressive form of periodontal disease can also occur in juveniles, although it is relatively uncommon.

The role of saliva in dental disease development

As discussed in Chapters 10 and 11, saliva is the watery secretion from the salivary glands that bathes the oral cavity to keep the tissues moist. It also protects against:

- caries by promoting remineralisation of early enamel caries
- periodontal disease by its cleansing and antibacterial properties

and promotes overall health of the mouth by its lubricating and cleansing effects.

People suffering from the condition of xerostomia (or dry mouth) do not benefit from these effects and are accordingly at much greater risk of both caries and periodontal disease. This disorder is covered in greater detail later.

Prevention of dental disease

As indicated previously, caries occurs due to a combination of certain types of bacteria being present within dental plaque that use NMEs to produce acids that cause enamel demineralisation, There are therefore three main areas of caries prevention available to the patient and dental team.

- **Increase the tooth resistance to acid attack** – by incorporating fluoride into the enamel structure.
- **Modify the diet** – to include fewer cariogenic foods and drinks, and to reduce their frequency of intake.
- **Control the build-up of bacterial plaque** – practise its regular removal by using good oral hygiene techniques.

The main cause of periodontal disease is consistently poor oral hygiene, along with contributory factors such as smoking, and in some cases an unfortunate genetic predisposition to periodontal problems.

The prevention of periodontal disease can be achieved in most patients, whereas it can only be controlled in others.

- **Control the build-up of bacterial plaque** –practise its regular removal by using good oral hygiene techniques.
- **Modify the contributory factors** – by giving advice on smoking cessation, for instance.
- **Control the host response** – in patients predisposed to periodontal problems, by more frequent dental attendance for monitoring and evaluation, and intervention where necessary.

It can be seen that controlling the build-up of bacterial plaque is a common requirement in the prevention of both dental caries and periodontal disease (including gingivitis). Educating patients in how to successfully remove bacterial plaque, on a daily basis and for the rest of their lives, is the most important aim of the dental team in helping their patients maintain a good standard of oral health.

Control of bacterial plaque

Plaque forms within hours on newly cleaned tooth surfaces, due to the action of oral bacteria on foods. Unless removed from these areas, the plaque will allow dental caries to develop, while that formed around the gingival crevice will be involved in the onset of gingivitis and eventually periodontitis.

Controlling bacterial plaque on a daily basis is the main method by which patients can promote their oral health. It is the role of the dental team to ensure that patients are taught the correct oral hygiene methods suitable to them, and that they carry them out on a frequent enough basis to avoid damage to their oral health.

Plaque can be easily removed by the patient at home by carrying out a combination of the following oral hygiene techniques on a daily basis.

- **Tooth brushing**, using a recommended **toothpaste**.
- **Interdental cleaning**.
- Using **suitable mouthwashes**.

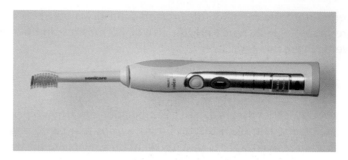

Figure 13.1   Sonicare toothbrush.

Tooth brushing

Tooth brushing is the method used to remove supragingival plaque and food debris from the smooth surfaces of the teeth – that is, the buccal, labial, lingual, palatal and occlusal surfaces, as well as the gingival crevice. Unless the patient has widely spaced teeth, the interdental areas will require special techniques of cleaning to remove plaque efficiently.

- Toothbrushes with a small head and multi-tufted medium nylon bristles are probably the most effective for the vast majority of patients.
- Good-quality, rechargeable electric toothbrushes take the need for consistently good manual techniques away from the patient, and are more likely to achieve prolonged high standards of oral hygiene (Figure 13.1).
- The brush is rinsed to wet the bristles and a portion of the recommended toothpaste added (see below).
- Each dental arch is divided into three sections: left and right sides, and front.
- Side sections are subdivided into buccal, lingual and occlusal surfaces; front into labial and lingual.
- When instructing patients, these areas should be referred to in terms the patient can understand – such as 'cheek side', 'tongue side', 'lip side', and so on.
- This amounts to eight groups of surfaces in each jaw, and at least 5 sec should be spent on each group.
- Egg timers or similar devices can give the patient an idea of how long the recommended 2-min brushing cycle actually is. Some electric brushes have a timer incorporated into their design.
- The patient should be encouraged to develop their own start and endpoint within the oral cavity and then follow it systematically at each brushing session, so that a methodical routine is developed; so perhaps lower left side (all surfaces) followed by lower front (all surfaces) and then lower right side (all surfaces), before moving to the upper arch.
- Each area is brushed in turn and the mouth is then cleared by spitting out the toothpaste and oral debris.
- The patient should be instructed not to rinse the mouth out, as this removes the residual toothpaste and prevents its chemical constituents from continuing to act in the mouth – this is particularly important with fluoridated toothpastes.
- Parents will need to perform effective tooth brushing on children up to the age of around 8 years, to ensure that all plaque is removed and to teach the child how to brush correctly (Figure 13.2).
- Brushes should be rinsed afterwards and allowed to dry, and they only have a limited life and need replacement every few months as the bristles curl down and render the brush ineffective (Figure 13.3).

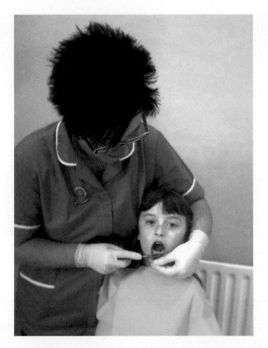

Figure 13.2   Supervised child tooth brushing.

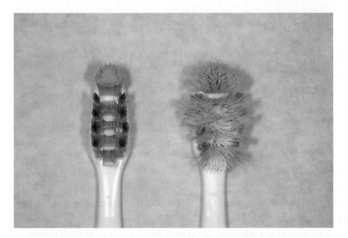

Figure 13.3   New and worn toothbrush.

Toothpastes

A huge variety of toothpastes is available, from shops' own brands to specialised ones from oral health product suppliers, with ingredients to fight all aspects of common oral disease. Individual recommendations should be given for any patient requesting advice from the dental team as to the most suitable product (Figure 13.4). This may vary from time to time as the patient may experience certain oral problems throughout life.

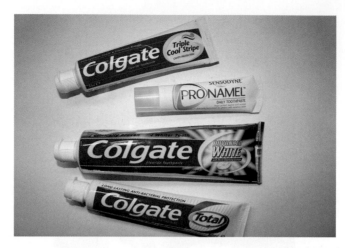

Figure 13.4   Types of toothpaste.

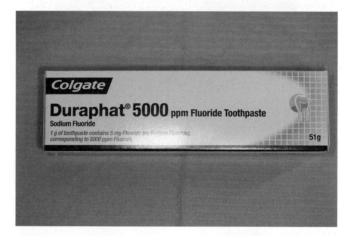

Figure 13.5   High fluoride toothpaste.

- Over 95% of toothpastes available in the UK contain **fluoride**, as sodium monofluorophosphate and sodium fluoride at 1000 parts per million (ppm).
- **High fluoride** toothpastes contain between 2800 ppm and 5000 ppm, for use by adult patients with an existing high caries rate or an excessive risk of developing caries (Figure 13.5).
- Several other toothpastes contain ingredients specifically to slow down **calculus** formation.
- Many now contain the substance triclosan combined with zinc, which acts as an **antiseptic plaque suppressant**.
- Some toothpastes are specifically formulated to help **relieve sensitivity**, and contain ingredients such as stannous fluoride (Figure 13.6).
- Others are advertised as '**whitening toothpastes**' and remove surface tooth staining by the use of abrasives or more recently by the use of biological enzyme systems.
- More recent developments have included toothpastes designed to help protect teeth against **acid erosion** (Figure 13.7).

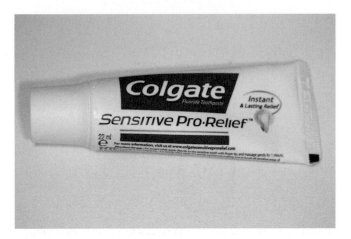

Figure 13.6   Pro-Relief toothpaste.

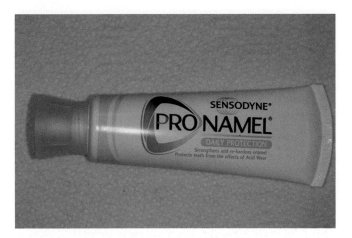

Figure 13.7   Pronamel toothpaste.

Interdental cleaning

However good the tooth-brushing technique, it is still impossible to clean interdental spaces perfectly with a toothbrush alone, unless a specialist electric brush is used. Consequently, the mesial and distal contact areas between adjoining teeth are more prone to developing caries and periodontal disease. To clean the interdental areas adequately, several oral health aids are available to assist patients to remove plaque that has formed here.

- **Dental floss** and **dental tape** are thread-like aids used to achieve interdental plaque removal; however, correct usage depends to some extent on the patient's manual dexterity and on receiving sound oral health instruction (Figure 13.8).
- '**Flossette-style**' handles hold the length of floss in place for the patient so that they can floss with one hand, therefore making the procedure less cumbersome, especially for posterior teeth where access is difficult for the majority of patients (Figure 13.9).

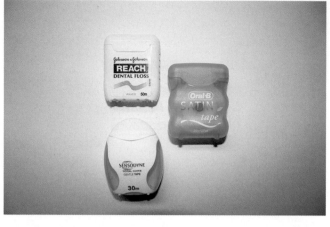

Figure 13.8   Dental flosses and tapes.

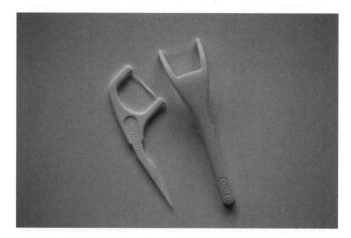

Figure 13.9   Interdental flossettes.

- **Interdental brushes** are a typical 'bottle-brush' design which are able to clean in spaced interdental areas, as well as around the individual brackets of fixed orthodontic appliances (Figure 13.10).
- **Woodsticks** (although they may also be plastic!) dislodge solid pieces of food debris from interproximal areas, as well massaging the gingivae area. However, their use should be restricted to competent adults whenever possible, as they can easily be stuck into the gum and cause problems if used incorrectly.

The aim of all these interdental aids is to dislodge food particles and accumulated plaque from the interdental areas of the teeth, so that the debris can be swallowed or removed from the oral cavity. As the plaque sticks to the tooth surface itself, the cleaning aids should be physically pulled across the mesial and distal tooth surfaces to remove this biofilm layer, so the majority of patients will require demonstrations in the correct technique by a member of the dental team. In particular, dental floss and tape needs to be 'wrapped around' the separate tooth surfaces to adequately clean them, and this requires a certain level of manual dexterity by the patient (see Figure 11.19).

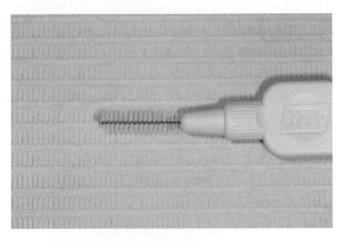

Figure 13.10   Interdental brush detail.

361

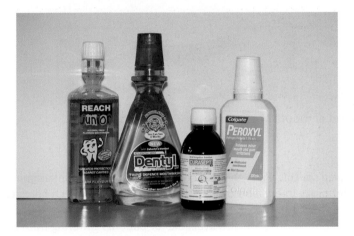

Figure 13.11   Types of mouthwash.

Even when used correctly, woodsticks are the least effective method of interdental cleaning available, and other techniques should be recommended to the patient wherever possible.

Mouthwashes

A wide range of mouthwashes is currently available, ranging from shops' own brands to specialised products from dedicated oral health product suppliers (Figure 13.11). Each patient should have specific products recommended for use by the dental team, once their particular oral health needs have been assessed.

- General-use mouthwashes contain various ingredients to promote good oral hygiene, including:
    - **sodium fluoride** – to provide topical fluoride application to the teeth
    - **triclosan** – a chemical that suppresses the formation of plaque in the oral cavity.
- Others are specialised for use on sensitive teeth (Figure 13.12).

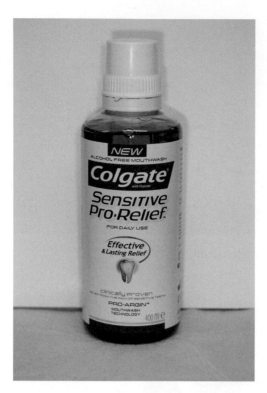

Figure 13.12   Pro-Relief mouthwash.

- Some are used specifically in the presence of oral soft tissue inflammation as a first aid measure, or after oral surgery, and contain **hydrogen peroxide** which helps to eliminate anaerobic bacteria (Figure 13.13).
- Specialised mouthwashes are also available for patients suffering from both acute and chronic periodontal infections, and contain **chlorhexidine** which is an **antiseptic plaque suppressant** (Figure 13.14).

Other methods of plaque removal

After eating a meal, tooth brushing may not always be possible until several hours later, by which time plaque will have formed and possibly started to cause damage. Obvious examples are after eating lunch at school or at work, or while out for a meal in the evening.

In these situations, loose food debris can be removed by using sugar-free chewing gum or finishing the meal with a *detergent food* and/or a piece of cheese. Detergent foods are raw, firm, fibrous fruits or vegetables, such as apples, pears, carrots and celery. By virtue of their tough fibrous consistency, they require much chewing and stimulate salivary flow, thereby helping to scour the teeth clean of food remnants. Although plaque is unaffected by detergent foods, they can remove some of the food debris which nourishes all plaque bacteria and enables some of them to produce acid. Although cheese at the end of a meal has no direct detergent effect, it stimulates salivary flow, neutralises acid and enhances remineralisation of enamel, due to its calcium content. Hard cheeses are more beneficial than soft cheeses.

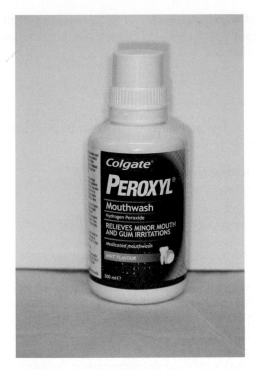

Figure 13.13   Peroxyl mouthwash.

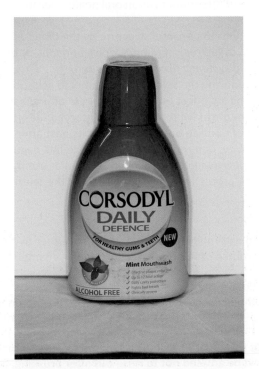

Figure 13.14   Corsodyl daily mouthwash.

The excessive use of chewing gum should be discouraged in all patients where evidence of attrition or bruxing appears. Its use should be confined to immediately after a meal only, and not continually throughout the day.

Prevention of dental caries

Two other factors were noted previously with regard to preventing dental caries, and they will both be discussed here.

- **Increase the tooth resistance to acid attack**.
- **Modification of the diet**.

Increase the tooth resistance to acid attack

The outer layer of the tooth, the enamel, is made up of inorganic crystals of calcium hydroxyapatite arranged as prisms running from the amelodentinal junction to the tooth surface (see Chapter 10). It was discovered many years ago that the incorporation of fluoride into and onto the tooth structure resulted in the replacement of the hydroxyapatite crystals by *fluorapatite crystals*. This new chemical structure of the tooth was found to be much more resistant to the damage caused by the weak organic acids formed by plaque bacteria – in other words, the fluoride protected the teeth from developing caries so easily.

Fluoride is therefore the single most important salt in the battle against dental caries. It occurs naturally in the water in some areas, and is added artificially to water supplies in other areas during the process of water fluoridation, as an oral health measure to aid in the reduction of caries incidence.

Fluoride can be taken into the enamel structure by the direct application of various oral health products onto the teeth, called *topical fluoride application*, or by being taken internally with food and drink products, called *systemic fluoride application*.

Besides its action of reducing the solubility of enamel to acids, by the formation of fluorapatite, fluoride also has an inhibitory effect on the *feeding rate* of oral bacteria. This effect results in the production of lesser amounts of weak acids and polysaccharides to initiate the carious attack.

The protective effect of fluoride on the teeth is at its best after they have formed and recently erupted into the oral cavity, before any carious damage has begun. Many oral hygiene products containing fluoride are now available, to allow their regular use by the general public throughout their lifetime, so that the protective effect of fluoride on the teeth is constantly 'topped up'.

Topical fluorides

These are administered externally to the tooth surface, either by the patient or the dental team, to provide a continual source of fluoride directly onto the enamel.

1. For use by the patient
   - **Fluoride toothpastes** containing the current recommended dose for all patients of 1000 ppm, up to 5000 ppm for use by adults at high risk of developing caries (see Figure 13.5).
   - A minimum of twice-daily brushing is advised to achieve maximum benefits.
   - Patients should be advised **not to rinse out** after brushing, as it washes the fluoride away and is therefore less effective.

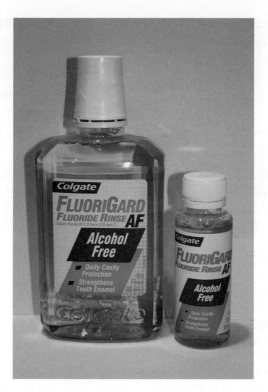

Figure 13.15   Fluorigard mouthwash.

- **Fluoride mouthwashes** for regular use by those with a high caries risk, and for those undergoing orthodontic treatment (Figure 13.15).
- **Dental floss** and tape impregnated with fluoride, for delivery directly to the interproximal areas.

2. For use by the dental team
   - **Fluoride gels** applied in trays over all the teeth for several minutes; they are administered at each examination appointment and are especially useful for patients with special needs and a high caries risk.
     - Children with rampant caries.
     - Patients with medical conditions such as haemophilia and heart defects which would make tooth extraction dangerous.
     - Patients who are too handicapped to achieve adequate oral hygiene.
   - The technique has two stages: first, a thorough polish to remove any plaque present, after which the teeth are washed and dried, and second, the gel is applied in the special applicator tray for a few minutes. On removal of the tray, patients are instructed not to rinse, drink or eat for half an hour. The gels are pleasantly flavoured and the procedure is usually well tolerated.
   - **Fluoride varnish** (such as Duraphat products; Figure 13.16) applied to individual teeth showing areas of previous acid attack, or to roots exposed by gingival recession or periodontal surgery. Registered dental nurses can undergo extended duties training to enable them to carry out this procedure on patients, under the prescription of the dentist.

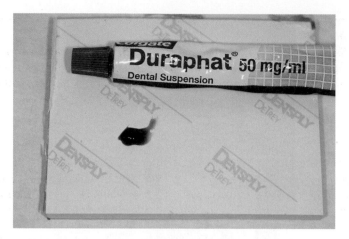

Figure 13.16   Duraphat varnish.

Systemic fluorides

These products are supplied in a form to be ingested and then incorporated into the enamel structure within the body.

- **Fluoridated water** supplies by the addition of the optimum concentration of **1 ppm** to drinking water.
- Naturally occurring fluoridated water supplies, in some parts of the world.
- Addition of fluoride to table salt, but this occurs in countries other than the UK.
- **Fluoride drops and tablets**, available on prescription for children, to be taken daily during the period of tooth development (up to 13 years); the doses required vary with the patient's age and the amount of fluoride in the local water supply.
- Usually reserved for those with medical or physical conditions which would make dental treatment difficult, or for those whose general health would suffer if caries occurred.

Water fluoridation is carried out as a public health measure in some areas of the UK, where fluoride at 1 ppm is added to the local water supply, is ingested by the local population and absorbed from their digestive tracts so that it can be incorporated into the enamel structure of their teeth.

Public health surveys have consistently proved the benefit of water fluoridation, by comparing the number of *decayed, missing and filled teeth* (DMF count) in various populations. In areas where systemic fluoride is present at the 1 ppm concentration, the incidence of caries is reduced by 50% compared to areas where there is no water fluoridation. However, the technique remains controversial as some opponents consider it to be a form of 'mass medication' of the population, carried out without necessarily having their approval as they can only avoid ingesting the drinking water by using bottled water instead.

Fissure sealing

Topical fluorides exert most of their effect on mesial and distal (proximal) surfaces of the teeth. Occlusal fissures and pits are just as vulnerable to caries but they are less well protected by fluorides. Fortunately they can receive extra, and even better, protection by the application of fissure sealants. These materials are composite fillings or glass ionomer cement, which are used to seal the naturally occurring stagnation areas of pits and fissures, therefore preventing damage from acid attacks and avoiding the onset of dental caries.

Successful fissure sealing should make an occlusal surface safe from caries. Like topical fluoridation, it can be carried out by hygienists and therapists as well as dentists and is of major importance in preventive dentistry as it can produce a significant reduction in the most common disease of children.

Enamel fluorosis

This is a condition which occurs when excessive fluoride is ingested during enamel formation. The teeth erupt with mottled white areas in the enamel surface which vary in severity but can be quite unsightly. Restorative techniques, such as veneers, are available to mask the areas but the condition is prevented by ensuring that parents receive the correct advice regarding fluoride.

- Children below the age of 8 years should have tooth brushing supervised by an adult, to prevent ingestion of the toothpaste.
- The amount of toothpaste should be kept to a minimum and allowed just twice daily.
- The parents must ensure that children spit the toothpaste out after use, rather than swallow it.
- All fluoride supplements should only be prescribed as necessary, and at the correct dosage which is dependent on the local water fluoridation levels.
- The dental team must therefore have knowledge of any local water fluoridation levels.

Modification of the diet

The single most important modification to the diet to help reduce the incidence of dental caries is the reduction (or ideally the elimination) of NMEs and dietary acids from the daily food and drink intake. It cannot be emphasised too strongly that even if teeth are thoroughly cleaned after meals, caries will still occur if NME sugary snacks and acidic drinks are taken between meals on a regular basis. This is because plaque persists in the inaccessible areas of fissures and tooth contact points after a meal, unless brushed away by the patient. Acid forms in this residual plaque within minutes of eating sugar, the pH of the oral environment is lowered, and the tooth enamel will be at risk of demineralisation until the pH balance is restored.

Then, as described in Chapter 11, a constant acid environment at the enamel surface allows demineralisation to proceed unchecked, and leaves insufficient time between intakes of sugar for the natural defence mechanism of remineralisation to occur. Although adequate tooth brushing and interdental cleaning twice daily may prevent supragingival periodontal disease, it cannot prevent caries unless accompanied by strict dietary discipline to eliminate NME snacks between meals.

If NME foods and acidic drinks (such as carbonated 'pops' and fizzy flavoured waters) are confined to mealtimes only, the acids involved are neutralised to some extent by the buffering action of saliva, and the extent of any demineralisation is reduced.

When giving dietary advice to patients, it helps if they are made aware of which food and drink products are safe or harmful, in relation to dental caries. This is especially important with what are known as 'hidden sugars' in foods – where NMEs have been artificially added to foods for taste and preservation purposes, very often in foods that patients would not expect to be harmful to their teeth.

A simple list of 'good' and 'bad' foods and drinks can then be used by the dental team when giving dietary advice to patients.

367

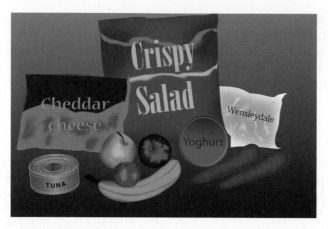

Figure 13.17   Examples of good snacks.

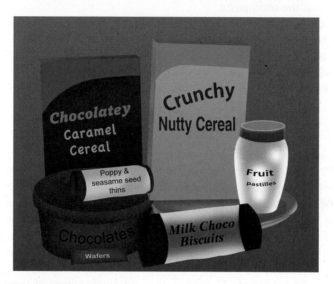

Figure 13.18   Examples of bad snacks.

Good snacks (Figure 13.17) include:

- non-citrus fruit, such as apples, pears and peaches
- fibrous raw vegetables, such as carrots and celery
- unflavoured crisps
- low-fat cheese
- unsweetened yogurt.

Bad snacks (Figure 13.18) include.

- sweets and other confectionery
- biscuits and cakes
- carbonated drinks
- pure citrus fruit juices
- tea and coffee with sugar.

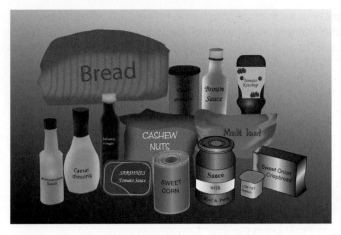

Figure 13.19   Examples of hidden sugar foods.

369

Care should be taken with excessive intake of citrus fruits such as oranges, lemons, grapefruits and limes between meals.

Those foods containing 'hidden sugars' can be identified by carefully reading the contents label of each product, and include the following (Figure 13.19).

- Cooking sauces, especially those with a tomato base.
- Table sauces, including ketchup.
- Flavoured crisps.
- Fruits tinned in syrup.
- Some tinned vegetables, including baked beans and sweetcorn.
- Some breakfast cereals.
- Jams, marmalades and chutneys.
- Some low-fat products, as sugar is often artificially added to improve their taste.
- Tinned fish and meat in tomato sauce.
- Soups.
- Savoury crackers and biscuits.
- Some processed ready meals.
- Energy drinks.

A universal system of clearly labelling food products so that contents such as hidden sugars are more readily identified is currently under discussion by politicians and food manufacturers. If enforced, bad snacks and unexpected sugar contents will be more obvious to the patient, and their ingestion can therefore be avoided or at least controlled more easily.

Although the incidence of caries is gradually reducing in this country, it remains a major health problem. It is most prevalent in younger age groups, so parental support is imperative if oral health messages are to be successful. The following dietary advice should be given.

- Eat a healthy diet with foods of low cariogenic (caries-causing) potential.
- Follow the 'good snacks' list given previously.
- Limit any cariogenic foods to mealtimes, so that they can be neutralised by the increased flow of saliva that occurs while chewing.
- Avoid carbonated drinks and confine fruit juices to mealtimes only.

- Use diet sheets to determine if any hidden sugars are being taken.
- Advise mothers on the damage caused by using cariogenic drinks in baby feeders.
- Parents should be encouraged to request sugar-free medicines for their children whenever possible.

Prevention of periodontal disease

Two other factors were mentioned previously with regard to preventing periodontal disease, and they will both be discussed here.

- **Modify the contributory factors**.
- **Control the host response**.

Modify the contributory factors

The contributory factors to be discussed do not, in themselves, cause periodontal disease – this is due to the presence of consistently poor levels of oral hygiene by the patient. The contributory factors just exacerbate (make worse) the periodontal disease that is already in existence – they aggravate it so that the extent of the disease is worse than it would be otherwise, and/or it progresses more easily and quickly than it would do otherwise.

The most common contributory factors include the following.

- Smoking.
- Unbalanced masticatory stress – such as when teeth have erupted out of alignment (especially when proclined) and normal chewing puts force on them in an abnormal direction.
- Excessive masticatory stress – such as when several posterior teeth are missing and the patient then 'nibbles' with their anterior teeth only, resulting in excessive chewing force on them.
- Hormonal imbalance that affects the reaction of gingival tissues to normal events such as plaque build-up – pregnancy and puberty are the usual examples.
- Open lip posture that allows the gingival tissues to dry out readily – such as occurs in various malocclusions or in patients who routinely breathe through their mouth rather than their nose (this may be a habit, or due to conditions such as having large adenoid glands).
- A history of radiotherapy treatment for cancer in the head and neck region will result in reduced saliva flow (as the salivary glands are damaged by the treatment), so that plaque is able to build up more easily (these patients also tend to experience a higher rate of dental caries).
- Certain medical conditions that alter the patient's ability to fight infection or to heal when attacked by pathogens – these patients are referred to as being *immune-compromised*.
  - Diabetes
  - Leukaemia and other blood disorders
  - Vitamin C deficiency
  - AIDS.
- Certain medicines that affect the normal reaction of the gingival tissues to the presence of plaque, often resulting in an overgrowth of tissue which makes plaque removal more difficult for the patient– the resultant tissue overgrowth is called *gingival hyperplasia*.
  - Phenytoin (Epanutin) used in the control of epilepsy
  - Antihypertensive agents, such as nifedipine
  - Immune-suppressant drugs to prevent transplant rejection, such as ciclosporin
  - Cytotoxic drugs used to treat various cancers.

- Certain medicines affect saliva production so that the patient suffers from xerostomia (dry mouth), resulting in loss of the natural cleansing effect of the saliva and a greater build-up of plaque.
  - Diuretics used to treat various heart conditions
  - Some antidepressants
  - Some antihypertensive medicines.
- Plaque retention factors that allow an increased local build-up of plaque, and/or prevent its ready removal by normal oral hygiene methods.
  - Tooth crowding in malocclusion
  - Unopposed teeth in one arch, so that there is no normal contact and self-cleansing action by friction of food or other teeth
  - Iatrogenic factors –those created by the dentist, including overhanging restorations, poor marginal fit of crowns, poorly designed dentures, etc.

Of this large list of contributory factors, the most obvious and relatively easiest ones for the dental team to overcome are those due to masticatory stress, and those due to localised plaque retention factors. Restorative dental treatments to restore the occlusion are discussed in detail in Chapters 15 and 16.

Of the remainder, patients can be informed of the effect of their various medications on their oral health and advised to discuss them with their doctor, who will be able to determine if alternative medications are available. Those patients suffering from medication-induced gingival hyperplasia can undergo a simple gingivectomy procedure to remove the excess tissue, so aiding plaque removal in the affected areas.

Little can be done for those patients suffering from hormonal imbalances and the various medical conditions that are an issue, except to ensure that they attend regularly for oral health assessment and treatment, and that the relevant oral hygiene messages are reinforced at each attendance.

As smoking has such a huge detrimental effect on both general and oral health, many patients are likely to have been given smoking cessation advice on numerous occasions by other healthcare workers besides the dental team. However, the team should still use every attendance by the patient as an opportunity to reinforce the health benefits of stopping smoking, and inform them of the various techniques that are currently available under the excellent NHS 'Quit Smoking' referral scheme.

Dental treatment is one of the few areas of the NHS where many patients are expected to pay for their health services, and while it may be an unusual tactic, the cost of dental treatment may be highlighted as an additional good reason for advising those patients who smoke to give up, especially where it can be shown that smoking has contributed to their treatment costs. The dentist should advise and lead the team in this technique, as skilful communication methods are required to ensure that the patient is helpfully advised and supported, rather than insulted and humiliated.

Control the host response

Some patients are prone to suffering from periodontal problems, often for genetic reasons. No matter how thorough their oral hygiene efforts become with help and support from the dental team, and even in the absence of any contributory factors, they may still go on to develop periodontal disease. As their genetic predisposition cannot be altered, the periodontal disease development is inevitable over time. These patients will require a high level of support and maintenance by the dental team to ensure that their disease does not spiral out of control and result in the loss of multiple teeth that could have been saved.

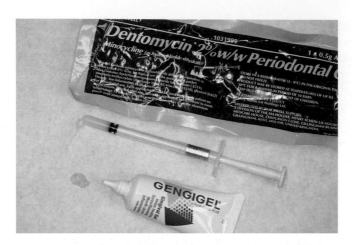

Figure 13.20   Periodontal pocket treatments.

These patients may therefore require interventional dental treatment on a regular basis.

- Any calculus that has built up must be removed by **scaling** and **subgingival debridement**, by a suitable member of the dental team (see Chapter 11).
- Advice should be given on suitable oral health products that act specifically to control calculus formation.
- Patients taking drugs that cause **gingival hyperplasia** may require the overgrown tissue to be surgically removed as a gingivectomy procedure, thereby eliminating these plaque retention areas.
- Once debrided, the periodontal pockets may have an antibiotic gel (Figure 13.20) inserted as an alternative to repeated courses of systemic antibiotics, in an effort to eradicate the bacteria involved in the disease process.
- Areas of persistent periodontal infection that fail to respond to treatment may require the **extraction** of the individual tooth involved, to remove the associated periodontal pockets as a source of the anaerobic bacteria.
- Patients who require a high level of periodontal maintenance are best referred to a **periodontal specialist** for their treatment.

Effective oral hygiene instruction

Communication skills

Good communication between the dental team and patients is crucial if they are to take an active role in managing their own oral health. Not only is it a necessity if any consent given for treatment is to be valid (see Chapter 3), but it will also lead to greater understanding between all parties, especially if the patient is unsure about treatment options or even refuses to have treatment as advised by the dentist.

An open relationship must exist at all times so that the patient feels they can ask for advice, query options given or explain why they do not wish to have certain treatments. All of this depends on the dental team showing good communication skills, and this is especially important for the dental nurse as patients often prefer to discuss matters with them rather than with the dentist.

Communicating means 'to give or exchange information' and this can be done both verbally and non-verbally.

- **Talking** – either directly with the patient face to face, or by telephone.
- **Written explanations** – which reiterate any verbal information given.
- **Information leaflets or posters** – which can be read and then discussed as necessary.
- **Body language** – which can be open and friendly, or defensive and 'stand-offish'.
- **Eye contact** – maintaining eye contact shows attentiveness, while breaking eye contact indicates that the patient is being dismissed by the listener.
- **Facial expressions** – again, these can be friendly or not.
- **Body position** – sitting to listen to the patient is more attentive than standing, especially if the body position of the listener is turned away from the speaker.
- **Touching** – this is sometimes used to reinforce points, although it is not acceptable in some situations and with some patients, and should only be used where there is a friendly and well-established rapport between the patient and the team member.

A friendly staff member will obviously appear more approachable to patients than one who seems unfriendly, but often an unfriendly demeanour occurs without the staff member realising it. When unexpected situations arise, such as an equipment failure or a very busy appointments session, staff can seem abrupt, harried or even dismissive towards patients as they try to deal with the unexpected situation.

Continuing to carry out tasks while being spoken to, especially if eye contact is not maintained, can appear extremely rude and dismissive to patients. On the other hand, standing too close to a patient ('invading their personal space') or making inappropriate physical contact may be construed as threatening or offensive by the patient. Some individuals have naturally good communication skills, but for other dental staff a training course or 'in-house' experiential learning, by following the lead of good communicators, is vital in the development of their own skills.

Communicating with ethnic groups

In our modern, multiracial society there are bound to be patients whose first language is not English, and communicating with them will present severe problems for the dental team in some circumstances, so wherever possible a family member or friend should be encouraged to attend and act as an interpreter. Full communication can then occur so that the patient is fully aware of the state of their oral health, and is fully informed of all risks and benefits before undergoing any dental procedure.

Valid consent cannot be given for treatment if the patient does not understand the language being spoken, and the relevant points have not been translated for them. The NHS issues patient information leaflets in various languages and it would be advisable for practices with a large ethnic minority patient base to have them to hand. They are free and can be delivered to the workplace.

Dental staff should also be aware of any cultural differences between ethnic groups, and accept and deal with them in an appropriate manner. Religious beliefs may prevent oral examination and dental treatment occurring at certain times, and these facts should be accommodated and handled sympathetically as far as possible, rather than being seen as an unnecessary hindrance to the running of the practice.

Religion probably plays the most important role in the differences encountered amongst many ethnic groups, both in their culture and in their daily lives, including their diet and eating habits. Several points of interest for dental staff around these cultural differences are summarised below.

Hindus

- Many are vegetarian, some vegan, and they take no beef in their diet.
- Fasting days for religious reasons are common.
- Their diet tends to be very high in saturated fats, and is often expensive.

Sikhs

- They eat more dairy products than other ethnic groups.
- They are often vegetarian.
- If meats are eaten, they tend to avoid beef and pork.

Moslems

- They have strict food laws, even including the methods used for animal slaughter.
- They avoid both alcohol and pork.
- They abide by Ramadan – a period of fasting during daylight hours for one month per year.
- They tend to eat a diet rich in fish.

All Asian groups tend to breastfeed their babies for up to 2 years, and sugar is routinely added to feeds, especially as milk-based additions that are therefore cariogenic and have low nutritional value.

All these issues are of relevance to both the oral and general health of these patient groups, but are unlikely to be altered because of their religious basis. The dental team must accept this and respect the wishes of each patient, while also advising them of the likely consequences to their oral (and general) health.

Patient evaluation and motivation in relation to age group

Each patient's knowledge and skills in relation to their own oral health are evaluated by adequate communication with them, and the aim of good communication is to identify their level of motivation, and if poor, what the actual problems are for them – what is preventing them from achieving and then maintaining a good standard of oral health?

During consideration of the issues, all the following points need to be looked at and taken into account.

- Do they just need direct advice, help and support to adequately achieve good oral health, such as one-to-one oral hygiene instruction with a member of the dental team?
- Are factors involved which prevent them from achieving good oral health, such as a disability or a diet- or habit-related problem?
- Are they simply uninterested in their oral health or are they unaware that they have a problem?
- Are general health factors involved which either exacerbate or actually cause the oral health problem?
- Is a serious general health problem present which over-rides their oral health problems?

Following the evaluation of each patient, their individual problems will have been identified and help can then be given by the dental team to aid the patient in achieving a better standard of oral health.

Any risk factors identified during the evaluation need to be discussed with the patient. These risk factors will vary, depending on the age group of the patient involved, and tend to be influenced by complex social attitudes and outside pressures.

Adults

- Smoking and drinking habits should be discussed in relation to oral health, but in a non-judgemental manner. Information should be given on the links between these risk factors and both the general and oral health problems associated with them, especially periodontal disease and oral cancer.
- Some patients may require referral to their dental or medical practitioner for individual advice on aids to stop smoking, such as nicotine patches and nicotine substitutes, and this is easier to arrange nowadays with the free NHS smoking cessation schemes available.
- Similarly, excessive alcohol intake should be discussed in relation to oral cancer and general health problems, but it is the patient's choice whether to act on the advice given.
- Diet should be discussed in detail, using accurate diet sheets filled in by the patient to identify any hidden dietary problems if necessary, such as a high NME sugars intake or frequent snacking episodes.
- The patient's diet should be assessed in relation to any general health effects.

Young people

This group of patients will require a quite different approach to support and motivation in relation to their oral health, for the following reasons.

- They have a different outlook on life and different priorities in their lives from adults; events that are important to adults are often of less concern to young people, and vice versa.
- They are likely to have little, if any, experience of long-term oral and general health problems and will therefore require some convincing that a problem actually exists.
- They are likely to require evidence for the existence of an oral health problem from the dental team, rather than just accepting their word for it, so the use of disclosing agents to stain bacterial plaque on their own teeth is often an invaluable aid in this situation.
- Some young people may be experimenting with alcohol and tobacco usage because of peer pressure, and this may already be having an effect on their oral health (and ultimately on their general health).
- Some may not wish to accept responsibility for maintaining their own oral health yet, and prefer to rely on their parents for this.
- Parental influence will be greater for some young people than others.
- Parental support will differ similarly, but is therefore of great importance – well-motivated parents tend to instil their attitudes and beliefs into their youngsters.

Children

The oral health of this group depends very much on parental influence and support, especially for the younger patients. Parents who have little interest in their own oral and general health are unlikely to instil their children with high levels of interest and motivation, although exceptions do occur.

- Wherever possible, parents should be included in their child's oral health education, and their support should be gained at an early stage.
- The oral health messages given by the dental team can then be reinforced at home by the parent, and will usually revolve around brushing techniques and dietary advice.
- A suitable vocabulary should be established for each child; if it is aimed too high they are unlikely to understand, but if too low they will be insulted by being treated childishly.

- A friendly, non-threatening approach is required so that their trust is gained.
- Ideally, the child should not be threatened by phrases such as 'if you don't brush your teeth you'll have to have a needle ...', as this will cause them to associate dental visits with fear and pain. Unfortunately, the team may sometimes find that this has already been threatened by a parent.
- The patient should also feel comfortable when asking questions, so the oral health team should maintain an open, frank manner with each child.
- Oral health messages need to be fun so that the interest of the child is maintained. Consequently, the use of games, drawings and competitions should be considered wherever possible.
- Again, the use of disclosing agents (either tablets or liquids) should be encouraged, both by the dental team and at home, to stain the bacterial plaque and make its removal easier.

Motivation can be thought of as the act of persuading people to do something for their own benefit. When there is a lack of motivation by patients to take an interest in their oral health, it needs to be established whether this is due to lack of knowledge, lack of interest or because of the presence of previously unrealised risk factors. Once these points have been understood, priorities and goals can be set out for each patient and the role of the dental team can be established.

Having established the different groups requiring oral health advice and the factors that can affect their motivation in relation to both their oral and general health, the various methods available to the dental team to improve that motivation can be considered in detail for each patient. Using this information, a plan of action can be developed in relation to the relevant oral and general health advice that is to be delivered, and how the various oral health messages should be communicated, especially in relation to caries and periodontal disease.

Successful communication with *adult patients* can be achieved in various ways.

- The use of specific oral health leaflets from dental suppliers.
- One-to-one discussions of relevant oral health issues with a member of the dental team, in a non-patronising manner.
- The non-use of dental jargon unless it is appropriate, but without condescension.
- The adoption of an attentive manner, so that the patient's own difficulties and problems relating to their oral health maintenance are listened to and understood.
- Any queries raised need answering at a level that the patient will understand, and may require referral to another member of the dental team by less experienced staff members.
- Eye contact should be maintained with the patient during the discussions, to ensure the correct level of attention is given.
- Reflective replies to their queries and concerns should be given, which relate to the patient's individual experiences.

The more mature *young people* can be approached in a similar fashion, but less mature patients will require an individual approach aimed at their level of understanding. Pubescent teenagers may even take offence at the implication that they have a 'dirty' mouth, and act quite negatively during attempts to discuss their oral health issues. This tends to be especially so for male teenagers.

A young person with a 'rebellious' nature will be determined not to make efforts to improve their oral health, enjoying the 'shock' effect that this has on both the dental team and their parents. Thankfully, most tend to grow out of this phase as they mature.

Oral health messages can be communicated to this group as follows.

- The use of relevant leaflets and dental literature, many of which are specifically aimed at this age group.

- Definitely a one-to-one approach to give oral health messages for those members of this age group who are easily embarrassed.
- Some will tend to react better in small groups, especially with similarly aged siblings or friends.
- Authority and control of the situation need to be maintained by the dental team throughout the session, but in a friendly manner.
- The dental team should never lose patience with these individuals, no matter how obstreperous they become.
- Good patient management by the dental team at this age should produce attentive and responsible adults in the future.

Children tend to respond best to a group approach when learning new information, but their interest in a subject can soon be lost or they can be easily distracted. Consequently, short interactive sessions are best, with plenty of opportunities for individual involvement by the children.

- The use of disclosing tablets to show the presence and position of bacterial plaque.
- Supervise individual attempts at tooth brushing, to determine how to improve plaque removal.
- Develop relevant games to play, especially any involving current TV or film characters.
- Encourage parental involvement in the oral health sessions wherever possible, as the parents need to maintain and promote the oral health messages at home.

Having received all of the available oral health advice given by the dental team, the patient should now be able to determine whether they are motivated and willing to improve their oral health.

A gentle and tactful reminder of the reasons why good oral health should be a personal goal for the patient can be given at this stage.

- To avoid the embarrassment of having halitosis (bad breath).
- To avoid the embarrassment and pain of having carious teeth.
- To avoid tooth loss due to periodontal disease or caries.
- To avoid the need for fixed or removable prostheses, and their expense.

Review of patient progress

The patient will need to be seen on a regular basis to determine whether progress with their oral hygiene has been made or not. The dental team's success or failure in promoting and maintaining oral health depends on an understanding of the determinants of oral health.

- Social factors.
- Environmental factors.
- Economic factors.
- Patient's knowledge.
- Patient's skills.

Oral health education should aim to modify any damaging behaviour, rather than unrealistically trying to reverse this behaviour, and oral health educators need to have an understanding of why any damaging behaviour occurs. In particular, the effects of being in a low socio-economic group need to be understood by the dental team, as many of these patients are entitled to free dental care under the NHS, and yet they often exhibit the worst standards of oral health. Some of the reasons identified for this anomaly are as follows.

- They are the group of patients least likely to attend for regular dental examinations, so there is little advice and preventive input from the dental team.
- Their associated poor diet, usually high in carbohydrates, predisposes them to general poor health.
- The high rate of smoking and alcohol use in this group tends to predispose them to periodontal disease and oral cancer.
- Dental ignorance, often compounded by low self-esteem, prevents their own oral health from being a high priority.
- Their high carbohydrate input tends to be related to the expected high caries incidence, and early tooth loss.
- Some of these patients feel intimidated by professionals, and are least likely to seek dental advice, especially in relation to information regarding lifestyle changes.
- Some people may also have difficulty understanding oral health advice, and this highlights the need for the dental team to develop good communication skills that can be adapted for various patients and situations as necessary.

Studies indicate that patients in lower socio-economic groups tend to have poorer general health overall, and advice given by the dental team must be sympathetic to this, as it is often related to the financial situation of these patients, in particular. All oral and general health advice should be given sympathetically and targeted at realistic outcomes. For example, parents in these groups tend to use sweets for their children as treats, or even bribes, because sweets are often cheaper to buy than books, toys or other presents. The finances of these families cannot be changed, so it would be totally unrealistic to try and stop the parents buying sweets for their children under these circumstances, and the delivery of the oral health advice and its promotion would fail. It would be more sensible in these circumstances to educate the parents to restrict sweets consumption to mealtimes, so that the frequency of acid attacks on their children's teeth is minimised, and hopefully their caries experience will be reduced or even eradicated.

Similarly, it would be unrealistic to expect older smokers to give up their nicotine habit without lots of encouragement and support from a smoking cessation scheme, as nicotine is addictive and the longer the patient has smoked, usually the harder they will find it to stop. Advice about current aids to help to stop smoking, such as nicotine patches or chewing gum, can be given, or a referral to the local cessation scheme.

Teenage smokers may be easier to re-educate, as they often only smoke to appear socially acceptable to their friends or because of peer pressure. Advice regarding the overall damage to health caused by smoking, given in an informed but friendly manner, is often the first step in their re-education.

With all the information collated with regard to the level of the patient's oral health at their assessment, the extent of their known risk factors to oral disease and their level of motivation to improve their oral health, the dental team is able to determine the outcome of their oral health promotion efforts on each patient at their review appointment. The outcome will fall into one of the following categories.

- Has progress been made, resulting in a higher standard of oral hygiene?
- Has the original oral hygiene status been maintained, but with no improvement?
- Has the oral hygiene status deteriorated, such that more damage has occurred?

When progress has been made, the patient should be congratulated and encouraged to maintain this raised standard of oral hygiene. Children can be given stickers, badges or certificates, all of which are available from oral hygiene product distributors. Many computer programs are available that can be used to design and print out certificates exclusive to the dental practice.

It should be remembered that oral health promotion is a long-term process, so regular monitoring will still be required for some time, although if the higher standard of oral hygiene becomes consistent, then review appointment intervals can be gradually lengthened.

When the oral health status has been maintained but not improved, the patient should still be congratulated on the fact that there has been no relapse, and they should be encouraged to try harder still before the next review.

These patients tend to have considered the financial and emotional costs and benefits to themselves of changing their oral hygiene status, and decided that the costs outweigh the benefits at the present time. All is not lost, as this decision may be transitory, due say to a particularly stressful period in their lives at the current time, so they feel unable or unwilling to attempt change now. Once this period is over, however, they may be receptive to further attempts by the dental team to promote oral health.

If patients feel that the goals set by the dental team are not achievable, or are unrealistic for now, they should be reviewed regularly and supported until they feel able to try again.

The patients who have undergone deterioration in their oral health may need referral to the dentist or hygienist for specialist input and reinforcement. However, reflection still needs to determine whether the goals set were completely unrealistic and unachievable for that particular patient. If so, then new ones will need to be discussed and agreed upon with the dental team.

Alternatively, and frustrating though it is, some patients really do not wish to change their lifestyle, nor do they accept the consequences to their oral health that may occur. Regular monitoring and review are all that the dental team can hope to achieve for these patients, although they should stay alert to any indication by the patient that they are willing to try again at any time.

The patient's right to choose not to accept the oral health advice given by the dental team should be respected and accepted by all.

With regard to oral health assessment recall intervals, these depend on various factors for each patient as shown below, and current guidelines issued by the National Institute for Health and Clinical Excellence (NICE) are used to determine the appropriate recall frequency in each case (Figure 13.21).

Effect of general health on oral health

It is essential that patients understand that their oral health is not a separate issue from their general health, as the two are very much linked together. The dietary and lifestyle advice that the dental team give to ensure good oral health will also be relevant to maintaining an overall high level of general health, if the patient chooses to follow that advice.

There are numerous medically related examples of the links between oral health and general health.

- Several chronic diseases have the **same risk factors** as oral diseases.
    - The association of **smoking** and other tobacco habits with heart and respiratory disease, periodontal disease, and cancers such as oral cancer.
    - Diets high in **NME sugars** and those containing many processed meals are linked to dental caries, obesity and an increased risk of heart disease.
    - **Excessive alcohol consumption** is associated with liver disease, periodontal disease, dental trauma (due to falls) and several cancers, including oral cancer.
    - **Eating disorders**, such as anorexia nervosa and bulimia, are associated with general ill health and acid erosion of the enamel of teeth, respectively.
    - **People with diabetes** suffer from poor wound healing generally, which also affects the oral soft tissues and makes the patients prone to postoperative complications, as well as to a higher incidence of oral infections (including periodontal infections).

NHS

National Institute for
Clinical Excellence

Issue date: **October 2004**

Quick reference guide

Dental recall

Recall interval between routine dental examinations

Guidance

- The recommended interval between oral health reviews should be determined specifically for each patient, and tailored to meet his or her needs, on the basis of an assessment of disease levels and risk of or from dental disease.

- This assessment should integrate the evidence presented in this guideline with the clinical judgement and expertise of the dental team, and should be discussed with the patient (see pages 2 and 3).

- During an oral health review, the dental team (led by the dentist) should ensure that comprehensive histories are taken, examinations are conducted and initial preventive advice is given. This will allow the dental team and the patient (and/or his or her parent, guardian or carer) to discuss, where appropriate:
  - the effects of oral hygiene, diet, fluoride use, tobacco and alcohol on oral health
  - the risk factors (see the checklist on page 2) that may influence the patient's oral health, and their implications for deciding the appropriate recall interval
  - the outcome of previous care episodes and the suitability of previously recommended intervals
  - the patient's ability or desire to visit the dentist at the recommended interval
  - the financial costs to the patient of having the oral health review and any subsequent treatments.

- The interval before the next oral health review should be chosen, either at the end of an oral health review if no further treatment is indicated, or on completion of a specific treatment journey.

- The recommended shortest and longest intervals between oral health reviews are as follows.
  - The shortest interval between oral health reviews for all patients should be 3 months.
  - The longest interval between oral health reviews for patients younger than 18 years should be 12 months.
  - The longest interval between oral health reviews for patients aged 18 years and older should be 24 months.

- For practical reasons, the patient should be assigned a recall interval of 3, 6, 9 or 12 months if he or she is younger than 18 years, or 3, 6, 9, 12, 15, 18, 21 or 24 months if he or she is aged 18 years or older.

- The dentist should discuss the recommended recall interval with the patient and record this interval, and the patient's agreement or disagreement with it, in the current record-keeping system.

- The recall interval should be reviewed again at the next oral health review, in order to learn from the patient's responses to the oral care provided and the health outcomes achieved. This feedback and the findings of the oral health review should be used to adjust the next recall interval chosen. Patients should be informed that their recommended recall interval may vary over time.

Clinical Guideline 19

Developed by the National Collaborating Centre for Acute Care

Figure 13.21   NICE guidelines for dental recall. © National Institute for Clinical Excellence. Reproduced from http://www.nice.org.uk/nicemedia/live/10952/29484/29484.pdf.

Checklist of modifying factors						
Name: Date of birth:						
Oral health review date:						
Medical history	Yes	No	Yes	No	Yes	No
Conditions where dental disease could put the patient's general health at increased risk (such as cardiovascular disease, bleeding disorders, immunosuppression)	☐	☐	☐	☐	☐	☐
Conditions that increase a patient's risk of developing dental disease (such as diabetes, xerostomia)	☐	☐	☐	☐	☐	☐
Conditions that may complicate dental treatment or the patient's ability to maintain their oral health (such as special needs, anxious/nervous/phobic conditions)	☐	☐	☐	☐	☐	☐
Social history						
High caries in mother and siblings	☐	☐	☐	☐	☐	☐
Tobacco use	☐	☐	☐	☐	☐	☐
Excessive alcohol use	☐	☐	☐	☐	☐	☐
Family history of chronic or aggressive (early onset/juvenile) periodontitis	☐	☐	☐	☐	☐	☐
Dietary habits						
High and/or frequent sugar intake	☐	☐	☐	☐	☐	☐
High and/or frequent dietary acid intake	☐	☐	☐	☐	☐	☐
Exposure to fluoride						
Use of fluoride toothpaste	☐	☐	☐	☐	☐	☐
Other sources of fluoride (for example, the patient lives in a water-fluoridated area)	☐	☐	☐	☐	☐	☐
Clinical evidence and dental history						
Recent and previous caries experience						
New lesions since last check-up	☐	☐	☐	☐	☐	☐
Anterior caries or restorations	☐	☐	☐	☐	☐	☐
Premature extractions because of caries	☐	☐	☐	☐	☐	☐
Past root caries or large number of exposed roots	☐	☐	☐	☐	☐	☐
Heavily restored dentition	☐	☐	☐	☐	☐	☐
Recent and previous periodontal disease experience						
Previous history of periodontal disease	☐	☐	☐	☐	☐	☐
Evidence of gingivitis	☐	☐	☐	☐	☐	☐
Presence of periodontal pockets (BPE code 3 or 4) and/or bleeding on probing	☐	☐	☐	☐	☐	☐
Presence of furcation involvements or advanced attachment loss (BPE code *)	☐	☐	☐	☐	☐	☐
Mucosal lesions						
Mucosal lesion present	☐	☐	☐	☐	☐	☐
Plaque						
Poor level of oral hygiene	☐	☐	☐	☐	☐	☐
Plaque-retaining factors (such as orthodontic appliances)	☐	☐	☐	☐	☐	☐
Saliva						
Low saliva flow rate	☐	☐	☐	☐	☐	☐
Erosion and tooth surface loss						
Clinical evidence of tooth wear	☐	☐	☐	☐	☐	☐
Recommended recall interval for next oral health review:	months		months		months	
Does patient agree with recommended interval? If 'No', record reason for disagreement in notes	Yes	No	Yes	No	Yes	No
BPE code * is used when attachment loss is ≥7mm and/or furcation involvements are present						

2

Figure 13.21   *(cont'd)*

- Certain commonly prescribed medicines have the unwanted side-effect of **reducing saliva flow**.
  - ○ Some antihypertensives.
  - ○ Some antidepressants.
- Some medical conditions may also result in a reduced salivary flow, such as Sjögren's syndrome.
- Other medicines have the unwanted side-effect of causing gingival overgrowth, **gingival hyperplasia**, which makes effective oral hygiene techniques more difficult.
  - ○ Phenytoin – used to prevent epileptic fits.
  - ○ Nifedipine – used to control heart problems.
  - ○ Ciclosporin – used in some autoimmune conditions, as well as to prevent organ rejection after transplant.

In addition to the above, the effects of patient disability (physical or mental) as well as old age have a huge influence with regard to oral health advice and promotion, and oral disease prevention.

Patients with disabilities

Disability comes in many forms, and can be either mental or physical in its effect on the patient. Mentally disabled patients range from those with minor learning disabilities, through the elderly suffering from various forms of senile dementia (such as Alzheimer's disease), to those with con-genital problems, such as Down's syndrome. Some patients have significant problems associated with learning and socialising with others, due to inherited disorders such as Down's syndrome, autism and Asperger's syndrome, or acquired but permanent disorders following severe head injury. Those with mild impairment are likely to access dental treatment via general practice, while the more severe cases are likely to be referred for specialist dental care in community special needs clinics.

The dental care of these patients can be very demanding and time-consuming for the dental team, but also challenging and rewarding, and those dental nurses with a particular interest in this area are advised to consider the postregistration qualification of Special Care Dental Nursing, run by the National Examining Board for Dental Nurses (NEBDN).

Often (but not always, as with autistic patients), those with some learning disabilities may exhibit a reduced level of general intelligence which presents the following problems to the dental team.

- They have a short attention span, so explaining treatment plans and gaining valid consent is often difficult.
- Poor memory retention means that information and advice have to be repeated many times.
- Reduced level of understanding may cause problems in gaining the trust of the patient before dental treatment can be provided.
- Careful explanations of treatment must be given, in basic and non-threatening terms.
- The link between diet, oral hygiene and dental disease is often impossible to explain satisfacto-rily, making co-operation in the management of their oral health very difficult.
- Some dental staff may slip into a type of 'baby talk' while communicating with these patients, and that is particularly offensive to those with acquired learning disabilities.

Those who have physical disabilities make up a wide-ranging group, from those who are paralysed and wheelchair bound, through those with visual or auditory impairments, to those who have acquired medical conditions which affect the level of dental care they are able to receive. Again, the more severely disabled patients tend to be treated in specialist units rather than general dental practice, the latter being able to accommodate the milder cases to varying levels of efficiency. Some of the more common problems that these patients present to the dental team are as follows.

- Hearing-impaired patients often rely on hearing aids or lip reading to understand when being spoken to, so the lowering of PPE masks and speaking face to face are very important in communicating with them.
- Visually impaired patients like to touch and feel, or listen to the sound of, dental equipment before it is used on them, and the dental team should accede to these requests at all times.
- Some physical disabilities will require the patient to be treated in downstairs surgeries only, with wheelchair access available.
- Any disabilities causing variations in muscle tone may restrict the ability of the patient to sit comfortably in the dental chair, and may also require the use of muscle relaxants to achieve adequate access to the oral cavity.
- Stroke victims may have difficulty communicating if their speech ability has been affected, and may rely on family members or carers to make themselves understood.
- Arthritic patients, and those with upper limb deformities (such as thalidomide victims or those with dwarfism), may find adequate oral hygiene impossible to achieve without special adaptations to toothbrushes, etc.

The dental team have a vital role to play in assisting disabled patients in the dental workplace, not only in adapting the level of oral health promotion given but also in the oral hygiene techniques that they teach. Effective oral hygiene measures may require adaptations to oral health products, such as adapting a toothbrush handle so that it can be gripped more firmly by an arthritic patient. The oral health of the patient may even be the responsibility of a carer, and it is vital that they also attend the evaluation, support and review appointments with the patient, so that they have the necessary access to the dental team.

Angled toothbrushes, or even children's sizes rather than adult size, can make access to the teeth so much easier, either for the patient themselves or their carer. Good-quality rechargeable electric toothbrushes, when used correctly, can ensure a good standard of oral hygiene, although battery-operated designs are not particularly recommended as they can lose their charge with time and become quite inefficient at plaque control.

Several floss holders are now available to allow efficient interdental cleaning; indeed, even manually dextrous patients may find these less cumbersome than the traditional method of wrapping floss around the fingers.

Elderly patients

The number of people living longer is steadily increasing in the UK as medical treatment improves and healthier lifestyles predominate. A greater proportion of the population is now made up of those over the age of 70 years – the elderly. Dentally, as oral health has become understood and methods of maintaining good oral health developed, these patients are also keeping their natural teeth for longer, but because of age-related changes to the oral tissues, their dental treatment is different in some aspects from those who are younger, and is classed separately as *gerodontology*.

The changes to the oral tissues with age, and their relevance to dentistry, are summarised below.

Skin

- Has less underlying fat and elasticity.
- This gives increased tissue fragility and the likelihood of soft tissue trauma and bruising postoperatively.

Bone

- Tends to be more brittle, especially in postmenopausal women who may have some degree of osteoporosis.
- The jaw bones are therefore at increased risk of fracture during extraction.
- In particular, elderly female patients who take bisphosphonates to counteract the debilitating effects of osteoporosis are likely to require referral for tooth extraction, as the risk of postoperative bone necrosis is high.
- The natural resorption of the jaw bones following tooth extraction makes denture retention more difficult to achieve.

Oral mucosa

- Is thinner and less elastic.
- It is therefore easier to traumatise during routine treatment.
- The ridge areas are less tolerant of bearing dentures, with discomfort and ulceration more likely.
- Gingival recession will be more pronounced, which increases the risk of root caries developing.

Salivary glands

- Undergo an alteration of the salivary components and volume, especially with certain drugs.
- More likely to suffer from a dry mouth (xerostomia).
- This leads to an increased caries rate, as the self-cleansing action of saliva is reduced.
- It may also cause problems with swallowing, speech and denture retention, as well as an increased incidence of localised periodontal conditions.

Teeth

- Undergo a gradual darkening in colour, making shade matching of anterior restoratives more difficult to achieve.
- Narrowing and sclerosis of the pulp chamber lead to difficulties in gaining access to the root canals during endodontic treatment.
- Have a reduced sensitivity.

Some of the reasons for these patients experiencing difficulties in accessing dental care are as follows.

- Immobility, or poor mobility, making regular attendance at a dental practice difficult or impossible.
- Poor mobility may restrict access to ground-floor surgeries only.
- Complicated medical problems, which may limit the dental treatments available to them.

- Complicated drug regimes, some of which may interact with dental anaesthesia and dental medicaments.
- Various degrees of senile dementia, which may make explanations of dental treatment difficult for them to understand or remember.
- Various degrees of visual impairment or hearing loss, which can again make explanations difficult.

Summary

Overall, there are many factors for the dental team to consider in relation to oral health advice and promotion, and oral disease prevention, but in summary the key points of global dental health education for all patients can be condensed into four simple messages.

- Reduce the frequency of consumption of food and drink containing sugar, and avoid acid drinks.
- Maintain adequate oral hygiene measures, including brushing twice daily with fluoride toothpaste.
- Regular dental attendance at least once a year.
- Do not smoke.

Further resources are available for this book, including interactive multiple choice questions and extended matching questions. Visit the companion website at:

www.levisonstextbookfordentalnurses.com

385

14

Pain and Anxiety Control

Key learning points

A **factual knowledge** of
- local anaesthetics in pain control

A **working knowledge** of
- local anaesthetic techniques in dentistry

A **factual awareness** of
- anxiety control techniques
- patient monitoring techniques

A **working understanding** of
- the role of the dental nurse during the use of anxiety control techniques

When a patient has dental disease, especially dental caries, the dental team will aim to treat and eradicate that disease by performing some type of dental or soft tissue surgery on the patient.

- Restorative treatment performed directly on the tooth involved by:
  - fillings
  - endodontics
  - fixed restorations (crown, veneer, inlay).
- Extraction of the tooth:
  - simple extraction
  - surgical extraction.
- Periodontal treatment involving the supporting structures of the tooth:
  - scaling and debridement
  - periodontal surgery.
- Other types of soft tissue surgery.

Levison's Textbook for Dental Nurses, Eleventh Edition. By Carole Hollins.
© 2013 John Wiley & Sons, Ltd. Published 2013 by John Wiley & Sons, Ltd. Companion website: www.levisonstextbookfordentalnurses.com

All these dental techniques are covered in later chapters.

As described in Chapters 9 and 10, the oral cavity has an excellent nerve supply to all areas and anyone who has suffered the misery of 'toothache' or even minor mouth ulcers will vouch for just how well developed pain reception in this area can be. To carry out any oral or dental surgical treatments without some form of pain control would be acutely painful for the patient, and the majority of procedures are therefore usually carried out under a technique of *local anaesthesia*.

Local anaesthesia

The term 'anaesthesia' is defined as 'the loss of all sensation' but in dentistry when local anaesthetics are administered, they produce the loss of pain sensation only – pressure can still be felt by the patient. Drugs used to produce the loss of pain sensation only would therefore be more correctly termed 'local analgesics'.

Teeth and their support structures are particularly well innervated with a sensory nerve supply that responds to temperature, pressure and pain. Local anaesthetics must be given by injection before dental treatment begins, so that the patient is comfortable and pain free throughout the procedure. As described in Chapter 5, all sensations felt by the body tissues are transmitted as electrical impulses along the length of the sensory neurones (nerve cells) to the brain, where the information is analysed and interpreted. Local anaesthetics act by blocking these electrical transmissions from the source of the stimulation (the tooth or its surroundings), so that the information that a painful procedure is being carried out does not reach the brain. The patient is conscious and fully aware of the treatment being carried out (unless they are sedated), but they feel no unpleasant or painful stimuli.

In addition, the sensations of hot and cold are also blocked as they would be interpreted as pain under these circumstances – the heat generated when a tooth is drilled with no cooling water spray is interpreted as pain by the brain, and similarly anyone with sensitive teeth will relate to the very uncomfortable sensation that occurs when cold drinks are taken.

The sensations of pressure and vibration will remain, so for example the patient will be aware of the pushing and wiggling sensations that occur during a tooth extraction procedure, but it should be completely painless if the local anaesthetic has been administered correctly.

Local anaesthetic drugs

Many local anaesthetics are now available for use in dentistry, and they are all supplied within glass or plastic cartridges for use in special dental syringes (Figure 14.1). The cartridges are available as either 2.2 mL or 1.8 mL sizes, and contain the following.

- **Anaesthetic** – to block the electrical nerve transmissions to the brain so that neither pain nor temperature changes can be felt.
- **Sterile water** – acts as a carrying solution for the other constituents, and makes up the bulk of the cartridge contents.
- **Buffering agents** – maintains the contents of the cartridge at a neutral pH, so they are neither acidic nor alkaline and do not irritate the soft tissues when they are injected.
- **Preservative** – to give an adequate shelf-life to the contents.
- **Vasoconstrictor** – present in some types of local anaesthetic (but not all), and acts to prolong the action of the anaesthetic by closing (constricting) local blood vessels so that the solution is not carried away so quickly in the bloodstream.

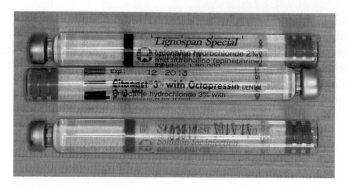

Figure 14.1   Local anaesthetic cartridges.

Both the anaesthetic agent and any vasoconstrictor present are classed as drugs, and are therefore subject to strict regulations with regard to their safe disposal. The topic of waste disposal is discussed in detail in Chapter 4, and used local anaesthetic cartridges are now classified as 'infectious hazardous waste'. Unused but out-of-date cartridges are classified as 'non-hazardous waste' as a medicine, although broken cartridges should be disposed of as sharps waste under the 'infectious hazardous waste' category.

The more common local anaesthetics currently in use in dentistry are as follows.

- **Lidocaine** – 2% lignocaine hydrochloride as the local anaesthetic with 1:80,000 adrenaline (epinephrine) as a vasoconstrictor (known as Lignospan and Xylocaine).
- **Articaine** - carticaine as the local anaesthetic with 1:100,000 adrenaline as a vasoconstrictor.
- **Citanest** – 3% prilocaine hydrochloride as the local anaesthetic, with 0.03 units/mL felypressin (Octapressin) as a vasoconstrictor.
- **Citanest plain** – 4% prilocaine hydrochloride as the local anaesthetic, with no vasoconstrictor present.
- **Mepivacaine** – 3% mepivacaine hydrochloride as the local anaesthetic, with no vasoconstrictor present (known as Scandonest).

Adrenaline (also called epinephrine) is the vasoconstrictor most commonly used in dental local anaesthetics, but it is a potent cardiac stimulant which increases the rate and depth of a patient's heart beat generally. This explains its usefulness as an emergency drug in various situations, such as during anaphylaxis when the blood pressure falls to such low levels that the heart can stop beating (see Chapter 6). Unfortunately, it also means that locals containing it cannot be used safely on patients with certain medical conditions.

- **Hypertension** – high blood pressure.
- **Cardiac disease** – poor functioning of the heart, whether due to valve defects or acquired problems such as coronary artery disease.
- **Hyperthyroidism** – an overactive thyroid gland, which tends to increase the overall metabolic rate of the patient, including the heart rate.

In addition, care should be taken with certain groups of patients or with those taking certain drugs.

- **Elderly patients** – as they may have complicated medical histories, be taking other drugs that could react with adrenaline, have undiagnosed diseases, or simply may not be able to excrete drugs efficiently due to their age.

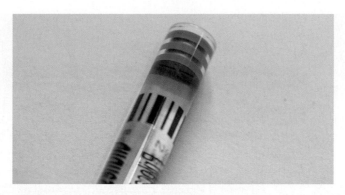

Figure 14.2   Close-up of cartridge details.

- **Hormone replacement therapy (HRT)** – given to women to counteract the adverse effects of the menopause and prevent the development of osteoporosis (thinning of the bones), but which may produce hypertension as a side-effect.
- **Thyroxine** – a drug given to patients suffering from hypothyroidism (an underactive thyroid gland), which increases their overall metabolic rate, including the heart rate.

Theoretical risks are also said to exist with patients taking certain antidepressants, including tricyclics and monoamine oxidase inhibitors (MAOIs).

The use of local anaesthetics containing no vasoconstrictor is an alternative in these groups of patients, but then the analgesic action would wear off more quickly and there is more risk of haemorrhage during surgical procedures. Alternatively, they can be given 3% Citanest – the only contraindications to its use being *pregnancy*, as felypressin is a potent drug used to induce labour due to its contractive action on the muscles of the uterus.

Local anaesthetic equipment

The equipment required to administer the local anaesthetic consists of the cartridge itself, the syringe and needle, and sometimes a topical anaesthetic is used.

The anaesthetic cartridge is a glass or plastic tube sealed at one end with a thin rubber diaphragm and at the other with a rubber bung (Figure 14.2). A special syringe and needle are used with dental cartridges. When a cartridge is inserted in the syringe, a double-ended needle pierces the diaphragm. Solution is injected when the syringe plunger engages the rubber bung and pushes it down the tube. As some patients are now known to have an allergy to latex, the rubber bung and diaphragm have been replaced by plastic alternatives in some types of specialised cartridges.

Various designs of local anaesthetic syringe are available, some being side-loading and some being breech-loading (from the back) (Figure 14.3). The majority are metallic so that they can be sterilised in an autoclave after each use, but single-use disposable ones are now also available.

In addition, the head of the plunger is adapted in some syringes so that the dentist can use an *aspirating technique* when administering the local anaesthetic, for patient safety reasons (Figure 14.4). The technique is designed to avoid the injection of the solution into a blood vessel, rather than around the nerve as is the required position. Once the needle has been positioned, the plunger is drawn back or pressed slightly and released, before injection, so that if a blood vessel has been pierced, blood will flow visibly into the anaesthetic cartridge. The needle tip can then be repositioned, the cartridge aspirated to check again, and then the contents safely injected into the correct position around the nerve.

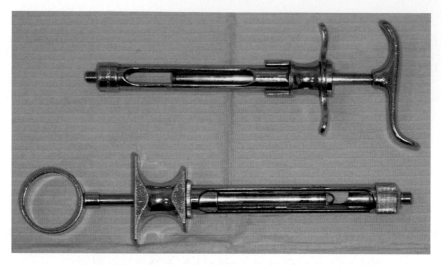

Figure 14.3   Local anaesthetic syringes.

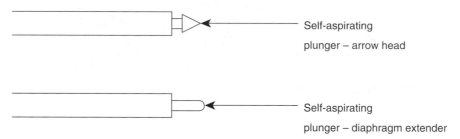

Self-aspirating
plunger – arrow head

Self-aspirating
plunger – diaphragm extender

Figure 14.4   Self-aspirating syringe plungers.

All syringes have a universal thread end for the needle to be positioned and attached. The needles are provided in various lengths and sizes, or gauges, depending on the type of injection to be given (Figure 14.5). Smaller sizes are less painful to use but are too fine to be used in some oral injection sites, especially where muscle tissue has to be penetrated to reach the target nerve.

Topical anaesthetics are used on the surface of the oral mucous membrane to provide localised anaesthesia in that area, so that a syringe needle can be inserted painlessly and the local anaesthetic can be administered. They are supplied as a paste, solution or spray which is applied to the appropriate site a few minutes before an injection is given. Commonly used surface anaesthetics are 5% lidocaine paste (Figure 14.6) or 20% benzocaine.

These products are also used to minimise the discomfort of superficial scaling, fitting matrix bands, and for preventing stimulation of the gag reflex when taking impressions.

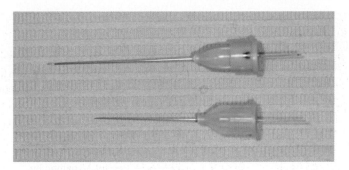

Figure 14.5   Local anaesthetic needles.

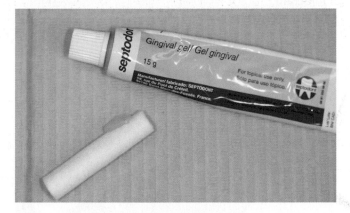

Figure 14.6   Topical anaesthetic gel.

Local anaesthetic administration techniques

Due to the variable anatomy of the jaws, the administration technique required to anaesthetise teeth is dependent on whether the relevant sensory nerve is deep within the bone or superficial to the surface. Other techniques can be used to anaesthetise individual teeth and their surroundings only, without causing any soft tissue effects. Generally, there are four basic methods of administering a dental local anaesthetic (Figure 14.7).

- Nerve block.
- Local infiltration.
- Intraligamentary injection.
- Intraosseous injection.

Nerve block

A nerve block is an injection which anaesthetises the nerve trunk as it runs in soft tissue, either before it enters the jaw bone or after it leaves it to reach the teeth and associated parts. Pain sensations from every part supplied by the nerve are blocked at the site of injection and cannot

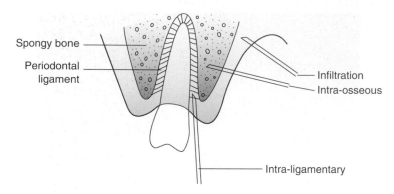

Spongy bone
Periodontal ligament
Infiltration
Intra-osseous
Intra-ligamentary

Figure 14.7   Types of injection.

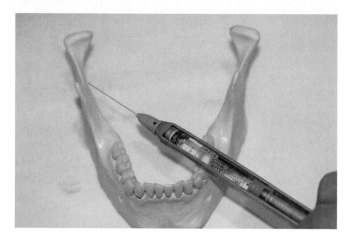

Figure 14.8   Inferior dental nerve block technique.

reach the brain. A nerve block is used when it is necessary to anaesthetise several teeth in one quadrant or where a local infiltration cannot work.

The most common example of this type of injection is the *inferior dental block*. For this injection, the anaesthetic solution is injected over the mandibular foramen, on the inner surface of the ramus of the mandible (Figure 14.8). At this site the inferior dental and lingual nerves are so close to each other that both nerves are anaesthetised together. Thus it has the effect of anaesthetising all the lower teeth and lingual gum on the side of the injection, together with that half of the tongue as well. Furthermore, it anaesthetises the lower lip and buccal gum of the incisors, canine and premolars as these are supplied by the mental branch of the inferior dental nerve. So once the patient confirms the numbness of the lower lip, the dentist knows that all the lower teeth on that side are numb too.

The only part unaffected by this injection is the buccal gum of the lower molars; this area of soft tissue is supplied by the long buccal nerve which is too far from the injection site to be affected. The nerve supply of the oral cavity is covered in detail in Chapter 9.

Other nerve block injections that may be administered by the dentist are as follows.

- **Mental nerve block** – to anaesthetise the end portion only of the inferior dental nerve, as it leaves the mandible through the mental foramen, so that only the anterior teeth and their buccal or labial soft tissues are affected (Figure 14.9).

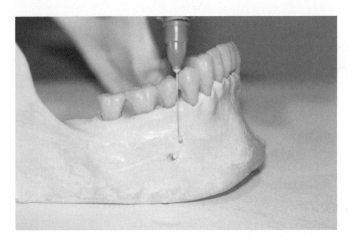

Figure 14.9   Mental nerve block technique.

- **Posterior superior dental nerve block** – to anaesthetise this nerve before it enters the maxillary antrum, so that both the upper second and third molar teeth are affected.

The nerve block technique is useful in situations where an infection is present around a tooth requiring dental treatment, as it can be anaesthetised without risking the spread of the infection by placing the injection at a distance from the tooth involved.

As stated previously, the nerves tend to run as neurovascular bundles and an aspirating technique should be used during a block injection, to prevent the inadvertent placement of the cartridge contents into a blood vessel.

Local infiltration

A local infiltration injection is given over the apex of the tooth to be anaesthetised. The needle is inserted beneath the mucous membrane overlying the jaw bone. The anaesthetic soaks through pores in the bone and anaesthetises the nerves supplying the tooth and gum at the site of injection. Thus the difference between these two types of injection is that a nerve block applies the anaesthetic to the nerve trunk, whereas an infiltration applies it to the nerve endings.

A local infiltration injection can only be used where the compact bone is sufficiently thin and porous to allow the anaesthetic to penetrate into the inner spongy bone. Thus it is usually effective for all upper teeth, and for the lower incisor teeth. The compact bone overlying the mandibular premolars and molars, however, is too thick and an inferior dental block or a mental block is necessary for these, respectively. A local infiltration can always be used to anaesthetise the local gingivae only, as will be required for procedures such as extractions.

Intraligamentary injection

The intraligamentary injection technique tends to be used in conjunction with either an infiltration or a nerve block, to produce deeper anaesthesia around hypersensitive teeth. Various specialised syringes are available, which hold the smaller 1.8 mL anaesthetic cartridge within a protective plastic sheath (Figure 14.10). The force required to administer the cartridge contents is considerable, so a ratchet design of plunger is used to maintain the pressure, and the plastic sheath prevents injury if a glass cartridge shatters during use, as sometimes happens.

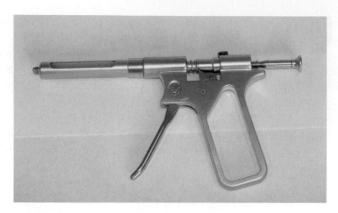

Figure 14.10   Ligmaject syringe.

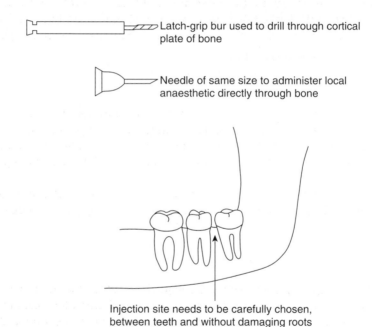

Latch-grip bur used to drill through cortical plate of bone

Needle of same size to administer local anaesthetic directly through bone

Injection site needs to be carefully chosen, between teeth and without damaging roots

Figure 14.11   Intraosseous system.

The anaesthetic is administered into the periodontal ligament of the tooth, and the surrounding gingivae can be seen to blanch as it takes effect. The technique is especially useful when a nerve block has failed to produce sufficient anaethesia of the tooth, but it cannot be used in the presence of gingival infection unless the tooth is being extracted. The force required for administration may also cause some postoperative soreness for the patient.

Intraosseous injection

An intraosseous injection is given directly through the outer cortical plate of the jaw and into the spongy bone between two teeth. A few drops of anaesthetic are first injected into the overlying gum to permit painless drilling of a small hole through the compact bone, to allow access for a needle to be inserted directly into the spongy bone (Figure 14.11).

This injection provides a relatively short duration, but profound depth, of anaesthesia for the tooth and buccal and lingual gum, on either side of the injection site, but it does not numb the cheek, lip or tongue. This makes it an excellent method for extractions. Other advantages are that it works immediately and rarely fails, thus making it useful where an infiltration or block has been unsuccessful. The disadvantages are that it cannot be used where gingival (gum) infection is present, nor should it be used in the region of the mental foramen of the mandible, as the nerve could easily be damaged while the access hole is being drilled.

The technique is very old but has gained a new lease of life with the introduction of the *Stabident* kit, containing a special drill for perforating the compact bone and a matching ultra-short needle for injecting directly into spongy bone.

Local anaesthesia for extractions

When a tooth requires extraction it is necessary to anaesthetise the surrounding periodontium as well as the tooth itself, as the periodontal ligament will be severed during the procedure. The injections required for each tooth will be more readily understood by referring back to the nerve supply of teeth.

Upper teeth

To anaesthetise any upper tooth for extraction, a local infiltration injection is given on both its buccal/labial and palatal sides. The buccal infiltration will anaesthetise the tooth and the buccal/labial periodontium, and the palatal injection will anaesthetise the palatal periodontium. It also helps to ensure sufficient anaesthesia of the tooth by infiltrating to the palatal root of the molars too.

For the second and third molars, some operators prefer to give a posterior superior dental block instead of a local infiltration on the buccal side. The nerve supply of the upper teeth and their gingivae is shown diagrammatically in Figure 14.12.

Lower teeth

An inferior dental block injection blocks the lingual as well as the inferior dental nerve. This single injection will therefore suffice for the extraction of premolars, canine and incisors, as their buccal/labial periodontium is supplied by the end section of the inferior dental nerve, the mental nerve.

For lower molars, whose buccal periodontium is supplied by the long buccal nerve, an additional local buccal infiltration is required for full anaesthesia.

The compact bone in the incisor region of the mandible is sufficiently thin to allow the use of a labial and lingual local infiltration, and many operators prefer this technique rather than an inferior dental block for anaesthetising lower incisors. The nerve supply of the lower teeth and their gingivae is shown diagrammatically in Figure 14.13.

Local anaesthesia for restorative treatments

It is unnecessary to additionally anaesthetise the palatal or lingual gingivae as well as the tooth and buccal/labial gingivae for restorative treatments, unless the gingivae in these areas need adjustment or removal as part of the restorative procedure. Examples of when this is necessary are when:

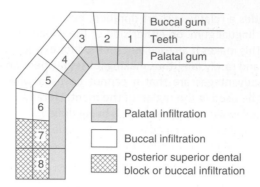

Figure 14.12   Injections for upper teeth.

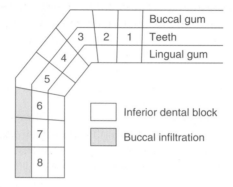

Figure 14.13   Injections for lower teeth.

- a cavity has been present for some time and the gingiva has grown into the space present – its removal is necessary to ensure that the filling material is fully adapted to the cavity walls
- a crown lengthening technique is required during tooth preparation for fixed prosthodontics – its adjustment is necessary to allow for a lengthened tooth preparation so that adequate retention of the restoration is achieved, or to achieve good aesthetics
- a crown has been lost and the remaining root face has been covered by gingival overgrowth – its removal is required to ensure an accurate impression is taken so that the new restoration fits the root face adequately.

Upper teeth

A local buccal/labial infiltration is enough for routine restorative treatments, although a posterior superior dental block is sometimes preferred for the second and third molars.

Lower teeth

An inferior dental block will anaesthetise every lower tooth, while a mental block may be used when treatment involves any tooth other than the lower molars. For restorative treatment involving just the lower incisors, a local labial infiltration will suffice instead of a full nerve block technique.

Preparation for local anaesthesia

All cartridges and needles are supplied by their manufacturers presterilised and ready for use. Reusable metal syringes are sterilised as usual in an autoclave.

A long needle of 27 gauge is used for a nerve block. For local infiltration, a short needle of 30 gauge is usually preferred. Although needles rarely break during an injection, precautions must still be taken to deal with such accidents immediately. A suitable pair of artery forceps (such as Spencer Wells or mosquito forceps) should always be available to grasp and remove the broken end.

A topical surface anaesthetic is applied for a few minutes on a cotton wool roll while the local anaesthetic equipment is prepared for use. The required cartridge is loaded into the syringe and then the smaller plastic guard at the syringe end of the needle is removed so that it can be screwed on to the syringe hub. When an aspirating technique is to be used, those syringes with a screw-type plunger will need the device screwing into the cartridge bung *before* the needle is attached, otherwise the cartridge contents will be partially ejected as it is screwed in with the needle already attached.

Injection of cold solutions can be painful, so cartridges should not be stored in a refrigerator but kept at room temperature. The injection site may be dried and disinfected by applying a suitable disinfectant, such as chlorhexidine or iodine, on a pledget of cotton wool for 15 sec. This disinfection procedure is not routinely carried out before administering a local anaesthetic for general dental treatment, but is more likely to be done during large surgical procedures, such as implant insertion or maxillofacial treatments. The injection is now given and the needle guard refitted immediately. Ideally, this should be carried out by the team member who administered the local anaesthetic, while they are still holding the syringe. The alternative is for them to lay down the syringe with its unsheathed needle onto the work surface, from where it then needs to be picked up by another team member for resheathing – increasing both the potential for a needlestick injury to occur, as well as the number of team members who may be injured during such an incident.

The used cartridge and needle are disposed of in accordance with the hazardous waste regulations – both are classed as infectious hazardous waste, subcategory 'sharps', so they need to be deposited in the sharps bin.

Inoculation injury

The used needle is a very real source of cross-infection, as it has pierced the patient's tissues and will be contaminated with blood (and possibly micro-organisms), no matter how small the amount. Resheathing of the needle is the most common cause of needlestick injuries to the dental team, and various needle guard devices have been designed to lower their incidence. Whatever the design, the needle sheath needs to be firmly held upright in a container, so that the syringe can be safely held by its back end while the needle is resheathed (Figure 14.14). In this way, fingers are kept away from the dirty needle and injury is unlikely. The team member who administered the local anaesthetic should always take responsibility for resheathing the needle personally, to reduce the number of potential injured persons involved.

If a contaminated needlestick injury does occur, the following actions must be taken.

- Stop working immediately, so that the patient and other team members are not contaminated and the potential for cross-infection to occur is minimised.
- The pierced area should be squeezed immediately to encourage bleeding, ideally under running warm water to slow down clotting at the wound site and increase the volume of blood expressed.

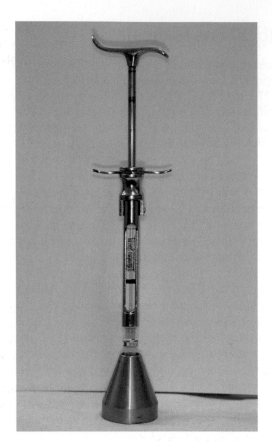

Figure 14.14   Needle resheathing device.

- Under no circumstances should the wound be sucked to encourage bleeding, as this will increase the chance of cross-infection by pathogens still further.
- The wounded area should then be cleaned with disinfectant soap, dried, and covered with a waterproof dressing.
- The senior team member should be informed of the incident.
- The patient's medical history form should be checked for known cross-infection risks, such as being HIV positive.
- If necessary, the matter should be reported to the occupational health advisor (OHA) at the local hospital, and any advice given should be followed immediately.
- The contact details of the OHA should be stored in the infection control policy documentation.
- The incident should be recorded in the accident book (low risk of serious infection) or a RIDDOR report should be written (high risk of serious infection) and the RIDDOR process followed.

Patient advice following local anaesthesia

Patients need to be informed of the expected effects they will experience after receiving a local anaesthetic, especially if it is their first injection. Otherwise, they may be unduly concerned at what they feel, or even inadvertently injure themselves.

- Sensation will be lost in the affected area for several hours – this varies between patients but is usually at least 2 h duration when a local anaesthetic containing a vasoconstrictor has been used.
- During this time, they should not attempt to eat, drink or smoke as they may bite or burn themselves without realising.
- Chewing food should be avoided directly onto the teeth restored that day, to prevent damaging the new restoration (unless the dentist has said otherwise).
- When the anaesthetic is wearing off, they will feel a 'pins and needles' sensation in the area – this is called **paraesthesia** and is perfectly normal.
- They should wait for this 'pins and needles' sensation to completely wear off before attempting to eat or drink.
- Nerve block techniques may cause a localised tenderness of the soft tissues.
- Intraligamentary techniques may cause soreness of the surrounding gingivae.
- Contact the surgery if any problems persist.

Anxiety control

Some patients exhibit high levels of anxiety at the thought of undergoing any form of dental treatment, often due to a previous 'bad experience' that may have occurred many years ago. The fear that all future dental treatment will be painful tends to stop these patients from attending for preventive care and regular treatment, and instead they usually book in as irregularly attending emergency patients with often serious oral problems.

Other patients will attend routinely for oral health assessment and preventive treatment, but will only undergo dental treatment (or at least certain aspects of it, such as an extraction) if they are able to have some form of anxiety control technique throughout the procedure. The two main types of anxiety control available are as follows.

- **General anaesthesia** – only performed in the hospital setting.
- **Conscious sedation** – can be performed in any suitably equipped dental workplace, as well as in dental hospitals and community clinics, and involves the following techniques.
    - **Oral sedation**.
    - **Inhalation sedation**.
    - **Intravenous sedation**.

General anaesthesia (GA) is a state of unconsciousness with complete loss of feeling and loss of the reflexes that normally protect and maintain the airway, such as the cough and gag reflexes. In the dental chair, the technique involved anaesthetic delivery via a nasal mask and was formerly used mainly for short procedures such as extractions (especially of the deciduous teeth in children), and the incision and drainage of abscesses.

Conscious sedation is a state of conscious relaxation which enables prolonged treatment to be carried out under local anaesthesia (LA). It is used for patients who are otherwise too nervous to tolerate dental treatment. The patient remains conscious and completely relaxed throughout and retains all their protective reflexes against blockage of the airway. It is used mainly for long procedures such as restorative treatments.

Some categories of special needs patients, and others who are too unco-operative to accept nasal mask general anaesthesia or sedation techniques, can be treated in suitably equipped hospital premises, with critical care facilities, under *endotracheal anaesthesia*. This is the general anaesthetic method normally used in hospitals.

Other methods of anxiety control that do not rely on drugs to alter the patient's state of mind are:

- **hypnosis**
- **acupuncture**.

Whichever method of anxiety control is used, the dental treatment performed will be as for any other patient, and a dental nurse will be required to assist and carry out their usual chairside duties throughout.

For those nurses with an interest in sedation and/or special care dental nursing, postregistration qualifications are available in both areas via the National Examining Board for Dental Nurses (NEBDN). Details are available at www.nebdn.org.

General anaesthesia

Endotracheal anaesthesia involves delivery of the anaesthetic gas mixture directly into the lungs through a *nasotracheal tube*. The anaesthetist passes the tube through a nostril, along the floor of the nose, into the nasopharynx. From here, using a special instrument called a *laryngoscope*, the tube is guided by direct vision through the larynx and into the trachea. The oropharynx can then be packed with gauze to prevent any foreign bodies, blood, saliva or debris entering the airway.

The advantages of endotracheal anaesthesia are that it gives the anaesthetist complete control over the airway, with no danger of obstruction, and allows use of any resuscitative measures which may be needed, while for the operator, it provides perfect anaesthesia with a clean, dry field of work for as long as required.

Referral for general anaesthesia

From time to time, some patients will need to be referred to the oral surgery department of the local hospital to undergo treatment under general anaesthetic. Special arrangements must be made for these patients that will vary according to the local facilities, but there are strict guidelines for referral cases that must be followed at all times. In particular, no referral will be accepted where attempts at providing treatment under local anaesthesia have not been offered initially in the dental workplace setting.

The referral guidelines are as follows.

- The referral letter must justify the use of GA and give the relevant dental and medical history of the patient.
- The hospital dentist treating the patient must be satisfied that GA is necessary and appropriate for the patient, and that a thorough and clear explanation of the risks and alternative options has been given.
- When the decision to provide such treatment has been agreed by the patient, the treating dentist and the anaesthetist, the patient's written consent must be obtained.
- Clear and comprehensive written pre- and postoperative instructions must be provided, and detailed records kept of all the dental procedures undertaken.
- The treating dentist must be satisfied that the facilities for such treatment, and the experience and training of the dental nurse, comply with the appropriate professional requirements.
- Adequate patient monitoring, emergency and critical care facilities and trained staff must be available in case of emergency, and these arrangements must be agreed and documented as available by all concerned.

- Adequate recovery facilities and trained staff must be provided for patients recovering from GA. They must be monitored continuously until pronounced fit for discharge by the anaesthetist, and provided with written postoperative instructions, before leaving with a responsible adult escort.
- All the team involved in dental treatment under GA must train together for dealing with emergencies, and practise such emergency procedures on a regular, and documented, basis.

The usual reasons for GA referral from a dental workplace to a hospital department are as follows.

- Young patients who require one or several extractions of deciduous or permanent carious teeth, and who will not co-operate under local anaesthesia or conscious sedation techniques.
- Older patients who require multiple third molar extractions, especially if a surgical technique is likely to be required for one or more teeth, due to impaction.
- Older patients with severe dental infection, where local anaesthesia cannot be used safely without risking the spread of the infection.
- Patient request – although this is for extraction only, not for restorative treatment.

Conscious sedation

Conscious sedation has replaced general anesthesia as a method of pain and anxiety control in general dental practice. Conscious sedation may be defined, in simple terms, as a technique that uses drugs to induce a state of relaxation that:

- is sufficient to allow the injection of local anaesthetic so that the required dental treatment can be carried out
- allows verbal contact with the patient to be maintained throughout the procedure
- allows the patient to remain conscious throughout the procedure, and able to understand and respond to commands from the dental team
- ensures that the patient retains their protective airway reflexes.

Normally in the dental surgery, long procedures such as multiple or complex restorations are done under local anaesthesia, but some patients are too nervous or otherwise unco-operative to tolerate this. In such cases, sedation techniques may be used to provide prolonged painless operating time on a relaxed patient. The three methods of conscious sedation available for use in dental practice are as follows.

- **Oral sedation** – a sedative tablet (of an anxiolytic drug such as temazepam or diazepam) is given the night before the dental appointment, and a second one 1 h before treatment begins.
- **Inhalation sedation** – formerly known as 'relative analgesia'; the patient breathes a controlled mixture of nitrous oxide and oxygen through a nasal mask, for the duration of the dental appointment.
- **Intravenous sedation** – a drug is injected into the patient's vein in a controlled manner, so that their anxiety is removed and dental treatment can be carried out.

The advantages of using sedation techniques with suitable patients are:

- patients remain conscious and co-operative throughout the session
- they retain their protective reflexes against blockage of the airway
- there is no need for a long period of starvation beforehand, as with a general anaesthetic
- a separate anaesthetist is not required, as the suitably trained dentist can act as both the sedationist and the dental operator.

INSTRUCTIONS FOR PATIENTS BEFORE UNDERGOING SEDATION BY INJECTION IN THE ARM

The technique of sedation by injection in the arm will relax you during your treatment. You will not go to sleep. You will be drowsy, but able to talk and reply to questions. You may not be able to remember much about the treatment afterwards.

The following advice will help you benefit most from this technique:

Make sure you advise your dentist of any changes in your medical history; any medicines you are taking; any recent visits to your doctor.

ON THE DAY OF TREATMENT

1. Please bring with you a responsible adult, who is able to wait and escort you home
2. At least 2 hours before have only light food prior to intravenous sedation
3. Take any routine medicines at the usual times
4. Do not drink any alcohol
5. Do not wear make up or nail varnish

DURING THE 12 HOURS FOLLOWING THE TREATMENT

1. Travel home with your escort, by car if possible
2. Stay resting quietly at home, supervised by your escort
3. Do not use any complex machinery, e.g. cooker, power tools
4. Do not drive a motor vehicle
5. Do not sign any legal or business documents, or make important decisions
6. Do not drink any alcohol

If you have any queries or questions regarding sedation, please do not hesitate to contact us at the surgery

I HAVE READ AND UNDERSTOOD THE ABOVE INSTRUCTIONS AND UNDERTAKE TO COMPLY BY THEM

Signed.. Date..

Figure 14.15   Example of an intravenous (IV) sedation consent form.

However, the General Dental Council (GDC) has issued strict guidelines concerning the levels of experience and training expected of all surgery staff involved in delivering dental treatment under sedation techniques, as well as the records that must be kept.

- A full medical and dental history must be taken before using or referring for conscious sedation.
- The type of sedation proposed must be explained to the patient, and appropriate alternatives given.
- Written pre- and postoperative instructions must be provided and written consent obtained, before the procedure is carried out; a suitable intravenous sedation consent form with instructions is shown in Figure 14.15.
- Adequate records must be kept during the procedure of the technique and drugs used; a suitable monitoring sheet for intravenous sedation is shown in Figure 14.16.

IV SEDATION PROCEDURAL RECORD

PATIENT NAME: **DATE:**

ASA: **RELEVANT MH?**   **YES**   **NO**

IV DRUG	EXPIRY DATE	BATCH NUMBER	INCREMENTS		TOTAL DOSE
			FIRST	LAST	

VENOUS ACCESS?	SITE	CANNULA
YES DIFFICULT NO		

MONITORING TIME	OXYGEN SATURATION	PULSE	BLOOD PRESSURE

RECOVERY SITE	SURGERY		
FIT FOR DISCHARGE	WALK	TALK	LISTEN
POST-SEDATION INSTRUCTIONS	TO ESCORT – VERBAL / WRITTEN		
TIME OF DISCHARGE			
CLINICIAN			
NURSE			

Figure 14.16   Intravenous monitoring sheet.

- As in all dental treatment, the dentist must only proceed within the limits of their own knowledge, training, skill and experience.
- A dentist who undertakes the dual responsibility of administering the sedation injection and providing the dental treatment must have completed relevant postgraduate education, training and continuing professional development (CPD).
- They must ensure that the most appropriate type of sedation is used, and that the minimum amount of drug is administered to achieve a suitable level of conscious sedation for the dental treatment to be carried out.
- A second appropriately trained person must be present throughout the procedure to assist the dentist and be capable of monitoring the condition of the patient, as well as assisting in any complication that may arise and acting as chaperone.
- Such a person would ideally be a dental nurse who holds the NEBDN Certificate in Dental Sedation Nursing, although a qualified and experienced dental nurse without this additional postregistration qualification is also currently acceptable in this role.
- Where a second medical or dental practitioner is administering the sedation, the treating dentist must ensure that the sedationist complies with the GDC guidelines already stated.

Conscious sedation guidelines and clinical governance (see Chapter 3) also require that:

- the technique must only be used when suitable equipment, facilities and drugs are immediately available at the chair side for treating complications
- all clinical staff are trained, practised and regularly updated to act as a team when using sedation techniques, monitoring patients and managing related complications
- supervision and monitoring of patients must be continued in the recovery area until the dentist decides they are fit for discharge, into the care of a responsible adult escort who has been provided with the written postoperative instructions.

Oral sedation

Some people are so frightened of experiencing pain while undergoing dental treatment that they are unable to sleep beforehand or to co-operate adequately in the dental chair. Such patients can be relieved of their anxiety by the use of anxiolytic drugs such as temazepam or diazepam, taken orally as a tablet. This is called *premedication* and may be used before any form of dental treatment, with or without local anaesthesia or conscious sedation. The sedation technique is particularly useful in reducing the 'gag' reflex when impressions are required.

Oral sedation is suitable for adults but not for children, and the drugs involved are addictive if they are overused. The patient is far less sedated than with other techniques, as the tablets are absorbed less by the body. However, a suitable escort must still be available for the patient, and a *pulse oximeter machine* should be used to monitor the patient if a prolonged appointment is required (Figure 14.17). This machine is connected to the patient by a finger probe, and records their pulse rate and oxygen concentration levels in the blood. If either goes outside the normal parameters, an alarm will sound and dental treatment must cease while the patient is attended to.

Inhalation sedation

This is the safest and best sedation method for children under the age of 16 years. It uses a gaseous mixture of *nitrous oxide* (N_2O) and *oxygen* (O_2). Nitrous oxide is a powerful analgesic gas that is supplied in light blue cylinders. Medical oxygen is supplied in black cylinders with a white top. These gases are administered through an autoclavable or disposable nose mask, called a *nasal*

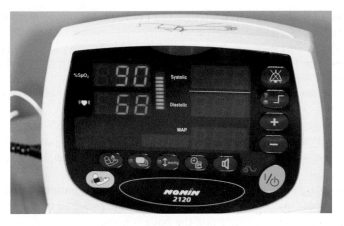

Figure 14.17   Pulse oximeter.

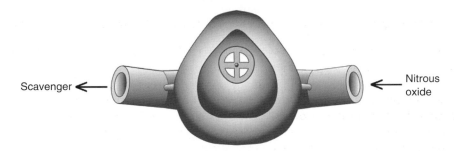

Figure 14.18   Nasal hood.

hood (Figure 14.18), from a special anaesthetic-type machine that prevents overdosage of nitrous oxide by limiting its maximum concentration to 50% and the minimum oxygen level to 30%. The technique was formerly known as relative analgesia (RA).

Sedation and analgesia are obtained by continuous inhalation of nitrous oxide and *at least* 30% oxygen. Apart from a small minority of cases, the degree of analgesia (lack of pain sensation) is insufficient to allow dental treatment without pain control, but the patient is sufficiently sedated to accept routine local anaesthesia.

Before the patient enters the surgery and the sedation session begins, the following checks are made.

- All the sedation equipment is working satisfactorily, with full gas cylinders, spare gas cylinders, resuscitation kit and the scavenging system ready for use.
- The patient's records have been read again, and the treatment plan is clear.
- An adult escort has accompanied the patient.
- All the preoperative instructions have been obeyed by the patient.
- The patient is not suffering from a cold or any other condition that may affect their ability to breathe through their nose.

The patient may then be shown into the surgery and seated, so that the treatment procedure can be explained and any questions answered. The patient is then lowered into the supine position and shown how to fit the nasal hood, and is then praised and encouraged throughout the whole of the following procedure.

- 100% oxygen is given at first, to allow the patient to familiarise themselves with wearing the nasal hood and breathing through it correctly.
- The flow gauge is adjusted to allow a first, 10% increment of nitrous oxide to be administered.
- The patient is told to expect pleasantly relaxing feelings as a 5% increment is then added; by altering the volume and tone of the voice while talking to the patient during the sedation, an element of hypnotic suggestion can be used to enhance the sedative effect of the nitrous oxide.
- Further increments of 5% nitrous oxide are added until the patient is relaxed enough to accept a local anaesthetic injection, and then to undergo the required dental treatment.
- When the treatment is complete and the patient is ready for sedation to be discontinued, the nitrous oxide is switched off and replaced by 100% oxygen for 2 min to allow the inhaled nitrous oxide to be fully dispelled from the lungs.
- During this stage the patient remains receptive to more praise and positive suggestion concerning future treatment.
- Finally the patient is asked to remove the nasal hood and the dental chair may then be gently raised to an upright position.

After 10–15 min the patient should be ready to leave the surgery, but must stay in the company of the escort for another 15 min before being discharged from the premises with the following instructions for the next 12 h.

- Do not drive.
- Do not operate machinery.
- Do not drink alcohol.
- Do not sign legal documents.

The advantages of inhalation sedation over other forms of conscious sedation or general anaesthesia are as follows.

- Patients may have a light snack up to 2 h beforehand.
- Patient recovery is rapid (about 15 min) because the sedative drug is exhaled out of the lungs and does not become absorbed into the body.
- Electronic monitoring equipment with a pulse oximeter is not required, but the pulse and respiration must still be checked by the team during the procedure.
- It is the safest and simplest form of conscious sedation, and is the best method for use with children.

The disadvantages of inhalation sedation are as follows.

- Safe delivery of the gaseous mixture requires a special inhalation sedation machine (e.g. Quantiflex MDM), which prevents less than 30% oxygen, and more than 50% nitrous oxide, from being given at any time. A normal general anaesthetic machine cannot be used instead.
- The technique necessitates a **scavenging system** for exhaled nitrous oxide, so that this is removed from the surgery area rather than being left to accumulate there, where it will be inhaled by the dental team during the working session.
- COSHH regulations must be followed with regard to the maximum number of hours that staff can work with the gases, as overexposure carries significant risks to their health.

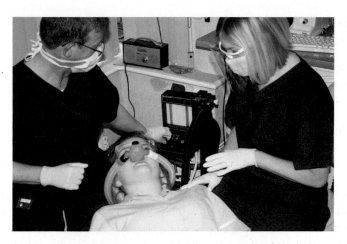

Figure 14.19   Inhalation sedation session.

- In common with most other types of drug treatment, neither inhalation sedation nor intravenous sedation should be given in the first 3 months (trimester) of pregnancy.
- However, inhalation sedation is suitable for most patients with heart disease and high blood pressure as it reduces their stress levels.
- Nitrous oxide is addictive, so overuse or drug abuse by members of the dental team may be a problem.

A typical treatment session under inhalation sedation is shown in Figure 14.19.

Intravenous sedation

This technique gives a more profound level of conscious sedation than is achieved with inhalation sedation, and is more suitable for extensive dental procedures and for those procedures that provoke high levels of patient anxiety, such as surgical extractions.

A single sedative drug such as midazolam (Hypnovel) is injected intravenously, that is, into the patient's vein, in a controlled manner. Although it does not produce anaesthesia or analgesia, the drug acts on special receptors in the brain to provide patient relaxation that is sufficient to allow them to accept the administration of a local anaesthetic. Intravenous (IV) sedation produces *amnesia* (loss of memory of the procedure) and is suitable for patients over 16 years of age. A light meal is allowed, but not less than 2 h beforehand.

The injection is usually given into a vein on the top (dorsum) of the hand or into one lying in the hollow of the elbow (antecubital fossa), and the needle (cannula) remains in the vein throughout the procedure, in case any emergency drugs have to be given. The procedure of injecting the drug directly into a vein is called *venepuncture*. Several types of cannula are available to carry out venepuncture, and Figure 14.20 shows a venflon and a butterfly cannula. An alternative 'Y-Can' is shown in Figure 14.21. The drug is administered to the patient in dose increments, so that the effect of each dose can be assessed for its sedative effectiveness before any more is given. This process is called *titration* and ensures that the patient does not become overdosed and fall into unconsciousness.

The patient signs that indicate the onset of sedation are slurring of speech and difficulty in touching the end of the nose with the finger.

Monitoring the patient's vital signs is essential throughout the procedure, and appropriate equipment should be available to do so, together with a resuscitation kit. Two specific requirements

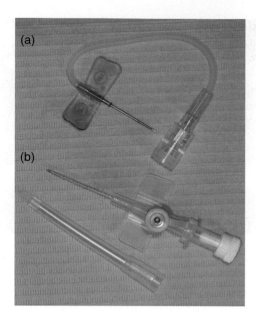

Figure 14.20   Cannulas. (a) Butterfly. (b) Venflon.

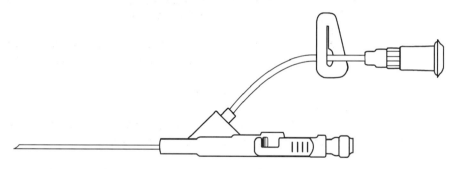

Figure 14.21   Y-Can cannula.

in such a kit for IV sedation are the drug flumazenil (Anexate) which is an emergency antidote to an overdose of the IV sedation agents, and a pulse oximeter machine (see Figure 14.17).

Recovery takes up to an hour and, as for inhalation sedation, the patient must not be left unattended in the recovery room. When the dentist has confirmed that the patient is fit to leave, verbal and written instructions are given for the patient not to drive, operate machinery, take alcohol or sign legal documents for 24 h.

The advantages of intravenous sedation over inhalation sedation are as follows.

- Better access to the patient's oral cavity for the dentist, as there is no nasal mask in the way.
- Rapid but controlled onset of sedation.
- Supportive hypnotic patter is not required during the sedation induction stage, although many operators still use it.
- Very effective degree of amnesia is produced, so no matter how difficult the dental procedure was during the session, the patient will not remember it. This is invaluable when trying to gain the patient's confidence to undergo procedures in the future.
- No nitrous oxide pollution of the surgery, and therefore no long-term risks to the dental staff.

The disadvantages of intravenous sedation are as follows.

- The drug does not produce analgesia, so the use of local anaesthetic is essential to enable all treatment to be carried out painlessly.
- The technique is unsuitable for children under 16 years of age, as their response to the drug is unpredictable.
- It should be used with caution in adults over 65 years of age, as some elderly patients may have an undiagnosed reduction of liver function, and be unable to metabolise and excrete the drug effectively.
- Overdose of the sedation drug may cause respiratory depression, and the patient's airway will need to be supported if this happens.
- Once injected, the drug and its sedative effects cannot be 'switched off'. Full recovery takes many hours and the patient will need to be supervised by a responsible adult for the rest of the day.
- There is the possibility of complications if the drug is accidentally injected into an artery instead of a vein, although a careful technique should prevent this from happening.
- Special monitoring equipment is required which is expensive to buy, but its use is essential in giving a wide margin of safety to the technique and it should always be available.

409

The dental nurse's duties

Dentists are only allowed to use sedation techniques *and* act as the operator if a suitably trained and experienced dental nurse is present throughout. Such dental nurses are:

- able to assist the dentist in the preparation and use of sedation agents and all relevant equipment
- required to monitor a patient's condition throughout the procedure and warn the dentist of any impending problems
- required to assist efficiently and speedily in any emergencies such as respiratory failure, cardiac arrest or other types of collapse
- required to know the uses of all the contents of an emergency kit so that no time is lost in successfully instituting whatever resuscitation measures are needed.

In detail, then, these duties are as follows.

For both inhalation and intravenous sedation

- Check that all preoperative instructions have been followed and that the patient is still fit for sedation.
- Have monitoring and resuscitation equipment ready and checked for its correct functioning.
- Use a soothing patter to reassure and calm the patient, but do not interrupt or contradict the operator.
- Throughout the procedure, regularly monitor and record the patient's pulse, respiration rate and skin colour.
- Inform the dentist immediately of any changes in the patient's condition.
- Be prepared, under the dentist's direction, to render immediate assistance in resuscitation procedures.
- On completion of treatment, assist the patient to the recovery area, then monitor and safeguard their recovery until the dentist allows the patient to return home with an escort.
- Before leaving, the dentist or sedation qualified dental nurse will remove any indwelling cannula, apply a dressing, and give verbal and written instructions: not to drive, operate

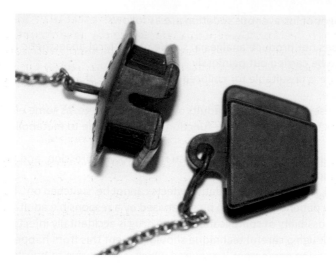

Figure 14.22   McKesson mouth props.

machinery, take alcohol or sign legal documents for 24 h, or the remainder of the day for inhalation sedation patients.
- At the end of the sedation procedure, ensure that all hazardous waste is disposed of in accordance with current regulations (see Chapter 4).

Duties specific to inhalation sedation

- Check the machine for correct functioning and cylinder labelling.
- Ensure spare oxygen and nitrous oxide cylinders are available.

Duties specific to intravenous sedation

- Have blood pressure monitoring equipment ready for use, and assist in its recording.
- Apply a surface anaesthetic to the intended injection site, if required.
- Lay out an arm board, drug syringe and needle, drug ampoules and labels, cannulae, wipes and dressings.
- Lay out the mouth props (Figure 14.22), local anaesthetic equipment, and all the dental instruments and materials required.
- Immobilise and prepare the patient's arm for venepuncture, and help to raise a vein where necessary.
- Have the pulse oximeter ready for use.

Although no special qualifications are currently necessary for adequately trained dental nurses to assist in conscious sedation, they can prove their competence by attending a course and passing the examination for the NEBDN's Dental Sedation Nursing award.

Care of the patient

Excessive fear of dental treatment is the most common reason for using sedation. Dental nurses should be constantly aware of such patients' anxiety and do everything possible to sympathise with their fears. A sympathetic and soothing manner will in itself make the whole procedure less stressful for the patient. Technical expertise alone is not sufficient for treating nervous patients.

They require the extra support of dental nurses who realise that what is a routine day's work for them is a terrifying ordeal for a frightened patient. The dental nurse must be caring, compassionate, calm and approachable, and at all times have the patient's interests at heart.

It is clear from this account that dental nurses have an extremely busy time during conscious sedation sessions, and up to three appropriately trained dental nurses may be required.

- One nurse assisting the sedationist and monitoring the patient during the procedure.
- A second nurse assisting the dentist to complete the dental treatment.
- A third nurse monitoring the previous patient in the recovery area.

Arrangements must also be made to ensure that messages, enquiries and telephone calls are dealt with by reception staff elsewhere, to prevent any interruptions or delays to proceedings in the surgery. Dental nurses have an indispensable role to play in ensuring that the entire session runs smoothly, efficiently and with the maximum consideration for the patient's comfort.

Monitoring patients

Throughout any conscious sedation procedure, it is essential to check that the circulation is adequately oxygenated. This is done by observing and recording the patient's vital signs: their skin colour, their breathing rate and depth, the quality and rate of their pulse, and their blood pressure. This is called monitoring and is made easier by the use of the pulse oximeter.

Full monitoring records must be kept at the time of the treatment, and stored in the patient's record card (see Figure 14.16).

Colour

A patient's skin colour can be observed by watching the face (especially the lips), the nailbeds of their fingers or their ears. The colour seen indicates the state of oxygenation of the blood – a pink colour is normal, whereas a purple tinge (called *cyanosis*) indicates deficient oxygenation, and pallor and sweating denote a more severe deficiency. Any such changes require immediate identification and treatment of the cause.

Breathing

Regular chest movements show that a patient is breathing, and it is also apparent by watching the movements of the reservoir bag on the inhalation sedation machine, or by feeling for rhythmic movements of the upper abdomen. The pulse oximeter will also record the blood oxygen saturation levels when in use, and this should normally be in the 95–100% range. The machine alarm will indicate if the oxygen saturation falls below 90%, and action must be taken to raise it above this level again, as it could be due to an airway blockage.

Pulse

The pulse can be felt where a superficial artery passes over underlying bone, and the usual sites are:

- the radial pulse in the inner wrist (see Figure 5.6)
- the carotid pulse in the neck (Figure 14.23).

The quality of the pulse indicates the rate, regularity and strength of the heart beats. The pulse oximeter machine will also automatically indicate the pulse, when it is attached to the patient by the finger probe.

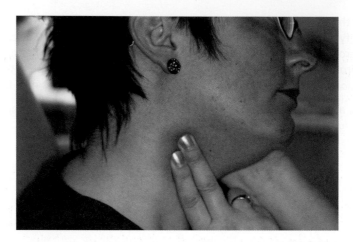

Figure 14.23   Taking the carotid pulse.

Blood pressure

The blood pressure is generally taken with an automatic machine (see Figure 5.5) rather than with the old technique of using a stethoscope and sphygmomanometer. Its measurement is usually taken before and after a sedation procedure, and gives an indication of the health of the patient's heart and circulatory system.

When the cuff device is inflated, it stops the flow of blood through the underlying artery. When the cuff is slowly deflated, blood starts flowing again (as the 'tap, tap' of the pulse) and this can be heard through the stethoscope or automatically sensed by the modern machine. The reading on the instrument scale at which the first sound is heard is noted – this is called the *systolic* pressure and denotes ventricular contraction. As deflation of the cuff is slowly continued, the sound increases to a maximum and then disappears completely. The reading at this point is called the *diastolic* pressure and denotes ventricular relaxation between heart beats.

Blood pressure readings are still measured in units of millimetres of mercury (mmHg), even though mercury is not used in modern equipment, and an average reading for a healthy young adult is 120/80 for systolic/diastolic pressures. However, it is quite usual for the preoperative systolic reading to be considerably higher than this in anxious patients, and is usually recorded at a more normal level postoperatively. Routinely, blood pressure readings above 140/90 would indicate some degree of cardiovascular problem, and the patient would be unsuitable for intravenous sedation. Inhalation sedation may still be used in the majority of these cases though.

The GDC requires dental nurses to be adequately trained and experienced for assisting with conscious sedation treatment, and this includes knowing how to monitor a patient's condition with the available equipment, and to understand the significance of their findings.

General anaesthesia and sedation emergencies

If breathing stops (respiratory failure), air cannot enter the lungs and death will occur within a short time. The heart continues beating during these critical first few minutes as there is still some residual air in the lungs, but once this has been used up, the heart itself stops beating (cardiac arrest) and death is imminent.

Respiratory failure can occur during general anaesthesia or conscious sedation procedures, and may be caused by blockage of the airway or an overdose of anaesthetic or sedation agent.

Blockage of the airway

Blockage of the airway is caused by an obstruction of the entrance to the larynx by the tongue or a foreign body. It is recognised by the following signs.

- Patient's face becomes very blue and congested.
- Clammy skin (appears with a sheen of sweat over it).
- Rise in pulse rate and blood pressure.
- Patient may also make snoring or wheezing sounds.

If the tongue is displaced backwards during general anaesthesia, it blocks the laryngeal entrance. Fortunately, this can be easily remedied by pulling the jaw forward, as the base of the tongue is attached to the mandible and moves with it. However, this type of obstruction is normally prevented by the anaesthetist's finger held behind the angle of the mandible, thus making it difficult for the jaw to be accidentally pushed backwards by the operator.

Blockage by a foreign body is an extremely serious matter as it must be located and removed before the patient is able to breathe again. Fortunately, it is rare under conscious sedation, as the normal protective reflexes that prevent such emergencies remain active. However, it may still occur, even with conscious patients. Before searching for a foreign body, the patient is laid flat with the head lower than the feet; this is called the head-down position. Then 100% oxygen is given.

In a patient undergoing general anaesthesia, the foreign body may be a mouth pack, mouth prop, extracted tooth, small instrument, clotted blood or vomited food. The purpose of a mouth pack is to prevent foreign bodies getting past it but these accidents do sometimes occur. Packs and props have a long piece of tape or chain attached which is left dangling out of the mouth, allowing them to be removed easily if they slip backwards and obstruct the airway. Any other foreign bodies are found by feeling behind the tongue with a finger or the anaesthetists's laryngoscope and removed immediately, using forceps or suction as necessary.

Whatever method is used to clear the airway, the essential factor is speed. Respiration cannot occur while the airway is blocked, so delay in removing an obstruction may be fatal.

Overdose of anaesthetic or sedative

An overdose of a powerful anaesthetic or intravenous sedation agent can cause respiratory failure by paralysing the respiratory muscles, so that the patient is unable to breathe in enough oxygen from the air or anaesthetic machine. This lack of oxygen is called *hypoxia* and its early stages are indicated by cyanosis (blue complexion). At this stage, intravenous injection of an antidote drug must be given, and in the case of sedation with midazolam, the antidote is *flumazenil* (Anexate). It reverses the action of midazolam and is an essential item for the emergency drugs kit in all workplaces using intravenous sedation techniques.

If these remedial measures are not taken, breathing will continue to weaken until it stops altogether. The face becomes ashen-grey and the pupils dilate. This will be followed by cardiac arrest unless oxygen can be introduced into the blood, by positive ventilation using emergency respiratory equipment. It is a legal necessity to have these items in any dental workplaces, whether conscious sedation techniques are carried out or not.

Resuscitation

If collapse (unconsciousness) occurs during conscious sedation in a dental workplace, the essentials of resuscitation are oxygenation of the blood and maintenance of the circulation. This is called *Basic Life Support* (BLS) and is covered fully in Chapter 6.

413

Emergency procedures

A state of preparedness is necessary for meeting dental emergencies associated with respiratory failure and cardiac arrest. A sterile, ready-for-use, emergency kit must be immediately available every time conscious sedation or any other treatment is undertaken. The kit must contain the following essential items.

- An efficient manual suction device for clearing a blocked airway, for use if the surgery suction unit is unavailable due to failure of the electric supply.
- Oropharyngeal (Guedel) airways (Figure 14.24).
- Manual pulmonary resuscitator, e.g. Laerdal pocket facemask (Figure 14.25).
- Resuscitation drugs, including flumazenil if intravenous sedation is used.
- Syringes and needles for drawing up and injecting emergency drugs.

A cylinder of oxygen with tubing and suitable attachments for use with a resuscitation mask and bag must also be part of the emergency equipment.

(a)

(b)

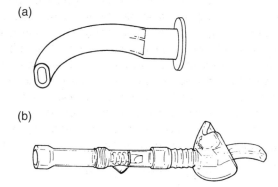

Figure 14.24   Airway tubes. (a) Oropharyngeal (Guedel) airway. (b) Brook airway.

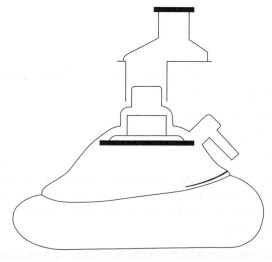

Figure 14.25   Laerdal pocket mask.

Other forms of anxiety control

Two other forms of anxiety control, which do not rely on the administration of drugs, have begun to play more of a role in dental treatment over the last few years. They are *hypnosis* and *acupuncture*. Although qualifications are not currently a legal requirement for dentists wishing to use them in practice, there are suitable qualifications already available in both techniques. A brief outline of each discipline is given.

Hypnosis

This is a technique of anxiety control that relies purely on the skill of the hypnotist to produce an altered state of mind in the patient, so that they are neither fully awake or asleep. It is achieved by verbally achieving hypnotic suggestion, to produce the altered state.

No clear definition of hypnosis is available but it can be described as 'an altered state of awareness in the patient, so that they are more amenable to suggestion'. When it is successfully suggested to them by the hypnotist that dental procedures are painless or pleasant or even happy experiences, this is a powerful tool in overcoming a dental phobia.

Full dental hypnosis is not currently practised by many dentists but with patients who are already consciously sedated using one of the conventional techniques involving drug administration, it is relatively easy for the depth of their sedation to be accentuated by using hypnotic suggestion as well. The easiest method is for the dentist to merely alter the tone and depth of their voice while talking to the sedated patient, so that a low and slow, monotone style of speech is used. The desired suggestions are then repeated to the patient in a calm, deep voice, often with key words dragged out in length, so for example the word 'slow' becomes 'sloooow'.

The technique requires lots of practice to be used successfully, and every dentist will develop their own favourite phrases and patter with time. Some examples are as follows.

- '... and any pain you feel will be just a tiny insect bite ...'
- '... and all the pain has been sucked away, and everything feels good now ...'
- '... and as you breathe in you can feel yourself becoming more and more relaxed ...'
- '... and you're lying on a nice sunny beach, and you can hear the waves gently lapping onto the shore ...'

Acupuncture

This is a branch of traditional Chinese medicine in which special needles are inserted into the patient's skin for the following reasons.

- As therapy for various disorders.
- To produce anaesthesia.
- To reduce anxiety.

Again, no qualifications are currently required, but the GDC would expect any dentist to have at least attended a validated training course before using the technique on patients.

The manner in which acupuncture works is not fully understood, but it is believed to be a combination of the following.

- The needle prick causes the patient's body to release its own painkillers (called **endorphins**) which act as local analgesics.

- The technique helps to induce a form of hypnosis in the patient.
- The needle prick acts as a distraction from the original source of pain.

However it works, acupuncture has been successfully used to carry out painless dental treatment, as well as to remove the 'gag' reflex in susceptible patients so that impressions can be taken. It is also used as a technique for long-term management of chronic dental pain in temporomandibular disorders. Although acupuncture can be used to reduce the anxiety associated with dental treatment, it is currently seldom used to do so.

Further resources are available for this book, including interactive multiple choice questions and extended matching questions. Visit the companion website at:

www.levisonstextbookfordentalnurses.com

15

Restorative Dentistry

Key learning points

A **factual knowledge** of
- cavity classification
- temporary and permanent filling materials

A **working knowledge** of
- cavity preparation and restoration using filling materials
- the instruments and equipment used in tooth restoration

A **factual awareness** of
- the causes of pulp death
- the various non-surgical endodontic techniques available to preserve a tooth
- the instruments and medicaments used in non-surgical endodontic techniques
- the technique of apicectomy

Following a dental examination during an oral health assessment, the dentist may often diagnose the presence of a cavity in a tooth. Cavities are caused by dental caries attacking the hard structure of the tooth, and if left untreated they will cause pain for the patient, and will develop into a more serious dental problem that may result in the loss of the tooth. A cavity will therefore require treatment and once its presence has been determined, a treatment plan will be decided upon based on the following information.

- **Cavity size** – is restoration of the tooth feasible with a restorative filling alone, or should a fixed restoration (such as a crown) be considered?
- **Cavity position** – which tooth surface or surfaces are involved, and do aesthetics need to be considered?

Levison's Textbook for Dental Nurses, Eleventh Edition. By Carole Hollins.
© 2013 John Wiley & Sons, Ltd. Published 2013 by John Wiley & Sons, Ltd. Companion website: www.levisonstextbookfordentalnurses.com

- **Tooth involved** – is a posterior chewing tooth involved, that will require a strong and long-lasting restoration, or is an anterior tooth involved where chewing forces are less but aesthetics have to be considered?
- **Extent of caries** – is it possible that full caries removal will cause pulp exposure, so that endodontic treatment will also be required?
- **Patient's wishes** – is the patient amenable to restorative treatment, or are they likely to be unco-operative, as may occur especially with younger children and some patients with special needs?

Taking into consideration all these points, restoration by filling may be on a temporary or a permanent basis.

- **Temporary restoration** – in less co-operative patients, and if a fixed restoration is being considered as the final restoration in the short term. The usual materials used are:
  - zinc oxide and eugenol cement
  - zinc phosphate cement
  - zinc polycarboxylate cement.
- **Amalgam restoration** – in posterior teeth, where restoration strength and longevity are more of an issue than aesthetics.
- **Composite restoration** – in anterior teeth for aesthetics, although more modern composite materials are suitable for use in restorations in posterior teeth too.
- **Glass ionomer restoration** – in deciduous teeth (because of its fluoride release) and in certain cavity sites where retention of the restoration is difficult.

The aims of good cavity preparation are the same, wherever the lesion has occurred and whatever restorative material is to be used.

- To remove all caries from the cavity.
- To remove the minimum amount of healthy tooth tissue while doing so.
- To avoid accidental pulp exposure, by poor dental technique.
- To protect the pulp after treatment by using linings or bases as necessary.
- To produce a retentive cavity for restoration, if necessary (some materials are adhesive to tooth tissue).
- To restore the tooth to its normal shape and prevent stagnation areas developing, as these would allow plaque retention and further carious attack to occur.
- To restore the function of the tooth, for adequate mastication.
- To restore the retentive shape of the tooth if it acts as a bridge abutment or denture retainer.
- To restore the aesthetics of the tooth (its correct appearance).
- To alleviate any discomfort or pain experienced by the patient, due to the initial presence of the cavity.

Fillings

Classification of cavities

Cavities are classified into five different types, depending on the site of the original caries attack. This is called *Black's classification* after the American dentist who devised the system. In general usage, his classification also applies to the naming of the shape of the fillings inserted in each class of cavity.

- **Class I** cavities are those involving a **single** surface, in a pit or fissure, so a class I filling could be an occlusal, a buccal or a lingual filling, for example.
- **Class II** cavities involve at least **two** surfaces of a posterior tooth, the mesial or distal, and the occlusal surface of a **molar** or **premolar**. Thus a class II filling could be a mesial-occlusal (MO) filling in a premolar, or a mesial-occlusal-distal (MOD) filling in a molar.
- **Class III** cavities involve the mesial or distal surface of an **incisor** or **canine**.
- **Class IV** cavities are the same as class III but extend to involve the **incisal edge** on the affected side.
- **Class V** cavities involve the **cervical margin** of any tooth. Thus a class V filling could be a labial cervical filling in an upper incisor or a lingual cervical filling in a lower molar.

This universal method of cavity classification enables their accurate recording on the dental chart so that a restoration can be placed, and an example of each type of cavity is shown in Figure 15.1.

Cavity preparation

A permanent filling cannot be inserted directly into a carious cavity. Instead, careful preparation of the cavity is required to ensure that:

- all plaque and soft carious dentine is removed from the cavity margins, although the deepest layer of dentine may be conserved to avoid exposure of the pulp
- as much of the enamel as possible is also conserved
- the filling will be as much a permanent fixture as possible, although its longevity will also depend on the standard of plaque control and good diet that the patient follows
- caries will not recur at its margins due to any restoration overhang or other defect.

Every dentist has their own personal preferences for the instruments used during restorative procedures such as the placement of fillings, and Table 15.1 shows the more usual items and an explanation of their function. They are usually set out on a tray for use, which is often referred to as a *'conservation tray'* (Figure 15.2).

The vast majority of tooth restoration carried out using fillings will require the administration of a local anaesthetic before proceeding, so that the patient does not have a painful experience. Techniques of local anaesthesia are discussed in detail in Chapter 14.

Retention of fillings

Permanent fillings are meant to stay put permanently and the cavity must be specially prepared to provide maximum retention. Before explaining how this is done, it is necessary to consider the types of filling materials used – plastic and preconstructed.

Plastic fillings are soft and plastic on insertion but set hard in the cavity. They include:

- all temporary cements
- amalgam
- glass ionomer cements
- composites.

Preconstructed restorations are called *inlays* and are made in the laboratory, after the teeth have been prepared, and then cemented into place.

- Gold
- Porcelain
- Other ceramic materials

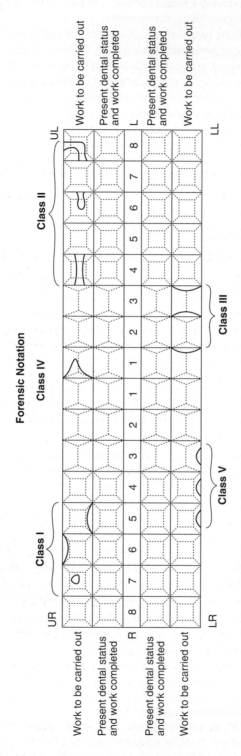

Figure 15.1 Completed chart with cavities recorded.

Table 15.1   Some of the instruments used during restorative procedures

Item	Function
Mouth mirror	To aid the dentist's vision To reflect light onto the tooth To retract and protect the soft tissues
Right-angle probe	To feel the cavity margins To feel softened dentine within the cavity To detect overhanging restorations
Excavators	Small and large spoon shaped, used to scoop out softened dentine
Amalgam plugger	To push filling materials into the cavity and adapt them to the cavity shape, leaving no air spaces and forcing excess mercury to the surface of the filling for removal during carving
Burnisher	Ball shaped or pear shaped, to press and adapt the restoration margins fully against the cavity edges so that no leakage occurs under the restoration
Flat plastic	To remove excess filling material and mercury from the restoration surface, and create a shaped surface that encourages food particles to flow off naturally, rather than becoming lodged around the restoration
College tweezers	To pick up, hold and carry various items such as cotton wool pledgets
Gingival margin trimmer	To trim the margin of the cavity to ensure no unsupported enamel nor soft dentine remains – their use is becoming obsolete with the wider range of burs available
Enamel chisel	To remove any unsupported enamel from the cavity edges – their use is becoming obsolete with the wider range of burs available

Retention for plastic fillings is obtained by simply cutting tiny grooves in the cavity walls to make the entrance smaller than its inside dimensions, as shown in Figure 15.3. As the materials are initially soft, they can be packed into the cavity easily to fill all the available space but cannot drop out of the cavity once set because they have hardened and are locked into position. For fillings involving occlusal and mesial surfaces, or occlusal and distal, a *dovetail* effect is produced by grooving the cavity walls to prevent the filling coming out mesially or distally (see Figure 15.3). Note that this diagram is deliberately exaggerated to show more clearly the principles of retention; in reality, sound tissue is not sacrificed for the sake of extensive undercuts. Tiny grooves in the cavity walls are sufficient to provide adequate retention.

Sometimes it is not possible to prepare cavities which are sufficiently undercut to retain a plastic filling. In such cases they may be made retentive in other ways.

- Self-tapping dentine pins for amalgam restorations.
- Acid etching for composites, to provide a microscopically rough surface on the enamel and allow mechanical locking of the material onto the enamel prisms.
- Chemical bonding for glass ionomer cement onto the dentine surface.

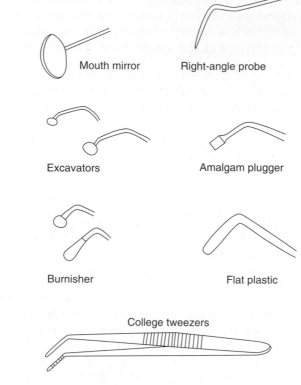

Mouth mirror   Right-angle probe

Excavators   Amalgam plugger

Burnisher   Flat plastic

College tweezers

Figure 15.2   Conservation tray instruments.

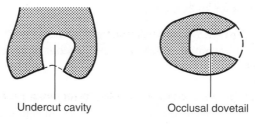

Undercut cavity   Occlusal dovetail

Figure 15.3   Undercutting of cavities.

These methods are covered in the appropriate section of this chapter, for each filling material.

Inlays are hard and rigid when inserted into the cavity, so the dentist would not be able to place and seat them fully if undercuts were present. To prevent them coming out occlusally, they rely on parallel cavity walls to provide maximum retention and the use of adhesive cement to 'glue' them into the prepared cavity. As with plastic fillings, a small dovetail effect may be used to prevent dislodgement mesially or distally.

Cavity lining

Before a permanent filling is inserted the cavity may need to be lined. A *lining* is an insulating layer of cement that is placed on the cavity floor and which has the following functions.

- Protects the pulp from temperature fluctuations that may be transmitted through metallic filling materials, and that are experienced as sensitivity or even pain in the tooth.
- Protects the pulp from chemical irritation of non-metallic materials.
- Seals the pulp from any residual caries bacteria, allowing secondary dentine to be laid down.

Dependent on how deep the cavity is, pain and possibly death of the tooth may occur through failure to protect the pulp tissue by the insertion of an adequate lining.

The linings used are zinc oxide and eugenol cement, zinc phosphate cement, polycarboxylate cement and calcium hydroxide.

The methods of insertion and techniques of finishing by polishing of fillings vary dependent on the material used, and are discussed in detail later.

Moisture control

Adequate moisture control during restorative procedures is one of the most important duties of the dental nurse. Control of moisture – from saliva, blood or instrument cooling sprays – is necessary for the following reasons.

- To protect the patient's airway from fluid inhalation, especially as the majority of procedures are carried out with the patient lying flat back in the dental chair (supine position).
- To ensure the patient is comfortable during treatment – so that they do not have a mouth full of fluids while lying in the supine position during dental treatment.
- To allow the dentist good visibility to the treatment area, therefore avoiding inadvertent patient injury by catching the soft tissues or the wrong tooth with the drill.
- To allow the restorative materials to set correctly, without moisture contamination.
- To allow the adhesion of cements and linings to the tooth, without moisture contamination.
- To avoid the uncontrolled loss of materials from the cavity during use, such as acid etchant which can burn the soft tissues.

The following methods are used to control moisture.

- High-speed suction.
- Low-speed suction.
- Use of absorbent materials – cotton wool rolls, cotton wool pledgets and oral inserts such as a 'Dryguard'.
- Use of rubber dam.
- Compressed air drying, using the triple syringe (3 in 1) of the dental unit.

High-speed and low-speed suction

This is provided by either high-speed aspiration (suction), for fast removal of moisture during drilling, or low-speed aspiration for continual moisture control without sucking at the soft tissues. In the case of high-speed suction, the dental nurse uses a wide-bore aspirator connected to the suction unit to rapidly remove fluids, blood and debris from the treatment area. This prevents the patient from choking, as well as emptying the oral cavity of volumes of fluid that would be uncomfortable for the patient to hold without feeling the need to spit out. With low-speed aspiration, the patient holds a *saliva ejector* attached to the suction unit or *aspirator* to slowly but continually remove any fluids that have pooled in the floor of the mouth, so that the patient does not have to constantly swallow during the treatment. Many different types of ejector are used but those with

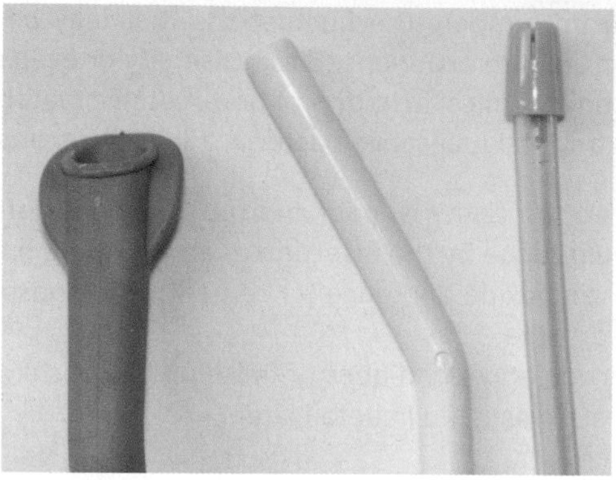

Figure 15.4   Aspirator and ejector tips.

a flange to keep the tongue away from the treatment area are particularly helpful. The dental nurse may also use the high-speed aspirator tube as a soft tissue retractor. Examples of aspirators and ejectors are shown in Figure 15.4.

Absorbent materials

Cotton wool rolls or absorbent pads are placed in the buccal or lingual sulcus to absorb saliva and keep the soft tissues away from the teeth. Cotton wool pledgets are used to dab the actual cavity dry, while excessive saliva contamination can be prevented by placing a 'Dryguard' over the parotid salivary gland duct. These pads contain an absorbent material similar to that used in babies' nappies, and can retain considerable volumes of fluid. The cavity itself can be further dried by blowing it with compressed air from the triple syringe of the dental unit. Examples of some of these materials are shown in Figure 15.5.

Rubber dam

This is the best method of moisture control of all and the various components are shown in Figure 15.6.

A rubber dam is a thin sheet of latex rubber or vinyl material which is placed over a tooth to isolate it from the rest of the mouth. A *rubber dam punch* is used to punch a small hole in the rubber sheet, which is then fitted on so that the tooth projects through the hole. The rubber dam is kept in place by a *rubber dam clamp* which is fixed on the tooth with rubber dam clamp forceps. Finally a *rubber dam frame* is used to support the sheet while in use, so that it remains taut and maintains a clear visual field. A napkin is placed between the patient's chin and the rubber to make it more comfortable and a saliva ejector may be provided to remove any pooled saliva. Dental floss or an additional piece of rubber dam material is used to work the sheet between the teeth.

A rubber dam may be applied to any number of teeth. It enables the operator to keep a tooth dry and maintain an uncontaminated field during dental treatment, and prevents pieces of filling material, debris or small instruments falling into the patient's mouth.

This moisture control technique is more comfortable for patients as it prevents water spray or irrigation fluids entering the mouth, and far better for the dentist, as it improves access and visibility by keeping the tongue, lips and cheek out of the way. It also helps prevent cross-infection of patients and chairside staff, by minimising the aerosol of infected debris spread by the use of compressed air and water spray.

424

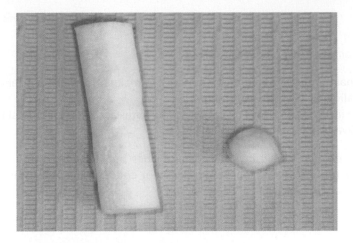

Figure 15.5 Cotton wool roll and cotton pledget.

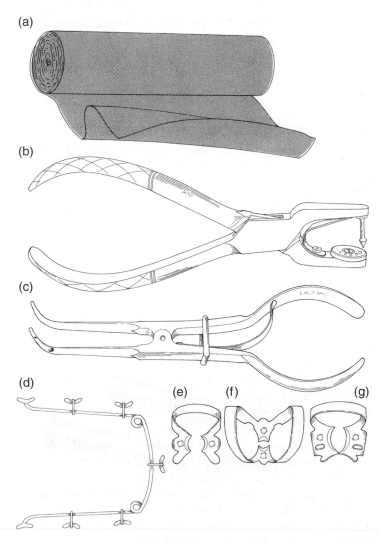

(a)

(b)

(c)

(d) (e) (f) (g)

Figure 15.6 Rubber dam instruments. (a) Rubber dam. (b) Rubber dam punch. (c) Rubber dam clamp forceps. (d) Rubber dam frame. (e) Premolar clamp. (f) Incisor (butterfly) clamp. (g) Molar clamp.

The two main uses of a rubber dam are:

- in root canal therapy (endodontic treatment), to maintain a sterile field and prevent inhalation or the swallowing of small instruments
- during the insertion of fillings (especially composites and glass ionomers) to avoid their failure due to saliva contamination.

Ideally, a rubber dam should be used for all fillings but most operators consider it too time-consuming for routine use in all procedures except endodontics. The technique is also not well tolerated by every patient.

Equipment

Handpieces

Cavities are cut by the use of dental burs fitted into the head of a handpiece. The speed of cutting depends on the type of handpiece and the purpose for which it is used. They have a built-in water spray to counteract the heat generated when cutting hard tissue and may also have fibre-optic illumination to aid cavity preparation.

Air turbine handpieces run at very high speeds of up to 500,000 revolutions a minute, and use friction grip *diamond* or *tungsten carbide burs* to cut easily through both enamel and dentine. There is a tiny air turbine motor in the head of the handpiece which is driven by compressed air. The advantages of air turbines are the ease and speed of cutting. The disadvantages are that they offer little tactile sensation to the dentist, so excessive tooth removal can occur, and their vibration may be associated with a condition called 'vibration white finger' when used over many years.

Slow handpieces run at around 40,000 revolutions per minute, and are driven by air or electric motors at the base of the handpiece. These are much more versatile in their range of speed and uses, varying from low-speed root canal treatment and removal of carious dentine to high-speed conventional cavity preparation. They use latch grip stainless steel or tungsten carbide burs when used on teeth or friction grip stainless steel acrylic trimming burs when used to trim dentures. They are more 'user friendly' for the dentist, as the tactile sensation provided is much better. Portable versions of the electric motors are particularly suitable for domiciliary dental treatment (that carried out away from the surgery, often in the patient's home). An air turbine and a slow handpiece are shown in Figure 15.7.

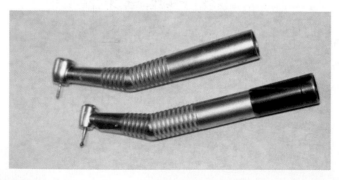

Figure 15.7 Handpieces.

All handpieces, however driven, and of whatever age, are made in two basic designs: *contra-angled* and *straight*. A contra-angle is used most often in the mouth as it provides access to every tooth. A straight handpiece is used to trim acrylic denture items.

Burs

Burs for low-speed procedures are made of steel. They are used for removing caries, cutting dentine (but not enamel), trimming dentures and other laboratory work. Examples are shown in Figure 15.8.

Burs for high-speed handpieces have diamond or tungsten carbide cutting surfaces and are used for rapid removal of enamel, dentine and old fillings. Examples are shown in Figure 15.9.

Straight handpiece burs have a long plain shank. Burs for low-speed contra-angle handpieces are short and have a notch in the shank which fits by a *latch grip*. Short burs are also used for air turbine handpieces but they have a plain shank which gives a *friction grip* (Figure 15.10).

Contra-angled low-speed handpieces with smaller heads, and using even shorter burs, are used on children. They are called *miniature* handpieces and burs.

The cutting ends of burs are made in many different shapes to allow different types of dental treatment to be carried out (Figure 15.11) but those most commonly used are as follows.

- Round – used for gaining access to cavities and at low speed for removing caries.
- Pear – used for shaping and smoothing cavities.
- Fissure – used for shaping and outlining the cavity.

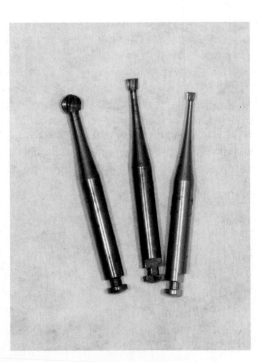

Figure 15.8   Slow-speed burs.

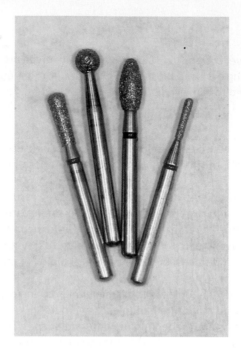

Figure 15.9 High-speed burs.

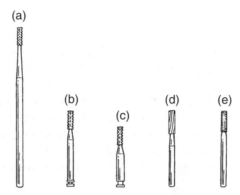

Figure 15.10 Burs. (a) Steel for straight handpiece. (b) Steel, latch grip, for low-speed contra-angle handpiece. (c) Steel, latch grip, for miniature contra-angle handpiece. (d) Tungsten carbide, friction grip, for air turbine handpiece. (e) Diamond, friction grip, for air turbine handpiece.

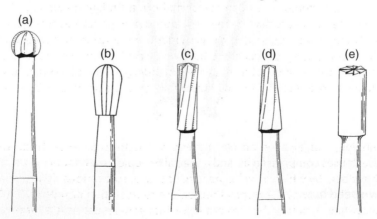

Figure 15.11 Bur shapes. (a) Round. (b) Pear. (c) Flat fissure. (d) Tapered fissure. (e) End-cutting.

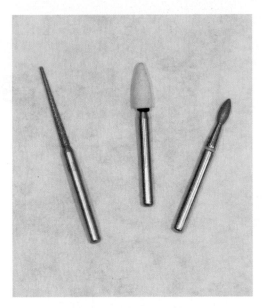

Figure 15.12   Polishing burs.

Polishing instruments

There is a great variety of polishing instruments but they generally comprise fine abrasive stones, wheels, discs and strips, finishing burs, brushes and polishing pastes. Apart from hand abrasive strips, they are all used with a handpiece. Finishing burs and stones are used for smoothing cavity margins and trimming fillings (Figure 15.12). Abrasive discs and strips are used for fine trimming and polishing.

Small abrasive stones, wheels and brushes are manufactured with a shank which fits the appropriate handpiece. Larger wheels, stones and abrasive discs require an independent mounting shank called a *mandrel*. Wheels and metal discs are fitted on a *Huey* mandrel, sandpaper discs with a metal centre and *Soflex discs* use a *Moore* mandrel, and plain sandpaper discs a *pinhead* mandrel (Figure 15.13).

Care of instruments

All cutting instruments must be kept sharp because blunt ones are inefficient and painful for the patient. Hand instruments such as chisels and excavators should be sharpened regularly on a small flat oilstone (*Arkansas stone*) or with an abrasive disc in a straight handpiece. Burs are cleaned in an ultrasonic cleaner and autoclaved after use, although any that become heavily contaminated during use or that are used on known high-risk patients are considered as single-use items and are discarded. These burs, along with all blunt burs, are discarded into the sharps container.

All handpieces must be lubricated regularly according to manufacturers' instructions before being decontaminated and sterilised. The methods used are described in Chapter 8.

Air abrasion

Modern technology has allowed an old method of tooth preparation to be reintroduced into dental practice. It uses compressed air and a special handpiece to convey a jet of abrasive particles on to a tooth surface, by which it can remove hard tissue, soft carious tissue or surface stains and even abrade metal or composite restorations before cementation or repairs. It is less painful than conventional cavity preparation but has not come into general use as it is rather expensive.

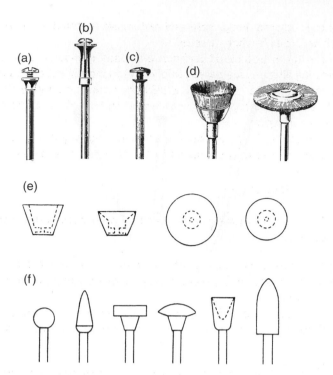

Figure 15.13   Mandrels and brushes. (a) Huey mandrel. (b) Moore mandrel. (c) Pinhead mandrel. (d) Polishing brushes. (e) Abrasive rubber cups and discs for Huey mandrel. (f) Mounted fine abrasives.

Role of the dental nurse during restorations

There are some duties that are specific to the preparation and placement of restorations, and others that are very similar in other areas of dentistry, but the good dental nurse must be competent and proficient in all. The role of the dental nurse during restorative treatment can be summarised as follows.

- Have a good understanding of the procedure to be carried out.
- Be aware of their position in the dental team for the procedure – this may be as the chairside nurse assisting directly with the procedure or as a second nurse available to mix materials as required.
- Have all the patient records, charts, radiographs and consent forms completed and available for the appointment.
- Communicate effectively with the patient throughout the procedure, inspiring confidence and trust.
- Monitor the patient throughout the procedure, ensuring their comfort and well-being and giving reassurance where necessary.
- Assist during the administsatration of local analgesia – having the correct syringe and needle loaded with the correct cartridge as directed, passing them safely to the dentist for use, then retrieving them after use and safely resheathing the needle using a hands-free device to avoid needlestick injury (unless this is done by the dentist).
- Provide careful but efficient moisture control and soft tissue retraction throughout the procedure, ensuring that no soft tissue trauma is caused.
- Anticipate and pass instruments, etc. to the dentist in the correct order of use during the procedure.

- Be aware of the required lining, base and restorative material to be used for the procedure, and mix each accordingly when directed.
- Be proficient in the four-handed technique of passing instruments, etc. to the dentist as required, ensuring all items are passed safely (and especially not across the patient's face).
- Follow the infection control policy to fully decontaminate the surgery after the appointment.
- Follow the health and safety policy with regard to hazardous waste disposal, especially in relation to waste amalgam.
- Ensure that all records, charts, etc. are correctly and securely stored for future use after being completed by the dentist, maintaining patient confidentiality at all times.

Temporary restorations

These are placed as a temporary measure, before the tooth is restored permanently, and are used for a variety of reasons.

- As an emergency measure to seal a cavity and prevent carious ingress.
- During endodontic treatment, as repeated access may be required to the pulp chamber over several appointments.
- During inlay construction to seal the preparation while the permanent inlay is constructed.
- To allow a symptomatic tooth to settle and become symptom free, before being permanently sealed.

There are several materials available for use as a temporary restoration, some of which have other uses in dentistry – they are multi-purpose materials. Overall, they are unsuitable for use as a permanent restoration because they are too soft to chew on, are too soluble in saliva, and would not remain intact for long periods.

The key features of all temporary restorations are as follows.

- Quick mixing and placement.
- Cheap compared to permanent restorative materials.
- Easily removed from the cavity when required.
- Not strong enough to be chewed on routinely.
- Have varying degrees of adhesiveness to the tooth.
- Some contain sedative ingredients to help settle inflamed pulps.

A variety of materials is available, under many trade names, but temporary restorations can generally be categorised into one of the following groups of materials.

- Zinc oxide and eugenol.
- Zinc phosphate.
- Zinc polycarboxylate.
- Gutta percha.

Zinc oxide and eugenol

Presented as zinc oxide powder and eugenol liquid ('oil of cloves'), the cement is made by mixing increments of the yellowy powder to a drop of the clear eugenol liquid on a glass slab with a spatula (Figure 15.14). Older varieties of the product can be thickened if necessary by squeezing in a napkin to remove some of the eugenol liquid, otherwise full setting of the cement produced takes a few hours.

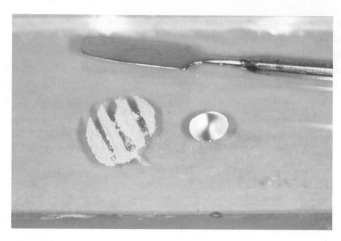

Figure 15.14   Zinc oxide and eugenol cement – to mix.

When ready for use, the cement should be able to be rolled into a 'sausage shape' with the spatula, without sticking to it or smearing across the glass slab.

Uses of the cement are:

- temporary filling
- non-irritant base for deep cavities
- sedative dressing for painful carious teeth and for dry sockets
- main constituent of some impression pastes, periodontal packs and root filling materials.

The main advantage of the cement over other temporary restorations is that it is soothing and non-irritant to the pulp and can be safely used in deep cavities. The main disadvantage is that it used to be too soft and slow-setting to use as a foundation for a permanent filling in one visit. However, this can now be overcome by using a strengthened quick-setting proprietary brand such as *Kalzinol*. In this form it is generally regarded as a satisfactory lining for metal fillings.

Other disadvantages are that the cement is not compatible with composite filling materials, and cannot be used as a lining beneath these types of restorations. Manufacturers' instructions must always be followed in selecting a suitable lining for any non-metallic fillings.

Also, some patients are allergic to preparations containing eugenol, although special eugenol-free alternatives are now available.

Zinc phosphate

Presented as zinc oxide powder and phosphoric acid liquid, the cement is prepared by mixing increments of the white powder to the clear liquid on a glass slab with a spatula (Figure 15.15). Two different mixes are used.

- A thick mix of putty consistency to use as a temporary filling or a base beneath a permanent filling.
- A thin creamy mix to use for crown and inlay cementation – this is called a **luting cement**.

Setting of the cement takes a few minutes depending on various factors.

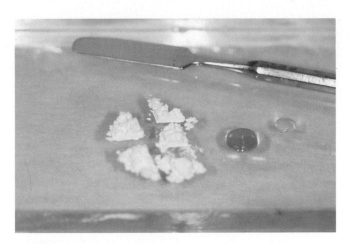

Figure 15.15   Zinc phosphate cement – to mix.

- A warm slab accelerates the setting time.
- A cold slab slows down the setting time.
- A thick mix sets more quickly than a thin mix.
- A dry slab must be used as moisture accelerates setting.
- Powder contaminated by moisture in the air will set too quickly for use, so it is most important to screw the cap on tightly, immediately after using the bottle of liquid.

These various factors can be used to advantage, depending on the particular use of the cement at the time. If a long setting time is required, such as when cementing a bridge, a cold dry slab can be used to give the maximum setting time possible, so that the cement can be loaded into each retainer and then fully positioning the bridge, before it begins to set.

This ability to control its setting time is the over-riding advantage of zinc phosphate cement.

Experience soon teaches a dental nurse how much powder and liquid to set out, but occasionally too little or too much powder will be put on the slab. In the former case, more powder can be added from the bottle, but the mixing end of the spatula must not be used for this purpose as it will contaminate and spoil the whole bottle. Excess unused powder may only be returned to the bottle if you are certain that it has not been contaminated by any liquid or mixed cement on the slab.

A cool *thick* glass slab should be used for mixing zinc phosphate cement. Thin slabs are warmed by the dental nurse's hand and can make the cement set too quickly.

Uses of a thick mix of the cement are:

- as a temporary filling
- as a cavity base
- for blocking out undercuts in inlay and crown preparations.

Uses of a thin mix of the cement are as a:

- luting cement to place inlays, crowns and bridges
- luting cement to place orthodontic bands.

The main advantage of the cement is that it sets very hard within a few minutes and therefore makes a sound base for permanent fillings, and also a more durable temporary filling than zinc oxide and eugenol materials. Furthermore, its adhesive nature to dentine makes it satisfactory as a luting cement for prefabricated restorations.

433

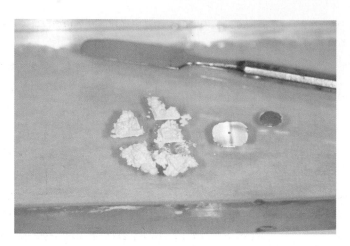

Figure 15.16   Zinc polycarboxylate cement – to mix.

The main disadvantage is that in deep cavities it may be irritant to the pulp, as the acidic nature of the liquid component produces a mixed material with a pH of 2. In these cases, a sub-lining of calcium hydroxide is inserted onto the cavity floor beneath the zinc phosphate base cement. The alternative is to use a different base material altogether. Zinc phosphate cement is also moisture sensitive and will not adhere to a damp cavity, so good moisture control is required during its use.

Zinc polycarboxylate

Presented as white zinc oxide powder and clear, viscous polyacrylic acid liquid, or as these two components combined in the powder and sterile water as liquid (Figure 15.16). In each case the cement is prepared by mixing increments of the powder to the liquid or sterile water on either a glass slab or a waxed paper pad, with a spatula. A measure is provided by the manufacturer for exact measurement of each increment.

The advantage of using the anhydrous system with sterile water is that only one bottle of material is needed and there is no liquid to deteriorate, to be used up too soon or left over when the powder bottle is empty. Furthermore, as the polyacrylic acid liquid is viscous (thick and 'gloopy' in consistency), it can be difficult to dispense from the bottle and also difficult to mix. Mixing with water is much easier and quicker.

Uses of the cement are:

- a thin mix for use as a luting cement with fixed restorations and orthodontic bands
- a thick mix for use as a cavity base
- therefore, an alternative to zinc phosphate cement.

The main advantages of polycarboxylate cement are that it is less irritant than zinc phosphate cement, and far more adhesive to dentine. For these reasons many operators prefer its use to that of zinc phosphate.

The main disadvantage is that it can be rather difficult to manipulate as it is adhesive to stainless steel instruments. Excess cement must be wiped off the spatula and instruments before it fully sets, as it is difficult to remove by manual scrubbing and unlikely to be removed by the action of the ultrasonic bath.

Table 15.2 The main categories of temporary restorative materials and their advantages and disadvantages

Material	Advantages	Disadvantages
Zinc oxide and eugenol	Cheap Sedative to inflamed pulp	Reacts with composites Eugenol can burn soft tissues
Zinc phosphate	Sets quickly Sets hard Adhesive to dentine	Irritant to pulp in deep cavity Moisture sensitive
Zinc polycarboxylate	Most adhesive cement	Sticks easily to instruments so difficult to place
Gutta percha	None over other cements listed	Messy to use Poor margin adaptation in cavity

Gutta percha

The final material in this category is gutta percha, which is presented as preformed cones or sticks (greenstick compound) of rubber material. It only requires heat to become plasticised, but is almost obsolete now as a temporary restoration, as the previous cements described are far superior in this role.

Its main use today is as a root filling material (see later), but it is also used during vitality testing and during border contouring of impression trays during denture construction.

The main categories of temporary restorative materials, with their advantages and disadvantages outlined, are summarised in Table 15.2.

Linings

These are materials placed in the deepest part of the cavity, over the pulp chamber, before a restoration is placed. Their aim is to protect the pulp from thermal and chemical shock, by providing a barrier between the permanent restoration and the living pulp tissue, so that temperature fluctuations in the mouth are not transmitted, nor is any adverse chemical stimulation from restorations.

Technically, thin layers of the zinc oxide materials discussed previously can be said to be linings in cavities, although realistically they are more correctly termed as 'bases' because they have to be of an adequate thickness to be placed, whereas a lining, by definition, is a very thin layer of a material used just to cover the inner surface of the cavity. The material universally referred to as a lining in dentistry is calcium hydroxide.

The material is presented in various forms to produce a calcium hydroxide paste on mixing, from a calcium hydroxide powder and resin in a solvent, or as two pastes to be mixed together (Figure 15.17), to a premixed single paste for light curing after placement.

Uses of the cement are as follows.

- Universal cavity lining, as it is non-irritant to the pulp and compatible with all filling materials.
- It promotes the formation of secondary dentine around the outer border of the pulp chamber, so allowing the tooth to attempt to protect the pulp and heal after a carious attack.

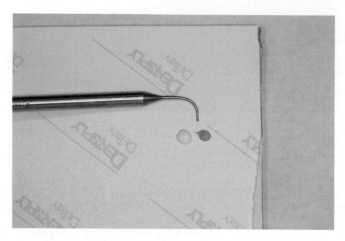

Figure 15.17   Calcium hydroxide liner with applicator.

- It promotes the remineralisation of hard tooth tissue, by allowing its calcium content to be incorporated as calcium hydroxyapatite crystals.
- Pulp capping (see later).
- Pulpotomy (see later).
- Other root treatment procedures (see later)

Calcium hydroxide is the best lining material for non-metallic fillings as it has no deleterious effect on them or the pulp. Its alkalinity counteracts the acidity of zinc phosphate, and also helps to kill the bacteria present in carious lesions.

The main disadvantage of the material is that in deep cavities, and especially those with metal fillings, it can only be used as a sublining as it forms too thin a layer to insulate the pulp against thermal irritation. Another base material must be inserted on top of the calcium hydroxide to provide a thicker layer of insulation against the conduction of heat or cold through metal fillings. In shallow cavities, calcium hydroxide alone is a satisfactory lining for metal fillings. A second disadvantage is that it is also soluble in water, unless a light cure product is used.

Permanent restorations

These are the materials used to permanently restore the tooth to its full function and appearance, and they must all have the following properties.

- Set to a hard enough degree to allow normal masticatory function to occur, without fracture of the material.
- Not to dissolve or otherwise deteriorate in saliva over time.
- To be biologically safe, by not reacting with the body's tissues or giving off any harmful chemicals.
- Capable of being applied to the tooth using normal conservation instruments, in a straightforward manner.
- Have a reasonable working lifespan of years, rather than of months.
- Ideally they should be aesthetically acceptable, although this limits the use of amalgam.

The three commonly used materials are *amalgam*, *composite* and *glass ionomer*.

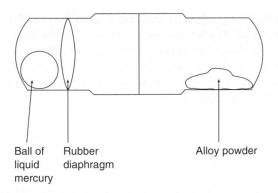

Figure 15.18   Amalgam capsule.

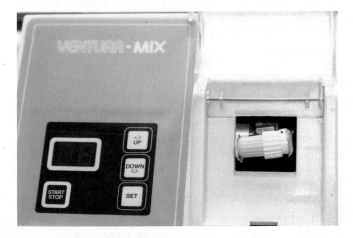

Figure 15.19   Amalgamator.

Amalgam

Amalgam has been in use for over 150 years and is probably still the most widely used permanent restorative material for posterior teeth in the UK. Despite advances in dental material science, it is still often cheaper to buy, more durable and easier to use than its tooth-coloured competitors – composite and glass ionomer.

Amalgam is prepared by mixing a powdered *alloy* with liquid *mercury*, usually provided as a preloaded capsule as illustrated in Figure 15.18. The two constituents are kept apart by a rubber separator diaphragm until mixing occurs, when the mixing vibration dislodges the separator and allows the powder and liquid to come into contact with each other. The mixture produced forms a plastic mass, which is packed into the tooth cavity and sets hard in a few minutes. The main constituents of amalgam alloy powder are:

- silver – up to 74%
- copper – up to 30%, in high copper alloys
- tin – variable quantities
- zinc – small quantities.

The preloaded disposable capsules are inserted into a special machine for automatic mixing, called an *amalgamator* (Figure 15.19).

Varying the alloy powder constituents produces an amalgam mix with different levels of marginal ditching and discolouration. Modern amalgams tend to have a 'high copper' content (up to 30% copper), to reduce these unwanted effects as much as possible.

As amalgam is a plastic filling and a good conductor, cavities are made retentive, lined to insulate the pulp against thermal injury, and the entire cavity may be varnished to give a good marginal seal before inserting the amalgam material.

Very large cavities may have too little crown structure left for adequate retention to be provided using undercuts and dovetails, and in these cases modern bonding agents (see later) or self-tapping dentine pins are used to provide retention instead.

Recommendations for providing the best long-term results of amalgam restorations are as follows.

- In shallow cavities, a calcium hydroxide lining or three coats of cavity varnish will suffice as a lining and marginal seal.
- Medium cavities are lined with either a zinc oxide and eugenol base or glass ionomer cement, and may also be sealed with three coats of varnish.
- Calcium hydroxide is used as a sublining in deep cavities, especially where zinc phosphate cement is used as a base.

Amalgam restoration procedure

The general technique for amalgam restoration of a tooth, and the instruments used, are as follows.

- All dental personnel and the patient wear the correct personal protective equipment throughout the procedure; in particular, the patient must be given safety glasses to wear.
- All caries is removed from the cavity using burs and excavators as described previously, and without breaching the pulp chamber.
- The cavity is **undercut** so that the amalgam restoration does not fall out.
- **Moisture control** techniques are used so that all fluids and debris are removed from the mouth, and so that the cavity remains dry during material placement.
- Adequate **soft tissue retraction** with aspirators or mouth mirrors is applied, without causing trauma to the patient.
- **A lining or base** is placed on the floor of the dry cavity to protect the pulp, if required.
- A **metal matrix band** in its holder will be adapted to the tooth to prevent amalgam spillage during placement, whenever a class II cavity is involved. This will either be a Siqveland (Figure 15.20) or a Tofflemire matrix outfit.

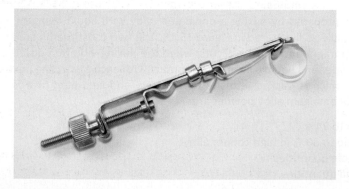

Figure 15.20   Siqveland matrix system.

- To ensure full adaptation of the band to the tooth in the interproximal area, a wedge may be pushed between the tooth and its neighbour to give a tight fit.
- The alloy and mercury are mixed in the amalgamator and the amalgam produced is inserted into the cavity in increments, using the amalgam carrier (Figure 15.21).
- Each increment load is fully pushed and **condensed** into the cavity, using the amalgam plugger.
- Once filled, any excess amalgam is carved off the tooth and the surface of the restoration is shaped so that food debris is naturally directed away from the interproximal areas, mimicking the normal occlusal fissure pattern of the tooth.
- The edges of the amalgam are adapted fully to the tooth surface by use of a burnisher instrument, so that no gaps or ridges remain.
- All excess amalgam and mercury are removed from the oral cavity through the **high-speed suction**.
- The matrix band is removed and the restoration is checked for **overhangs**.
- The **occlusion** is checked and adjusted as necessary.

A summary of the materials and instruments involved is shown in Table 15.3.

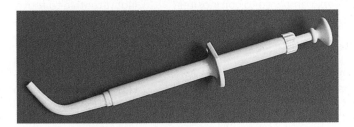

439

Figure 15.21   Plastic amalgam carrier.

Table 15.3   Amalgam restoration procedure: materials and instruments

Item	Function
Liner and/or base material	To protect the pulp from thermal shock Various available including calcium hydroxide and some of the temporary cements, all suitable under amalgam restorations
Matrix system	To prevent overspill in cavities of two or more surfaces Usual systems are Siqveland or Tofflemire; the bands are single use
Wedges	Placed interdentally with matrix system, to tightly adapt the band to the tooth Both wooden wedges and plastic wedges are available
Amalgam carrier	Autoclavable 'gun' used to pick up and carry the amalgam to the cavity, where it is squeezed out
Amalgam plugger	Instrument to pack and condense the amalgam into the cavity so that no air spaces remain
Finishing instruments	To ensure the restoration is adapted to the tooth and is not high in occlusion Various items used – Ward's carver, flat plastic instrument, burnisher, greenstone drills

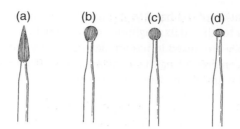

Figure 15.22 Finishing bur shapes. (a) Flame. (b) Pear. (c) Round. (d) Oval.

Table 15.4   The advantages and disadvantages of amalgam

Advantages	Disadvantages
Easy to use	Mercury is toxic
Relatively cheap, compared to composites and glass ionomers	Not retentive to tooth, so cavities have to be undercut
Good set strength	Can transmit thermal shocks, so liners and bases are required in deeper cavities
Able to withstand normal occlusal forces	Has to be mixed very accurately to be dimensionally stable
Excellent longevity, lasts for many years under normal conditions in well-maintained mouths	Aesthetics are poor, so its use is limited to posterior teeth

Although the initial set of the amalgam takes only a few minutes to occur, it is not complete for several hours. The patient is therefore instructed not to attempt to eat or drink until the effects of the local anaesthetic have worn off, or for at least 2 h post treatment if no anaesthetic was used. If considered necessary, the filling may be polished at a subsequent visit using water-cooled *finishing burs*, brushes and pumice paste. Amalgam finishing burs are made of steel for use in low-speed handpieces, and come in a variety of shapes but are distinguished from other burs by having far more cutting blades than usual (Figure 15.22).

The advantages and disadvantages of amalgam are shown in Table 15.4.

Mercury poisoning

Despite the many advantages of amalgam over other permanent restorative materials, its one big disadvantage is the fact that it contains mercury, which is known to be toxic. It was formerly believed that mercury poisoning could only occur after several years of mishandling. However, it is now known that it can occur within a few months if a large quantity of mercury is spilled. There is also debate about the safety of the material within the oral cavity, to patients. The risks are considered so great that some countries are currently considering a ban on the use of amalgam as a dental restorative material, although this does not include the UK yet. In the meantime, every dental nurse must therefore understand the risks involved and the methods of preventing hazards associated with the use of mercury and amalgam.

Mercury poisoning can occur in the following ways.

- **Inhalation** of the vapours.
- **Absorption** through the skin, nailbeds, eyes and wounds on the hands.
- **Ingestion** by being swallowed.

Although the possibility of skin contamination is obvious when handling mercury or amalgam, the risk of inhaling mercury vapour is not. Both mercury and amalgam release mercury vapour at ordinary room temperature – and the higher the temperature, the more vapour is released. Mercury vapour is odourless and invisible, so it is of the utmost importance to keep all mercury and waste amalgam in sealed containers in a cool, well-ventilated place – not near a hot steriliser or radiator, or even in sunlight. In particular, amalgam carriers must be dismantled and fully emptied of any residual amalgam before they are autoclaved, not only to prevent the release of mercury vapour but also to prevent blockage of the carrier by hardened amalgam residue.

Another source of mercury poisoning is the removal of old amalgam fillings. This releases a cloud of minute amalgam particles which can be inhaled or contaminate eyes and skin. It can be prevented by combining the use of copious water spray and an efficient aspirator, which is sealed to prevent the release of vapour in the clinical area. The use of a rubber dam and safety glasses is the best protection available for patients during filling removal.

Apart from very rare cases of allergy, there is currently no evidence of danger to patients from the presence of their amalgam fillings, as a well-placed restoration should have had all excess mercury removed during the procedure. However, it has been advised that removal or insertion of amalgam fillings in pregnant patients should be deferred until after the baby is born, if clinically reasonable to do so. Pregnant chairside staff involved in such procedures may also be concerned, but regular urine tests for mercury contamination of staff can be carried out to show if any risk is present.

The symptoms of mercury poisoning are as follows.

- Early symptoms may include headache, fatigue, irritability, nausea and diarrhoea.
- At this stage it is unlikely that mercury poisoning would be suspected.
- Later symptoms are **hand tremors** and **visual defects** such as double vision.
- The final stage is **kidney failure**, and then death.

Precautions to be followed by all staff

The routine use of personal protective equipment (PPE), such as gloves, mask and safety glasses, or visors worn for protection against cross-infection, will provide protection against mercury hazards. Dental nurses can be reassured that no danger exists if the following precautions are taken. However, they are so important that they are repeated here, having been previously covered with other occupational hazards in Chapter 4.

To avoid absorption of mercury through the skin, the basic rules of cross-infection control should be followed.

- Always wear disposable gloves when handling mercury, mixing amalgam and cleaning amalgam instruments.
- Do not wear open-toed shoes in the clinical area, as the floor may be contaminated by spilled mercury or dropped amalgam.
- Do not wear jewellery or a wrist watch as they may harbour particles of amalgam.
- Incidentally, gold jewellery can be spoiled by contact with mercury or amalgam.

To avoid pollution of the air by mercury vapour, the following precautions must be taken.

- Ideally, a preloaded capsule system should be used, rather than the old-fashioned system of bottled mercury and alloy powder being manually loaded into the amalgamator.
- If the latter system is still in use, containers of mercury must be tightly sealed,. and stored in a cool, well-ventilated place.
- When transferring mercury from a stock bottle, great care must be taken not to spill any. It is very difficult to find and recover mercury which has dropped on the floor or working surface as it is a liquid metal and rolls away easily (see Figure 4.24).
- For removal of old amalgam fillings, the use of a high-speed handpiece with diamond or tungsten carbide burs, water spray and efficient aspiration helps to reduce the aerosol of amalgam dust and mercury vapour while the use of a rubber dam will protect the patient.
- Surgery staff must wear full PPE throughout such procedures, as they should for all chairside procedures.
- All traces of amalgam must be removed from instruments before autoclaving, otherwise vapour will be released as the autoclave heats up – this is especially pertinent with amalgam carriers.
- Keep the surgery well ventilated.
- Amalgamators and the capsules used therein should be checked after use as cases have been reported of mercury leakage from capsules during mixing.
- Amalgamators must be stood on a tray lined with aluminium foil so that any droplets can be easily collected and disposed of as hazardous waste, using a disposable syringe (see Figure 4.25).
- The machines must also have a lid over the capsule holder, so that leaking capsules do not throw their dangerous contents into the surgery.
- All premises using amalgam must have a **mercury spillage kit** so that any accidents can be dealt with swiftly and correctly (see Figure 4.27).

Surgery hygiene

Much can be done to minimise any dangers of working with mercury by adopting the following rules, many of which would be common sense anyway.

- Smoking, eating, drinking and the application of cosmetics must not take place in the surgery. Any of these actions could permit absorption of mercury – from mercury vapour in the air or from contaminated hands.
- The storage and handling of mercury must be confined to one particular part of the surgery, away from all sources of heat.
- Any spillage of mercury *must* be reported to the dentist or other senior staff member.
- Mercury spillage kits must be used for the safe recovery of all spillages greater than a few droplets.
- Vacuum cleaners must never be used for this purpose as they vaporise any mercury they pick up and discharge it back into the surgery.
- Floor coverings must not have any cracks or gaps in which mercury or amalgam can be trapped, and carpets must not be used as a surgery floor covering.
- Surgery equipment and plumbing must have easily accessible filter traps to collect particles of waste amalgam flushed through spittoons, aspirators or other suction apparatus. This waste must be collected and transferred to the surgery waste amalgam containers.
- Modern aspirators must be fitted with an amalgam trap, so that no waste material enters the drains (Figure 15.23).

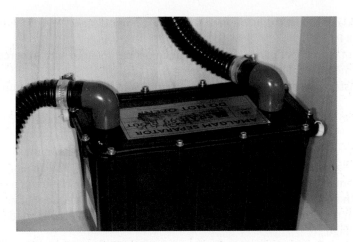

Figure 15.23   Waste amalgam separator trap.

- Waste amalgam must be saved in sealed tubs containing a mercury absorption chemical, and taken for collection by specialist waste contractors for recycling (see Figure 4.18).
- Efficient ventilation is essential at all times of the year, and high surgery temperatures should be avoided.
- The Environmental Protection Agency must be notified of any large spillage that may result in mercury poisoning, under RIDDOR.

Safe disposal of waste amalgam

All amalgam waste and extracted teeth with amalgam fillings present must only be collected for disposal by authorised *hazardous waste contractors* (see Chapter 4). The reason for this is that most other hazardous waste is incinerated, and if that containing any amalgam waste was included, the incineration process would pollute the air with mercury vapour. Before collection by the authorised contractor, the amalgam waste must be stored in special containers, which they supply and which prevent the escape of mercury vapour (see Figure 4.19). The contractors may also arrange periodic testing of the workplace mercury vapour levels and the checking of amalgamators for mercury leakage. If these tests show an unexpectedly high concentration of mercury vapour in a workplace with no report of a spillage occurring previously, expert advice can be sought from the Environmental Health Agency in tracing the source and resolving the problem. As stated previously, urine tests can also be carried out on staff to ensure that they have not been exposed to high levels of mercury vapour, although unfortunately these tests are not routinely carried out by occupational health departments at the moment.

Mercury spillage

Accidental spillage of mercury or waste amalgam must always be reported to the dentist or other senior staff member. If a spillage occurs, globules of mercury can be drawn up into a disposable intravenous syringe or bulb aspirator and transferred to a mercury container (see Figures 4.24, 4.25) while small globules can be collected by adhering to the lead foil from x-ray film packets. Waste amalgam can be gathered with a damp paper towel. For larger spillages, the following protocol should be undertaken.

443

- Stop work and report the incident to the dentist immediately.
- Put on full PPE.
- Globules of mercury or particles of amalgam must be smeared with a **mercury absorbent paste** from the mercury spillage kit (see Figure 4.27).
- This consists of equal parts of **calcium hydroxide** and **flours of sulphur** mixed into a paste with **water**.
- It should be left to dry and then removed with a wet disposable towel and placed in the storage container.
- Risk assess the incident to determine if protocols require amendment.
- Larger spillages still require the evacuation of the premises, the sealing of the area and the involvement of **Environmental Health** to remove the contamination as a specialist procedure.
- The **Health and Safety Executive** will be notified under RIDDOR, so that an investigation can be carried out to determine if the practice procedure needs to be changed to prevent a recurrence of the spillage.

Composite restorations

Composites are tooth-coloured restorative materials that are presented in a wide range of shades, to match the darkest or lightest tooth. Modern systems are set quickly by exposure to a blue curing light, rather than the older systems that relied on a chemical reaction for setting to occur. Composites were initially developed for the aesthetic restoration of anterior teeth but specialist products can also be used for restoring posterior teeth but they do not tend to wear as well here as amalgam fillings.

Composite materials consist of an *inorganic filler* in a *resin binder*. The inorganic filler, which acts as a strengthener, may consist of *powdered glass*, *quartz*, *silica* or other *ceramic particles*. This is incorporated into the resin binder to produce the composite material, which then requires a catalyst to produce setting. The particle size of the filler can be varied to produce the following range of materials.

- **Microfine composites** – very small particle size, giving superior polishing and a gloss finish for anterior restorations.
- **Hybrid composites** – various size particles to give higher strength and better wear resistance for posterior restorations.
- **Universal composites** – combination of microfine and hybrids, to be used for both anterior and posterior restorations.

Composite filling materials

The composites used for permanent restorations contain a filler, resin binder and catalyst. When the catalyst is activated it makes the filling set. The original composites, such as *Adaptic*, were supplied as two pastes: one containing a resin binder and filler, the other containing a catalyst. Mixing the two together activates the catalyst and makes the filling set. This method of mixing two components to produce setting is called a *chemical-cure* (self-curing) system. However, it has been almost superseded by materials containing a catalyst activated by exposure to light (e.g. *Tetric, Filtek, Heliomolar*). This setting method is called a *light-cure* system. However, there is still a need for chemical curing in situations where metallic restorations (crowns, bridges and inlays) are cemented into, or on to, prepared teeth. The blue curing light cannot penetrate metal, so a special type of *dual-cure* composite material has been developed, which can be set at the margins by a curing light and then will set chemically beneath the metallic restoration.

Light-cure system

Unlike chemical-cure composites, which cannot set until two components are mixed together, light-cure materials (e.g. *Filtek, Solitaire, Helioseal*) have introduced an ideal setting system. A single component contains the resin binder, filler and a special catalyst which is only activated when exposed to a very bright light. The spot of intensely bright blue light activates the catalyst and makes the material set in less than a minute. No mixing is required. The unique advantage of this system is that the dentist has more control over the setting time of the restoration, although the material will eventually begin to harden under the influence of the overhead dental light.

The single component of light-cure composites enables manufacturers to supply their product in multidose dispensing syringes, or single dose capsules called *compoules* (Figure 15.24) with an injector gun (Figure 15.25), thereby allowing the dentist to inject the filling directly into a prepared cavity. The dentist then has as much time as necessary to adapt, contour and trim the filling

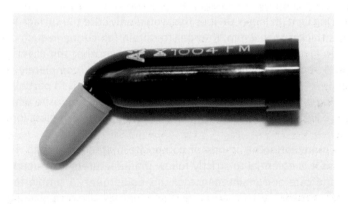

Figure 15.24   Composite compoule.

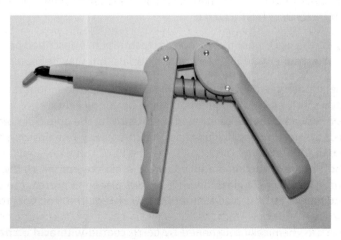

Figure 15.25   Compoule in gun.

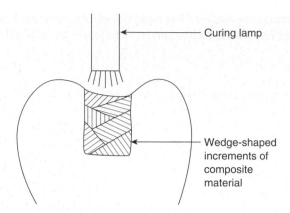

Curing lamp

Wedge-shaped
increments of
composite
material

Figure 15.26   Composite curing technique.

material before commanding it to set. In this way, the time-consuming removal of excess material which has set rock-hard can be avoided.

Just a thin layer of composite is needed to fill a shallow cavity and this only requires one application of the curing light. In larger cavities this would only cure the surface layer as the light cannot penetrate layers thicker than 2 mm. In order to obtain full curing in such cases, the composite is inserted in a thin layer, then light-cured before adding another thin layer and light-curing again. This sequence is repeated *incrementally* until the cavity is completely filled with fully cured composite (Figure 15.26). One way of saving time in such cases is to partially fill a large cavity with a thick layer of lining material, followed by a surface layer of composite which can be cured in one application of the light. The usual lining material for this purpose is glass ionomer cement which is described later.

There are so many different brands of composite materials, and so many different types of curing lights, that it is essential to strictly follow manufacturers' instructions for the curing time, light bulb life, and care and maintenance of this equipment. A simple test of the curing light's effectiveness is to cure a small measured portion of composite on a glass block or mixing pad and then check that it has set hard throughout its full thickness.

Composite restoration procedure

The procedure for the placement of a composite restoration is described below, along with a table of the additional instruments, equipment and materials that may be required for the procedure.

- All dental personnel and the patient wear the correct PPE throughout the procedure, especially orange-tinted safety glasses to counteract the blue curing light.
- All caries is removed from the cavity, without breaching the pulp chamber.
- Moisture control techniques are used so that the cavity remains dry; this may involve the placement of a rubber dam.
- Adequate soft tissue retraction is applied, without causing trauma to the soft tissues.
- Calcium hydroxide lining, or glass ionomer base, is placed to protect the pulp if required.
- **Transparent matrix strip** is placed interdentally if required, to separate the tooth from its neighbours (Figure 15.27).
- Cavity edges are chemically roughened by being coated with **acid etchant** for about 15 sec– this is 33% phosphoric acid (see Figure 4.28).

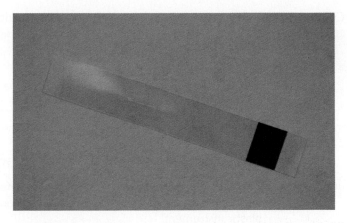

Figure 15.27   Transparent matrix strip.

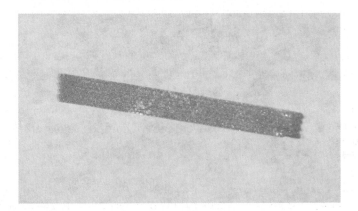

Figure 15.28   Finishing strip.

- Microscopically, this roughens the enamel surface by dissolving the interprismatic substance and leaving the prisms projecting from the tooth surface.
- This is thoroughly and carefully washed off and collected by the high-speed suction, and the cavity is wiped dry.
- **Dentine primer** may be placed at this point.
- **Resin bond** is wiped over the etched enamel and cured for about 10 sec.
- This adheres to the prisms and provides tags for the composite to stick to when placed.
- Shade is determined and the composite material is pumped into the cavity in increments of 2 mm, and cured with the curing light.
- The cavity is gradually fully filled and cured, while the matrix strip is adapted tightly to avoid any overhangs.
- Restoration is finished using a variety of finishing strips (Figure 15.28) and/or finishing burs (see Figure 15.12).
- Occlusion is checked using articulating paper and adjusted as necessary.

A summary of the materials and instruments involved is shown in Table 15.5 and the advantages and disadvantages of composite restoratives over others are shown in Table 15.6.

Table 15.5 Composite restoration procedure: materials and instruments

Item	Function
Liner or base material	To protect the pulp from chemical shock Calcium hydroxide lining, and glass ionomer base in deep cavities
Matrix system	Transparent matrix strips, to allow curing of the composite through it Various holder systems available, or held in place manually
Plastic instruments	To place the composite and remove excess before curing Various designs available, the most common one being a flat plastic instrument Ceramic-tipped instruments to avoid sticking of the material to the instrument are available
Finishing instruments	To ensure no overhangs are left and that the surface of the restoration is smooth Various items used – specially shaped plastic instruments, abrasive strips, polishing discs, polishing burs of various designs

Table 15.6 The advantages and disadvantages of composite restoratives

Advantages	Disadvantages
Excellent aesthetics with a wide range of shade choice	Technique sensitive
Adhesive to tooth, using acid etch and bond	Longer procedure than for amalgam restoration
Little marginal leakage occurs, due to their adhesion to enamel	More expensive material than amalgam
Sufficient strength in smaller posterior restorations	Not as strong and hard-wearing as amalgam in posterior teeth
Usually only require lining of calcium hydroxide	Possible safety issue with resin bond
Indirect inlay technique possible for larger restorations	Can only use glass ionomer as a base, as composites react with other bases
Fast set with curing light	Acid etchant can burn soft tissues if used carelessly
Available in premixed compoules for easy insertion into cavity	Safety issue with curing light causing eye damage; orange-tinted safety shield must always be used

Safe handling and usage of composite

Great care is required when using the acid etch liquid or gel during the placement of a composite restoration, to prevent soft tissue damage to the patient or the dental team. It consists of a 33% concentration of phosphoric acid, and this is more than sufficient to cause acid burns and permanent scarring of the patient's soft tissues, including their facial skin.

Also, the blue curing light used to fast-set the restoration can cause damage to the retina of the eyes if looked at directly, so the patient must wear correctly tinted safety glasses during treatment (orange tinted are best). An orange-tinted protective shield should also be held over the fibre-optic end of the light during use, to prevent the dental team from having to look at the light without eye protection too.

Other uses of composite materials

These materials have a variety of other uses besides tooth restoration, the most usual of which are discussed below.

Restoration of fractured incisors

Before acid etching techniques were introduced, the most satisfactory way of restoring fractured incisors was by fitting a porcelain jacket crown. Unfortunately, this is unsuitable for children as the pulp chambers of immature teeth are too large and crown preparation may cause pulp damage. This, together with the fact that incisor fractures most commonly occur during childhood, meant that some other form of temporary crown had to be used – and these were of relatively poor appearance.

Composite filling materials and acid etching have transformed the treatment of fractured incisors. Small fractures in children and adults can be permanently restored in this way. Although porcelain jacket crowns may remain the best treatment for extensive fractures, acid-etched restorations provide children with a satisfactory alternative until such time as the tooth, and the patient, are ready for a more suitable restoration.

Enamel margins are acid etched and lined with a bonding agent. A hybrid composite filling material is applied in a clear plastic crown form, such as an *Odus pella* crown form (Figure 15.29). When it has set, any excess is trimmed off and the restoration is polished where necessary.

449

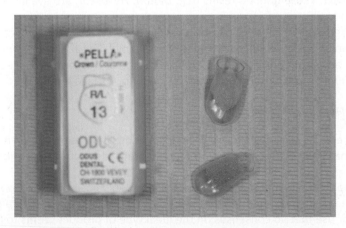

Figure 15.29   Odus pella crown form.

The acid etch/composite filling technique is also used for building up malformed or misshapen teeth to improve their appearance; for the direct bonding of orthodontic brackets, porcelain veneers and small bridges (see later); and for the construction of temporary splints. The latter are involved in stabilising loosened teeth due to trauma or periodontal disease, and are made by bonding a length of wire or fibre-glass tape to the loose tooth and its neighbours with a light-cure composite.

Fissure sealing

As mentioned in Chapter 13, fissure sealing is used as a caries prevention measure. Occlusal fissures and buccal pits are natural stagnation areas where caries commonly occurs. If these fissures can be filled soon after eruption of a permanent posterior tooth, the occlusal surface and buccal pit should then stay free of caries.

The advent of new materials, such as composites and glass ionomer cements, allows fissure sealing to be done with minimal (if any) cavity preparation, because they are adhesive to the tooth structure itself. Retention is obtained by acid etching the fissures or pits. Whichever material is used, any existing caries is removed and the cavity is filled at the same time as the sound fissures. It is hoped that in the vast majority of cases, the procedure is carried out as a preventive measure on a caries-free tooth anyway, rather than as a treatment for existing disease.

The application of fissure sealants should be done as soon as possible after eruption but requires a completely dry occlusal surface. This is difficult to achieve in young children but may be overcome by applying a fluoride varnish (e.g. *Duraphat*) as a temporary seal, until a child is co-operative enough to permit the attainment of a dry field for sufficient time.

Unfilled resins

All the composite filling materials described so far consist of a resin binder incorporating an inert inorganic filler. They are accordingly called *filled resins*. A catalyst makes the resin set, while the filler remains unchanged throughout. This gives the unset material its paste consistency and the set filling its hardness and durability.

Thus it is only the resin and catalyst which are actually involved in the setting process. Several brands of composite make use of this fact by providing a liquid base containing just the resin without a filler. This is called an *unfilled resin* and sets in the same way as all the others by using the same catalyst. These unfilled resins (e.g. *Delton, Helioseal*) are available in chemical-cure or light-cure brands.

The advantage of an unfilled resin is its liquid consistency. Both resin and catalyst are liquids and the mixture can be easily flowed over acid-etched enamel, into fissures or mixed with a filled resin paste to give any desired consistency. Unfilled resins are accordingly used as fissure sealants (although coloured materials are also available), and for surface glazing.

Dentine bonding agents

Although acid etching can satisfactorily bond older composite materials to enamel, it cannot bond them to dentine. Small undercuts are therefore required for adequate retention of some composite restorations.

A new group of dental materials are now available which can bond composites to dentine and enamel. There is such a bewildering range of products available, with such a confusing pattern of instructions for use that no consensus on the ideal type of product seems to have been achieved. However, the simplest product would be one that is a single-component, one-stage application to

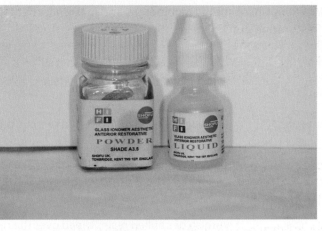

Figure 15.30 Glass ionomer cement material.

enamel and dentine, without any need to keep the prepared tooth dry. Some light-cured products that approach these ideals are already available, e.g. *Optibond Solo Plus*, *Solobond M*. The material used will be an individual choice by the dentist, based on previous experience and knowledge of dental materials.

Glass ionomer cements

Glass ionomers are tooth-coloured restorative materials that are adhesive to all the hard tissues of the teeth, so they tend to be used in situations when little natural retention of the restoration is available, especially in class V cavities. They are composed of a powdered glass-like mixture of aluminosilicate particles and polyacrylic acid mixed with water (Figure 15.30), and although they have a range of shades available, their aesthetics are inferior to composites.

Various other forms are available, such as mixed with silver to produce a harder wearing posterior restoration, mixed with composite (as a compomer) to achieve a restoration with the advantages of both materials, or mixed with other metals (as cermets) for use in tooth core build-ups (for example, *Vitremer*).

Some products set chemically, others by exposure to the blue curing light as for composites.

Glass ionomer restoration procedure

The procedure for the placement of a glass ionomer restoration is described below. Additional instruments, equipment and materials that may be required for the procedure are shown in Table 15.7.

- All dental personnel and the patient must wear the correct PPE throughout the procedure, especially orange-tinted safety glasses if a light cure material is to be used.
- All caries is removed from the cavity, without breaching the pulp chamber.
- Moisture control techniques are used so that the cavity remains dry; this may involve the placement of a rubber dam.
- Adequate soft tissue retraction is applied, without causing trauma to the soft tissues.
- **Calcium hydroxide lining** is placed in deep cavities; this is not necessary in shallower cavities.

451

Table 15.7   Additional instruments, equipment and materials that may be required for the glass ionomer restoration procedure

Item	Function
Liner	Calcium hydroxide, if any is required, to protect the pulp from the acrylic acid
Plastic instruments	To place the glass ionomer and remove any excess material
Cervical matrix	Foil coated and preshaped for use when restoring class V abrasion cavities Cannot be used if the glass ionomer is a light-cured type of material
Finishing materials	Varnish or unfilled resin, wiped over the restoration surface to prevent moisture Contamination

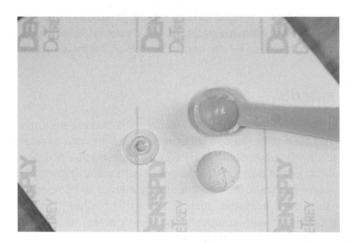

Figure 15.31   Glass ionomer powder, scoop and liquid.

- The cavity has a '**conditioner**' applied, which increases the adhesion of the material to the tooth and improves the marginal seal – the conditioner is either polyacrylic acid or tannic acid.
- This is washed off after about 20 sec and collected by the high-speed suction, then the cavity is dried.
- Shade is determined and the material is carefully apportioned (using the scoop provided) and mixed, ideally using a waxed paper pad and plastic spatula to do so (Figure 15.31).
- The aluminosilicate particles of the powder are very abrasive, and tend to score glass blocks and some metal spatulas during mixing, so these items should be avoided.
- Some materials are presented in capsules which are mixed in a conventional amalgamator and then light cured, once placed (Figure 15.32).
- Material is placed into the cavity and allowed to achieve its initial set, or is light-cured.
- **Cervical foil matrix** is used when restoring class V abrasion cavities, to produce a smooth surface (Figure 15.33).

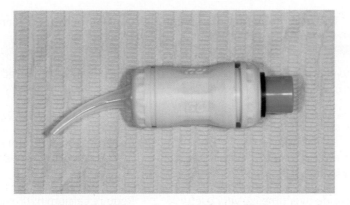

Figure 15.32 Glass ionomer capsule.

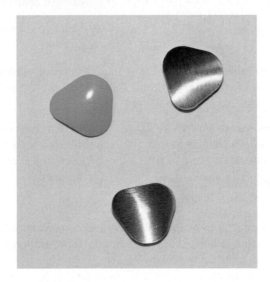

Figure 15.33 Glass ionomer class V matrix system.

- Excess material is carefully removed, without touching its surface as this will produce a chalky appearance – glass ionomer materials cannot be 'finished' immediately after placement as other permanent restorations can, unless they are a light-cure type.
- Surface is coated with **varnish** or **unfilled resin** while fully setting, to prevent moisture contamination.

The advantages and disadvantages of glass ionomer restoratives over others are shown in Table 15.8.

Other uses of glass ionomer materials

Glass ionomer cement has many different uses which depend on two outstanding properties.

- It releases fluoride and thereby prevents the recurrence of caries in and around the cavity, making it the ideal restorative material in deciduous teeth and especially younger children, where poor co-operation may prevent full caries removal.

Table 15.8   The advantages and disadvantages of glass ionomer restoratives

Advantages	Disadvantages
Adhesive to enamel, dentine and cementum, so minimal cavity preparation is required	Low strength compared to amalgam or composite
Ideal for use with class V abrasion cavities	Very technique sensitive
Good marginal seal, preventing leakage This can be improved further with the use of conditioners	Exact proportions of material and liquid must be used to produce the ideal mix
Release fluoride over time, so very useful when restoring deciduous teeth	Require calcium hydroxide lining in deep cavities, to avoid pulpal damage by polyacrylic acid
Better aesthetics than amalgam	Moisture contamination causes failure of restoration
Addition of metals to some products produces cermets, which are strong enough for use as core build-ups	Require protection from moisture during full setting
Addition of glass ionomer to composites produces compomers, which have better aesthetics plus fluoride release and better adhesion than composite alone	Produce a chalky surface if any attempt at finishing occurs before the material has fully set, and then the restoration has to be replaced

- It chemically bonds directly to enamel, dentine and cementum without acid etching, so that adhesion is excellent and undercuts are not essential for retention of the material in the cavity, therefore making it suitable for the following uses.
  - Unprepared deciduous cavities.
  - Prepared deciduous cavities, where the reduced strength of the material is irrelevant as the teeth will be shed anyway.
  - Fissure sealing.
  - Cavity base.
  - Luting cement for fixed restorations and orthodontic bands.
  - Dentine substitute where excessive loss of tooth substance has occurred, avoiding the use of pinned amalgam restorations.
  - Core build-ups.

Non-surgical endodontics

As discussed above, when a tooth is attacked by bacterial caries a cavity eventually forms. For whatever reason, not all patients will seek dental treatment at this stage so the cavity is allowed to progress, and eventually the bacteria will come close to, or breach, the pulp chamber of the tooth. Once the pulp is involved, the tooth cannot be saved by caries removal and filling alone, but must undergo some form of root canal therapy or *endodontic treatment*. The only other alternative is to extract the tooth.

Endodontics is the term used for all forms of root canal therapy. Non-surgical endodontics includes all of the following procedures.

- Pulpectomy – conventional root filling.
- Pulpotomy.
- Pulp capping.

The procedure of surgical endodontics is correctly called *apicectomy*, discussed in a separate section below.

Caries is not the only reason for endodontic treatment– any event that causes significant inflammation of the pulpal tissues, or a breach of the pulp chamber, is likely to need some form of endodontic treatment. Other reasons for endodontic treatment are as follows.

- **Thermal injury**, by heat transmission through unlined restorations or inadequate cooling of the air turbine during restorative treatment.
- **Chemical irritation** from restorative materials.
- **Tooth fracture** following trauma, possibly causing pulp exposure.
- **Severe impact injury** without causing tooth fracture.
- **Irritation** from very deep fillings, over time.
- **Accidental pulp exposure** during restorative procedures, especially during restoration of deep cavities.

Any of these events will result in inflammation of the pulp tissue, and as it is confined within the closed root canal chamber of the tooth, any swelling that occurs will squeeze the pulp contents, cutting off the blood supply to the tooth and ultimately resulting in its death.

The correct term for inflammation of the pulp is *pulpitis*, and this can occur as either of the following events.

- **Reversible pulpitis** – not causing pulp death and treated by a restorative filling of the tooth only.
- **Irreversible pulpitis** – causing partial or full pulp death and requiring one of the non-surgical endodontic techniques listed above to save it.

Any tooth can be affected by irreversible pulpitis at any age, and the tooth involved and when it erupted, as well as the severity of the pulpitis, will determine which of the three non-surgical techniques is used to try to save it.

Deciduous teeth will eventually be resorbed and exfoliate, as a natural progression to the eruption and development of the permanent dentition, so full root canal therapy is not required to treat them and either pulp capping or pulpotomy is adequate. When permanent teeth erupt, it can take up to 3 years for the root apex to close, so these teeth will have a good blood supply during this time and can also be maintained by either a pulp capping or pulpotomy procedure. Once the root end has closed, and in the full adult dentition, pulpectomy is required to treat the tooth in an attempt to save it from extraction.

Diagnosis of irreversible pulpitis

The dentist's decision on whether to treat a carious tooth by an ordinary filling, endodontics or extraction depends on the state of the pulp. If it is dead, endodontics or extraction is necessary. If it is alive and unexposed, an ordinary filling will suffice.

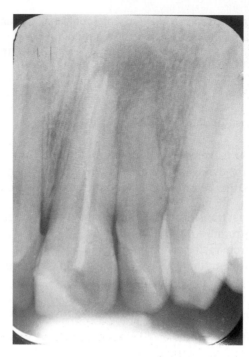

Figure 15.34   Radiograph showing periapical area.

The state of the pulp is not always apparent and vitality tests are often required to determine whether it is alive, dying or dead. These tests depend on the painful response of the pulp to temperature extremes or electrical stimulation, and are fully discussed in Chapter 12. If the pulp responds to these stimuli it is vital or dying; if not, it is probably dead.

In addition, a periapical radiograph can also be used as an indicator of the health of the tooth.

- A widened periodontal ligament space indicates some level of inflammatory response present, although it may not always result in tooth death.
- A crown fracture or deep cavity may be seen to be in contact with the pulp chamber, or very close to it.
- A root fracture will be visible as a black line across the root.
- A periapical abscess will appear as a radiolucent area around the apex of the tooth (Figure 15.34).

Often, a tooth will have been giving symptoms for some time before deteriorating into irreversible pulpitis, and this is especially true when caries is the cause as it is a progressive infection of the dental hard tissues, rather than a sudden event such as trauma.

The patient usually experiences symptoms that gradually increase in severity until the tooth dies.

- Occasional sensitivity to cold, then to hot and sweet stimulation.
- Develops into spontaneous intermittent spasms of pain.
- Becomes a continous throbbing pain with time, which prevents use of the tooth.
- Eventually not affected by hot, cold or sweet stimulation.
- Becomes hypersensitive to vitality testing as the pulp is dying, and then becomes unresponsive as it dies.
- No longer tender to percussion (TTP) when tapped.

Treatment option considerations

There are many factors to be considered by both the dentist and the patient (or their guardian) when discussing treatment involving non-surgical endodontics.

- **Usefulness of the tooth in occlusion** – if the tooth stands alone and is not routinely used for mastication or involved in the retention of a prosthesis, then it could be argued that there is little point in trying to save it from extraction.
- **Tooth restoration possibilities** – if the tooth is badly broken down with little structure remaining for restoration, the possibility of restoring it to full function is lessened.
- **Dental health of the patient** – if this is poor generally, with a lack of good oral hygiene and poor diet control, the tooth is unlikely to survive for any reasonable length of time.
- **Patient co-operation** – both child and adult patients may refuse the treatment offered for whatever reason, and their right to do so has to be respected by the dental team.
- **Medical history of the patient** – some medical conditions contraindicate endodontic treatment due to the risk of a residual infection occuring.
  - Diabetes.
  - Acquired valvular heart disease and other heart conditions.
  - Congenital heart defects.
- Other medical conditions contraindicate extraction.
  - Epilepsy – dentures should be avoided in these patients if possible, to avoid their fracture and choking risk during a seizure.
  - Bleeding disorders – especially haemophilia where haemostasis may be difficult to achieve.
  - Cleft palate.
- **Cost of treatment** – successful endodontic treatment usually culminates in the tooth being crowned eventually to preserve it for as long as possible, and both treatments can be too expensive for some patients to consider.

All these considerations need to be fully and clearly discussed with the patient, or their guardian in the case of children, before the decision can be made whether to proceed or not. Dental terminology may have to be avoided with some patients, to modify the necessary explanations to their level of understanding or language. However, this must never result in full information not being given, nor the patient being patronised. It is possible to issue patient leaflets in various languages nowadays to help explain dental treatment, and their availability should be investigated in your local area.

In addition, some specific information about possible complications and procedure details must be given to the patient or guardian to enable them to be fully informed, and therefore give consent to endodontic treatment.

Complications

- The procedure carries a 70–80% chance of success, so extraction may ultimately be necessary in some cases.
- Endodontically treated teeth become brittle with time, so long-term restoration is likely to involve a crown to protect the tooth and prevent future fracture.
- If the root apices are close to underlying nerves (especially lower molars), there is a possibility of nerve damage from overinstrumentation or from the medicaments used.
- If the root apices of upper molars are close to the floor of the maxillary antrum, there is a risk of creating an oroantral fistula.

Procedure

- Often involves one or two long appointments, where full mouth opening will be necessary.
- Local anaesthesia will usually be required initially.
- A rubber dam may be used, which may be a new experience.
- Antibiotics may be required to control any infection.
- Temporary dressings may be used, and care will be required not to dislodge them.
- Postoperatively, anti-inflammatories may be recommended.
- Patient may experience some tenderness postoperatively and may need to contact the surgery if this worsens.

Pulpectomy – conventional root canal therapy

This is the non-surgical endodontic procedure carried out to try and save a fully formed permanent tooth from extraction, once it has suffered irreversible pulpitis. The aim of the treatment is to remove all of the pulpal tissue from the pulp chamber and root canal, and replace it with a sterile root filling material. This must be placed to fully seal the whole root canal system and prevent any contamination from causing a recurrent infection at the root apex, so the material used must be insoluble in saliva and tissue fluids.

The aim is achieved by following the treatment principles summarised below.

- Complete removal of the pulpal contents – **extirpation**.
- Shaping of the root canal to allow thorough irrigation.
- Irrigation with antibacterial disinfectants such as sodium hypochlorite or chlorhexidine.
- Removal of these irrigants and any residual bacteria from the root canal.
- Filling of the root canal with a non-irritant, impermeable material – **obturation**.
- This seals any further bacteria off from the periapical tissue fluids.
- Restoration of the tooth to full function, either by filling or by cementing a crown or inlay.

The same procedure provides drainage and complete cure of an existing abscess. The root-filled tooth will then function just as well as one with a normal pulp. Success depends on achieving a leak-proof seal at each end of the root canal, thereby preventing micro-organisims from entering or leaving it.

Pulpectomy is often carried out in two stages: the first to remove the infective material and prepare the canal, the second to insert the root filling. However, if no difficulties arise during the first stage, the dentist may choose to complete both stages in one visit.

Although the dentist will use many hand instruments during the endodontic procedure that are multifunctional and used in other dental disciplines, there are several instruments used exclusively for root canal therapy which are detailed in Table 15.9. Their functions are similar whether used as hand instruments or as rotary instruments in the dental handpiece.

At the first visit:

- the pulp is extirpated, using a **barbed broach**
- the root canal is reamed and filed to enlarge and shape it using **reamers** and **files**, then cleaned and disinfected to prepare a dry, smooth, empty canal which tapers gradually from the pulp chamber down towards the apex
- an **antiseptic dressing** and temporary filling are inserted to seal the entrance to the empty root canal to kill any residual bacteria and prevent contamination of the canal between visits.

Table 15.9   Specific instruments for root canal therapy

Item	Function
Broach	Plain broach to help locate the entrance to each root canal Barbed broach (Figure 15.35a) to remove (extirpate) the pulpal contents from the canal
Reamer (Figure 15.35b)	Hand or rotary – to enlarge the root canals in a circular shape laterally, down to the root apex
File (Figure 15.35c)	Hand or rotary – to enlarge the canal in its actual shape laterally, smooth the root canal walls, and remove any residual debris from them
Irrigation syringe (Figure 15.36)	Blunt ended with a side bevel, to irrigate and wash out debris from the root canal without injecting the syringe contents through the root apex Solutions used include chlorhexidIne, sodium hypochlorite, local anaesthetic solution
Metal ruler	Used with a file in place, to work out the full length of each root canal by comparing a periapical radiograph view of the tooth to the established working length
Apex locater (Figure 15.37)	To determine the working length electronically
Spiral paste filler (Figure 15.35d)	Used with the slow dental handpiece to spin sealant material into the root canal
Lateral condenser or finger spreader (Figure 15.38)	Used to condense the root filling points laterally into each root canal, so that no space remains for micro-organisms to return Not required if root filling material used is inserted while hot and flowable

459

At the second visit:

- the temporary filling and dressing are removed
- if the root canal is still clean and dry, it is **obturated** with **gutta percha** (GP) to seal off the entire canal to within a millimetre of the apex.

Instrument details

Barbed broaches are single-use disposable hand instruments for removing the pulp. They consist of a fine wire with multiple barbs. When the broach is inserted in a root canal and rotated, its barbs snag into the pulp tissue and pull it out of the canal as the broach is removed.

Root reamers resemble wood drills and are used for enlarging root canals in a circular fashion so that a filling can be inserted. They are made in standardised sets – all of the same length but with an increasing range of widths. Each reamer is numbered or colour-coded to indicate its size. The reamer is inserted in the canal and advanced by hand or by specially adapted handpieces for use

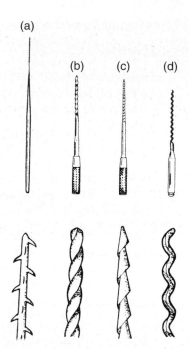

Figure 15.35   Root canal instruments. (a) Barbed broach. (b) Root canal reamer. (c) Root canal file. (d) Rotary paste-filler.

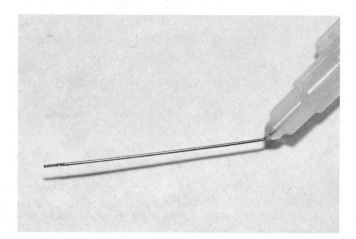

Figure 15.36   Monoject syringe needle end.

with rotary endodontic instruments. As very few root canals are exactly circular in shape, reamers have largely been superseded by files.

Root canal files are hand or handpiece instruments which are similar to reamers but are flexible, and can be engaged around the walls of any canal shape present in the tooth. They are also made in the same standardised range of sizes and colours as reamers. Their function is to smooth and clean the walls of enlarged root canals and remove debris, and their flexibility allows them to negotiate curved root canals as well as the more typical oval shape of root canals (rather than circular). They are inserted in the canal and used with a down-twist-and-up filing action against the canal walls. Many practitioners use files exclusively instead of reamers, but in the same sequence of sizes.

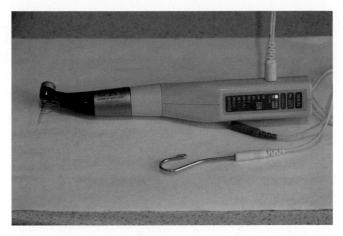

Figure 15.37   Endodontic apex locator handpiece.

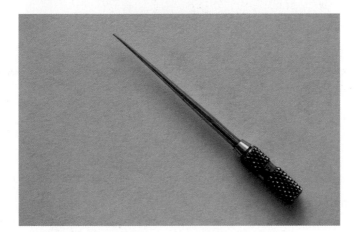

Figure 15.38   Finger spreader.

Reaming and filing root canals by hand is laborious and time-consuming. However, the introduction of flexible nickel-titanium root canal instruments used with modern variable speed handpieces allows dentists to undertake these procedures far more easily and precisely. They are particularly useful for the curved canals of multirooted teeth.

In addition, some of these specialised handpieces are also electronic apex locators, and can be set to give an audible alarm when the tooth apex has been reached – this is called the working length. Once determined, all other files used can then be premeasured to this length so that the root canal is fully obturated. When used correctly, the apex locator is far more reliable at determining the accurate working length of the tooth, and this can be confirmed with a postoperative periapical radiograph.

Root canal pluggers or *spreaders* have a long, tapered smooth point used to condense the gutta percha filling points against the canal walls and obliterate any gaps. These may also be referred to as lateral condensers, but they all have the same function.

Rotary paste fillers are engine instruments for inserting pastes into a root canal. They consist of a spiral wire which fits in a slow-running hand-piece and propels the required material to the full length of the root canal.

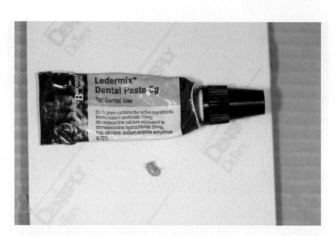

Figure 15.39   Ledermix paste.

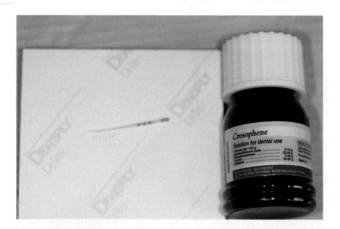

Figure 15.40   Cresophene antiseptic.

As with the use of some specific instruments for endodontic treatment only, there are materials and medicaments used exclusively in non-surgical endodontic treatment too, all of which will have been risk assessed in accordance with COSHH regulations Their potential to cause both the patient and dental personnel harm if misused must be fully appreciated and understood by the whole dental team. Consequently, working safely as a member of the dental team throughout chairside procedures should be second nature to the dental nurse, ensuring that there is no potential for accidents nor mistakes during any treatment session.

The materials and medicaments used in root canal therapy treatments are as follows.

- **Irrigation solution** – used during root canal preparation to lubricate the instruments and wash out any debris. The solution used is an individual choice between sodium hypochlorite (bleach), chlorhexidine (although some patients may be allergic to this), and local anaesthetic solution.
- **Antiseptic paste** – non-setting and containing antiseptic anti-inflammatories, and used to dress infected root canals for a time before root filling – an example is *Ledermix paste* (Figure 15.39).
- **Cresophene** – medical-grade creosote used to dress infected root canals for a time, soaked onto paper points before insertion (Figure 15.40).
- **Lubricating gel** – for use with engine files and reamers (those used with a handpiece) to ensure the instruments do not snag on the canal walls and snap during use – an example is *Glyde* (Figure 15.41).

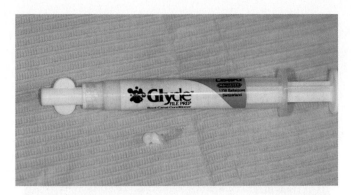

Figure 15.41   Glyde endodontic lubricant.

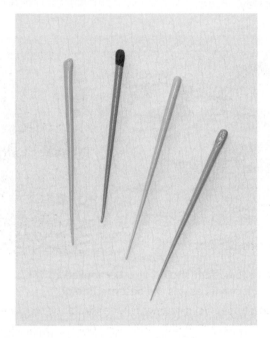

Figure 15.42   Gutta percha points.

- **Gutta percha (GP) points** – varying diameter tapered rubber points used to fill (obturate) the root canal system, with the same colour-coded width system as files and reamers (Figure 15.42), so if a 'red' (size 25) file or reamer is used as the final canal preparation instrument, then a red GP point must be used to obturate the root canal.
- **Sealing cement** – setting cement used to aid the insertion of the GP points and to seal off any residual spaces in the root canal; some contain antiseptics and anti-inflammatories.
- **Restorative materials** – used to restore the tooth to full function and appearance after root filling, as discussed earlier.

Pulpectomy preparation

As the root canal must be disinfected before it is filled, all instruments and dressings used must be sterile. A convenient arrangement is to keep a sealed container holding a complete sterilised root canal therapy kit ready for immediate use (Figure 15.43).

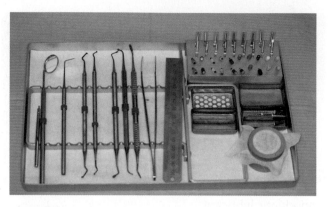

Figure 15.43   Endodontic tray.

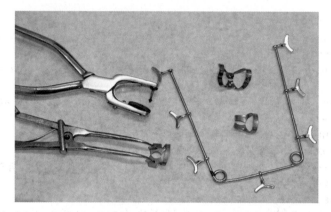

Figure 15.44   Rubber dam instruments.

Wherever possible, a rubber dam should also be applied to the tooth under treatment before access to the root canal is made, as it is the best method of:

- preventing ingress of micro-organisms from the mouth into the root canal
- preventing accidents such as inhalation or swallowing of small root canal instruments
- improving access and visibility for the dentist.

The items required for the application and use of rubber dam are illustrated in Figure 15.44.

A non-latex purple or blue rubber dam should be available for use on patients who are, or may be, sensitive to latex, otherwise the regular green latex dam sheets are used. If, for whatever reason, use of a rubber dam is impractical, small root canal hand instruments must have a length of dental floss or a *parachute chain* attached, to allow them to be retrieved if they accidentally slip out of the dentist's hand. Engine reamers and files will be locked into the handpiece by their latch grip device, in the same way as dental burs are for restorative treatment.

Procedure

Modern infection control practice stipulates that all endodontic instruments inserted into a root canal must be considered as single use and safely disposed of in the sharps box. A new set of instruments must then be used on the next patient, and disposed of in a similar fashion.

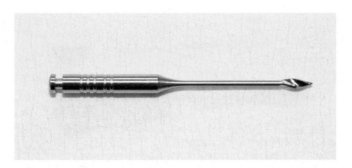

Figure 15.45   Gates Glidden drill.

As mentioned earlier, more than one visit may be necessary. The following description is for a two-visit procedure carried out under ideal conditions.

- Local anaesthetic is used if the pulp is still vital.
- A rubber dam is applied, then the area of the tooth is swabbed with a disinfectant such as chlorhexidine.
- Access to the pulp chamber is gained by drilling through the tooth with conventional diamond burs.
- Access to each root canal is gained by drilling at the base of the pulp chamber, using a stainless steel bur or a Gates Glidden drill (Figure 15.45).
- Any intact pulp tissue can be extirpated with a barbed broach.
- The length of the root canal must be measured before any further instrumentation is undertaken – this is called the **working length**. This is done by taking a diagnostic periapical radiograph with a root reamer or file of known length inserted in the canal, and using a paralleling technique, or by the use of an electronic apex locator.
- Once the radiograph shows the required length of canal preparation (1 mm short of the apex), all subsequent reaming and filing are kept to this length by fitting a stopper to each instrument before insertion. This prevents penetration of the apical foramen or too short a preparation of the canal.
- The walls of the root canal are smoothed and cleaned with files to produce a smooth-bordered canal which tapers from a wide entrance to a narrow apical end. It is achieved by using a wide file at the root canal entrance followed by successively narrower files until the preparation reaches its end point, 1 mm short of the apical foramen. This results in a wide entrance to the root canal, with adequate visibility and access for instrumentation, and a progressively narrower taper towards the apex.
- Throughout reaming and filing, the canal is irrigated with a disinfectant such as sodium hypochlorite or chlorhexidine to remove debris and disinfect the canal. A special sterile disposable syringe, with a blunt end and a side bevel (*Monoject syringe*), is used for this purpose. The side bevel prevents the irrigation solution from being injected through the apex into the surrounding tissues – this is especially undesirable when sodium hypochlorite is used.
- The canal is then dried with absorbent **paper points** (Figure 15.46) and its entrance covered with dry sterile cotton wool, or if infection was present before cleaning, an antiseptic-soaked paper point can be left in the canal.
- The pulp chamber is sealed off with a temporary filling to prevent contamination of the empty, clean, dry root canal between visits – suitable materials are *Cavit* or *Kalzinol*.

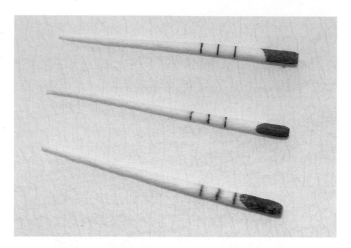

Figure 15.46   Paper points.

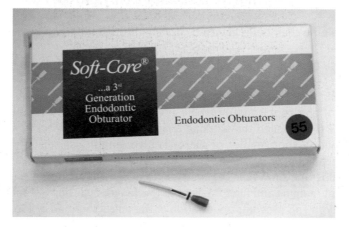

Figure 15.47   Thermafil system.

- At the next visit, if the root canal is still clean and dry, or all signs of infection have gone, it is ready for insertion of the permanent filling. A **gutta percha point** of the same colour code as the last file or reamer used is selected. This is called the master point and has to be sealed to the apical end of the canal with cement.
- Various proprietary brands of root canal sealers are available, many being based on a modified zinc oxide-eugenol cement, such as *Tubliseal*. The canal walls and the end of the master point are coated with sealer and the point inserted into the root canal.
- The gap between the canal walls and the master point is filled by **condensing** successive GP points against the canal walls with a **finger plugger or lateral condenser** until no space is left.
- Warming the spreader softens the GP points and assists condensation against the canal walls. The use of self-locking tweezers facilitates handling of paper and GP points.
- Alternatively, flowable GP can be used before inserting the master point, so that the liquid material is pushed into any lateral canals as the point is inserted.
- Another alternative technique uses preheated GP and pluggers to provide easier and effective sealing by vertical condensation – examples are *Thermafil* (Figure 15.47) and *Alphaseal*.

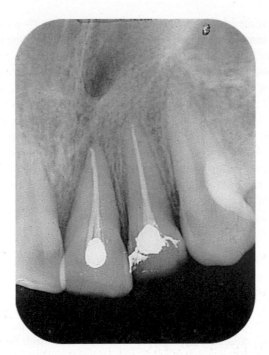

Figure 15.48   Radiograph showing root-filled teeth.

- Whichever method is used, it must ensure that each end of the root canal has a leak-proof seal once obturation is completed.
- A periapical radiograph is taken to ensure that the root filling is satisfactory and to check the subsequent progress of the tooth (Figure 15.48).
- Having completely filled the root canal with GP, the access cavity and pulp chamber are lined with glass ionomer cement and filled with composite or amalgam.

If, at step 10, the root canal is not dry, it means that apical infection is still present. In that case the canal is debrided again and irrigated with disinfectant, dried with paper points and another temporary dressing is inserted in the access cavity. It should then be ready for a permanent root filling at the next visit. If not, a temporary root dressing of non-setting calcium hydroxide paste is inserted until the next visit. The paste is available as materials such as *Hypocal*, or it can be made by mixing calcium hydroxide powder with sterile water or local anaesthetic solution. The paste is inserted into the canal with a rotary paste filler.

Pulpotomy

In adults, the conservative treatment of an exposed vital pulp in a permanent tooth is by conventional root filling, as described above. But in the permanent teeth of children, growth of the root is not complete until up to 3 years after eruption, so an exposed tooth may still have a wide open apex, instead of the minute apical foramen. Root filling is unnecessary for these teeth as pulp death does not always occur, because the wide open apex allows blood circulation through the pulp to continue, without being cut off by a build-up of inflammatory pressure. Instead of total removal of the pulp from the chamber and the root, followed by root filling, it is only necessary to remove the infected part of the pulp in the pulp chamber itself – a procedure known as *pulpotomy*. The very rich blood supply through an open apex allows healing to occur. The radicular pulp (that within the root) survives and root growth continues to its natural completion. In fully grown teeth, such healing is rarely possible and that is why the entire pulp must be removed and a root filling inserted.

The procedure in pulpotomy is similar to root filling only insofar as a sterile technique is necessary. The pulp tissue is removed from the pulp chamber within the crown of the tooth only. The amputated pulp stump at the entrance to the root canal is then covered with a calcium hydroxide dressing. This stimulates the radicular pulp in the root canal to form a layer of secondary dentine over itself. The pulp is thereby completely sealed off again, as it was before the exposure occurred, and normal growth continues until apical formation is complete. In some cases, it may still then be necessary to do a full root filling.

The procedure is as follows.

- All the necessary PPE is placed.
- Local anaesthetic is administered and allowed to take full effect.
- The tooth is isolated from saliva contamination, ideally by the use of a rubber dam but in younger patients this is often not possible.
- The pulp chamber is opened through the exposure site, using a dental bur and handpiece.
- Any potentially contaminated pulp tissue is removed from the pulp chamber only, using sharp sterile hand instruments, such as excavators, to separate it from the pulp lying in the root canal – the radicular pulp.
- All bleeding of the pulp stump is stopped using sterile cotton wool pledgets and pressure.
- Once bleeding has stopped, the stump is covered with a calcium hydroxide material to encourage dentine repair.
- Any material used as a calcium hydroxide cavity lining is suitable, although there are specific products also available. The essential feature is that the calcium content is used by the tooth to lay down a calcific barrier of secondary dentine over the radicular pulp exposure, isolating it from possible oral contamination and allowing root growth to continue.
- The calcium hydroxide layer is sealed beneath a base material and then the restorative material used to restore the tooth to function is placed over that.

The tooth will be regularly monitored by the dentist to ensure that tooth development continues.

Open apex root filling

The technique of pulpotomy is only successful if the exposed radicular pulp is vital and can separate itself from the exposure site by laying down a secondary dentine bridge. A dead tooth with an open apex must be root filled as no secondary dentine will form, but this cannot be done in the same way as one with a closed apex, because the gutta percha points will be too small to seal the open apex and will perforate the apical foramen and pass through it instead. In these cases of an open apex, an endodontic technique is used that seals the open apex over time, before filling the rest of the root canal conventionally at a later date.

The procedure used is illustrated in Figure 15.49, and is as follows.

- Antibiotic cover and local anaesthesia are given where necessary.
- A rubber dam is applied and the working length of the canal is determined.

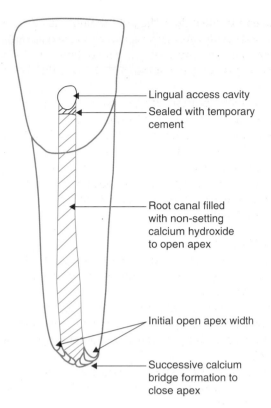

Lingual access cavity

Sealed with temporary cement

Root canal filled with non-setting calcium hydroxide to open apex

Initial open apex width

Successive calcium bridge formation to close apex

Figure 15.49   Open apex root filling.

- The dead pulp is removed with barbed broaches.
- The root canal is cleaned with hand files and irrigated with sterile saline, taking care not to proceed with any instruments beyond the open apex.
- The prepared canal is dried with paper points.
- A spiral root canal filler is then used to fill the entire canal with a special **non-setting calcium hydroxide paste** (for example, *Hypocal*). This disinfects the canal, shows up on radiographs, and does no harm if it goes slightly beyond the open apex.
- The material must be non-setting so that it can be fully and easily removed and replaced at subsequent appointments, while the tooth is under treatment.
- After confirmation of adequate filling of the canal by radiograph, a reinforced zinc oxide-eugenol temporary filling is inserted to seal the root canal entrance.
- After a pulpotomy procedure, the calcium hydroxide in the pulp chamber forms a hard tissue bridge that seals off the root canal entrance but in the open apex root-filled tooth, it only seals off the apex, gradually closing down the size of the apical foramen. This may take 6 months or more to achieve, after which the calcium hydroxide filling is removed and replaced with a conventional root filling.

Pulp capping

This can be carried out in either deciduous or permanent teeth, as a temporary measure before tooth exfoliation in the former or before pulpotomy or pulpectomy in the latter. It is carried out in the following instances.

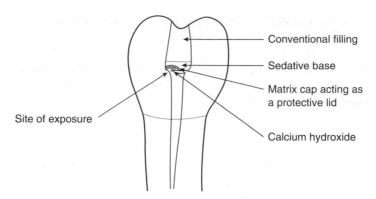

Conventional filling

Sedative base

Matrix cap acting as
a protective lid

Site of exposure

Calcium hydroxide

Figure 15.50   The pulp cap procedure.

- When routine restorative treatment produces a small, unexpected pulp exposure in an otherwise healthy tooth.
- When a patient attends as an emergency with a small pulp exposure following trauma.

The aim is to *seal the exposed pulp* from the oral cavity so that no oral micro-organisms contaminate the tooth and cause an infection. This buys time for either the tooth to exfoliate naturally or for the patient to be reappointed so that either pulpotomy or pulpectomy can be carried out without them developing pain and/or an infection in the interim.

The procedure used to pulp cap the tooth is illustrated in Figure 15.50, and is as follows.

- All dental personnel and the patient wear suitable PPE.
- Local anaesthesia is administered.
- The tooth is isolated from saliva contamination using moisture control techniques suitable for the situation, and for the patient.
- The pulp exposure is dried with sterile cotton wool, and carefully covered with **calcium hydroxide paste** to promote dentine repair.
- A cap made from a glass ionomer cervical matrix is placed over the calcium hydroxide paste, to prevent excess pressure being applied to the exposure site while the tooth is dressed.
- If a permanent tooth is involved and pulpectomy is planned at a later date, the exposure can be covered with an antiseptic dressing (for example, *Ledermix*) instead.
- The cavity or fracture site is temporarily sealed with a sedative dressing of zinc oxide and eugenol.

If a deciduous tooth is pulp capped, it can then be left to painlessly exfoliate naturally. If a permanent tooth is involved, it can be left for some time before any second procedure is carried out, or even just kept under observation by the dentist at 3-monthly intervals, as often no further endodontic treatment is required because the dentine bridge that forms successfully protects the pulp from further damage.

Surgical endodontics

Apicectomy

Apicectomy is a surgical endodontic procedure carried out to remove an infected apex of a tooth, and its surrounding infected tissue. The purpose of apicectomy is to save the tooth in cases where root filling is either unsuccessful or impossible. It is the final alternative to extraction and is carried out for the following reasons.

- Root filling unsuccessful – attempts have been made to save the tooth by root canal therapy, but the treatment has been shown to have failed by:
  - incomplete filling of an inaccessible canal
  - continued pain and infection after pulpectomy
  - continued presence of a chronic sinus tract
  - an enlarging periapical area on subsequent radiographs.
- Root filling is impossible to complete, due to one of the following events.
  - Canal blocked by broken instrument
  - Canal blocked a pulp stone
  - Alveolar abscess on tooth with post crown, so the site of the infection cannot be reached by conventional orthograde access
  - Persistent periapical area following re-root filling, so the infection source requires direct removal
- Removal of excess root filling material from the periapical area, which has occurred during root canal treatment and is acting as a source of inflammation.
- Elimination of curved or fractured root apices, which cannot be root filled and which will act as a source of infection.

The procedure is carried out less frequently in general practice nowadays, but is still to be seen in specialist dental practices and hospital departments and is an important method of saving a tooth from extraction. The technique is classed as a type of minor oral surgery procedure (see Chapter 17), as a mucoperiosteal flap is raised and the jaw bone is drilled to gain access to the root apex.

The procedure is as follows.

- The procedure is carried out under sterile surgical conditions, as for other minor oral surgery procedures.
- The patient and all dental personnel must wear suitable PPE.
- Local anaesthesia is administered so that the tooth and all its surrounding soft tissues are numb.
- An incision is made through the gingiva and a mucoperiosteal flap is raised off the bone with a periosteal elevator.
- Using a straight handpiece and surgical burs, a window is cut in the exposed bone to gain access to the infected root apex.
- The apex is separated from the tooth using burs, and removed from the bone cavity.
- All infected soft tissue (which will be that forming the chronic abscess present) within the bone cavity is scraped out using a **Mitchell's trimmer** or a **surgical curette**, which resembles a large excavator.
- The cut end of the root is then sealed using a permanent filling material, although new materials are currently being developed specifically for this purpose too.
- Debris is removed by syringing with sterile saline using high-speed aspiration and a surgical suction tip.
- The mucoperiosteal flap is sutured exactly back into place.
- Sutures are removed 7 days later and a radiograph is taken for record purposes. By comparing this radiograph with future ones, the progress of healing can be observed.

471

Use of antibiotics in endodontics

The aim of endodontic treatment is to attempt to save the tooth from extraction. When a patient presents with obvious signs of an acute infection, a course of antibiotic therapy may be required before treatment of the tooth can commence. The signs of an acute infection are as follows.

- The presence of pus.
- A raised body temperature (**pyrexia**).
- Obvious debilitation of the patient.
- Severe pain and loss of function of the affected tooth.
- Swelling, either intraorally or extraorally.

The dentist will attempt to begin treatment and alleviate these symptoms if possible, by either *lancing* the intraoral abscess or opening the root canal and placing the tooth on *open drainage*. At the same time, antibiotics will prescribed.

- **Amoxicillin 250 mg four times daily**, or **erythromycin** if the patient is allergic to penicillin derivatives.
- **Metronidazole 200 mg three times daily**, given at the same time if a severe infection is present which may involve other types of bacteria too.

 Further resources are available for this book, including interactive multiple choice questions and extended matching questions. Visit the companion website at:

www.levisonstextbookfordentalnurses.com

16

Prosthodontics

Key learning points

A **factual knowledge** of
- the various prosthodontics techniques available to restore a damaged tooth
- the various prosthodontics techniques available to replace a missing tooth

A **working knowledge** of
- the various impression materials and techniques used in prosthodontics
- fixed prosthodontics techniques, including instruments and materials used
- removable prosthodontics techniques, including instruments and materials used

A **factual awareness** of
- other removable prosthetic procedures
- fixed and removable orthodontic appliances, including instruments and equipment used
- the use of dental implants in tooth replacement

Prosthodontics is the branch of dentistry that involves the restoration or replacement of damaged or missing teeth by the use of artificially constructed devices. In this specialty, teeth that have been damaged (whether by dental caries, trauma or some other means) are restored by dental techniques other than fillings – namely, inlays, crowns and veneers – or they are extracted and replaced. Missing teeth are replaced by the use of dentures, bridges or implants.

Tooth restorations or replacements that are permanently cemented to existing teeth are also referred to as fixed prostheses, while those that can be removed from the mouth by the patient are referred to as removable prostheses. Implants are a stand-alone category of tooth replacement that are provided by dentists who have undergone additional training and are overviewed here for the sake of completeness.

Levison's Textbook for Dental Nurses, Eleventh Edition. By Carole Hollins.
© 2013 John Wiley & Sons, Ltd. Published 2013 by John Wiley & Sons, Ltd. Companion website: www.levisonstextbookfordentalnurses.com

All the artificial devices used to restore or replace the teeth are constructed outside the oral cavity by a technician, rather than within it by the dentist or therapist, as for fillings. For this reason, accurate copies of the prepared teeth and/or the dental arches must be taken and provided to the technician for them to create the artificial restoration or replacement. This is then returned to the dentist for placement or fitting in the patient's mouth, at a later date. These accurate copies are made by taking impressions of the teeth, after the necessary tooth preparation has been carried out by the dentist beforehand.

In addition, the occlusion of the individual patient's dental arches must also be recorded accurately, as any disruption to the normal occlusion will be uncomfortable for the patient, sometimes to the point of being painful. This is because the musculature surrounding the temporomandibular joint, especially the lateral pterygoid muscles, will become strained as the teeth attempt to bite in their correct positions, and the patient will experience facial pain as the muscles are stretched, as well as dental pain due to premature contacts on the teeth.

The skill of the dental technician involved in fixed prosthetic dentistry is to construct the restorations with the same tooth morphology as the original tooth, and to fit the restoration into the occlusion of that individual patient. So each restoration is consequently constructed by hand as a unique artificial device. An inlay or crown made for one specific tooth in one dental arch would therefore fit no other tooth accurately in any other patient. Although the teeth used in denture construction are preformed, the technician involved in removable prosthetic dentistry is equally skilled in constructing prostheses that accurately fit the individual oral anatomy of the patient, as well as sitting comfortably in the correct occlusion. Again, each removable artificial device is hand-made and unique to that patient.

The techniques used to cement fixed prostheses to teeth are similar to those used with fixed orthodontic appliances, while the construction of removable prostheses is the same for removable orthodontic appliances. Consequently, orthodontic appliances are overviewed at the end of this chapter. Occlusion and malocclusion are discussed in detail in Chapter 12.

Impression materials used in prosthodontics

As mentioned above, all prosthodontics devices are constructed outside the patient's mouth, and impression materials are used to record an accurate copy for that construction to take place. An impression is also taken of the opposing arch of the patient (the dental arch that does *not* contain the tooth to be restored or replaced), and this may involve a different impression material.

The variety of impression materials available for use in dentistry is vast, but they must all have the following properties.

- To be easily mixed – if their correct mixing is too difficult to achieve by the average member of staff, their use will be limited.
- To be cost effective – certainly within the NHS where treatment costs are fixed, materials that are overly expensive to use routinely will not be cost-effective and are likely to be avoided by the profession.
- To have an adequate working time before setting – the working time is that available to correctly mix the material before it begins to set; if this is too short then the impression will not be in place before it begins to set, and the mix will be unusable.
- To have a relatively short setting time – the setting time is that taken for the material to fully set so that it can be removed from the mouth without any tearing or distortion, and needs to be as short as possible for the patient's comfort.

- To record the tooth details accurately – a high level of accuracy must be achieved with every impression, so that tooth morphology, tooth preparation and occlusion can be reproduced correctly.
- To be stable when set – models cast from the impression must be accurate and not distorted, so the material must not deteriorate in normal room temperature and conditions before before it arrives with the technician and the models are cast up.
- To be elastic – this property ensures that tearing of the impression on removal from the mouth does not occur, while any distortion that does occur as the impression is pulled out of any undercuts is not permanent, and the impression 'bounces' back into its original shape and maintains the recorded details accurately.
- To be able to be disinfected without affecting the accuracy of the details recorded – this is to avoid cross-infection from the patient to the dental staff and the technician, and the impression must be able to withstand the use and concentrations of any recommended disinfectants.

Where no undercuts are present in the mouth, such as in some edentulous patients (those with no remaining teeth), non-elastic impression materials may be used, but they have been largely superseded by the more modern elastic materials. The more commonly used elastic types of impression materials fall into one of the following categories.

- **Irreversible hydrocolloids** – alginate.
- **Addition silicones**, from heavy-bodied putty to light-bodied paste.
- **Polyethers**.

A far less commonly used impression material is agar, which is a *reversible hydrocolloid*.

Details of the more common materials available are shown in Table 16.1, but some of the more modern ones can be mixed automatically in special machines, rather than by hand. However, impression material mixing is a daily task of the dental nurse in the vast majority of dental workplaces, and all should be proficient in the hand mixing of all commonly used materials. The techniques and skills required should be covered in all good training courses.

Alginate impression material

This is the impression material most commonly used in the dental workplace, as it is easy to mix and relatively cheap. It is suitable for producing impressions for models for the following.

- Opposing arch models for crown, bridge, inlay and veneer construction.
- Models for the construction of full and partial acrylic dentures.
- Models for the construction of removable orthodontic appliances.
- Study models, for any purpose.
- Models for the construction of special trays, bleaching trays, orthodontic retainers.
- Reproduction of models, as more than one cast can be made from a single impression.

However, the set material is not accurate enough to be used to take the working model for crown, bridge, veneer or inlay construction.

It is presented as a coloured dry powder of *calcium salt*, *alginate salt* and *filler*, with a measured scoop, which is mixed with water at room temperature using a similar measuring cup (Figure 16.1). Once the container has been shaken to ensure even distribution of the constituents, and then measured out into the flexible mixing bowl using the scoop provided, a 1:1 proportion of water is added and the constituents are mixed together with a large spatula. Correct mixing is achieved by

Table 16.1   Common impression materials used in prosthodontics

Name	Type of material	Mixing components and technique
Alginate	Irreversible hydrocolloid	Powder and room-temperature water in equal portions, mixed by spatulating in a bowl
Addition silicone	Elastomer	Base and catalyst, as putty and liquid or two pastes, mixed in equal portions by spatulation, or in preloaded tubes, or in a mixing machine
Polyether	Elastomer	Base and catalyst pastes, mixed in equal portions by spatulation, then loaded into a syringe for direct application
Agar	Reversible hydrocolloid	Gel in a sealed tube, becomes fluid by heating the tube and is mixed by manipulation within the tube before use Used in the laboratory to produce duplicate models

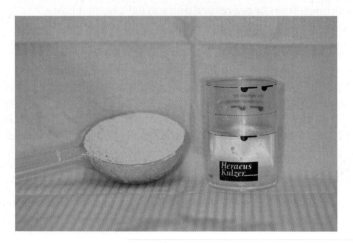

Figure 16.1   Alginate scoop and water measurer.

folding the powder into the water initially, then vigorously spreading it against the bowl side – this is called *spatulating* (Figure 16.2). The mix needs to be spatulated thoroughly to be free of air bubbles, and to create a stiff and creamy consistency.

The mix is then loaded into an impression tray before insertion into the patient's mouth (see later). A set impression is shown in Figure 16.3.

The working time of alginate is affected by the temperature of the mixing water used, and the setting time is affected by the room temperature. In both cases, the higher the temperature, the less time is required. Room temperature water and surroundings provide the optimum conditions of use but are not always possible, such as on cold winter days and hot summer days. Some alginates are presented as 'chromogenic' materials which change colour during the mixing and setting stages, so that the tray can be loaded and the impression taken at the optimal points

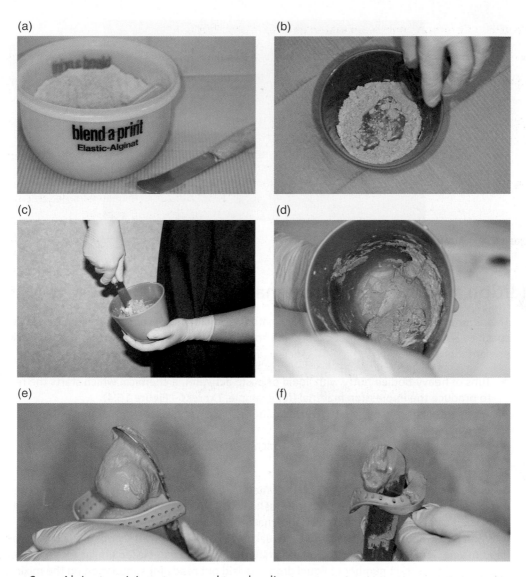

(a)

(b)

(c)

(d)

(e)

(f)

Figure 16.2   Alginate mixing stages and tray loading.

of the procedure. So an initial white powder changes to pink during the working time, and the tray is loaded and inserted into the patient's mouth. Once the material has changed to a purple colour it is set, and the impression can be removed from the patient's mouth.

The uses and advantages of alginate are listed above. Its disadvantages are as follows.

- Can undergo dimensional changes in the presence or absence of water.
  - If left immersed in water, the impression expands.
  - If allowed to dry out, the impression shrinks.
- Ideally, then, the model should be cast immediately.
- When this is not possible, the impression should be wrapped in a damp gauze and sealed in an airtight plastic bag before sending to the laboratory.

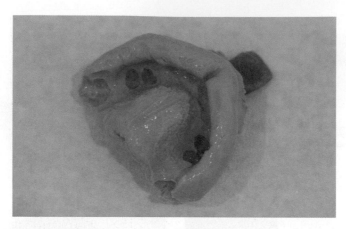

Figure 16.3   Alginate impression.

Addition silicone impression material

This is one of the elastomer impression materials and is highly accurate when set. It is used specifically for all fixed prosthetic work and some removable prosthetic work. It has a variety of presentations.

- Tubs of heavy-bodied putty with liquid or paste activator, a chemical which starts the reaction to produce the impression material (for example, *Express* – Figure 16.4).
- Tubes of light-bodied paste with liquid or paste activator (for example, *Xantopren* – Figure 16.5).
- More recent preloaded gun syringes which mix the constituents automatically (for example, *Express* – Figure 16.6).

As with alginate, measuring scoops are provided for accurate mixing, but it should be noted that it is possible for the mixing and setting times to be affected by some types of rubber PPE gloves. If mixing is to occur by hand, it is advisable that vinyl gloves are worn.

When putty materials are being mixed, equal numbers of measured scoops are laid out ready for hand mixing, and when lighter bodied materials are being mixed, either similar measured lengths of paste or the correct number of liquid drops are laid out ready for spatulation on the mixing pad. Many of the materials can also be measured out and mixed in an automatic mixing machine. As each component is usually highly coloured, adequate mixing can be seen to have occurred when a non-streaky mix is produced. Unlike alginates, silicones are not affected by temperature.

The silicones can be used either in a one-stage technique (the most widely available, and using addition cured silicones) or a two-stage technique (using condensation cured silicones).

With the former, both the heavy-bodied putty and the light-bodied paste are mixed at the same time. The putty is loaded into the impression tray while the paste is either syringed onto the prepared tooth or placed onto it using a flat plastic instrument. Both materials then set and are removed together.

With the latter, the putty is mixed, loaded into the tray, inserted into the mouth and allowed to set first. It is then carefully removed and spaced in the area of the preparation, while the mixed paste is syringed or wiped onto the tooth. The set putty and tray are reinserted and the whole is removed when the paste has set.

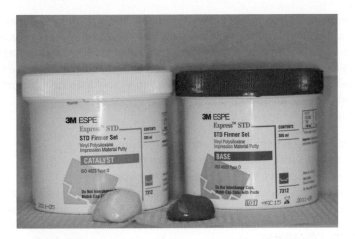

Figure 16.4   Express putty material.

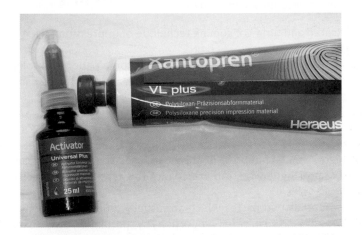

Figure 16.5   Xantopren wash material.

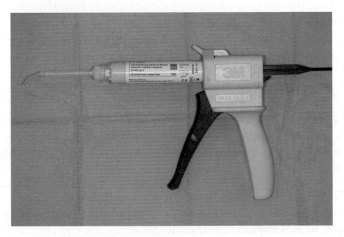

Figure 16.6   Express soft body material in delivery gun.

While the one-stage technique is obviously quicker, the two-stage ensures that adequate paste remains around the prepared tooth during tray insertion and gives a very accurate impression, whereas it can be displaced by the putty during tray insertion in the one-stage method. Adhesive is usually supplied by the manufacturer, but perforated trays can also be used.

Setting time for the silicones is usually 4 min or more, so adequate moisture control to maintain patient comfort is of great importance during this period.

The advantages of silicones are as follows.

- Are dimensionally stable in the presence of moisture.
- Have excellent elasticity, strength and accuracy that allow for:
  - use in deep undercuts, without tearing of the impression
  - undistorted final impression for model casting, as their elasticity allows the material to 'bounce back' to its original shape once it has been removed from the mouth
  - several tooth preparations to be recorded accurately in one impression, without tearing.
- Suitable for use for all types of denture construction, as well as for fixed prostheses.

The disadvantages of silicones are as follows.

- More complicated and time-consuming technique of impression taking than for alginate.
- More expensive materials.
- Longer setting time may be too uncomfortable for some patients to tolerate.
- Paste materials are particularly sticky before setting, and need to be carefully handled to avoid causing an unnecessary mess.

Polyethers

These are also highly accurate impression materials, used specifically for fixed prosthetic work and certain removable prosthetic work. An example of this type of impression material is *Impregum* (Figure 16.7).

They are presented as two pastes which are usually different colours to ensure that uniform mixing occurs. They are mixed in equal proportions by spatulation on a waxed paper pad, and then collected into special syringes for administration to the prepared tooth (Figure 16.8).

The remaining material is loaded into the impression tray. Again, adhesive is supplied by the manufacturer. Polyethers have a similar setting time to silicones but set more stiffly than other elastomers, and therefore need to be removed with a sharp displacing action from the mouth, otherwise they can be difficult to remove. Their advantages and disadvantages are as for silicones, except that they are slightly less dimensionally stable when moist.

Impression handling

As all the impressions taken have been inside the patient's mouth, they will obviously be contaminated by their saliva and perhaps even their blood. To avoid cross-infection from the patient to either staff or the technician, the impressions (and bite records) must be disinfected immediately after their removal from the mouth. This is done as follows.

- Rinsed under cold running water to remove any visible debris.
- Fully immersed in a disinfectant bath of a recommended impression disinfectant, such as a solution of up to **10% sodium hypochlorite** (bleach).
- Immersed for up to 10 min.

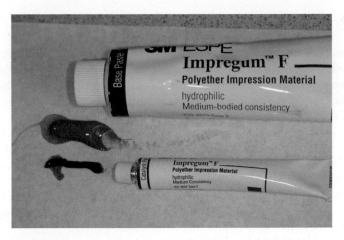

Figure 16.7   Impregum material.

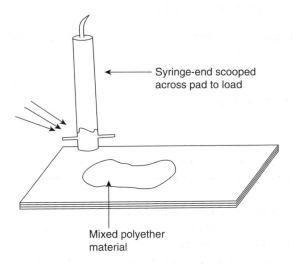

Figure 16.8   Polyether collection technique.

- Rinsed under cold running water again, to remove the disinfectant solution.
- Alginate impressions – covered with wet gauze and sealed in an air-tight bag.
- Elastomer impressions – blown dry using the triple syringe and then sealed in an air-tight bag.
- All stored at room temperature or below before transportation to the laboratory.
- Work ticket enclosed, detailing dentist, patient name and age, prosthesis to be constructed, material to be used, shade, additional features, date of delivery for fitting, disinfection details. The work ticket details should also be recorded onto the patient's record card or computer notes.

As indicated, the majority of impressions are sent away to a laboratory and this can take some considerable time, especially if they are posted. During this period, they must remain stable so that the cast models eventually produced are accurate, otherwise the fixed prostheses will not fit onto the patient's tooth or into their mouth accurately. For this reason, impressions should not be exposed to any heat sources or chemicals, and alginate impressions must be kept moist and not be allowed to dry out, otherwise they will distort and any models cast from them will be useless.

481

Impression trays

Impression trays are devices used to hold the semi-solid impression material in the shape of a dental arch, so that it can be inserted into the patient's mouth and held in place without dripping, while it sets over the teeth and other oral structures. The tray then holds the set impression in a horse-shoe shape while it is removed from the mouth, inspected and disinfected, then sent to the laboratory for model casting.

The trays are available for use with edentulous patients (Figure 16.9) and dentate patients (Figure 16.10), the latter examples being referred to as 'box trays'. They can be plastic and single use, or metal and autoclavable for reuse. As many impression materials are not adhesive to plastic or metal, the trays are either perforated so the set material locks itself into the tray, or are unperforated and require the use of an adhesive so that the impression sticks to the tray. Obviously, the shape of upper and lower trays differs by the inclusion of the palatal coverage required in the upper trays.

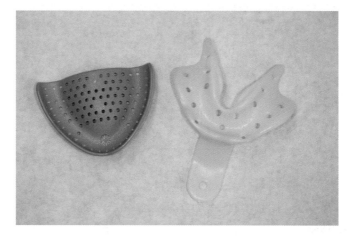

Figure 16.9   Edentulous impression trays.

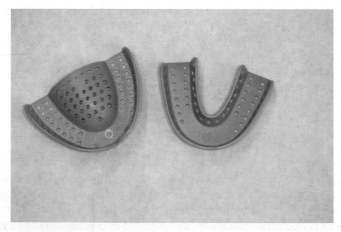

Figure 16.10   Boxed impression trays.

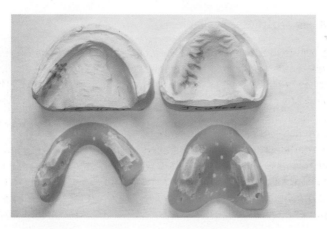

Figure 16.11   Special trays with models.

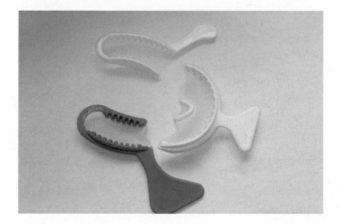

Figure 16.12   Triple trays.

Those impression trays available in a variety of child and adult sizes and preformed by the manufacturer are called 'stock trays', while those hand-made in acrylic by the technician from an initial study model are called 'special trays' (Figure 16.11). These are custom-made and individual to the patient, and are used when a high level of accuracy is required, such as when chrome-cobalt dentures are being constructed.

A final type of tray is that used for fixed prosthodontic work, which records a partial section of both dental arches and the occlusion of the area in one impression. Examples are the *triple trays* shown in Figure 16.12, which are discussed later.

Fixed prosthodontics

These tooth restorations or replacements are cemented within, or onto, a tooth and include the following prostheses (Table 16.2).

- **Temporary or permanent crown** – a cap or shell-like device made to cover three-quarters to the whole surface of a single tooth.

Table 16.2   Types of fixed prostheses available

Fixed prosthesis	Purpose of prosthesis	Construction materials
Temporary crown (Figure 16.13)	To cover the prepared tooth while awaiting a permanent crown As an emergency restoration	Preformed acrylic or polycarbonate Cold-cure acrylic
Permanent crown (Figure 16.14)	To protect a heavily filled or root-filled tooth from fracture during chewing Aesthetics Tooth shape change	Porcelain ceramic Bonded porcelain to metal Precious metal alloy Non-precious metal alloy
Temporary bridge	To cover prepared teeth and replace missing teeth while awaiting the permanent bridge To replace missing teeth after extraction while resorption occurs	Acrylic Resin-based materials
Permanent bridge (Figure 16.15)	To replace missing teeth Aesthetics	Ceramic Bonded porcelain to metal Precious metal alloy Non-precious metal alloy
Veneer (Figure 16.16)	Aesthetics, to cover the labial surface of an anterior tooth when it is discoloured or misshapen	Porcelain
Inlay (Figure 16.17)	To restore a cavity in a tooth with a material stronger than conventional filling materials	Porcelain Precious metal alloy Non-precious metal alloy

- **Temporary or permanent bridge** – two or more crown-like units joined together as a single device, at least one of which is to replace a missing tooth.
- **Veneer** – a facing made to fully cover the labial surface of a tooth.
- **Inlay** – an insert into a tooth cavity that has been constructed in a laboratory.

All are provided for varying reasons but involve the use of similar impression and cementation materials, and similar instruments. The material used depends on the following considerations.

- Tooth involved – are high chewing forces likely to occur?
- Aesthetics – is an anterior tooth involved?
- Longevity – is the prosthesis temporary or permanent?
- Occlusion – is the patient's bite unusual in any way?

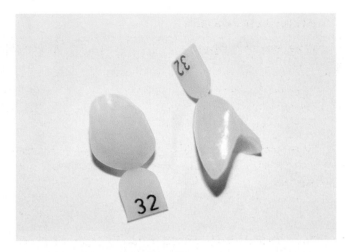

Figure 16.13   Temporary polycarbonate crown forms.

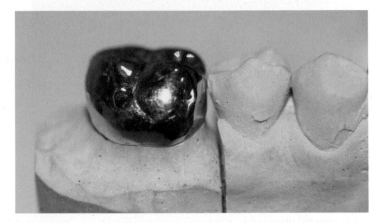

Figure 16.14   Full gold crown on model.

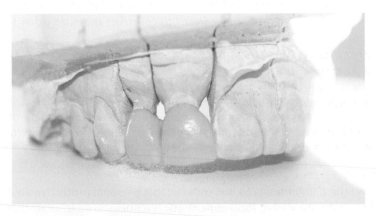

Figure 16.15   Permanent bridge on model.

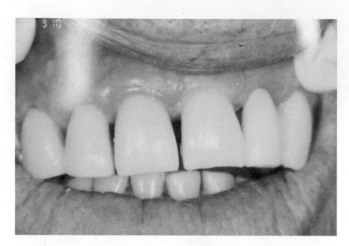

Figure 16.16   Porcelain veneers.

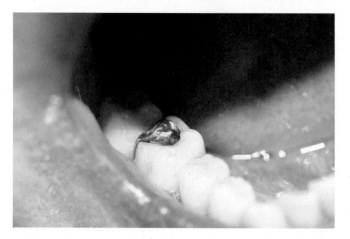

Figure 16.17   Cemented gold inlay.

Although some temporary crowns and bridges can be constructed at the chair side, using either stock crown-forms or preoperative impressions to construct them, all other fixed prostheses are sent to a laboratory for construction by the technician.

Crowns

A crown is a laboratory-constructed artificial restoration which replaces at least three-quarters of the natural crown surface of the tooth. There are various types, made of various materials, and they require at least two visits for the tooth preparation, crown construction and fitting to be completed.

The surgery procedure for the tooth preparation is summarised below.

- All staff and the patient are provided with suitable personal protective equipment.
- Unless the tooth is non-vital, **local anaesthetic** is administered to anaesthetise the tooth to be prepared.

- An **alginate impression** of the opposing arch is taken, using the appropriate impression tray.
- An **occlusal registration** is often taken, especially in complicated cases, using softened wax which the patient bites into, a specific occlusal recording material such as *Blu-Mousse* or a face bow technique for articulation of the models at the laboratory.
- The **tooth is prepared** by reducing its overall dimensions by 1 mm for metallic or ceramic crowns or 1.5 mm for bonded crowns, using diamond burs which produce near-parallel sides to provide optimum retention, but without producing undercuts (Figure 16.18).
- The prepared tooth shape to be achieved is illustrated in Figure 16.19.
- To ensure accurate recording of the crown preparation margins, **gingival retraction cord** can be pushed into the gingival crevice and removed immediately before the impression is inserted. This is cord soaked in either adrenaline or alum, both of which cause the gingivae to retract and pull away from the tooth, thus allowing impression material to flow into the crevice created and accurately record the prepared tooth margins.
- An **elastomer impression** is then taken of the working arch, using a silicone or polyether material.

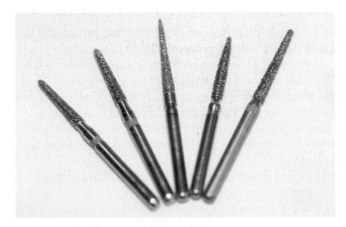

Figure 16.18   Tapered diamond crown preparation burs.

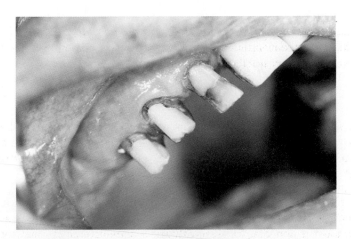

Figure 16.19   Crown preparations.

- When satisfactory impressions have been produced, a **temporary crown** is made at the chair side and cemented temporarily to the prepared tooth (see later).
- A **shade** of the tooth is taken by comparing the adjacent teeth to a suitable shade guide (Figure 16.20), and ensuring that any surface characteristics such as root darkening or hypomineralised spots are mimicked too – this stage may be carried out at any point in the procedure.
- All relevant details are **accurately recorded** on the laboratory slip, which is sent to the laboratory with the disinfected impressions and occlusal registration for construction of the permanent crown.
- A correct return date should be given, to coincide with the patient's next appointment for fitting of the crown.

Laboratories vary in the time required for the crown to be custom made, and the period may range from a few days to 2 weeks. Accurate and detailed information provided on the laboratory slip will ensure that unnecessary delays are avoided, and a professional and trusting relationship between the practice and the laboratory technician often allows for a speedier completion on occasion.

The surgery procedure for the fitting of the crown is summarised below.

- Provide suitable personal protective equipment for the patient and all staff.
- Local anaesthesia is administered, unless the tooth is non-vital.
- At this point, some dentists may choose to apply a rubber dam to the prepared tooth, so that it is isolated from possible oral contamination.
- Removal of the temporary prosthesis, using specific crown removal instruments or a bur in the high-speed turbine to cut the temporary prosthesis off the tooth.
- Try-in of the permanent prosthesis onto the tooth (or teeth).
- The marginal fit of the crown will be checked for accuracy, along with the occlusion and the shade of the prosthesis.
- Occlusion will be checked using articulating paper – high spots will leave a coloured mark to indicate the point that needs reducing.
- Reduction is carried out using burs in the high-speed handpiece, and polishing burs or stones to smooth the area afterwards.

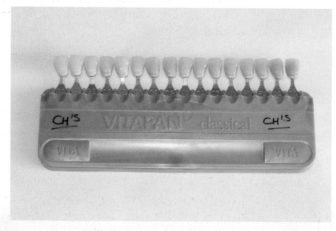

Figure 16.20   Shade guide.

- When the dentist and patient are happy with the fit, the prosthesis can be cemented into place using one of a variety of luting cements – these materials are summarised below, and discussed in detail in Chapter 15.
- If the fit is poor or the occlusion is completely incorrect, the dentist will take new impressions and bite registration and request a remake of the prosthesis.

Instruments and materials required

The majority of dentists have a normal 'conservation tray' set up as the basic instruments required for crown preparation and fitting, and some may work under a rubber dam too. The additional equipment and materials specifically required are shown in Table 16.3.

The fixed prosthesis is permanently cemented to the prepared tooth using a luting cement. These are adhesive to the dentine of the tooth, and are mixed to a creamy consistency so that the prosthesis can be seated fully onto the tooth before the cement sets. Types available are discussed fully in Chapter 15 and summarised in Table 16.4.

Modern types of cement tend to be provided in double syringe form with no mixing necessary, but older types (such as phosphate, polycarboxylate and glass ionomer cements) require correct proportioning and thorough mixing before use.

All can be mixed on a cool glass slab with a small spatula, by incorporating increments of powder into the relevant liquid and spatulating thoroughly until a smooth, creamy mix is produced.

489

Table 16.3   Crowns: additional equipment and materials

Item	Function
Diamond burs (see Figure 16.18)	Tapered so that no undercuts are produced on the prepared tooth or teeth, otherwise the fixed prosthesis will not seat fully onto the tooth
Retraction cord	Cord soaked in an astringent solution (adrenaline or alum) that is then packed into the gingival crevice to cause shrinkage of the gingiva away from the prepared tooth. This provides a definitive tooth margin which is reproduced in the impression and also the cast model
Impression trays (see Figures 16.10 and 16.12)	Variety of plastic or metal boxed trays, sized to fit fully over the dental arch – upper and lower styles. Also triple tray system
Crown former (see Figure 16.13)	Preformed plastic or polycarbonate tooth-shaped formers, in a variety of sizes and available for each tooth shape
Beebee crown shears (see Figure 16.21)	Short beaked shears for cutting and shaping the margins of temporary crowns
Shade guide (see Figure 16.20)	Shaded teeth in holder, to determine the required shade of the prosthesis by comparing each example to the adjacent teeth and determining the best match available

Table 16.4   Types of luting cement

Type	Action	Mixing
Zinc phosphate	Mechanically adhesive to rough inner surface of prosthesis, and surface of tooth	Glass slab and spatula
Zinc polycarboxylate	Chemically adhesive to tooth and inner surface of prosthesis	Glass slab and spatula
Glass ionomer	Chemically adhesive to tooth and inner surface of prosthesis	Waxed pad and spatula
Polyester resin	Chemically adhesive, and inert in saliva	Waxed pad and spatula
Self-cure resin	Chemical bonding between tooth and prosthesis	Double syringe mix
Light-cure resin	Light-cure bonding between tooth and prosthesis	Double syringe mix
Dual-cure resin	Combination of self-cure and light-cure bonding between tooth and prosthesis	Double syringe mix

Temporary crowns are provided for aesthetic reasons, to prevent overeruption of the prepared tooth, and to avoid sensitivity problems in the prepared tooth while the permanent crown is being constructed. They can be hand made at the chair side on the day of crown preparation, or prefabricated types can be adjusted to fit the individual tooth.

Those hand made on the day are created as follows.

- An alginate impression of the tooth is taken before crown preparation begins.
- A cold cure acrylic material is then mixed and placed in the impression after crown preparation, and reinserted into the mouth over the prepared tooth.
- This takes just minutes to set, and produces a temporary crown of exactly the shape of the original tooth.
- Shades are rather restricted, so colour matching is as accurate as can be expected.

Temporary crowns can also be provided by mass production in various sizes, for each tooth shape. These can be cut and trimmed at the chair side to fit any prepared tooth, using either acrylic trimming burs or 'Beebee' crown shears to ensure an accurate marginal fit (Figure 16.21). They are then temporarily cemented to the tooth, using a zinc oxide and eugenol temporary cement such as *Temp Bond*, while awaiting the permanent crown construction.

The types of permanent crown available can be summarised as follows.

- Porcelain jacket crown (PJC) – an early type of all-porcelain crown used for anterior teeth only, to provide good aesthetics when the only other alternatives were metal crowns.
- Ceramic crown – the modern successor to PJCs, constructed of stronger ceramic materials than porcelain alone (such as zirconia), and therefore able to be used both anteriorly and posteriorly to give a more 'tooth-like' appearance than other crowns.

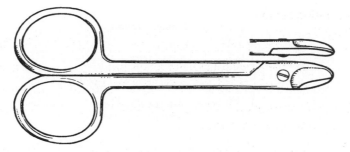

Figure 16.21   Beebee crown shears.

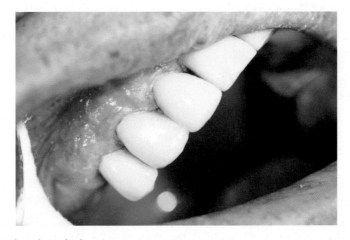

Figure 16.22   Porcelain bonded crowns.

- Porcelain bonded crown (PBC) – these consist of a substructure of metal for strength with a buccal or labial face of porcelain for better aesthetics than an all-metal crown (Figure 16.22); these crowns are currently popular although the porcelain can be cracked off the underlying metal in patients with a heavy bite.
- Full gold crown (FGC) – these can be made of yellow gold (see Figure 16.14) or a mixture of precious or non-precious metals to give a silvery appearance, and are the strongest of all crowns available, making them ideal for posterior teeth, especially in patients with a heavy bite.
- These can be made as full coverage crowns or three-quarter crowns which leave the buccal or labial surface of the tooth intact but cover the rest of the tooth – this gives better aesthetics while still providing adequate coverage of the tooth cusps, so providing strength to the device.
- Three-quarter crowns have tended to be superseded by bonded crowns, which provide both good aesthetics and strength in the same situations.

Post crowns

As discussed in Chapter 15, when teeth die and are preserved by root filling and restoration, the remaining tooth structure often becomes brittle with time and fractures. Sometimes the fracture is so extensive that there is not enough tooth structure left to restore it without the use of additional support. This support is often achieved by the placement of a metallic post and core

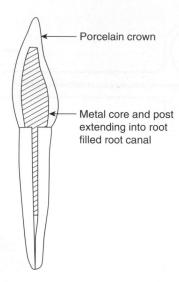

Figure 16.23   Post crown.

structure which is then shaped to hold a conventional crown – these restorations are called post crowns (Figure 16.23).

The metallic post and core system can be constructed from preformed posts, such as *Paraposts* or *Dentatus* posts with a core constructed at the chair side, or the prepared root forms part of the crown preparation impression, and the post and core are hand made by the technician, along with the crown.

The chairside procedure differs only in the preparation of the post hole in the root, and the chairside post and core placement or impression technique, as follows.

- The root face margins of the fractured tooth are shaped as for a conventional crown preparation.
- The root filling material in the root canal is carefully removed to a suitable depth using Gates Glidden drills (see Figure 15.45).
- The post needs to be as long as possible to provide adequate support for the new crown, but drilling should not be so deep that there is a risk of root fracture.
- The canal is then prepared widthways, using drills specific to the type of post to be placed, so that a parallel-sided hole is produced – this will give the maximum retention for the post, once cemented.
- A prefabricated post is then either screwed into the canal (*Dentatus* system) or cemented into the canal (*Parapost* system, *Composipost* system) using one of the usual luting cements. Examples of the post systems are shown in Figure 16.24.
- Alternatively, a wax post is placed in the hole and forms part of the impression to be sent to the technician for post crown construction.
- Using this technique, the post hole must then be retained as an unblocked channel while the post crown is under construction, often by the insertion of a temporary post.
- If a prefabricated post has been placed at the chair side, its top end is then used as the retainer for the core to be suitably shaped to hold the eventual crown itself.
- Suitable materials for core construction are hardened glass ionomer cements such as *Vitremer*.

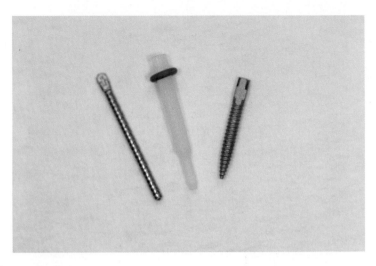

Figure 16.24   Post systems.

- Once the impression has been taken, the core then holds the temporary crown in place while the final crown is under construction.
- Otherwise the technician will construct the post and core as a single structure, and then the crown as a separate structure to be cemented onto it at the fitting appointment.

Temporary crowns

Temporary crowns are placed for a limited time only while the permanent crown is being constructed, and are used for the following reasons.

- To maintain the appearance.
- To prevent sensitivity of the prepared teeth between the preparation and fitting visits.
- To maintain the correct space between adjacent teeth so that the permanent crown fits – sometimes the adjacent teeth tend to tip into the space once the crown preparation has been carried out, as the contact points between the teeth are removed during the procedure.
- To maintain the correct occlusion between opposing teeth – the opposing tooth to the prepared tooth will have no occlusal contact after the crown preparation procedure, and may therefore tend to overerupt.

Temporary crowns are made by fitting a *crown form* over the prepared tooth. For anterior teeth a clear plastic crown form such as an *Odus pella* (see Figure 15.29) may be used. It is trimmed with crown scissors (see Figure 16.21) and filled with a material which matches the teeth, such as composite. Alternatively, tough tooth-coloured *polycarbonate* crown forms are used, such as *Directa* (see Figure 16.13) and these only need trimming with slow burs.

Metal crown forms made of aluminium, nickel-chromium or stainless steel are used on posterior teeth (Figure 16.25).

Trimmed temporary crowns are cemented with a material which is adhesive but easily and cleanly removed for fitting the permanent crown, for example *Temp Bond* or *ProTemp*.

Stainless steel crown forms, cemented with glass ionomer cement, are also used as the best restoration for large cavities in deciduous molars instead of a conventional filling.

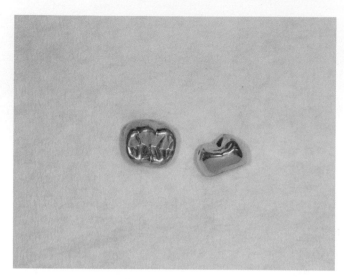

Figure 16.25   Metal temporary crowns.

Bridges

A bridge is a laboratory-constructed artificial device which is composed of two or more units, one of which will replace a missing tooth. Essentially, they are composed of one or more units which are each exactly the same as a single crown, but as a bridge they are all joined together to make one structure. Within that structure will be one or more units that lie over the dental ridge where a tooth is missing, while the other units sit over the prepared teeth that will hold the bridge in place. The unit replacing the missing tooth is called a *pontic*, the units holding the bridge in place are called *retainers*, and the teeth that they are cemented onto are called *abutments*. A conventional bridge is illustrated in Figure 16.26.

Bridges have several advantages over removable prostheses (dentures), which may also be used to replace missing teeth.

- There is no embarrassment of a loose prosthesis falling out, as bridges are fixed to the teeth permanently.
- On the whole, their aesthetics are superior to dentures.
- They are more hygienic than dentures, because there is no involvement of any teeth except the retainers and therefore fewer stagnation areas.
- Usually only two appointments are required for their provision, while denture construction may require up to five visits.
- The materials used in their construction are better able to resist occlusal forces than the acrylic used to construct many dentures.
- The shades available can be customised in any way by the laboratory technician to mimic the patient's other teeth, whereas those available for dentures are mass produced and unalterable.
- They solve the problem of patients with a strong gag reflex who require tooth replacement, and who usually cannot cope with a denture.
- They are also better tolerated because of the minimal amount of soft tissue coverage involved.

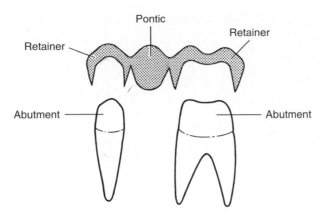

Figure 16.26   Bridge components.

However, good oral hygiene control postoperatively is of paramount importance with bridges, as they produce stagnation areas unlike any others in the mouth (that is, under the pontics), and therefore require special techniques for effective cleaning to be carried out. Due to the complexity of their design and construction, as well as the cost of the materials used in their manufacture, bridges also tend to be far more expensive than dentures.

Several different types of bridges have been developed, but all designs rely on retaining teeth (abutments) to hold the bridge permanently in place, and they are joined to the missing teeth (pontics) in one structure as follows.

- **Fixed-fixed bridge** where retaining teeth are involved to either side of the missing teeth, as one solid design (Figure 16.27).
- **Fixed-moveable bridge** where a joint is incorporated in the design to allow some degree of flexibility to the bridge (Figure 16.28).
- **Cantilever bridge** where the retaining tooth or teeth are to one side of the pontic only.
  - ○ **Simple cantilever** design where retaining teeth are those immediately to one side of the pontic only (Figure 16.29).
  - ○ **Spring cantilever** design where the retaining teeth are to one side but several teeth away from the pontic (Figure 16.30).
- **Adhesive bridge** where the retaining teeth undergo minimal tooth preparation and retention is provided by lingual or palatal metal wings only (Figure 16.31).

The choice of which type of bridge is used depends on several factors.

- Whether an anterior or a posterior tooth is being replaced, as the latter usually experience heavier occlusal forces, so full crown retainers are generally required.
- Like crowns, bridges can be constructed of all-metal or ceramic materials and obviously the former would not be provided anteriorly.
- Fixed-fixed bridges tend not to be used so frequently nowadays, as their inflexibility during use can cause damage to retaining teeth – their solid structure, especially with long bridge spans, allowed occlusal forces on one end of the bridge to gradually loosen the other end from the abutment tooth. While undetected, this would allow caries to seep under the retainer and eventually destroy the abutment tooth.

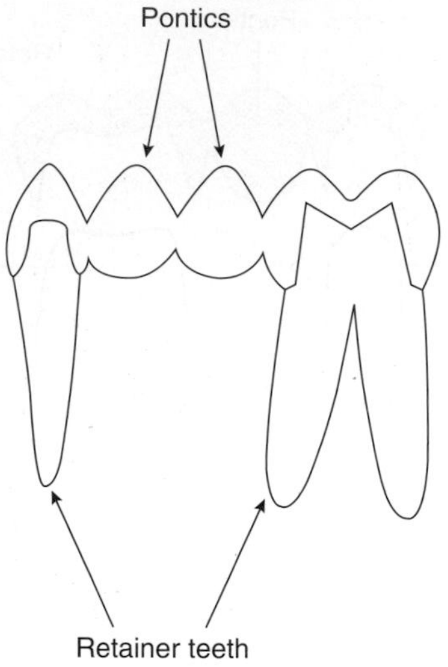

Pontics

Retainer teeth

Figure 16.27 Fixed-fixed bridge.

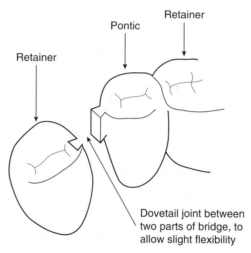

Retainer

Pontic

Retainer

Dovetail joint between
two parts of bridge, to
allow slight flexibility

Figure 16.28 Fixed-moveable bridge.

- Wherever possible, adhesive bridges are used, as they involve minimal tooth preparation.
- If a patient has natural spaces between the teeth, only a spring cantilever design can be used so as to maintain the spaces and give good aesthetics.
- The health of the abutment teeth is of paramount importance to the success of the bridge, and if there is any cause for concern, an adhesive type of bridge is advisable so that any problems would result in its dislodgement rather than causing damage to the abutments.

All types of bridge except adhesive ones rely on the retaining teeth being of full crown coverage. Indeed, the tooth preparation is exactly the same as for a single crown, as are the instruments and impression materials used.

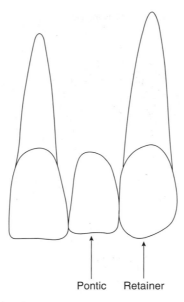

Pontic   Retainer

Figure 16.29   Simple cantilever bridge.

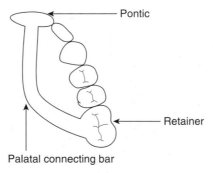

Pontic

Retainer

Palatal connecting bar

Figure 16.30   Spring cantilever bridge.

Some additional procedures and techniques are used when constructing and fitting a bridge.

- While radiographs are always taken to determine the health of any tooth involved in fixed prosthodontics, study models are often also taken before bridge construction, so that:
  - the occlusion can be checked from all angles
  - the bridge design can be visualised and decided upon
  - any potential undercuts of adjacent teeth can be identified.
- With bonded bridges, the metal substructure is often tried onto the abutment teeth before proceeding with the porcelain work so if the fit is then found to be incorrect, a full remake will not be required.
- Ensuring the correct occlusion is present with a multiunit bridge is a complicated process, and needs to be checked and finalised before the bridge is cemented onto the abutments. It is best carried out as follows.
  - High spots are identified by the patient closing onto a fine film of articulating foil or Mylar (shimstock).

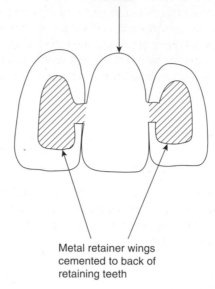

Figure 16.31 Adhesive bridge.

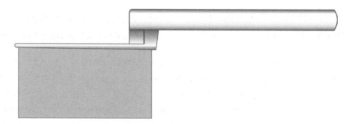

Figure 16.32 Miller forceps and articulating paper.

- ○ Alternatively, fine, coloured articulating paper may be used – that used for removable prosthodontics is too thick.
- ○ The foil or paper can be held in place using Miller forceps (Figure 16.32) which can be slid gently into the buccal or labial sulcus without compromising the occlusion.

Adhesive bridges

These bridges are used to replace just one or two front teeth. The pontic has a porcelain-bonded facing while the metal backing has wing-like flanges which rest against the palatal or lingual surface of the abutments, and are bonded directly to their acid-etched enamel.

These Maryland-type bridges (see Figure 16.31) conserve tooth tissue, as the only preparation required is to roughen the palatal/lingual enamel where the flanges will adhere, and possibly prepare a defining ridge in the enamel to help the technician to determine the margins of the flanges. Adhesive bridges are accordingly ideal for younger patients, who are more likely to have few if any restorations present. They are far quicker to make and can be replaced much more easily than conventional bridgework, as they do not have to be cut off the abutment teeth. However, they will not withstand heavy occlusal forces without becoming dislodged, so suitable cases have to be chosen carefully. The ideal cases are younger patients with a minimal overbite, or even an open bite, where the pontic is likely to experience little if any occlusal loading.

The adhesive bridge requires special dual curing resin cements with primers, to provide a strong chemical bond between the retaining teeth and the metal wings of the bridge. The fitting surface of the flanges is made retentive by acid etching and sand blasting, and a chemical-cure adhesive resin, such as *Panavia Ex*, which bonds to both metal and enamel, is used as a luting cement.

Temporary bridges

A temporary bridge is necessary between the bridge preparation and fitting visits to prevent tooth sensitivity, space closure and tipping or overeruption of the abutment teeth. It may be made directly in a similar fashion to that of a chairside constructed temporary crown.

- Before the abutment teeth are prepared, the gap of the missing tooth is filled with a piece of cotton wool roll, to mimic the presence of the missing tooth.
- A putty or heavy-bodied elastomer impression of the bridge area is then taken, the cotton wool discarded, and the impression put aside.
- The abutments are then prepared and an impression for the permanent bridge is taken.
- The first impression is now used to make a temporary bridge.
- A composite-type resin (such as *Temphase* or *Protemp*) is placed in the part of the impression containing the abutment teeth and pontic area, and the impression is then reinserted until the resin sets.
- On withdrawal of the impression, the temporary bridge is removed, trimmed and cemented back into place with a temporary cement until the permanent bridge is cemented at another visit.

499

Alternatively, temporary bridges may be used as tooth replacements for up to 6 months after the extraction of a tooth, to allow bone resorption to occur before a permanent bridge is constructed. The abutment teeth are prepared in the same way and the impression is taken and sent to the technician. The abutment teeth have a temporary crown-like covering placed. The technician then removes the tooth to be extracted from the working model and constructs the temporary bridge to replace it, using composite-type resin materials or acrylics.

Once the temporary bridge is returned, the abutment covers are removed, the tooth is extracted and the prosthesis cemented to the abutment teeth. Bone resorption can then progress without leaving unsightly gaps beneath the pontic of a permanent bridge. Any gaps that do become apparent under the temporary bridge can be closed using composite materials, until the risk of further resorption is over – usually around 6 months post extraction. The permanent bridge can then be constructed to replace the temporary bridge.

Oral hygiene instruction for crowns and bridges

No matter how well fitting the crown or bridge is to the tooth, microscopically the junction between the two is a potential stagnation area for plaque to gather. Thorough brushing at the margins of the crown will ensure that plaque does not accumulate and cause recurrent caries or periodontal problems.

The general oral health messages to be relayed to the patient following crown or bridge cementation are:

- regular and thorough tooth brushing daily
- use of fluoride toothpaste and medium-textured toothbrush

- regular flossing to clean crown margins interproximally
- careful use of floss so as not to dislodge crown
- attend for dental examinations so that margins can be checked professionally
- sensible diet, low in non-milk extrinsic sugars
- regular use of good-quality mouthwash, to reinforce plaque control.

In addition, bridges provide a challenge to the patient with regard to adequate oral hygiene, as they are fixed prostheses producing stagnation areas actually beneath the pontics.

As well as the oral hygiene instructions for crowns, patients with bridges need to be instructed in the use of *Superfloss* (Figure 16.33). This is a type of dental floss with a stiff end, which can be threaded under the pontic and then drawn through to a sponge part which is used to clean beneath the pontic. When used regularly, it keeps this region of the bridge plaque free and prevents caries undermining the retainers, with catastrophic consequences.

More recently, the use of sonic toothbrushes has been shown to provide excellent cleaning in these areas, without dislodging the bridge, and these are being recommended more frequently in these cases.

Veneers

Conventional crown preparation requires the removal of a significant amount of dentine from the tooth, involving all of the tooth surfaces. While this may be harmless in fully developed adult teeth, it could result in pulpal damage in younger patients as the pulp chambers are larger in recently erupted teeth. In other cases, it may be felt that labial enamel defects in incisors that require a restoration to improve appearance do not justify a full jacket crown preparation, and the teeth are more suitable for restoration by veneers.

Veneers are either a composite or porcelain facing made to cover the labial surface of anterior teeth. Where composite is used, the dentist carries out the restorative procedure at the chair side, as for a routine filling with this material. Porcelain veneers require the input of a technician to construct each one by hand, in the laboratory. They are used in the following situations.

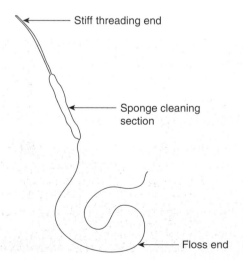

Stiff threading end

Sponge cleaning section

Floss end

Figure 16.33   Superfloss.

- To mask a **discoloured tooth** (such as with tetracycline staining).
- To mask a root-filled tooth that has become darkened with time.
- To **close diastemas** between teeth, and improve the appearance.
- To **change the shape** of rotated teeth so that they appear aligned.
- To change the shape of malaligned teeth so that they appear aligned.
- To **correct poorly shaped teeth**, such as peg laterals.
- As a **cosmetic procedure**, to lighten the whole labial segment, although this has been largely superseded by the use of tooth-whitening techniques.

Porcelain veneers are fragile once constructed, and can break if the patient is careless with them. Ideally, they are only fitted to patients with low incisal edge forces and they are sometimes constructed so as not to cover the incisal edge of the tooth at all, but finish just in line with it.

The instruments and impression materials used for porcelain veneer construction are the same as for crowns and bridges, but often no opposing arch impression is required as veneers rarely encroach on the occlusion.

The surgery procedure for veneer preparation is as follows.

- Unless the tooth is non-vital, local anaesthetic will be required.
- On the rare occasion that an opposing arch impression is required, this is taken in a stock tray using alginate.
- The labial surface of the tooth is prepared by removing enough enamel to allow the technician to construct the veneer; this is especially important if the veneer is to give the appearance of an improved alignment to the tooth (Figure 16.34).
- An impression is taken of the labial segment using one of the highly accurate elastomer materials, as for crowns and bridges.
- The prepared tooth is covered temporarily for appearance and sensitivity reduction, using composite material etched just to the centre of the tooth, so that it can be removed easily at the veneer fit appointment. This stage may not always be necessary when minimal tooth preparation has been carried out.
- An accurate shade is taken, recording all tooth characteristics for the technician, as for crowns and bridges.

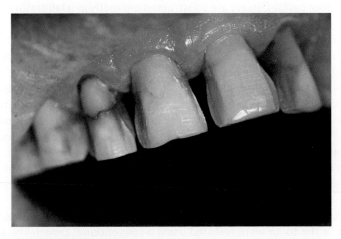

Figure 16.34   Veneer tooth preparations.

As with all fixed prostheses, veneers are custom made in the laboratory by a highly skilled technician. The shades taken in the surgery will be accurately replicated as the veneer is constructed by hand from porcelain, before the final firing in an oven to produce the surface glaze. The fitting surface of the veneer will be abraded and chemically roughened using hydrofluoric acid in the laboratory, to produce a rough surface for cement adhesion. The finished product is then returned to the surgery for fitting.

The veneer fitting procedure is as follows.

- Again, local anaesthetic may be required.
- The temporary veneer is removed, by flicking it off carefully with a hand instrument, such as a flat plastic or an excavator.
- The veneer is carefully tried onto the tooth and the fit and shade are checked.
- Special light-cure or dual-cure luting cements are used for veneer cementation, such as *RelyX*. They contain little filler content and are often available in different shades so that the final veneer appearance can be further matched to the adjacent teeth.
- If the fit and shade are satisfactory, the fitting surface of the veneer is coated with a **silane agent**, which allows the luting cement to chemically bond to it for good adhesion.
- The tooth is isolated with either a rubber dam or celluloid matrix strips, and then etched, washed and dried.
- The dual-cure resin bond and cement are applied to the tooth and the veneer is carefully pushed onto it with a paddling action, in the correct position.
- Excess cement is carefully removed before light curing occurs, without disturbing the position of the veneer.
- Flecks of cement trapped interproximally can be removed using abrasive diamond strips, otherwise they will act as stagnation areas and hold plaque.

The final appearance possible is shown in Figure 16.16.

Inlays

These are fixed prostheses used to restore a cavity in a tooth, rather than to cover the whole or part of the surface of a tooth, as the other fixed prostheses do. Unlike fillings, though, which are also used to restore cavities, inlays are constructed indirectly in a laboratory by a technician rather than placed directly into the tooth.

They are constructed of gold alloy, porcelain or a special type of composite which contains more filler than usual, and is therefore stronger than conventional composite filling materials that are placed at the chair side.

The purpose of using an inlay rather than a filling is to produce a restoration of higher strength than that possible with plastic materials, and of a more permanent nature, although with the continual improvement of filling materials, gold alloy inlays are being provided less frequently nowadays. They are generally confined to teeth which have lost cusps, undergo heavy occlusal forces or are otherwise too weak to be satisfactorily restored with amalgam. Small uncomplicated cavities do not usually warrant the extra time and expense of restoring them with inlays. Their use in anterior cavities has also declined with the development of better aesthetic anterior filling materials.

As the inlay is inserted into the tooth rather than cemented onto it, less tooth preparation is also necessary than if the tooth were restored using a conventional crown. The equipment, materials and impression techniques are the same as for other fixed prostheses.

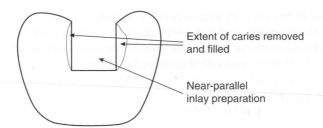

Extent of caries removed
and filled

Near-parallel
inlay preparation

Figure 16.35 Inlay preparation.

Inlay preparation is as for a conventional filling, with the full removal of all carious tooth tissue to sound dentine, but then the resultant cavity preparation is adjusted to ensure that the sides are not undercut but *parallel* (Figure 16.35). This may involve any undercut walls being filled in with plastic materials, such as glass ionomer cements. This allows the inlay to be inserted fully, without becoming stuck on an undercut. The maximum retention possible is produced, by ensuring that the inlay fits snugly against all the cavity walls. Only a fine cement layer will then be required, which reduces the risk of cement dissolution in saliva with time, and the gradual loosening of the inlay.

Once the cavity has been suitably prepared, the necessary impressions and occlusal registrations are taken. Gingival retraction cord may be used to ensure that deep cavity margins are sufficiently exposed for an accurate impression to be taken. The tooth is restored with a temporary filling while the inlay is being constructed.

At the fit of the inlay, the occlusion is checked as for crowns and when correct, the inlay is cemented into place using any one of the luting cements available.

Gold alloy inlays have their margins well adapted to the tooth by *burnishing* at the fit stage, so that the wafer-thin edge of the gold is pressed firmly against the cavity wall. This prevents ingress of saliva and reduces the possibility of the cement being dissolved out (*dissolution*), with subsequent loss of the inlay.

503

Removable prosthodontics

Removable prostheses are all types of dentures – appliances that are made in the laboratory in various stages to replace missing teeth. They can be removed from the mouth by the patient, for example for cleaning, and reinserted again easily, without the use of cements. Generally, removable prostheses are made to replace several missing teeth rather than just one or two, as bridges do, or even to replace all the teeth in some patients.

When there are no teeth left in a jaw, it is said to be *edentulous* (edentate) and the artificial replacement is called a *full* or *complete denture*; if some teeth are still present, the replacement is called a *partial denture*. The majority of dentures are made completely of acrylic, although many may also be constructed with a base of chrome-cobalt metal.

Teeth may need to be replaced by a removable prosthesis (or indeed by a bridge or an implant) for the following reasons.

- Prevent excessive masticatory forces on the remaining teeth, which may cause their eventual fracture.
- Prevent overeruption of the opposing teeth, which may cause occlusal problems.

- Prevent tilting of the adjacent teeth into the edentulous spaces, causing stagnation areas.
- Prevent soft tissue trauma of the alveolar ridges during mastication.
- Allow adequate mastication and avoid digestive problems and malnutrition, especially in the elderly.
- Provide good aesthetics, especially if anterior teeth are missing.

Not all patients are suitable for tooth replacement by the use of dentures, and the following points are considered for every case before treatment commences.

- Is there any previous denture experience, and was it successful or not?
- If not, is there a cause which can be remedied?
- Is the shape of the patient's mouth naturally retentive for full dentures, with good ridges and a high palate, or might preprosthetic surgery be necessary?
- Are there any potential retention problems for partial dentures and if so, can they be remedied by tooth shape adjustment?
- Might the patient's occlusion cause problems with the provision of a denture; is there enough clearance without premature contact onto the denture?
- Are there any medical contraindications to dentures, such as epilepsy or an adverse reaction to the acrylic material?
- Are there other dental problems which need addressing first, such as caries or periodontal disease?
- If the teeth have been lost within the previous 6 months, bone resorption is likely to occur and this will affect the fit of a denture adversely.
- Good co-operation and perseverance by the patient are paramount to the success of dentures. If there is any doubt about these then the treatment is likely to fail.
- Can the patient afford the treatment?

Full and partial acrylic dentures

These are the most common types of denture – full ones (Figure 16.36) for edentulous patients and partial ones (Figure 16.37) for patients with any number of missing teeth up to one tooth short of being edentulous. The material used for their construction, and that of removable orthodontic appliances too, is either pink or transparent acrylic.

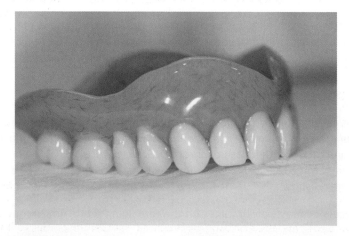

Figure 16.36 Full denture.

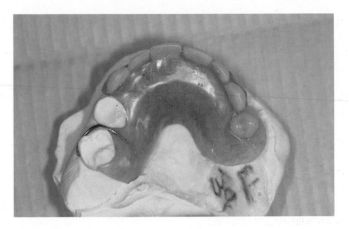

Figure 16.37   Partial denture on model.

Acrylic consists of a powder called a *polymer* and a liquid called a *monomer*. When mixed together, they form a plastic mass which has the consistency of dough. This sets into a hard acrylic by a process called *curing*. Curing is effected by heating the dough slowly in a special flask in an oven, or by adding a catalyst which allows it to cure at room temperature. These two methods of curing are known respectively as *heat curing* and *cold curing*.

Heat-cured acrylic is used for dentures and orthodontic appliances, and the curing process is carried out by a technician in the laboratory. Cold-cured acrylic (also called self-cured or autopoly-merised acrylic) can be used by the dentist at the chair side to make temporary crowns, and to carry out denture repairs. It is also used by the technician for the construction of special trays to take accurate second impressions.

As dentures are removable prostheses, their retention must be adequate to keep them in position in the mouth during speech and chewing, but weak enough so that the patient can easily remove the device from their mouth as they wish, say for cleaning purposes. The level of retention achieved relies on the following factors.

- A **suction film** of saliva developing between the denture and the patient's soft tissues.
- A **post-dam** along the back border of the denture, to help the suction film to develop.
- An **accurate design and fit** of denture, to allow the film to develop adequately.
- Use of any **natural undercuts** in the patient's mouth, such as the alveolar ridges or any suitably shaped natural teeth.
- Use of **stainless steel clasps** around standing teeth with partial dentures, to increase the retention of the denture by the clasps gripping the teeth and preventing it from being dislodged by normal soft tissue movements (Figure 16.38).

Sometimes no natural undercuts are present so the patient's own teeth are adjusted to provide them, in the following ways.

- Use of a crown to change the overall shape of the tooth.
- Use of composite build-ups to provide a retentive area for clasps to engage.
- Shape change of an existing restoration for similar reasons.

With edentulous patients, the alveolar ridges can be changed surgically, to improve retention and comfort.

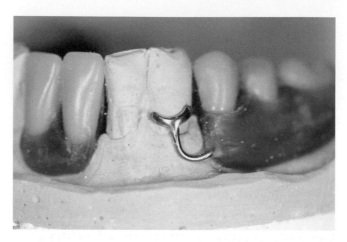

Figure 16.38   Denture clasp example.

- **Alveoplasty** – changing the shape of the existing ridge, such as by the removal of gross undercuts which would prevent the denture being seated.
- Flat ridges can be built up by the addition of **artificial bone substitutes** under the mucoperiosteum, to increase natural retention by creating a ridge that the denture can sit on.
- **Alveolectomy** – the surgical removal and smoothing of sharp ridges to allow comfortable wearing of the denture.

Denture construction

Usually, acrylic dentures are made in four or five stages, with each stage being returned to the technician at the laboratory between patient appointments. The dentist prepares and records the details of the patient's oral cavity, and the technician uses these records to construct the dentures to fit that patient's mouth. Each laboratory stage is returned to the dentist for the next clinical stage to be recorded in the patient's mouth, until the end result – the acrylic dentures, with or without clasps, are produced for fitting.

The stages are as follows, although not every stage is required in every case.

- **First impressions** – using stock trays and alginate impression material (see Figure 16.3); the tooth shade and shape (mould) are often decided at this stage too. The impressions are correctly disinfected, as described previously, and suitably wrapped for dispatch to the laboratory.
- **Laboratory** – study models are cast in plaster of Paris from the impressions, and special acrylic impression trays are custom made from them if required – in simple cases, the first impression may be accurate enough for denture construction to proceed.
- **Second impression** – using special trays and either alginate or elastomer impression material to produce a very accurate impression, and the tooth shade and mould may be chosen at this stage if not already recorded.
- **Laboratory** – working models are cast in dental stone and wax occlusal rims are constructed on them.
- **Bite registration** – the existing, or required, occlusal face height of the patient is measured using a Willis bite gauge (Figure 16.39), and recorded on the occlusal rims by warming them or

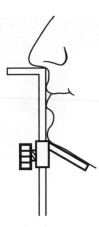

Figure 16.39 Willis bite gauge in position to record occlusal face height.

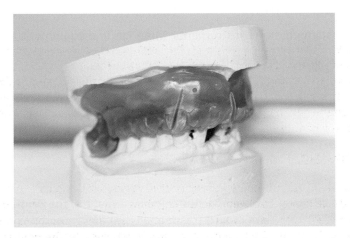

Figure 16.40 Wax rims on working models.

using bite registration paste to stick them together. The rims then hold the models in the correct position and angulation for the dentures to be constructed (Figure 16.40).

- **Laboratory** – models in their recorded face height positions are mounted onto an articulator, so the technician can construct the wax try-in dentures in these correct horizontal and vertical positions.
- **Try-in** – wax try-ins with the actual acrylic teeth mounted in them (Figure 16.41) are inserted and checked for accuracy of fit and occlusion, as well as shade; any major inaccuracies will result in new records being taken and a retry being requested.
- **Laboratory** – stainless steel clasps are added as necessary, then the try-ins on their models are sealed into flasks and the wax is replaced by heat-cured acrylic to form the final dentures, which are then cleaned and polished to provide a shiny outer surface to the denture.
- **Fit** – acrylic dentures are inserted in the patient's mouth and checked for comfort, fit and aesthetics, then specific denture care information is given.

Each stage of the denture construction in the surgery involves the use of specific instruments, materials and equipment which the dental nurse must be able to recognise and lay out at each appointment. They are summarised in Tables 16.5–16.9.

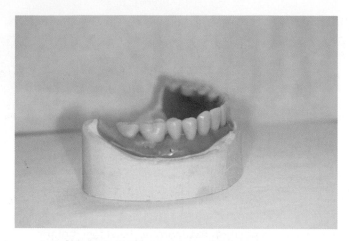

Figure 16.41   Try-in stage of lower full denture.

Table 16.5   First impressions: instruments, materials and equipment

Item	Function
Stock impression trays	To be sized and used to take the initial impressions, so that special trays can be constructed – they may be upper and/or lower, and edentulous or dentate
Alginate impression material and room - temperature water	To be mixed, loaded into the trays and inserted to produce the initial impressions
Shade and mould guides	To determine the colour and shape of the denture teeth, to be as close in appearance to any remaining teeth as possible
Work ticket or docket (Figure 16.42)	To record the patient and dentist details, the denture design and base material to be used, the tooth shade and mould, the type and position of any clasps, and the return date

The work ticket information must be duplicated onto the patient record card or the computerised notes, so that if the ticket itself is ever lost or misplaced, the relevant details are still available.

The handling and aftercare of the impressions are as for fixed prostheses.

Table 16.6   Second impressions: instruments, materials and equipment

Item	Function
Study models and special trays	To take the more accurate second impressions where required, to produce the working models
Alginate or elastomer impression material	To take the more accurate second impressions
Work ticket	To record the next stage request and the return date

Table 16.7   Bite registration: instruments, materials and equipment

Item	Function
Wax bite rims	Adjusted in height so that correct face height of the patient can be recorded
Heat source (Figure 16.43a)	To warm the hand instruments and rims for adjustment
Wax knife (Figure 16.43b)	To remove or add additional wax to the rims, as necessary
Bite registration paste (optional)	To be mixed and applied to the rims, so that they are held in the correct position once set
Pink sheet wax (Figure 16.43c)	For addition to the rims, as necessary
Willis bite gauge (see Figure 16.39)	To record the desired occlusal face height in edentulous patients, where no natural teeth remain as a guide
Work ticket	To record the next stage request and return date

Table 16.8   Try-in

Item	Function
Try-in prostheses	To determine if fit, occlusion and aesthetics are correct before finishing the dentures
Heat source	To warm the wax and make adjustments, as necessary
Le Cron carver (Figure 16.44)	To make fine adjustments to the try-in, as necessary
Wax knife	To warm and smooth the wax after adjustments, as necessary
Shade and mould guides	To check or alter the shade or mould, as necessary
Pink sheet wax	For addition to the try-in, as necessary
Patient mirror	To allow the patient to view the try-ins and decide if they are happy with the appearance, before completion of the dentures
Work ticket	To record any changes required for a retry, or to record the fit return date

If changes are required to the prostheses they must be requested at this point, as once the flasking process has been carried out, no further changes can be made and the whole construction process would have to be started again.

Any concerns that the patient may have must be identified and discussed at this point, and resolved to the satisfaction of both the patient and the dentist.

Table 16.9 Fitting

Item	Function
Completed removable prostheses	To fit, to the patient and dentist's satisfaction
Straight handpiece and selection of trimming burs and carborundum polishing stones (Figure 16.45)	To remove any acrylic pearls or occlusal high spots before polishing and smoothing the adjusted area for comfort
Patient mirror	To allow the patient to view the completed prostheses
Articulating paper	To identify occlusal high spots, for adjustment as necessary
Pressure relief paste	To identify high spots on the denture fitting surface, for removal as necessary

510

Instructions are given on the wear, care and cleaning of the new dentures, as follows.

- A demonstration of how to insert and remove the dentures is given, with the patient then practising the techniques in front of the mirror and under the dentist's supervision.
- Do not wear them overnight if possible, to avoid the development of oral fungal infections (thrush).
- Store them overnight in a denture pot containing water or ideally a soaking agent such as *Steradent* or *Dentural*.
- Clean after each meal if possible, using a denture brush and denture toothpaste – some ordinary toothpastes may be too abrasive for use on the acrylic teeth.
- Clean over a bowl of water, to avoid damage to the denture if it is dropped.
- Avoid soaking in bleach-based cleansers if any metal components are included in the design.
- Eat soft foods initially, while the oral soft tissues acclimatise to the prostheses.
- Take time to chew foods thoroughly, to avoid causing indigestion by swallowing large food particles.
- Harden oral soft tissues by carrying out hot salt water mouthwashes initially, otherwise the new dentures are likely to rub the soft tissues and make them sore.
- Return to the surgery if any ulceration occurs beneath the dentures, as further adjustments are likely to be required to remove high spots and deep flange edges.
- Dentate patients must continue to attend for oral health assessment at their regular recall interval, and edentulous patients are advised to attend at least once every 2 years, but ideally annually.

Patients are also told that new dentures do not last forever, and their fit and appearance will be checked at each recall. Alveolar bone gradually changes its shape following the loss of teeth and the denture will eventually become too loose as resorption spaces develop beneath the fitting surface. By that time, most patients will have learned how to control a loose denture using a combination of their soft tissues and denture adhesive products such as

ACME DENTAL LABORATORIES LTD. M.H.R.A. REF. CA 008044

136 WATERLOO ROAD, BURSLEM, STOKE-ON-TRENT ST6 3HB

Telephone: 01782 817621 Fax: 01782 824142

DAMAS
Dental Appliance Manufacturers
Audit Scheme

DAMAS
Dental Appliance Manufacturers
Audit Scheme

Dentist _____ Job No. _____

Surgery Address _____

THIS IS A CUSTOM MADE DEVICE FOR THE EXCLUSIVE USE OF

Patient Mr./Mrs. _____

Special U ☐   Acrylic ☐   Shade ☐   Mould ☐   Teeth ☐

Trays   L   ☐

<u>RETURN DATES</u>   *Please tick box*

Bite _____   Received _____   PVT ☐

Try in _____   Received _____   IND ☐

Retry _____   Received _____   N.H.S ☐

Finish _____   Received _____

<u>DENTURES</u>

Notes   I.D.Names

NON STERILE DEVICE   LABORATORY FEE _____

STATEMENT.   This device conforms to the relevant requirements set out in

Annex I of the Medical Devices Directive

Inspected and Signed by

Figure 16.42   Denture laboratory docket.

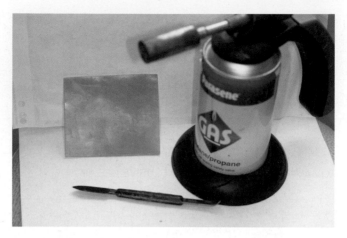

Figure 16.43   Pink wax, wax knife, burner.

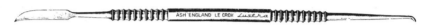

Figure 16.44   Le Cron carver.

(a)   (b)

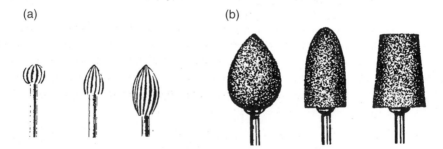

Figure 16.45   Acrylic burs (a) and stones (b).

Polygrip and *Fixodent* (Figure 16.46), but the alveolar bone changes can adversely affect appearance as the loose denture may no longer provide adequate support for the lips and cheeks. It is consequently necessary to *reline* the fitting surface of a denture from time to time and perhaps make other adjustments (see later). Ultimately, the denture will need to be replaced.

If the denture cleaning advice is not followed, the soft tissues covered by a denture may become inflamed and develop into a condition called *denture stomatitis*. This is treated with antifungal drugs such as nystatin or fluconazole, and the reiteration of suitable oral hygiene instructions. Similarly, the dentures may become stained by products such as tea and coffee, and calculus may form on them in the same regions as for natural teeth. Patients with these problems are advised to clean the dentures by soaking in hypochlorite (for example, *Milton solution*) for 20 min, rinsing

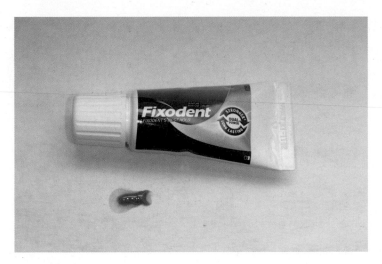

Figure 16.46   Denture adhesive.

thoroughly and then immersing in water overnight. Dentures with metallic components should be soaked in non-hypochlorite disinfectants, such as *Dentural*, instead, otherwise the bleach-based products will cause metal corrosion.

Full and partial chrome-cobalt dentures

The metallic alloy chrome-cobalt can be used as the base of the denture, rather than acrylic, but the teeth still need to be attached to this metal base by acrylic on the ridges. Chrome-cobalt can form the base of both edentulous and partial dentures. Metal-based dentures are more difficult to construct than acrylic ones, as the metal is rigid and provides no room for adjustment once made, so the impression and working model must be perfectly accurate. They also cost more than acrylic dentures to construct, but still have several advantages.

- A much **thinner palatal covering** is possible with chrome-cobalt, which makes the whole denture more tolerable to patients, especially those with a strong gag reflex.
- Overcomes any tissue reaction to acrylic monomer, which some patients are sensitive to.
- Denture base is **far stronger** and less likely to break, even in thin section.
- Allows patients with deep overbites onto their palate to be able to wear a denture, as the bite point can be completely avoided or have just a very thin metal coverage.
- Can design partial dentures as '**skeletons**', giving minimal tissue coverage and making the denture more tolerable for the patient (Figure 16.47).
- As less tissue coverage is involved, especially around the teeth, chrome dentures tend to be more hygienic than acrylic ones.

If the whole palate is covered by a chrome base, then retention is provided by the saliva suction film, as for acrylic dentures. However, if a skeleton design is used then chrome-cobalt clasps must be incorporated into the design of the denture for retention, so an adequate number of healthy and well-positioned teeth are required for this purpose.

The clasps will be part of the chrome base, and tooth adjustments can be carried out to provide undercuts, as for stainless clasps on acrylic dentures.

513

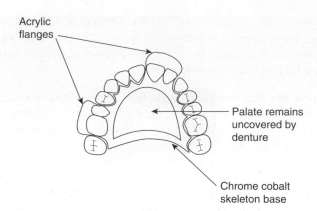

Figure 16.47   Chrome skeleton denture design.

Denture construction

The surgery stages are as for acrylic dentures, with the following exceptions.

- Final impressions are often taken in a highly accurate **elastomer** material, rather than alginate, to ensure that a good working model is produced for the metal casting.
- The chrome-cobalt base is then made on the final model as a wax pattern by the technician, before being cast in a special furnace.
- The casting of the metal base is sometimes carried out at specialised laboratories, so extra time between appointments may be necessary.
- A try-in of the metal base only is often carried out, to ensure it is accurate before proceeding to add the teeth to the design.
- A second try-in is then performed, with the teeth added and held by wax to the metal base.
- No adjustment of the metal base can be made in the surgery once it has been constructed, except for minimal easing using a pink stone in the slow handpiece.

Additional instructions are given to the patient at the fitting stage to ensure that they never use bleach-based denture cleaning products, because they will corrode the metal. A suitable alternative is the cleaning solution *Dentural*. Otherwise, the same post-fitting instructions are given to the patient.

Some designs of partial chrome-cobalt dentures can be quite intricate, and adequate time must be spent ensuring that the patient is competent in both the fitting and removal of the denture before they leave the premises.

Immediate replacement dentures

Dentures are usually made some months after the teeth have been extracted, as this allows time for completion of the initial alveolar bone resorption and gum healing to occur. Many patients, however, are not prepared to wait that long for the replacement of missing front teeth, and do not wish to have unsightly extraction gaps present, even for a few days. In such cases, the patient can be provided with an *immediate replacement denture*, which is made before the anterior teeth are extracted and fitted on the day of extraction, immediately after haemostasis has been achieved in the extraction sockets.

Obviously, there can be no try-in stage for this technique, but otherwise the procedure for construction is the same as for conventional dentures, until the final stage when the technician removes the teeth to be extracted from the model and replaces them with the the new denture teeth. The construction procedure is as follows.

- The dentist provides the technician with final impressions, the occlusal registration and the required shade for the new teeth, before any anterior extractions are carried out.
- In the laboratory, the anterior teeth to be extracted are cut off the working model by the technician, and the artificial ones fitted in their place as a wax-up on the model.
- This cannot be tried in the patient's mouth, as the teeth are still present, so the technician proceeds to tidy the wax-up and then processes it as a heat-cured acrylic.
- The final denture is trimmed and polished, then returned to the dentist.
- In the surgery, the anterior teeth are extracted and the denture is fitted at the same visit.
- Only minimal adjustments are made at this stage, as the oral soft tissues will be swollen from the local anaesthetic injections and the accuracy of the fit will not be obvious.
- The patient is given an appointment to attend the next day, and is instructed not to remove the denture before then.

The patient must be made aware that following the fitting of the immediate denture, alveolar bone resorption will occur and this could result in the prosthesis becoming loose quite quickly. Patients tend to accept this phenomenom readily, as the alternative is to have extraction spaces visible for months before a conventional denture is provided.

As chrome-cobalt cannot be adjusted once cast, immediate dentures are always constructed from acrylic only, although the replacement denture made after resorption has occurred can be a metal-based one.

If just one anterior tooth is to be replaced, the denture is usually designed in a 'spoon' shape, so that the gingival margins of other teeth are not covered by the denture, making it less likely to retain food debris around the teeth, and therefore more hygienic (Figure 16.48).

The aftercare instructions given to the patient on the day of extraction and fitting are as follows.

- Leave the denture in place overnight, to protect all the extraction sockets from food debris and the loss of any blood clots.
- Return to the surgery the following day, when the local anaesthetic has worn off and any high spots will be obvious. Any adjustments necessary can then be carried out.
- From then on, remove the denture after meals and carry out hot salt water mouthwashes to help heal the extraction sockets.
- Return to the surgery when bone resorption has caused significant loss of retention, so that adjustments can be made or a permanent denture provided – this may take between 3 and 6 months to occur in some patients.

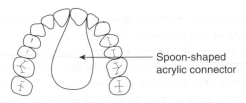

Figure 16.48   Spoon denture.

Other removable prosthetic procedures

From time to time, other procedures may be carried out to existing removable prostheses to improve their fit or extend their period of wear, without having to resort to the construction of a new denture.

- Relines or rebases.
- Additions of teeth or clasps.
- Use of tissue conditioners as:
  - soft linings
  - functional impression materials.

Relines and rebases

These may be required as alveolar bone resorption occurs beneath the denture with time, and the retentive fit is lost as a space develops beneath the fitting surface of the denture and it becomes loose. The bone lost during this natural process can be replaced with the addition of a new layer of acrylic within the fitting surface of the denture, as follows.

- The denture is thoroughly cleaned at the surgery, ensuring that no food debris is present.
- The patient is asked to carry out a vigorous mouthwash at the surgery, and tooth brushing if necessary, to also remove any food debris from their mouth.
- An accurate impression (**wash impression**) is taken within the denture itself, using an elastomer impression material.
- Alternatively, an alginate impression is taken of the mouth itself (without the denture in place).
- The impression and the denture are sent to the technician.
- The technician makes a cast within the denture, so that the alveolar bone is recorded where a wash impression has been taken, or casts a model of the arch from the alginate impression.
- Wash impression is removed from the denture and the space present between it and the model is filled with acrylic, or the denture is placed over the new model and the space between the two is filled with acrylic.
- This creates a new base fitting surface to the denture, which will then sit accurately against the oral soft tissues again and improve the retention of the denture.

Additions

The addition of either a tooth or a clasp to an exisiting denture may be necessary from time to time, as the patient loses a natural tooth or the retention of the prosthesis deteriorates with time. The procedure is very straightforward and can often be completed by the technician within the day, as follows.

- An aginate impression is taken over the denture while in place in the mouth.
- The impression and denture are sent to the technician.
- The technician casts the model with the denture *in situ*.
- The position of the denture is then accurately recorded on the model.
- The denture can now be removed and repositioned exactly in place on the model, so that the new tooth or clasp can be fitted accurately to the exisiting denture, and will then fit perfectly into place when returned to the patient.

Tissue conditioners

These are special materials used in two circumstances.

- As a **soft lining** when the soft tissues beneath the denture are continually sore, for whatever reason, so that the denture cannot be worn routinely without causing great discomfort to the patient.
- As a **functional impression** material which sets over several hours and therefore records the soft tissues and denture extremities more accurately than conventional impression techniques.

Persistent soreness beneath a denture is often a problem with elderly patients, and can cause medical problems due to them being unable to eat sufficiently well. The soft lining construction procedure is similar to that used to place a hard reline into a denture, in that an impression is taken inside it using an elastomer material, so that the technician can cast up a working model. The base of the denture is then cut out by the technician, and replaced by a soft tissue conditioner which acts as a cushion between the alveolar ridge and the denture. When the patient bites with the revamped denture, the cushioning 'bounces' and dissipates the occlusal force so that it is not transmitted onto the alveolar ridge as pain and discomfort. The conditioner requires regular replacement every 12–18 months though, as it deteriorates in saliva over time, gradually becoming hardened and losing its 'bounce'.

Functional impressions are required in complicated cases of removable prosthesis construction, where conventional impression techniques fail to record the oral anatomy in sufficient detail to produce an adequately retentive denture.

Normal impressions record the hard alveolar ridge and any standing teeth, with the soft tissues pushed out of the way and held stationary while the impression is setting. The natural situation in the mouth is one of continual movement and change. Recording this real situation in an impression requires a material which takes hours to set while the denture is being worn and used.

The oldest functional impression material is black gutta percha but this has been superseded by modern materials which are a type of slow-curing acrylic resin, for example *Visco-gel* and *Coe Comfort*. They usually consist of a powder and liquid which are mixed together and applied to the fitting surface of the denture, reinserted into the patient's mouth, and worn for up to 6 h. The patient must take no food or drink during this time. When found to provide a comfortable and satisfactory fit, the denture and its incorporated impression is sent to the laboratory for the casting of a working model. The impression material is then removed and replaced with heat-cured acrylic, producing a well-fitting and functional prosthesis.

Obturators

These are specialist removable prostheses that will be provided to a patient via a hospital dental department, rather than from a general dental workplace.

They are appliances used to seal off an abnormal cavity in the maxilla, such as that due to a cleft palate or the space left after significant oral surgery for tumour or cyst removal. The abnormal cavity requires sealing off from the oral cavity to allow proper speech, as well as to prevent food and drink collecting in the maxilla. The denture area of the obturator is constructed in the usual way, but an elastomer material is also used to record the cavity accurately, before being incorporated into the denture design. As elstomers can record undercuts accurately, the impression material can be inserted into the cavity, allowed to set, then withdrawn without tearing and distorting.

Where large abnormal cavities require closing over, the extension area is made to be hollow so that the obturator is not too heavy to wear.

Overdentures

An overdenture is a full denture which is fitted on top of standing teeth or retained roots in the dental arch. The advantage of an overdenture is the presence of natural roots remaining in the alveolar bone. These have the effect of greatly reducing the absorption and shrinkage of alveolar ridges which normally occur after tooth extraction. When teeth are extracted, the alveolar bone becomes redundant, as it has lost its natural function of providing support for the teeth, and consequently diminishes in size as the bone resorbs. This loss of bone may be so great that it becomes very difficult to make a denture which is not perpetually loose, and lower dentures pose the most awkward problems in this respect.

As long as any roots remain, there is hardly any loss of alveolar bone and these problems of difficult lower dentures are far less common. However, dentures cannot be fitted directly on top of retained roots or teeth. In most cases, a certain amount of preparation of these abutment teeth is required to remove undercuts and prevent caries.

Retained roots are root filled and ground to a dome shape level with the gum. If the root surface is irregular because of previous caries, the dome shape can be restored by fitting an appropriately shaped post crown. Teeth which still have intact crowns are usually treated by reducing the crown to a small tapered stump and fitting a full gold veneer thimble over the top. Having prepared the remaining teeth or roots, the overdenture is then made in the usual way of a full denture.

Overdentures are usually made as full dentures but they can be used as partial dentures in rare cases where some of the remaining teeth are unsuitable for the full denture design. They may also be used for patients with cleft palates and for those who have undergone surgical removal of part of their jaw, during treatment for oral cancer. In such cases the alveolar ridges may be so misshapen that properly fitting conventional dentures cannot be made.

More recently, or where there are no remaining roots anyway, *dental implants* can be used to support an overdenture. They are covered later in the chapter.

Orthodontic appliances

As mentioned previously, both fixed and removable orthodontic appliances share many common features with fixed and removable prosthodontics, especially in the materials used to construct and fit them. Consequently, they are included here for ease of reference.

Orthodontic appliances are used to align (straighten) crooked teeth, so that the patient is able to carry out effective oral hygiene techniques and prevent caries or periodontal disease from developing.

Two basic types of appliance are used.

- **Fixed appliance** – composed of individual metal or ceramic components bonded onto each tooth and connected together by an archwire, they cannot be removed from the mouth by the patient and are therefore similar to fixed prostheses.
- **Removable appliance** – composed of an acrylic base with stainless steel clasps and springs, and able to be removed from the mouth for cleaning, eating and adjustment, these appliances are therefore similar to removable prostheses.

Greater and more complicated forces can be applied to the teeth using fixed appliances, and the range possible for both types of appliance is as follows.

- Movement of teeth forwards or backwards in each arch – removable and fixed.
- Movement of jaws in relation to each other – functional and fixed.
- Alignment of slightly misplaced teeth in arch – removable and fixed.
- Alignment of severely misplaced teeth in arch – fixed.
- Derotation of teeth – fixed.
- Guided eruption of unerupted teeth – fixed.
- Guided reduction of deep overbite – removable and fixed.

Fixed orthodontic appliances

These consist of separate stainless steel or ceramic components called brackets that are individually bonded onto each tooth, using an orthodontic light-cured resin material. Molar teeth often have a circular metal device, called an orthodontic band, placed instead and these can be cemented with any type of luting cement.

The fitting procedure, called bonding, is carried out in the surgery with no laboratory input required except to cast up the preoperative and postoperative study models required. A bonded arch using metal brackets is shown in Figure 16.49. Bonding of the components causes no tooth damage, and they are 'snapped off' at the end of the treatment harmlessly, using special orthodontic instruments.

The equipment and instruments required for the monitoring and adjustment of the fixed appliance once it has been initially bonded are shown in Table 16.10.

Patient advice for fixed appliances

Every tooth is incorporated into a fixed appliance, so the number of stagnation areas and the potential for oral damage to occur are far greater than for individual fixed prostheses. Routine twice-daily tooth brushing alone is insufficient to maintain adequate standards of good oral hygiene, and special instructions and techniques are recommended for patients undergoing fixed orthodontic therapy.

- Careful manual tooth brushing should be carried out after each meal.
- Good-quality electric tooth brushes, such as *Sonicare* and *Oral B*, may be used instead.
- Use of fluoridated toothpaste.

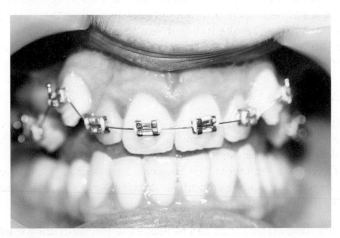

Figure 16.49   Bonded arch using metal brackets.

Table 16.10   Equipment and instruments required for the monitoring and adjustment of the fixed appliance once it has been initially bonded

Item	Function
Archwire (Figure 16.50a)	Flexible nickel titanium or stainless steel wires, to fasten into the brackets or bands
End cutters	Right-angled cutters to trim the ends of the archwire after replacement
Alastiks	Rubber bands to hold the archwire into the slots of each bracket
Alastik holders	Ratcheted holders (similar to artery forceps) to apply the alastiks to the brackets
Brackets (Figure 16.50b)	Metal or ceramic components to attach to each tooth, if any have been lost since last appointment
Bands (Figure 16.50c)	Metal rings to attach to molars especially, although bands are available for all teeth and were the only attachments available before brackets were developed
Bracket holders	To hold and position each bracket to the centre of the tooth, if any replacements are required
Bracket and band removers (Figure 16.51)	To remove brackets, bands and any residual bond material before replacing, if necessary
Bonding materials	Acid etch and orthodontic resin bond material, to hold brackets onto the tooth
Band cement	Any luting cement material, to hold bands onto the molar teeth

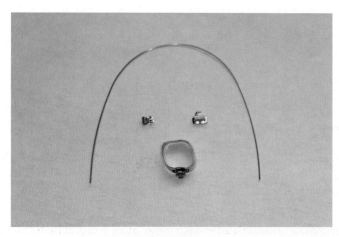

Figure 16.50   Archwire, bracket, molar band and tube.

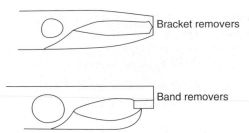

Figure 16.51   Bracket and band removers.

- Daily use of **interdental brushes** to clean around each bracket individually.
- Avoidance of cariogenic and acidic food and drinks, for the full period of treatment.
- Avoidance of sticky foods, for the full period of treatment.
- Use of **fluoride mouthwash** daily, to minimise the risk of decalcification.
- Regular use of **disclosing tablets**, to highlight problematic areas where plaque is being retained, to minimise the risk of decalcification.

Removable orthodontic appliances

These are similar to dentures in construction, in that alginate impressions of both arches and a wax bite registration are taken and sent to the laboratory, along with a work ticket detailing the exact design of appliance required. Usually, the technician involved in the appliance construction specialises in orthodontic devices, as some of the components used are specific to this dental discipline and are not used with other prostheses.

A set of both study models and working models are cast from the impressions, and the latter set are used to construct the acrylic bases for each appliance, or for just one appliance if treatment is being carried out in one arch only. The additional components that can then be added to the acrylic base are as follows.

- **Adam's cribs** to retain the appliance in the mouth, usually to fit onto molar or premolar teeth and made of stainless steel (Figure 16.52).
- **Springs** in a variety of designs, to move the teeth along the arch as required (Figure 16.53).
- **Retractors** to push one or several teeth backwards (Figure 16.54).
- **Expansion screws** to move several teeth or each half of the upper arch outwards.

The equipment and instruments required for the monitoring and adjusting of the appliance are shown in Table 16.11.

Patient advice for removable appliances

As with removable prostheses, orthodontic appliances are capable of acting as stagnation areas and holding food debris and plaque against the teeth and gingivae, unless a good standard of oral hygiene is maintained.

Although some dentists prefer patients to wear appliances during meals, it is possible that more acrylic breakages will occur if this is the case. The instructions for patients wearing removable appliances are as follows.

- Wear as directed by the dentist.
- Clean the appliance and teeth after each meal, using a toothbrush and toothpaste.
- Avoid cariogenic and acidic foods and drinks, as advised.

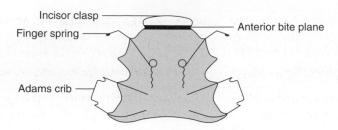

Figure 16.52   Removable upper orthodontic appliance.

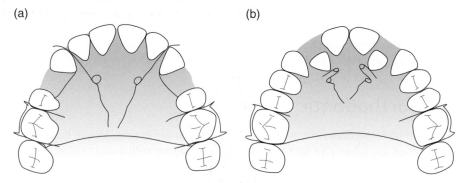

Figure 16.53   Types of spring. (a) Palatal finger spring. (b) 'Z' spring.

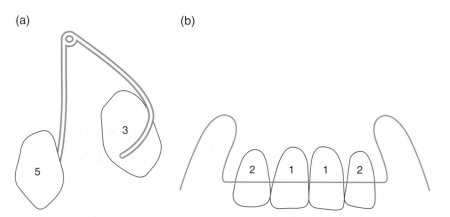

Figure 16.54   Types of retractor. (a) Buccal canine retractor. (b) Roberts retractor.

- Attend all dental appointments for the necessary adjustments.
- Contact the surgery immediately if any breakages or loss of the appliance occur.
- Expect the appliance to feel tight initially after each adjustment.
- Contact the surgery if any prolonged or excessive symptoms occur.
- If the appliance is to be removed for meals, ensure it is placed safely in a rigid container to avoid breakages during mealtimes.

Table 16.11   Equipment and instruments required to monitor and adjust the appliance

Item	Function
Adam's crib pliers (Figure 16.55)	To adjust all metal springs and retractors, as necessary
Straight handpiece and acrylic trimming bur (Figure 16.56)	To adjust all acrylic areas of the appliance, as necessary
Measuring ruler	To record any measurable tooth movement, such as the overjet
Expansion screw key	To count the number of turns applied to the screw between visits, to ensure compliance by the patient

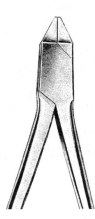

Figure 16.55   Adam's universal pliers.

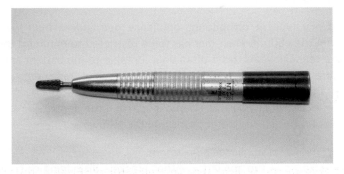

Figure 16.56   Acrylic trimming bur in straight handpiece.

Functional appliances

These are a specialised type of removable orthodontic appliance made of acrylic and stainless steel components, and worn in both arches at the same time, the most common one currently being a *Twinblock* (Figure 16.57).

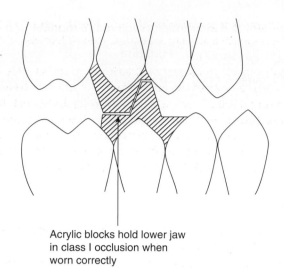

Acrylic blocks hold lower jaw
in class I occlusion when
worn correctly

Figure 16.57   Functional appliance.

They are used to correct skeletal class II discrepancies, where the mandible is further back from the ideal position, and work by holding the mandible forwards in the ideal class I position and allowing mandibular growth to occur and correct the malocclusion naturally. As their success depends on the growth of the mandible, they can only be used while the patient is still growing but after the premolars have erupted (these teeth are required for retention of the appliance), so the ideal age is up to 14 years old.

The materials, instruments and patient advice are as for removable orthodontic appliances.

General patient co-operation and motivation with orthodontic appliances

The wearing of any type of orthodontic appliance demands a high level of motivation and co-operation from the patient. Their diet has to be restricted to minimise the risk of caries developing, and in the teenage years this is often unacceptable to the patient and their motivation will wane. This is more likely to happen with prolonged courses of treatment.

Co-operation and levels of motivation need to be assessed at each adjustment appointment, and reinforced as necessary by both the dental nurse and the dentist.

Warning signs of reducing co-operation include the following.

- Failed appointments for appliance adjustment.
- Recurrent breakages of the appliance, either brackets dislodging or springs and acrylic being fractured.
- Continual reporting of problems wearing appliances which cannot be detected by the dentist, which have resulted in non-wear.
- Falling standards of oral hygiene or evidence of carious damage.
- Obvious lack of interest during adjustment appointments.
- Requests for early removal of fixed appliances, before treatment has been completed.
- Failure to wear removable or functional appliances during the daytime, so that when only worn at night little improvement is achieved.

Any combination of these signs should alert the oral health team that the treatment may fail, so co-operation must be reinforced and improvement seen to happen, otherwise the decision must be taken to abandon the treatment.

A system of discontinuation of treatment must be in place, so that patients are aware that failure to comply will result in early removal of the appliance and incomplete treatment. This may mean that malocclusions remain as they were for life, with all the consequences that that will mean to the patient. If a patient persistently fails to wear the appliance or to attend appointments for adjustment and review, treatment is best discontinued at an early stage before too much surgery time has been wasted.

Patients who have discontinued treatment once and then re-present for continuation should be treated with great caution, as the likelihood of a second failed course is greater still.

Dental implants

The use of dental implants over the last 20 years or so has provided a technique for improving the life and masticatory efficiency of many patients.

Previously, when a tooth had to be extracted it could only be replaced by a denture or a bridge. Both of these techniques have their own advantages and disadvantages as discussed earlier in the chapter, but a reminder of the main disadvantages of each is summarised below.

- **Dentures** – poor retention, making chewing and successful wear very difficult.
- **Bridges** – permanent loss of tooth tissue while preparing abutment teeth, and overloading of remaining teeth causing the eventual failure of the bridge.

The development of dental implants as an alternative to the replacement of missing teeth has helped to overcome these disadvantages.

An implant is effectively a titanium double-screw cylinder that is inserted into a hole drilled into the alveolar bone of either jaw, to replace one or several teeth. Unlike when posts are cemented into tooth roots when placing post crowns, the implant is not 'glued' into place. Instead, the alveolar bone gradually grows around it and into its hollow screw structure so that it is eventually locked into the bone itself. This is called *osseointegration* and takes several months to occur.

Once the implant is firm within the bone structure, the top section can have the tooth replacement screwed onto it, and this can be any of the following devices.

- Single crown tooth.
- Multiple crowns to form a bridge.
- Metal bar to act as a locking device beneath a denture.
- Metal ball to act as a locking device beneath a denture (Figure 16.58).

525

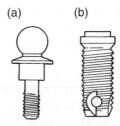

(a)   (b)

Figure 16.58   Implant components. (a) Ball abutment for overdenture. (b) Implant fixture.

The success of the use of implants depends on many factors.

- **Bone** – there must be a deep enough section of alveolar bone to screw the implant into, without it damaging other structures such as dental nerves or the maxillary antrum (although techniques are being developed to replace bone using synthetic alternatives, and an operation can be performed to 'raise' the floor of the antrum to provide more space).
- **Patient selection** – not all patients will be suitable for such an extensive surgical procedure; some medical conditions may also contraindicate the use of implants (such as osteoporosis, haemophilia, diabetes due to poor wound healing).
- **Oral health** – patients with poor oral health are unsuitable for implants, as their success depends very much on being kept clean of dental plaque. The presence of plaque allows periodontal disease to develop around the implant, and the resultant pocketing will allow the titanium cylinder to become loose and the implant will fail – this condition is called *perimplantitis*.
- **Lifestyle factors** – factors such as smoking and poor dental attendance may lead to failure of an implant in the same way that they are associated with higher levels of dental disease (especially periodontal disease) in dentate patients without implants.

Implant and prosthesis placement procedures

- A team consisting of an implantologist, a specialist technician and a hygienist examine and assess the patient, helped by study models, radiographs or even three-dimensional computer scans.
- They can then plan the preparation, construction and maintenance of an implant procedure for the patient.
- Depending where the placement procedure is carried out, local anaesthetic (with or without conscious sedation) or general anaesthetic is given to the patient.
- The oral surgery procedure of inserting the titanium implants into the alveolar bone is carried out under the usual surgical conditions of other minor oral surgery procedures.
- A mucoperiosteal flap is raised to expose the bone and special low-speed drills are used to prepare holes for the implants, or the extraction socket of the tooth itself is used and prepared in a similar fashion.
- The implants are screwed into the prepared holes and the tissue flap is then sutured back into place to completely bury the implant (Figure 16.59).
- After a suitable time period, which can be up to several months, the implants become firmly embedded in the bone by osseointegration, and the prosthesis can be placed.
- Under local anaesthetic, a small incision is made in the overlying gingiva to expose the top of each implant, and the artificial abutments are then screwed into the inner surface of the implants. Abutments may be in the form of stumps for fitting single crowns or bridge pontics (Figure 16.60) or a ball or bar for clipping on a removable overdenture.

Obviously, the succesful placement of implants in dentistry depends on the surgical skill of the dentist or oral surgeon involved. Training available ranges from weekend courses, through module type diplomas, to full surgical specialty and qualification. The more complicated cases should only ever be handled by those with adequate training in the more complicated techniques, and specialist implantologists.

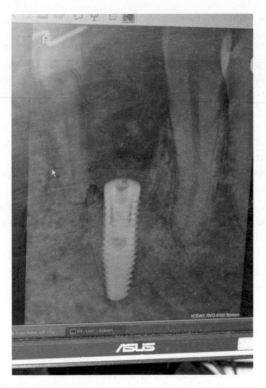

Figure 16.59   Radiograph of implant placement.

527

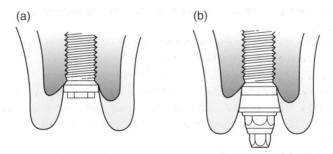

Figure 16.60   Implant procedure. (a) Stage 1: implant fixture. (b) Stage 2: crown or bridge abutment fitted.

In addition, the laboratory stages of the top section of the appliance have to be carried out by specialist technicians, although the chairside preparation stage is no different from that for a conventional crown or bridge preparation. The use of denture locking devices requires special impression techniques to be used.

The need for specialist training in dental implants, as well as all the necessary equipment required, means that implants are very expensive to place. The simplest case of a single tooth implant is usually in the region of £1500–2000 (at 2013 prices), and the more complicated cases will run into tens of thousands of pounds each. Their only availability on the NHS is as teaching cases in dental hospitals.

However, their use is on the increase as they provide succesful dental treatment options to patients who were previously untreatable, as well as offering less invasive techniques in simpler cases, such as single tooth replacements. Training courses are currently being developed for qualified dental nurses, so that they are able to assist in specialist implant clinics and hospital departments.

In the meantime, the dental nurse has an important role in helping to provide oral hygiene instruction and reinforcement for implant patients, in a similar way to that given for crowns, dentures and bridges.

 Further resources are available for this book, including interactive multiple choice questions and extended matching questions. Visit the companion website at:

www.levisonstextbookfordentalnurses.com

17

Extractions and Minor Oral Surgery

Key learning points

A **factual knowledge** of
- simple extraction techniques
- surgical extraction techniques

A **working knowledge** of
- the instruments and equipment used in simple tooth extractions
- the instruments and equipment used in surgical extractions and minor oral surgery procedures

A **factual awareness** of
- the complications of extraction and their avoidance
- other minor oral surgery procedures

Many procedures carried out daily in the vast majority of dental workplaces can be collectively termed as 'minor oral surgery' (MOS), as opposed to major oral surgery procedures such as treatment and reconstructive surgery for oral cancer, orthognathic surgery to correct skeletal problems, and head and neck trauma surgery. Those minor surgical procedures to be discussed here are the following.

- **Simple extractions** – of roots or whole teeth, where no soft tissue or bone removal is required.
- **Surgical extractions** – of roots or whole teeth, where soft tissue alone, or with bone, has to be removed to gain access to the root or tooth.

Levison's Textbook for Dental Nurses, Eleventh Edition. By Carole Hollins.
© 2013 John Wiley & Sons, Ltd. Published 2013 by John Wiley & Sons, Ltd. Companion website: www.levisonstextbookfordentalnurses.com

- **Operculectomy** – the surgical removal of the gingival flap overlying a partially erupted tooth, especially a lower third molar.
- **Alveolectomy** - the surgical adjustment and removal of bone spicules from the alveolar ridge after tooth extraction, to produce a smooth base for denture seating.
- **Gingivectomy and gingivoplasty** – periodontal soft tissue surgery to adjust the shape of the gingivae to aid oral hygiene measures.
- **Periodontal flap surgery** – the surgical raising and replacing of surgical flaps, to enable subgingival debridement to be carried out.
- **Soft tissue biopsies** – the partial or complete removal of soft tissue oral lesions, for pathological investigation and diagnosis.

Arguably, these surgical procedures constitute those most worrying to the patient, as bleeding and possible postoperative pain are quite likely to occur. The dental nurse has a very important role in the reassurance and monitoring of the patient during these procedures, so that the patient remains less anxious and more co-operative throughout.

As always, Health and Safety and infection control procedures must be strictly adhered to before, during and after the surgical procedure.

Extractions

These procedures involve the removal of teeth, or their roots if the crown of the tooth has disintegrated, to leave a section of the alveolar ridge bare and ready for tooth replacement by:

- the pontic of a bridge
- a denture
- an implant.

Reasons for tooth extraction

Both deciduous and permanent teeth may require extraction at some point. This is usually due to infection and pain being present following caries, periodontal disease or trauma, but may also be due to the following reasons.

- The tooth is unrestorable, whether pain and infection are present or not.
- The position of the tooth prevents the placement of a fixed or removable prosthesis.
- The tooth is too poorly positioned to be aligned orthodontically.
- The tooth may be selectively extracted to provide space in a crowded dental arch.
- Attempts to save the tooth by root filling have failed.
- The tooth may be partially erupted and impacted, and suffer from recurrent painful infections (pericoronitis) due to food trapping.
- Deciduous teeth can be selectively extracted to encourage the timely eruption of their permanent successors into more favourable positions.
- The patient's choice, where attempting to save the tooth by root filling is not the preferred option.

To ensure that any tooth is extracted painlessly and successfully, the dentist has an in-depth knowledge of the anatomy and physiology of the head and neck region, as well as the oral cavity and its nerve supply. An efficient and supportive dental nurse must also have a background knowledge of these subjects, to be able to provide the level of preparation, chairside support and help required during any likely complication that may arise.

When the dentist has no choice and decides that a tooth has to be extracted, it will be for one or more of the following reasons.

- Unless successful treatment to save it can be carried out, a carious or periodontally involved tooth is a continual source of infection in the patient's oral cavity.
- Any infection may be intermittent, but often there are acute and very painful episodes that may require analgesic and antibiotic treatment.
- Infection can spread into the bloodstream (**bacteraemia**) and the patient can become generally unwell – this can be a serious event in elderly and medically compromised patients.
- Repeat prescriptions of antibiotics to treat infection without tooth removal are considered poor practice.
- No replacement of the tooth can be carried out to restore oral health until the tooth has been extracted.

Once it has been determined that a tooth or root requires extraction, the complexity of the procedure depends mainly on which tooth is involved, how much tooth or root is present, and its position in the jaw bone. The options available for the extraction procedure will then fall into one of the following categories.

- Simple extraction.
- Surgical extraction involving soft tissue removal to expose an unerupted tooth or buried root.
- Surgical extraction involving dissection of the tooth in its socket and removal in sections.
- Surgical extraction involving the raising of a mucoperiosteal flap and bone removal to gain full access to a tooth or root.

If the tooth involved is a deciduous one, the following points need to be considered.

- **Resorption** – has root resorption occurred so that effectively just the crown of the tooth remains, attached merely to the gingivae?
- **Permanent successor** – is the underlying permanent tooth present, and likely to be damaged during the extraction procedure?
- **Infection** – is any dental infection present, that may make the procedure unnecessarily painful?
- **Age and co-operation** – younger patients are usually less willing to undergo extraction procedures than older patients and, along with some of those with special needs, are less able to understand the need for the procedure nor the consequences if it is not carried out.
- **Medical history of the patient** – some medical conditions contraindicate extraction.
- **Tooth status** – a grossly carious deciduous tooth may be difficult to extract simply and quickly, but a surgical procedure is not usually feasible in conscious younger patients, so some form of anxiety control will have to be considered.

If the tooth involved is a permanent one, the following points need to be considered.

- **Infection** – is any dental infection present, that may make the procedure unnecessarily painful?
- **Medical history of the patient** – some medical conditions contraindicate extraction.
- **Medications** – some adult medications will mean hospitalisation for extractions or MOS, because of possible serious side-effects.

- **Co-operation** – some adults and some patients with special needs will require some form of anxiety control to undergo these types of procedure.
- **Age** – older patients have more friable soft tissues which are more easily traumatised during surgical procedures, and their jaw bones will be more brittle and more easily fractured.
- **Tooth status** – a grossly carious tooth is more likely to require a full surgical procedure to complete its removal.
- **Post extraction** – will the missing tooth require replacement, and if so what are the options and cost implications?

Simple extractions

Simple extractions are so called because the tooth or root is removed whole from the dental arch without involving tooth sectioning, flap raising or bone removal. Any or all of these additional techniques may be required during a surgical extraction. Whether the tooth is still vital or has died from any associated infection, local anaesthesia will always be required to numb the surrounding gingivae at least, even for a simple extraction.

The specific instruments, equipment and medicaments that may be required for a simple extraction are shown in Table 17.1.

Forceps are the instruments most frequently used to extract a tooth, and are handled by being pushed along the sides of the root to sever the periodontal membrane. Once a reasonable position has been achieved, the root is gripped and gentle wrist movements are employed to gradually loosen the tooth in the socket. The forceps are gradually worked further towards the apex of the tooth until it is loose enough in the socket to be removed. In effect, then, a tooth is actually extracted by being *pushed out* of the socket, rather than being pulled out of it, as most people would assume.

Table 17.1   Specific instruments, equipment and medicaments that may be required for a simple extraction

Item	Function
Forceps	Range of sterile hand instruments used to grip a tooth or root at its neck before applying appropriate wrist actions to loosen the tooth/root in its socket during the extraction procedure. Various designs are available for use on upper or lower teeth, and for each individual tooth
Luxators	Sterile hand instruments used to widen the socket and sever the periodontal ligament attachment
Elevators	Sterile hand instruments used to prise the tooth/root out of the socket. Various patterns are available – Cryer's, Warwick James', Winter's
Fine-bore aspirator	Disposable suction tip used to suck away all blood and maintain good moisture control during the procedure; also useful for sucking and holding tooth debris so that it can be removed from the mouth safely
Haemostats	Gelatine sponges or oxidised cellulose packs, which are inserted into the socket after extraction to aid blood clotting and achieve haemostasis – can be used with or without a suture

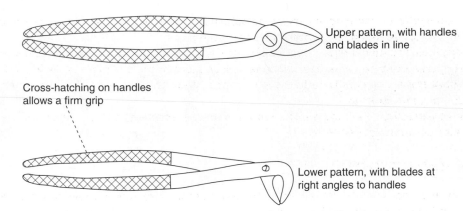

Figure 17.1   Upper and lower pattern of forceps.

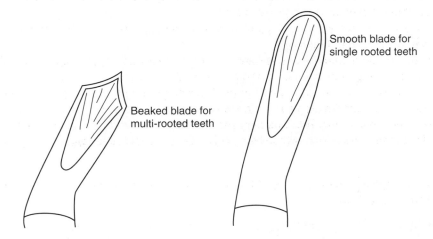

Figure 17.2   Blade detail of forceps.

Unnecessary force during extractions often results in tooth or root fracture, although this can also occur anyway with grossly carious teeth.

Forceps are designed in various patterns, to be used individually for each type of tooth. Upper tooth forceps tend to have their handles and blades roughly in line with each other, whereas lower tooth forceps tend to be at right angles to each other for ease of access to the lower arch (Figure 17.1). Multi-rooted molar tooth forceps have blades which are shaped like beaks so that they can grip the *furcation* area between the roots, but single-rooted tooth forceps are smooth (Figure 17.2).

The most common patterns of forceps are shown in Figure 17.3.

- **Upper incisor and canine forceps** are straight with single rounded blades and have both wide and narrow patterns.
- **Upper root forceps** are similar in appearance, with narrow, straight blades.
- **Upper premolar forceps** have slightly curved handles and single rounded blades.
- **Upper left molar forceps** have curved handles and a beaked blade to the right of the instrument, and a rounded blade to the left to grip the buccal roots and the palatal root respectively (many dental nurses identify upper molar forceps by the mantra 'beak to cheek').

533

(a)   (b)

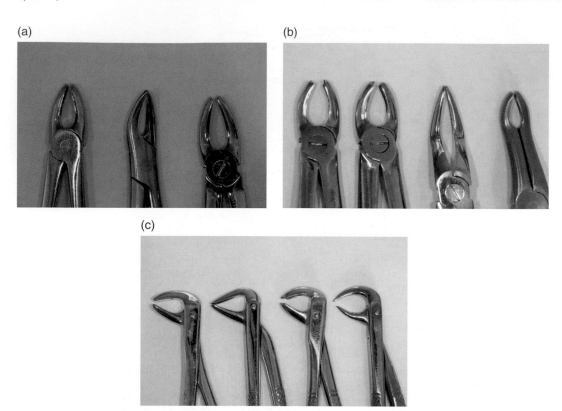

(c)

Figure 17.3   Extraction forceps. (a) Upper straight, root, premolar. (b) Upper left and right molar, bayonets. (c) Lower anterior, root, molar, cowhorns.

- **Upper right molar forceps** have curved handles and the beaked blade is to the left of the instrument.
- **Upper bayonet forceps** have extended handles and angled blades to gain access to third molars, or have angled pointed blades to gain access to fractured roots.
- **Lower anterior forceps** have single, rounded blades at right angles to the handle that are particularly useful for extracting lower premolars.
- **Lower root forceps** are similar, with narrow and straight blades that are also particularly useful for extracting small or crowded incisors.
- **Lower molar forceps** have beaked blades at right angles to the handles, to grip the furcation of the two roots.
- **Lower 'cowhorn' forceps** have curved and pointed blades at right angles to the handles, to grip the furcation of lower molar teeth.
- **Smaller versions** of most patterns exist, for deciduous tooth extractions.

Similarly, elevators are available in a variety of patterns and are used to gradually sever the periodontal membrane and loosen the tooth in the socket (Figure 17.4). They are specifically used to elevate retained roots and impacted teeth, where adequate access to the root or tooth is not possible with conventional forceps, or where the angle of elevation required to loosen the root or tooth is not possible with forceps.

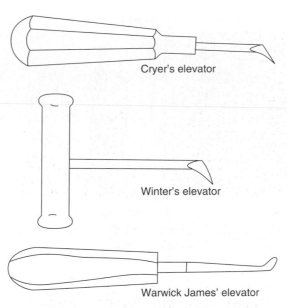

Figure 17.4   Types of elevators.

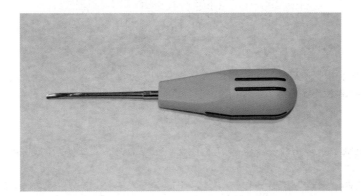

Figure 17.5   Luxator.

The more common types are as follows.

- **Cryer's elevators** are available as left and right patterns, but can be used on either side of the mouth, depending whether they are engaged mesially or distally – the tips are triangular shaped and pointed.
- **Winter's elevators** have a similar blade design as Cryer's, but have a corkscrew style handle to give more leverage.
- **Warwick James' elevators** are available as left, right and straight patterns – the tips are a similar shape to the round blade of forceps.

Alternatively, the dentist may choose to use one of a variety of *luxators* (Figure 17.5) that are available and are used in a similar fashion to an elevator but with greater effect, as the tips are sharper and finer

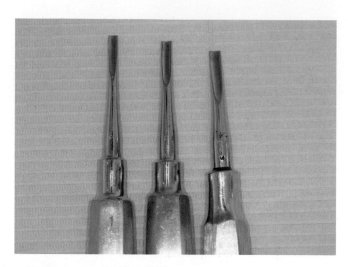

Figure 17.6   Coupland's chisels – sizes 1, 2, 3.

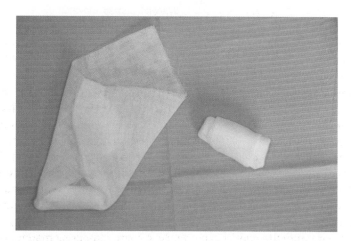

Figure 17.7   Bite pack construction.

and therefore more easily pushed into the periodontal space between the root and the bony socket. It is possible to extract practically any tooth using a luxator alone, and many dentists are able to do so.

A single-bladed chisel is also available for splitting multi-rooted teeth, called a *Coupland's chisel* and available in sizes 1, 2 and 3 (Figure 17.6).

Difficult extractions can be quite exhausting for the dentist and the patient, and it often helps both for the dental nurse to actually support the patient's head or mandible during the extraction. In this way, the dentist is not wasting energy by rocking the patient's head rather than loosening the tooth, and it also allows the patient to relax more, rather than trying to hold their head still for the dentist.

Upon removal of the tooth, the dentist squeezes the socket walls together, places a bite pack over the socket, and instructs the patient to bite on it for 10 min to help to achieve haemostasis (stop the bleeding). After treatment, the patient is not dismissed until the bleeding has ceased and postoperative advice has been given. A suitable bite pack can be made from a cotton wool roll and gauze sheets, as shown in Figure 17.7.

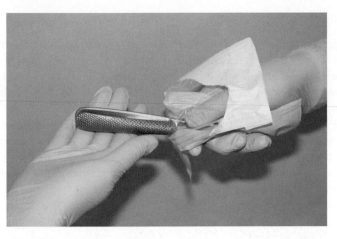

Figure 17.8   No-touch technique of passing forceps.

Role of the dental nurse during the procedure

The dental nurse should have a full working knowledge of each instrument likely to be used, including the full range of forceps available, to ensure the ability to provide close support and assistance to the dental team during the procedure.

Each instrument will be sterile and bagged, and should be carefully opened without touching it and then handed to the dentist handles first, while holding the tips still within the sterile pouch – this is the 'no-touch' technique (Figure 17.8). In this way, infection control is maintained.

As with any dental procedure, all the required instruments and equipment will have been made ready before the procedure begins and laid out in their bags, close to the dental chair for easy access but not in full view of the patient – this is likely to increase their anxiety.

The dental nurse will anticipate the dentist with regard to the instruments required and their order of need, and safely pass them as required using the 'no-touch' technique described above.

Throughout the procedure, the dental nurse will monitor the patient for any signs of distress (such as feeling pain) and notify the dentist accordingly. A calm, reassuring manner is required to put the patient at their ease and this must be adapted for the various types of patient that may be treated – whether a child, an adult or elderly person, or a patient with special needs. When treating patients from different ethnic backgrounds, it is very useful to have a friend or family member present to interpret as necessary.

As the forceps, luxators and elevators used have to be pushed into the tooth socket, the dental nurse may also be required to stabilise the patient's head or mandible so that the dentist's efforts are not wasted. The purpose of the support should be briefly explained to the patient beforehand.

Surgical field considerations

Whichever technique is used to extract a tooth or root, the procedure is considered a surgical one, as bleeding will definitely occur and the tissues of the patient's oral cavity will be breached by the instruments used. If the working area is not treated as a sterile field during the procedure, there is a potential risk of cross-infection occurring and this is more likely with oral surgery procedures than with any other in dentistry.

537

Consequently, the following special precautions are taken.

- **Sterile bagged instruments** – all instruments to be used must have been individually sterilised and bagged before the procedure, unlike restorative instruments that are bagged together.
- **PPE for the dental team** – over and above the usual PPE requirements for dental procedures, surgical gowns or single-use plastic aprons should be used to prevent blood contamination of the uniform.
- **Disposable items** – wherever possible, disposable items should be used to prevent cross-infection, including aspirators, scalpel blades, needles, suture needles, etc.
- **Contamination policy** – any single-use items and materials that are opened but not used during the procedure should be disposed of anyway, to avoid their possible contamination and then spread of infection by resealing and using at a later date.
- **Suction equipment** – must be run through immediately after the procedure with the required disinfectant solution to remove all traces of blood from its inner workings, rather than at the end of the session as usual.
- **Operative field** – should be assumed to be blood contaminated and wiped down thoroughly with sodium hypochlorite (bleach) or another accepted decontaminant.
- **Equipment coverage** – items such as the dental chair will obviously be reused and are not sterilisable, so they must be covered before the procedure with a single-use impervious membrane, to prevent blood contamination.
- **Sterile field** – the oral cavity and its immediate vicinity will be regarded as a sterile field during the procedure, and any team member who is not wearing suitable PPE should not enter it nor pass instruments into it without using a 'no-touch' technique.

The aspects of infection control and Health and Safety that are relevant to these procedures, especially cleaning methods, infection control and sterilisation, are fully discussed in Chapters 4 and 8. They are summarised below.

- All sharps are carefully disposed of in the sharps box – this includes local anaesthetic needles.
- All autoclavable items are placed in a washer-disinfector unit or an ultrasonic bath, and decontaminated thoroughly before being placed in the autoclave for sterilisation.
- All contaminated waste is placed in hazardous waste sacks – this includes all the impervious covers used as barriers on equipment items.
- All surfaces are disinfected using the correct solution.

Pre- and postoperative instructions

Often, the patient will request information regarding the procedure itself in advance, and the dental nurse is ideally suited to allay their fears by giving advice beforehand as follows.

- Local anaesthesia will always be necessary for an extraction.
- The procedure will not be painful, as adequate local anaesthesia will be given.
- If a surgical procedure is being undertaken, sutures will be necessary.
- Patient must take all medication as normal before the procedure unless the dentist informs them otherwise, except for aspirin which prevents blood clotting and could cause postoperative bleeding.
- Patient must have a light snack 2 h before the procedure, to avoid fainting.
- Full postoperative instructions will be given in writing, so the patient does not have to remember them.
- If the patient is a nervous adult or child, they should be escorted by a reassuring and competent adult.

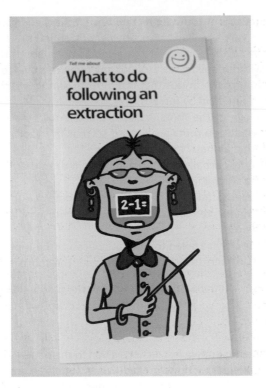

Figure 17.9   Postoperative instruction leaflet.

After the procedure a full list of postoperative instructions should be given verbally and in writing (Figure 17.9). It is important that the patient understands that most postoperative complications occur because of disturbance to the blood clot which forms in the area, and that they should avoid this happening wherever possible. Postoperative instructions should include the following points.

- Pain, swelling or bruising may occur after the procedure.
- Analgesics (**except aspirin**) may be taken as required.
- Alcohol, hot drinks and exercise should be avoided for 24 h after the procedure.
- No mouth rinsing should be carried out on the day of the procedure.
- Hot salt water mouthwashes should be carried out after each meal, from the day after the procedure for up to 1 week.
- If bleeding does occur, bite onto a cotton pack for up to 30 min.
- Give an emergency telephone number for care and advice if problems occur.
- Give details of further appointments if necessary, including suture removal.

Surgical extractions

Under certain circumstances, a simple extraction cannot be carried out to remove a tooth, and either soft tissue alone or soft tissue and alveolar bone have to be removed so that the dentist can gain access to a tooth or root. These procedures are referred to as surgical extractions, and may be necessary for any of the following reasons.

- When previous attempts at tooth extraction have left a significant section of retained root in the alveolar bone – very small apical sections are often left *in situ*, as they cause no problems and sometimes rise to the surface of the alveolar bone some time later, when they can be simply extracted without having to carry out any bone removal to do so.
- When a tooth is so grossly carious that attempts at simple extraction are impossible, as the tooth is too rotten to be held by forceps.
- When the morphology of the roots makes it unlikely that the whole tooth can be removed simply, especially when the roots are curved so that the tooth cannot be pushed out of the socket in one direction alone.
- When the tooth is only partially erupted and impacted, so that full eruption cannot occur and the tooth becomes a stagnation area.
- When the tooth is unerupted and has associated pathology, such as a cyst.
- When the tooth is unerupted and likely to cause future problems with either prostheses or orthodontic treatment.
- When a deciduous tooth has failed to exfoliate because the root has become cemented to the alveolar bone and natural exfoliation cannot occur – the tooth is said to be ankylosed.

Consequently, surgical extractions will fall into one of the following categories.

- Extraction involving tooth sectioning.
- Extraction involving the raising of a mucoperiosteal flap.

The preoperative and postoperative instructions given to the patient have been detailed previously, as is the dental nurse's role during these procedures. What differs from simple extractions is the list of instruments that may be necessary to allow the dentist to gain access to the tooth or root.

Extraction involving tooth sectioning

Tooth sectioning is effectively a variation on the simple extraction technique for multi-rooted teeth that cannot be extracted whole. This is often due to unfavourable root curvature or gross root caries that prevents a simple forceps removal of the roots. The dentist can cut the tooth into a number of sections equal to the number of roots present, and then effectively extract each one as a separate root in the usual way, using forceps, elevators or luxators.

Sometimes, it may be necessary to remove some of the septal bone that lies between the roots and forms the individual socket walls. The only differences in the tooth sectioning technique from that of simple extractions are as follows.

- Use of high-speed turbine and a suitable diamond bur (usually a crown preparation bur, for its greater length) to cut the tooth into sections down towards the furcation area.
- Use of a Coupland's chisel to achieve the final separation of the roots, by inserting the chisel into the drilled slot between the tooth sections and twisting to snap them apart.
- Use of a surgical handpiece and bone burs to remove any septal bone.
- Use of high-speed suction to remove the water coolant of the handpieces.
- Careful retraction and protection of the patient's soft tissues during the cutting and sectioning procedures.

Extractions involving mucoperiosteal flaps

There are certain cases when successful extraction cannot be carried out without gaining full access to a tooth or root by raising a mucoperiosteal flap.

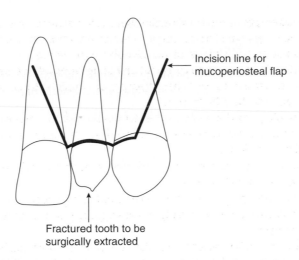

Incision line for
mucoperiosteal flap

Fractured tooth to be
surgically extracted

Figure 17.10 Surgical flap design.

- Unerupted or impacted tooth.
- Buried retained root.
- Root curvature is excessive and requires extensive bone removal.
- Gross root caries prevents adequate instrumentation to extract the tooth in any other way.

541

Teeth lie in sockets of alveolar bone, with a covering of mucoperiosteum over the bone which runs into the gingivae around each tooth (see Chapter 10). The mucoperiosteum is tightly held onto the bone, and has to be cut and separated to its full thickness before bone removal can be carried out – this is the *mucoperiosteal flap* (Figure 17.10).

The flap thus raised has to have a wide base to ensure a good blood supply, so that full healing occurs once the procedure has been completed. It then has to be sutured accurately back into place for long enough so that reattachment can occur.

This is a full surgical technique so all the surgery and instrument preparation as described for simple extractions apply but more specific surgical instruments are required. These are detailed in Table 17.2.

The principle of the sterile field and the maintenance of thorough infection control are of great importance in preventing any contamination complications during the procedure. Patients with a compromised medical history may require the surgical procedure to be carried out in a hospital or dental clinic environment.

The dental nurse has specific roles to perform during the flap procedures, over and above all those previously identified.

- Correct and accurate use of suction equipment to remove water coolants and irrigation solutions.
- Correct and accurate use of fine-bore surgical aspirator to remove blood and debris from the immediate surgical site.
- Careful retraction of soft tissues for their protection and to provide a clear operative field, but without being so forceful that tissue damage occurs.
- Assisting during the placement of sutures, which may include holding the flap taut and cutting the suture ends.
- Preparation of bite packs to aid haemostasis.
- Assisting in the placement of haemostats, such as oxidised cellulose or gelatine sponge.

Table 17.2   Surgical instruments for flap procedures

Item	Function
Scalpel blade and handle (Figure 17.11)	To make the initial incision through the full-thickness mucoperiosteum and around the necks of the teeth to create the flap
Osteotrimmer (Figure 17.12)	To raise the corners of the flap off the underlying alveolar bone
Periosteal elevator (Figure 17.13)	To complete the elevation of the flap off the bone, by pushing the instrument over the bone surface beneath the flap and effectively peeling it off the bone
Handpiece and surgical burs	To remove any alveolar bone necessary to gain access to the tooth or root
Irrigation syringe	To irrigate the surgical field with sterile saline or sterile water, although the handpiece often has its own irrigation supply from the bracket table bottle
Austin and Kilner retractors	To protect and retract cheeks, lips and tongue from the surgical field, providing clear access for the dentist
Rake retractor	To retract the mucoperiosteal flap itself
Bone rongeurs	To nibble away bony spicules and produce a smooth bone surface for healing
Dissecting forceps (Figure 17.14)	To hold the loose flap edges taut during suturing
Needle holders (Figure 17.15)	To hold the prethreaded needle firmly while suturing
Suture pack (Figure 17.16)	Half-moon needle, prethreaded with either black braided silk or a resorbable suture material such as vicryl, to suture the flap back into position over the alveolar bone
Suture scissors (Figure 17.17)	To cut the suture ends after each stitch

Again, full verbal and written postoperative instructions are given before the patient is discharged, and then the surgery is decontaminated as previously described.

While the records are being written, the number of sutures used is specifically recorded so that all can be accounted for if they are of the non-resorbable type, at the suture removal appointment.

Tooth impaction

The most usual teeth to become impacted are the lower third molars, or 'wisdom' teeth. These are the last permanent teeth to erupt and are often short of space to do so. The type of impaction that occurs will affect the difficulty of the removal of the tooth.

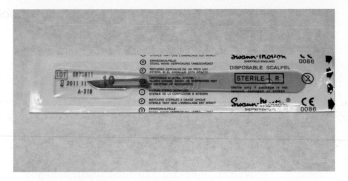

Figure 17.11   Sterile scalpel blade and handle.

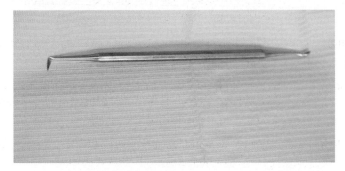

Figure 17.12   Mitchell's trimmer.

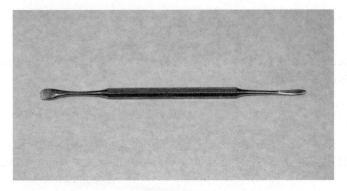

Figure 17.13   Periosteal elevator.

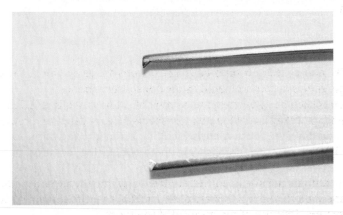

Figure 17.14   Tissue dissecting forceps – end detail.

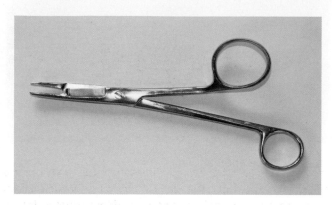

Figure 17.15   Example of needle holders.

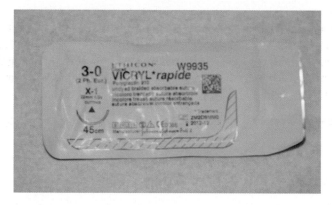

Figure 17.16   Suture pack.

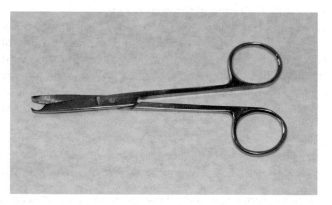

Figure 17.17   Suture scissors.

- **Vertical impaction** – the tooth is upright but impacted into the ramus of the mandible.
- **Horizontal impaction** – the tooth is lying on its side, facing forwards, backwards or across the dental ridge.
- **Mesio-angular impaction** – the tooth is tilted forwards into the second molar tooth (Figure 17.18).
- **Distoangular impaction** – the tooth is tilted backwards into the ramus of the mandible.

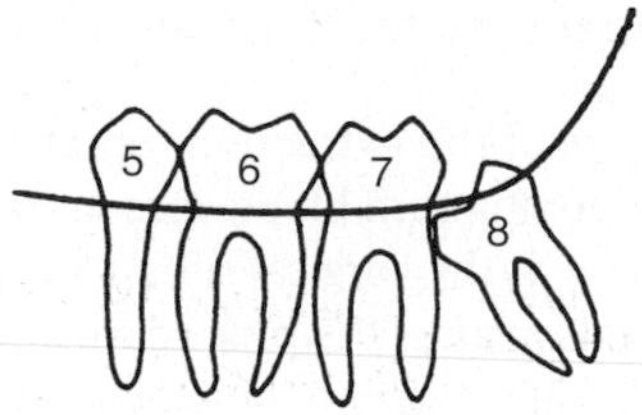

Figure 17.18   Mesio-angular impacted lower third molar.

Some dentists will refer patients with the more difficult types of impaction to a specialist oral surgeon for extraction, if the teeth are persistently infected or are causing food trapping and caries in adjacent teeth. However, if the impacted tooth is causing no problems (that is, it is *asymptomatic*) then it is usual for it to be left *in situ*, as there are risks involved in having the tooth surgically extracted.

- Extensive bone removal can weaken the mandible.
- Postoperative pain and swelling are very likely to occur after a full surgical procedure.
- The inferior dental nerve and lingual nerve lie close to the operation site, and can be temporarily or even permanently damaged if they become traumatised or severed during the surgical procedure.
- Limited mouth opening (**trismus**) can occur temporarily after surgery, and this will make eating and talking difficult.

Patients must be warned of all these possible complications before undergoing the surgical extraction procedure.

Complications of extractions

Complications that may occur during extraction include damage to adjacent nerves, fracture of the tooth, perforation of the maxillary sinus and loss of a tooth. Complications that may occur after extraction are bleeding and infection of the bony socket.

Some complications can be highlighted as potential risks that may occur during the extraction procedure, the most common being the possibility of damage to one of the trigeminal nerve branches during the procedure. This risk can be identified by good preoperative dental radiography and accurate planning of the procedure beforehand. Where there is potential for nerve damage to occur, such as when the roots of lower molars lie very close to the inferior dental nerve, the patient should be referred to a specialist for the procedure and warned of the possibility of it happening beforehand, so that informed consent may be given.

Similarly, those medically compromised patients with conditions that may cause problems during extractions (such as haemophiliacs) should also be referred to specialist clinics or hospitals for treatment. Reasons for the occurrence of the other possible complications listed above are as follows.

- **Unexpected tooth fracture** – especially if the tooth is heavily filled or root filled, and this may result in a simple extraction becoming a more complicated one.
- **Oroantral fistulas** – due to a perforation of the maxillary sinus, this can occur while extracting the upper premolar or molar teeth, as the maxillary sinus lies over their roots and is often only separated by a membrane, so perforation of the sinus is not difficult.
- **Loss of the tooth** – either into the respiratory or digestive tracts or out of the mouth, and due to it slipping out of the dentist's grip while pushing the tooth out of the socket or lifting it out of the mouth.

Complications that can occur after the patient has left the surgery are as follows.

- **Bleeding** – either within hours of the extraction (**reactionary haemorrhage**) due to the blood clot being disturbed and reopening torn blood vessels, or after 24 h (**secondary haemorrhage**) due to an infection developing at the surgical site.
- **Infection** – between 2 and 4 days after the procedure and following loss of the blood clot from the socket, the bony socket walls become infected – the condition is called **localised osteitis** (dry socket).

Tooth fracture

A grossly carious or heavily filled tooth is likely to fracture during extraction attempts, and the dentist should be aware of the possibility and warn the patient regarding progression to a surgical procedure if necessary. This progression is likely to occur when the tooth fracture extends subgingivally, as adequate access to the roots may then be difficult without bone removal. Alternatively, root fracture may occur during extraction, especially where the roots are fine or curved, and then require a surgical procedure to remove them.

However, if small apical pieces of root fracture off during extraction, they can be left *in situ* to either rise to the alveolar ridge surface by themselves over time, and be more easily removed, or to remain buried and cause no further problems. Whichever occurs, the patient must always be informed and a full explanation given.

Oroantral fistula

This is a complication of the extraction of upper premolar and molar teeth only, as the maxillary sinus lies over and between their roots. An inappropriate extraction technique can sometimes push the root into the sinus, where it will act as a foreign body and cause infection. The patient is best referred to a specialist oral surgeon for its removal.

Long-rooted upper molar and premolar teeth sometimes impinge into the sinus naturally, and when they are extracted an opening will be created between the antrum and the oral cavity. This is called an oroantral fistula and if small, it will close naturally within a week, although the patient should be instructed not to blow their nose during this healing period. Indeed, the presence of a fistula can be confirmed by the appearance of air bubbles in the socket when the patient pinches their nose closed and blows.

Large openings require surgical repair either by direct suturing or by raising a gingival flap off the palate and swinging it across to seal the fistula.

Loss of the tooth

The tooth can be dropped during its removal from the mouth, or the force exerted during extraction can cause it to dislodge rapidly from the socket, before a firm grip has been achieved with the forceps.

If the tooth is swallowed, it poses no problem and should be allowed to pass naturally. However, if the tooth is likely to have been inhaled (especially likely if the patient has a coughing fit as the tooth disappears), the patient should be sent to hospital immediately for chest and abdominal radiographs, to locate the tooth, as it could cause a serious respiratory infection. It may be removed using a bronchoscope if lodged in the main bronchi but if it has descended further into the respiratory tract, thoracic surgery may be necessary to remove it.

Bleeding

Haemorrhage during extraction is a natural occurrence, as blood vessels in the periodontium are torn during the procedure. This usually stops within 5 min of completion of the extraction with the use of a bite pack, and is called **primary haemorrhage**.

When there is no history of previous haemorrhage, sutures may still be required if excessive bleeding occurs. This may even be carried out in elderly patients and those with hypertension, as a precautionary measure. In all cases, however, the patient must not be dismissed from the premises until bleeding has ceased.

The blood clots in the following way.

- Torn blood vessels constrict to slow the blood flow.
- **Platelets** circulating in the blood are exposed to air at the wound site. This causes them to become sticky, and clump together.
- Two complicated **clotting mechanisms** ensue, resulting in the protein fibrinogen being converted to fibrin.
- **Fibrin** chemically seals the cut vessels, and the haemorrhage ends.

Bleeding which occurs several hours after the extraction is called **reactionary haemorrhage**, and is usually caused by the patient not following the postoperative instructions accurately and disturbing the blood clot, either by using a mouthwash or taking alcohol or exercise.

In healthy patients, it is easily controlled by reapplication of pressure to the socket, reiteration of the postoperative instructions or by suturing of the socket to compress the wound edges and promote clotting again, possibly with the insertion of a haemostatic sponge too.

An additional cause of primary haemorrhage is failure of the blood-clotting process so that uncontrolled bleeding occurs. This is an uncommon but very serious matter, occurring in patients taking anticoagulant drugs, those with liver disease, and with some rare blood diseases such as haemophilia. Patients with such conditions should have been identified by the completion of a thorough medical history beforehand, or they may carry a warning card for presentation to any practitioner they attend. In particular, patients with certain heart conditions may be prescribed the anticoagulant drug *warfarin*. The effectiveness of their blood clotting will be regularly monitored by undergoing a blood test to determine their international normalised ratio (INR) score and this will indicate whether extractions can be safely carried out in a dental practice or whether the patient requires a hospital referral. Current practice is for patients with an INR score of more than 4 to be treated in hospital for surgical procedures, including extractions.

Patients taking aspirin to prevent a stroke should be treated carefully when undergoing surgical procedures in the practice, and the use of a haemostatic sponge and suture may be required as a matter of routine to avoid complications.

The third type of bleeding complication is **secondary haemorrhage**, where the blood clot is lost early and the socket subsequently becomes infected, with breakdown of the healing mechanism. This occurs after 24 h from the extraction being carried out. Cleansing of the socket, then pressure and the insertion of a haemostatic sponge should solve the problem.

Infection

The condition of infection of the extraction socket is called localised osteitis (dry socket) and is a very painful condition which develops 2–3 days after extraction. It is an acute inflammation of the bone (*osteitis*) lining the socket and is caused by microbial invasion. The natural protective barrier against such invasion is the blood clot which fills the socket immediately after an extraction, so anything which prevents formation of an adequate blood clot can give rise to a dry socket, such as:

- infection of the blood clot
- failure of formation of a blood clot
- disturbance of the blood clot.

Infection of the blood clot may occur in neglected mouths where gingival or periodontal infection is already present, and also is particularly likely to occur in patients who smoke. Hordes of micro-organisms invade the socket, overwhelm the defending white cells, disintegrate the blood clot and set up an acute inflammation of the unprotected bare bone of the socket. Pre-extraction scaling of the teeth reduces gingival infection and may prevent a dry socket. Alternatively, application of chlorhexidine to the gingival crevice just before extraction helps to reduce the risk of infection.

Failure of formation of a blood clot may occur in difficult extractions, as pressure on the bone during such an extraction crushes the blood vessels and results in insufficient bleeding to produce a protective blood clot. It is more common in the mandible than maxilla as the former has a thicker layer of compact bone.

Disturbance of the blood clot is caused by too much mouth washing soon after extraction or by the patient poking at the extraction socket, especially with dirty fingers. This breaks away the blood clot and leaves the socket bare, and introduces micro-organisms to the immediate vicinity.

To treat the condition, any food debris or necrotic clot tissue is removed with gentle irrigation and the use of tweezers, and then a sedative dressing (such as *Alvogyl*) is carefully placed in the socket. The pain experienced by the patient can be relieved with the usual anti-inflammatory analgesics, and it is best if the postoperative instructions are reiterated, in particular the use of hot salt water mouthwashes.

The dental nurse's duty

Sometimes the dentist is away from the workplace when a patient returns with postextraction haemorrhage. In such a case it is the dental nurse's duty to reassure the patient that the condition is not likely to be serious and should be easily remedied. After obtaining full details about the patient and the extraction, the dental nurse must contact the dentist for instructions.

Meanwhile, the patient is made more comfortable by the provision of a mouthwash to remove the unpleasant taste and clean the mouth. Then, unless instructed to the contrary, the dental nurse may give the patient a pressure pad to bite on until the dentist arrives. While awaiting the arrival of the dentist, the dental nurse should switch on the autoclave and prepare the surgery for a possible suture procedure. Mouth mirror, tweezers, cotton wool, swabs, suction, haemostatic drugs, local anaesthetic and suture equipment may be required.

If the dental nurse is unable to contact the dentist, and a pressure pad is ineffective, help may be sought from an emergency dental service, the patient's doctor or a local hospital.

Accidental extraction

This is the term used to describe the unplanned situation where a tooth is lost from its socket unexpectedly, and can occur for several reasons. One example is the removal of an unerupted premolar while extracting its deciduous predecessor. As a premolar crown is surrounded by the deciduous molar roots (Figure 17.19), it can be dislodged or completely extracted together with the deciduous tooth.

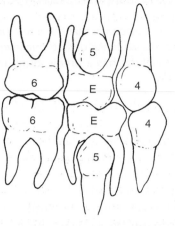

Figure 17.19   Deciduous second molars and premolar successors. (*A Textbook of Orthodontics*, 3rd edn, T.D. Foster, Blackwell Science, Oxford. Used with permission.).

Fortunately, the accidentally extracted premolar can be saved by immediately replanting it in its socket. The periodontal membrane and pulp should retain their vitality and the tooth subsequently erupts normally. Success is accomplished by immediate replacement, which gives no time for the periodontal membrane to become infected or dried out.

549

The same procedure can be adopted if a child's tooth – usually an incisor – is knocked out by a fall or a blow. Such a tooth is said to be *avulsed*. As long as the periodontal membrane remains vital, the tooth can be pushed back into its socket, with complete success in many cases. This type of accident constitutes a dental emergency and it is essential that correct first aid treatment is applied before the child reaches the dental workplace. The following advice should be given to the person reporting the accident.

- Reassure the child (and the parent) that successful treatment is possible.
- Retrieve the tooth and, holding it by its crown, rinse it gently in warm water.
- Instruct them not to use any type of disinfectant or mouthwash solution to rinse the tooth.
- Put the tooth back into its socket, it they feel able to do so.
- If that is not possible, let the tooth lie loose in the child's own mouth to keep it moist in saliva, although care should be taken with younger patients to avoid choking.
- If that is impracticable, immerse the tooth in a container of milk.
- The tooth must not be wrapped in anything, but should be left bathing in the milk.
- Come to the surgery immediately.

Once the tooth has been replanted in its socket and an x-ray taken, no further treatment may be necessary, but a splint is sometimes required to immobilise it for a week or so, followed by root filling if the tooth becomes non-vital.

Use of antibiotics with minor oral surgery

As previously stated, many extractions are carried out because the patient presents with the pain of an acute infection. Previously, antibiotics were often prescribed for these patients as the first line of treatment (especially if the patient attended without an appointment), and the dental problem would be dealt with at a later date. Current thinking is that antibiotics:

- are an adjunct to treatment only so are to be used as a back-up to treatment, not as a replacement for it
- should only be given if there is evidence that the infection is spreading locally
- should only be given if there is evidence of systemic involvement (raised body temperature is a good indicator) or if the patient has a predisposing medical condition which necessitates antibiotics during treatment.

The routine use of antibiotics is contraindicated for the following reasons.

- The source of the infection is better removed by extracting the tooth or by lancing any abscess present and draining as much pus as possible from the area.
- Resistant strains of bacteria are more likely to develop if antibiotics are overprescribed.
- A single course of antibiotics can have long-term consequences for the normal bacterial flora in the body, possibly lasting for months.
- The dangerous potentiating action that antibiotics have on several drugs, especially oral anticoagulants – they increase the blood-thinning effect of the anticoagulants so that haemostasis cannot be achieved.
- The possibility of other drug interactions, especially with oral contraceptives and alcohol.
- The development of hypersensitivity to the antibiotics by the patient, preventing their use in future.
- All drugs should be avoided wherever possible during pregnancy.

If antibiotics do need to be prescribed, the following regimes are currently recommended.

- First choice – amoxicillin 250 mg, four times daily for 5 days.
- Second choice – metronidazole 200 mg three times daily for 3 days.
- Third choice – erythromycin 250 mg four times daily for 5 days, for patients who are allergic to penicillin and its derivatives.

In severe infections and where more than one type of micro-organism may be involved, the first and second choices can be given together.

Other minor oral surgery procedures

Operculectomy

This procedure is the surgical removal of the gingival flap (operculum) overlying a partially erupted tooth, especially a lower third molar.

As teeth begin to erupt, the overlying gingiva is pushed up into the mouth and bulges over the tooth until its incisal or occlusal surface breaks through into the oral cavity. However, in some patients, this gingival bulging over the lower third molars means that the area is constantly bitten and traumatised by the upper teeth when the mouth is closed, causing pain and inflammation in some cases.

As the area becomes more painful, the patient often reduces their oral hygiene efforts, which then compounds the issue by allowing plaque and food debris to collect further, and eventually an infection will develop – this is called *pericoronitis*. In severe cases, the patient develops *trismus* and is unable to fully open their mouth.

Treatment is as follows, in order of lesser to greater severity of the symptoms.

- Oral hygiene instruction, to ensure the removal of food debris and plaque.
- Irrigation of the underside of the flap to remove debris, using chlorhexidine or an oxygen-releasing solution, such as *Peroxyl* mouthwash.

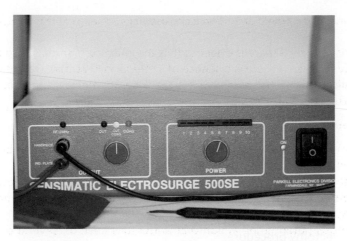

Figure 17.20   Electrosurgery unit.

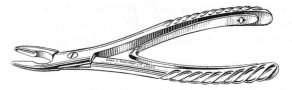

Figure 17.21   Bone rongeurs.

- The use of anti-inflammatory analgesics, such as *ibuprofen*, to reduce the inflammation and ease the symptoms.
- The surgical removal of the operculum if the problem recurs, ideally using an electrosurgical cautery unit (Figure 17.20) rather than conventional techniques, as the control of haemorrhage is far superior.
- A 3-day course of metronidazole antibiotics, to destroy the anaerobic bacteria involved.

Alveolectomy and alveoplasty

These are procedures carried out to remove pieces of the alveolar ridge or smooth and alter its shape, respectively.

When teeth have been extracted, the edges of the sockets can sometimes remain as sharp spicules of bone which make the wearing of dentures impossible without discomfort to the patient. The quality of the alveolar ridge can easily be seen on a radiograph and where appropriate, the spicules and sharp edges can be removed, so that dentures can be worn. A mucoperiosteal flap must be raised to gain access to the ridge, and then bone rongeurs (Figure 17.21) or surgical burs are used to remove all the bony projections.

Alveoplasty is carried out to alter the shape of the ridge so that deep undercuts are removed and dentures can seat correctly and comfortably.

Gingivectomy and gingivoplasty

These are periodontal surgery techniques that are carried out to adjust the shape of the gingivae and aid oral hygiene measures, so that more effective plaque removal is possible.

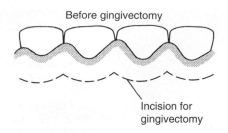

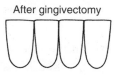

Figure 17.22   Gingivectomy procedure.

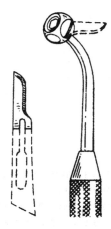

Figure 17.23   Blake gingivectomy knife.

Sometimes, successful treatment of periodontal disease is hindered by failing to eliminate established false pockets, and they can be surgically removed by the technique of gingivectomy. This is the removal of a strip of gingival margin level with the the point of the epithelial attachment (Figure 17.22). It is mainly confined to cases with excessive overgrowth of gum (*gingival hyperplasia*) caused by certain drugs used for medical conditions: phenytoin (for epilepsy), nifedipine (for hypertension) and ciclosporin (following organ transplant).

The excess gum is removed with a *gingivectomy knife* or one used for periodontal flap surgery (see later). There are many different types of gingivectomy knife available with various angled handles and blades for ease of access, the most common being Blake's gingivectomy knife (Figure 17.23). The strip of incised gum is removed with tweezers and the raw area covered with a zinc oxide-eugenol *periodontal pack*, such as *Coe-Pak*, to protect the gum and promote rapid painless healing. The pack is removed about a week later and thorough scaling is then performed.

A technique similar to gingivectomy may also be necessary for exposing more root surface prior to crown preparation, in cases where there would otherwise be insufficient retention for a crown. This procedure is called *crown lengthening*.

Surgical recontouring of the gingiva can also be carried out once periodontal health has been established, to help the patient in their effort to thorough cleanse the area. This technique is called

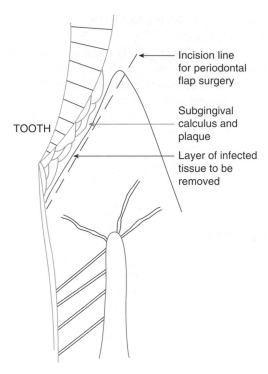

Figure 17.24   Flap incision.

gingivoplasty, and is often carried out using an electrosurgical cautery unit which cuts and coagulates bleeding tissues at the same time.

Following gingival surgery, patients are given or prescribed analgesic drugs to relieve afterpain, given an appointment for removal of sutures or pack a week later, and instructed to avoid smoking, eating hard food and using a toothbrush on the operative area meanwhile. A soft diet and chlorhexidine mouthwashes are advised instead.

Periodontal flap surgery

Periodontal conditions which do not respond to plaque control procedures, such as meticulous oral hygiene by the patient and subgingival scaling by a dental operator, may require treatment by minor oral surgery procedures. They are performed under local anaesthesia and may be undertaken by the patient's own dentist or by referral to a periodontal specialist.

Periodontal flap procedures use techniques and instruments similar to some of those described previously for the surgical extraction of an unerupted tooth, but they do not involve the raising of a full mucoperiosteal flap. They cover a variety of procedures to remove inaccessible subgingival plaque and facilitate subsequent plaque control. Teeth with irregular gingival pocketing, a complex and uneven pattern of bone loss or involvement of the *furcation* (the branching of roots of multi-rooted teeth) are those most likely to need such operations (Figure 17.24).

- The incision is made through the gingival papilla of the tooth, down to the tooth surface, so that the layer of gingiva in contact with the tooth and forming the inner wall of the periodontal pocket is separated from the remainder of the gingival tissues.
- This severed piece of tissue is removed from the area.

- The remaining gingival flap is then reflected to expose the underlying bone, root surface and all the hidden subgingival calculus.
- Alveolar bone surfaces may then be trimmed and contoured to eliminate bony pockets.
- All subgingival plaque and calculus are removed, using curettes or an ultrasonic scaler.
- In addition, all contaminated cementum and any toxin-impregnated granulation tissue are removed.
- Local delivery antibiotic systems such as *Gengigel*, *Dentomycin* or *Periochip* may then be placed in these inaccessible areas, to help the healing process (see Figure 13.20).
- The flap is then sutured back into place.
- There is no removal of full-thickness gingival tissue but the gingival margin may be repositioned more apically, and thus permanently expose more of the root to make cleaning easier in future.

Soft tissue biopsies

These are procedures carried out to remove a soft tissue lesion from the mouth, to be sent away for pathological examination and diagnosis. Large lesions may have just a section of tissue removed and these are referred to as *incisional biopsies*. Ideally, and certainly with smaller lesions, the whole of the tissue lesion is removed, and these are referred to as *excisional biopsies*.

It is usual for the patient to be referred to a hospital dental department for these types of procedure to be carried out by an oral surgery specialist, as incomplete removal of a sinister lesion (such as oral cancer) may make its treatment ultimately more difficult or even risk spreading cancerous cells more widely.

Cyst removal

A cyst is a fluid-filled sac confined within a soft tissue lining. There are many different types found in various parts of the body. In dental practice, they are most commonly seen as an abnormal cavity in the bone, at the apex of a dead tooth (*dental* or *apical cyst*) or surrounding and preventing eruption of an unerupted tooth (*dentigerous* or *follicular cyst*). If left untreated, a cyst gradually enlarges, causing swelling of the jaw and displacement of other teeth. Whenever possible, they are removed, complete with their lining, and invariably by a specialist oral surgeon within the hospital.

Frenectomy

This means the removal of a frenum, which is a band of fibrous tissue, covered with mucous membrane, which attaches the tongue and lips to the underlying bone. If the lingual frenum restricts the movement of the tongue so that speech is affected, a lingual frenectomy is performed. If the upper labial frenum is too large it may allow a wide gap to persist between the upper central incisors – this gap is called a *median diastema*. It can also affect the fit of an upper denture. In such cases an upper labial frenectomy is often undertaken.

Patient monitoring during minor oral surgery procedures

Any type of extraction or minor oral surgery procedure can be a worrying prospect for the patient, and this is especially so for younger patients and some of those with special needs – when it may be difficult for them to appreciate why the procedure must be carried out – as well as those patients with an abnormal fear of the procedure (a *phobia*).

A friendly, supportive and calming attitude throughout by the dental nurse will help to pacify the patient to some extent, as will talking to them and encouraging them when appropriate.

Actual monitoring of the patient to determine signs of any complications include the ability to notice the following.

- **Pain** – signs of pain in the patient may be seen as them grimacing, wincing or crying and should be pointed out to the dentist, as the local anesthetic administered may not be sufficient.
- **Colour** – the patient may feel faint and become pale and clammy, so the procedure must be stopped while action is taken to restore their cranial blood flow (usually by dropping the dental chair so their head is below their feet).
- **Choking** – debris or a tooth may be lost to the back of the mouth, causing choking, and immediate action is required to prevent a serious medical emergency.
- **Medical emergency** – anxiety can precipitate angina or a cardiac arrest in vulnerable patients, so patient response levels and vital signs should always be monitored by the whole team.
- **Tooth complications** – unexpected complications can occur, and the dental nurse should maintain a calm manner while assisting during the complication, especially by using suction and aspiration to retrieve debris, or applying pressure during primary haemorrhage.
- **Bleeding** – immediately after the extraction, primary haemorrhage is quite normal but should stop after up to 5 min of pressure with a suitable dressing, so any recurrent bleeding must be reported to the dentist immediately, and the patient must not leave the surgery until all bleeding has stopped (this may involve assisting in placing haemostats or sutures).

555

Further resources are available for this book, including interactive multiple choice questions and extended matching questions. Visit the companion website at:

www.levisonstextbookfordentalnurses.com

Index

Index